The Little
ICU
Book
of Facts and
Formulas

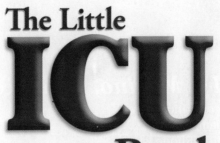

Paul L. Marino, MD, PhD, FCCM

Director of Critical Care
The Miriam Hospital,
Providence, Rhode Island

Associate Professor
Brown University School of Medicine
Providence, Rhode Island

With contributions from:
Kenneth M. Sutin, MD, FCCM

Department of Anesthesiology
Bellevue Hospital Center

Associate Professor of Anesthesiology & Surgery
New Yrok University School of Medicine
New York, New York

Illustrations & Page Layout by Patricia Gast

The Little
ICU
Book
of Facts and
Formulas

 Wolters Kluwer | Lippincott Williams & Wilkins
Health
Philadelphia · Baltimore · New York · London
Buenos Aires · Hong Kong · Sydney · Tokyo

Acquisitions Editor: Brian Brown
Managing Editor: Nicole Dernoski
Project Manager: Bridgett Dougherty
Senior Marketing Manager: Benjamin Rivera
Creative Director: Doug Smock
Production Services: Nesbitt Graphics, Inc.

Library of Congress Cataloging-in-Publication Data
9-780-7817-7823-7
0-7817-7823-9
Marino, Paul L.
  The little ICU book of facts and formulas / Paul L. Marino ; with contributions from
Kenneth M. Sutin.
     p. ; cm.
  Based on: The ICU book / Paul L. Marino. © 2007.
  Includes bibliographical references and index.
  ISBN-13: 978-0-7817-7823-7
  ISBN-10: 0-7817-7823-9
  1. Critical care medicine--Handbooks, manuals, etc. 2. Intensive care units--Handbooks,
manuals, etc. I. Sutin, Kenneth M. II. Marino, Paul L. ICU book. III. Title.
  [DNLM: 1. Critical Care--Handbooks. 2. Intensive Care Units--Handbooks.
WX 39 M339L 2008]
  RC86.8.M3864 2008
  616.02'8--dc22

                                                    2008018875

Care has been taken to confirm the accuracy of the information presented and to describe
generally accepted practices. However, the authors, editors, and publisher are not responsible for errors or omissions or for any consequences from application of the information in
this book and make no warranty, expressed or implied, with respect to the currency, com-
pleteness, or accuracy of the contents of the publication. Application of the information in
a particular situation remains the professional responsibility of the practitioner.

The authors, editors, and publisher have exerted every effort to ensure that drug selection
and dosage set forth in this text are in accordance with current recommendations and practice at the time of publication. However, in view of ongoing research, changes in govern-
ment regulations, and the constant flow of information relating to drug therapy and drug
reactions, the reader is urged to check the package insert for each drug for any change in
indications and dosage and for added warnings and precautions. This is particularly important when the recommended agent is a new or infrequently employed drug.

Some drugs and medical devices presented in the publication have Food and Drug Administration (FDA) clearance for limited use in restricted research settings. It is the responsibility of the health care provider to ascertain the FDA status of each drug or device planned
for use in their clinical practice.

To purchase additional copies of this book, call our customer service department at (800) 638-
3030 or fax orders to (301) 223-2320. International customers should call (301) 223-2300.

Visit Lippincott Williams & Wilkins on the Internet: at LWW.com. Lippincott Williams &
Wilkins customer service representatives are available from 8:30 am to 6 pm, EST.

RRS1208

                                                    1 1 10 9 8 7 6 5

To Daniel Joseph Marino,
my 20-year-old son,
who is raising his sails,
and waiting for that breeze.

A wise man recognizes the convenience of a general statement, but he bows to the authority of a particular fact.

OLIVER WENDELL HOLMES
(1872)

Preface

As the title implies, *The Little ICU Book* is a smaller, more condensed version of its older sibling, *The ICU Book*, and is intended as compact reference for the bedside. A majority of the chapter titles in *The ICU Book* have been retained in the "little book", but each chapter has been completely rewritten to include only the most essential information, and the content is presented in outline form for easy access. Although small in stature, *The Little ICU Book* is densely packed with facts and formulas that represent the essentials of patient care in the (adult) ICU.

Acknowledgments

This work owes its existence to the considerable efforts and expertise of Patricia Gast, who is responsible for all the illustrations, tables, and page layouts in this book. Her patience and capacity for exhaustive work are exceeded only by her talent.

Also to Brian Brown and Nicole Dernoski at Lippincott Williams & Wilkins, for their trust and enduring support.

And finally to Vivienne DeStefano, who has become so important to this author and his work in so many ways.

PLM

Contents

I. PREVENTIVE PRACTICES IN THE CRITICALLY ILL

1   Infection Control in the ICU   1
2   Stress-Related Mucosal Injury   19
3   Venous Thromboembolism   31

II. VASCULAR ACCESS

4   Vascular Catheters   53
5   Establishing Venous Access   61
6   The Indwelling Vascular Catheter   77

III. HEMODYNAMIC MONITORING

7   The Pulmonary Artery Catheter   97
8   Cardiac Filling Pressures   113
9   Systemic Oxygenation   125

IV. DISORDERS OF CIRCULATORY FLOW

10 Hemorrhage and Hypovolemia   139
11 Colloid and Crystalloid Resuscitation   157
12 Acute Heart Failure(s)   173
13 Cardiac Arrest   189

V. CRITICAL CARE CARDIOLOGY

14	Acute Coronary Syndromes	209
15	Tachycardias	233

VI. COMMON PULMONARY DISORDERS

16	Acute Respiratory Distress Syndrome	255
17	Asthma and COPD in the ICU	269

VII. MECHANICAL VENTILATION

18	Basics of Mechanical Ventilation	283
19	Modes of Positive-Pressure Breathing	299
20	The Ventilator-Dependent Patient	315
21	Discontinuing Mechanical Ventilation	333

VIII. ACID-BASE DISORDERS

22	Acid-Base Interpretations	349
23	Organic Acidoses	363
24	Metabolic Alkalosis	379

IX. RENAL AND ELECTROLYTE DISORDERS

25	Oliguria and Acute Renal Failure	391
26	Hypertonic and Hypotonic Conditions	409
27	Potassium	427
28	Magnesium	443
29	Calcium and Phosphorus	457

X. TRANSFUSION PRACTICES IN CRITICAL CARE

30	Anemia and Erythrocyte Transfusions	477
31	Thrombocytopenia and Platelet Transfusions	493

XI. INFLAMMATION AND INFECTION IN THE ICU

32	Fever in the ICU	505
33	Infection, Inflammation, and Multiorgan Injury	521
34	Pneumonia in the ICU	535
35	Sepsis from the Abdomen and Pelvis	549

XII. NUTRITION AND METABOLISM

36	Nutritional Requirements	563
37	Enteral Tube Feeding	577
38	Total Parenteral Nutrition	591
39	Adrenal and Thyroid Dysfunction	603

XIII. CRITICAL CARE NEUROLOGY

40	Disorders of Mentation	613
41	Disorders of Movement	627
42	Acute Stroke	641

XIV. PARENTERAL DRUG THERAPIES IN THE ICU

43	Analgesia and Sedation	653
44	Antimicrobial Therapy	671
45	Hemodynamic Drugs	689

XV. TOXICOLOGY

46	Pharmaceutical Toxins & Antidotes	705

XVI. APPENDICES

1	Units and Conversions	719
2	Selected Reference Ranges	725
3	Additional Formulas	731
Index		735

Chapter 1

INFECTION CONTROL IN THE ICU

This chapter describes the patient care practices that are designed to prevent the growth and spread of pathogenic organisms in the hospital setting.

I. SKIN HYGIENE

Common organisms isolated from the skin of ICU personnel are (in order of decreasing prevalence): *Staphylococcus epidermidis* (over 90% of people cultured), gram-negative aerobic bacilli (20%), Candida species (15%) and *Staphylococcus aureus* (5 – 10%). Eradicating these organisms from the skin is a major concern of infection control.

A. Soap and Water

Soaps are detergents that can disperse particulate and organic matter, but they lack antimicrobial activity. Cleaning the skin with plain soap and water will remove dirt and grease but will not eradicate the microbial flora on the skin. The eradication of microbes (called *decontamination*) requires the application of agents that have antimicrobial activity.

B. Antiseptic Agents

Antimicrobial agents used to decontaminate the skin are called *antiseptics*, and those used to decontaminate inanimate objects are called *disinfectants*. The antiseptic agents used most commonly are described below (see Table 1.1) (1-3).

TABLE 1.1 Common Antiseptic Agents

Agent	Major Advantage	Major Disadvantage
Alcohol	Broad coverage	Little residual activity
Iodophors	Broad coverage	Inconsistent residual activity
Chlorhexidine	Good residual activity (≥ 6 hrs)	Limited coverage

From References 1–3.

1. *Alcohols*

   The alcohols (ethanol, propanol, isopropyl alcohol) are germicidal against most bacteria, fungi, and viruses (including HIV).

   a. Alcohols have a rapid onset of action, but have little persistent (residual) activity.

   b. Repeated use of aqueous alcohol solutions can cause drying and irritation of the skin. This effect is minimized when a waterless alcohol gel is used.

   c. The alcohols are less effective in the presence of dirt and organic matter, so skin that is dirty or soiled with body fluids should be cleaned before applying alcohol.

2. *Iodophors*

   Iodine has broad-spectrum germicidal activity (like the alcohols), but it is irritating to the skin and soft tissues. Skin irritation is reduced by employing a carrier molecule to release iodine slowly. Iodine preparations that use a carrier molecule are called iodophors. The most popular iodophor in the United States is povidone-iodine.

   a. Since the active ingredient in iodophors (iodine) is released slowly, iodophors must be left in contact with the skin for a few minutes to achieve maximum antisepsis. Prolonged contact with iodine can be irritating, so iodophors should be wiped from the skin after drying. This removal limits the persistent (residual) antiseptic activity.

b. Iodophors are neutralized by organic matter, so skin that is soiled with blood and body fluids should be cleaned before applying an iodophor.

3. *Chlorhexidine*

Chlorhexidine gluconate is a germicidal agent that is effective against gram-positive bacteria, but has less activity than alcohol and iodophors against gram-negative bacilli and fungi.

a. The major advantage of chlorhexidine is its prolonged activity, which can last for 6 hours or longer (2). This activity is reduced by soaps and hand creams.

b. Chlorhexidine is available in 0.5% to 4% aqueous solutions. The 4% solution is most effective, but repeated use can cause skin irritation. Chlorhexidine is also an ocular irritant, and care should be taken to avoid contact with the eyes.

4. *Spore-Forming Organisms*

Antiseptic agents are not effective against spore-forming organisms like *Clostridium difficile* and *Bacillus anthracis* (1). Proper use of gloves is required to prevent the spread of these organisms.

C. Handwashing

Appropriate handwashing is the cornerstone of infection control, and Table 1.2 presents the guidelines for handwashing issued by the Centers for Disease Control.

1. *General Recommendations*

a. Antiseptic soaps and gels are preferred to plain soap and water for handwashing.

TABLE 1.2 Recommendations for Handwashing

I. Handwashing with soap (plain or antiseptic) and water is recommended:

  1. When hands are dirty or soiled with blood or body fluids.
  2. Before eating.
  3. After leaving a restroom.

II. Handwashing with an antiseptic preparation* is recommended:

  1. Before direct contact with a patient.
  2. After contact with a patient's skin (intact or non-intact).
  3. After contact with body fluids, secretions, excretions, mucous membranes, wound dressings, and contaminated items.
  4. Before donning sterile gloves to insert central intravascular catheters or other invasive devices that do not require a surgical procedure.
  5. Before inserting urinary catheters, peripheral venous catheters, or other invasive devices that do not require a surgical procedure.
  6. After removing gloves.
  7. When moving from a contaminated to a clean body site.
  8. After contact with inanimate objects in the immediate vicinity of the patient.

*A waterless alcohol gel is preferred to antiseptic soaps, but the hands must be clean prior to application.

From References 2 and 3.

  b. If the hands are not visibly soiled, a waterless alcohol gel is recommended for handwashing (alcohol has proven more effective than iodophors or chlorhexidine for reducing bacterial counts on the hands) (3). The gel should be rubbed into the hands until the hands feel dry.

  c. Antiseptic soaps are recommended when the hands are dirty or soiled with body fluids. The soap should be rubbed over the entire surface of the hands for at least 30 seconds (2,3). The soap is then removed with a tap water rinse, and the hands should be dried completely (residual moisture on the skin will promote microbial growth).

d. Hot water is not recommended for handwashing (3) because it is not more effective than warm or cold water for removing skin microbes (4), and it can be irritating to the skin.

e. During handwashing, special attention should be given to the subungual areas under the fingernails, where microbes tend to congregate.

Despite the importance of handwashing, surveys reveal that only a small percentage of ICU personnel adhere to the handwashing guidelines, and physicians are consistently the worst offenders (1-3).

II. PROTECTIVE BARRIERS

Protective barriers like gloves, gowns, masks, and eye shields provide a physical impediment to the transmission of infectious agents in blood and body fluids.

A. Gloves

1. *Indications*

   The tasks that require gloves (sterile and nonsterile) are listed in Table 1.3.

   a. Sterile gloves are required when catheters are placed in arteries, large central veins, and closed spaces (including the epidural and subarachnoid spaces).

   b. Nonsterile gloves are used for contact with blood, body fluids, secretions, excretions, nonintact skin, and mucous membranes.

   c. Nonsterile gloves can be used for insertion of peripheral vein catheters as long as a "no touch" technique is used (i.e., the gloved hands do not touch the shaft of the catheter).

2. *Gloves and Handwashing*

   a. The use of gloves does not eliminate the need for handwashing.

   b. Handwashing is recommended both before donning gloves, and again after the gloves are removed.

3. *Latex Allergy*

Latex is a natural rubber product that is used in the manufacture of several medical products, including gloves, face masks, blood pressure cuffs, and catheters. Repeated exposure to latex can promote hypersensitivity reactions.

   a. Latex hypersensitivity is reported in 10% to 20% of hospital workers, compared to 1% of the general population (8). It is particularly prevalent in patients with spina bifida (up to 40% of patients), for unclear reasons.

   b. The clinical manifestations of latex allergy can include atopic dermatitis (urticaria or eczema), anaphylaxis, rhinoconjunctivitis, or asthma (8,9).

   c. The diagnosis of latex allergy can be elusive because the clinical presentation is nonspecific, and some of the manifestations (rhinoconjunctivitis and asthma) do appear without direct contact with latex. Allergic reactions that are work-related (i.e., appear when at work and disappear when away from work) should raise suspicion of latex allergy.

   d. There are two tests for latex hypersensitivity: a skin test, and an assay for latex-specific IgE levels in the bloodstream. Both have shortcomings. The latex-specific IgE assay is currently the favored test, but the sensitivity can be low (10).

TABLE 1.3 Recommendations for Glove Use in the ICU

I. Sterile gloves must be worn for the following procedures:
1. Central venous catheterization.
2. Peripherally-inserted central catheters.
3. Arterial catheterization.
4. Placement of drainage catheters in a closed space (pleural, pericardial. or peritoneal cavities).
5. Insertion of epidural or intraventricular catheters.

II. Nonsterile gloves are recommended for the following situations:
1. When there is contact with blood, body fluids, secretions, excretions, nonintact skin, and mucous membranes.
2. Insertion of peripheral venous catheters (the gloved hands must not touch the catheter).

III. General recommendations:
1. Handwashing is recommended before glove use, and again after gloves are removed.
2. Gloves should be changed between tasks involving the same patient if there has been contact with potentially infectious material.
3. Gloves should be removed immediately after use. before contact with noncontaminated objects in the environment, and before going to another patient.

From References 5–7.

e. The treatment of latex allergy includes symptom relief and removal of latex from the subject's environment. Latex-free (vinyl) gloves are available in most hospitals, but complete removal of latex from the hospital environment is often not possible because of the large number of medical products that contain latex (it is even found on tongue depressors).

B. Masks & Other Barriers

Face masks, eye shields, and gowns are also used as physical barriers to infectious agents. These barriers are recommended for any procedure or patient care activity that could generate a splash of blood, body fluids, secretions, or excretions.

1. *Face Masks*

   There are two general types of face masks: surgical masks and respirators.

   a. Surgical masks do not provide an effective barrier for airborne pathogens, and they should not be used as a preventive measure for airborne illnesses. The popularity of these masks in the ICU is unfounded.

   b. Respirators are devices that protect the wearer from inhaling a dangerous substance. Particulate respirators block particulate matter, and can block the inhalation of airborne pathogens, especially the tubercle bacillus. The most effective of these devices is the N95 respirator (11): the "N" indicates that the mask will block non-oil based or aqueous aerosols (the type that transmits the tubercle bacillus), and the "95" indicates the mask will block 95% of the intended particles.

2. *Airborne Illness*

   Infectious particles that are capable of airborne transmission are divided into two categories: those greater than 5 microns ($> 5\mu$) in diameter, and those that are 5 microns or less ($\leq 5\mu$) in diameter. The organisms and airborne illnesses in each category are shown in Figure 1.1.

   a. The larger airborne particles ($> 5\mu$ in diameter) usually travel no farther than 3 feet through the air, and to prevent transmission of these particles, a surgical mask is recommended (despite lack of proven efficacy!) when hospital staff or visitors are within 3 feet of the patient (5).

b. The smaller (≤ 5µ in diameter) infectious particles can travel long distances in the air. To prevent transmission of these particles, patients should be isolated in private rooms that are maintained at a negative pressure relative to the surrounding areas.

c. For patients with infectious tuberculosis (pulmonary or laryngeal), all hospital staff and visitors should wear an N95 respirator mask while in the room (5,12).

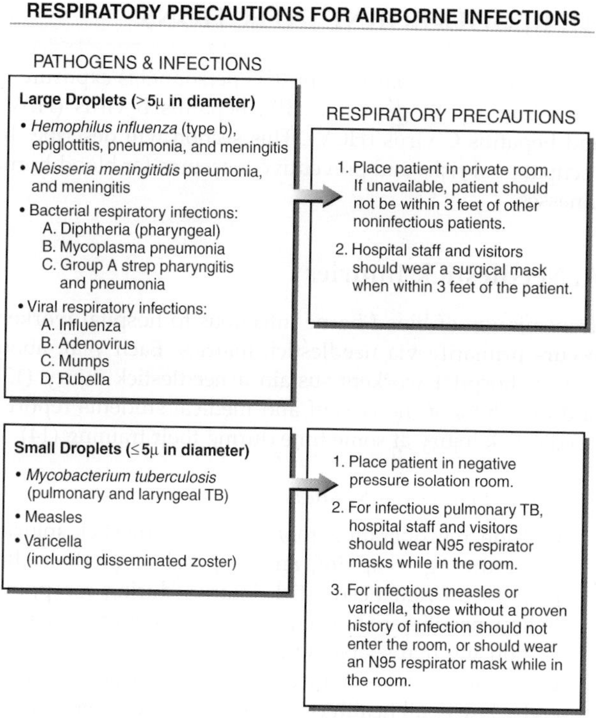

RESPIRATORY PRECAUTIONS FOR AIRBORNE INFECTIONS

PATHOGENS & INFECTIONS

Large Droplets (> 5µ in diameter)

- *Hemophilus influenza* (type b), epiglottitis, pneumonia, and meningitis
- *Neisseria meningitidis* pneumonia, and meningitis
- Bacterial respiratory infections:
  A. Diphtheria (pharyngeal)
  B. Mycoplasma pneumonia
  C. Group A strep pharyngitis and pneumonia
- Viral respiratory infections:
  A. Influenza
  B. Adenovirus
  C. Mumps
  D. Rubella

RESPIRATORY PRECAUTIONS

1. Place patient in private room. If unavailable, patient should not be within 3 feet of other noninfectious patients.
2. Hospital staff and visitors should wear a surgical mask when within 3 feet of the patient.

Small Droplets (≤ 5µ in diameter)

- *Mycobacterium tuberculosis* (pulmonary and laryngeal TB)
- Measles
- Varicella (including disseminated zoster)

1. Place patient in negative pressure isolation room.
2. For infectious pulmonary TB, hospital staff and visitors should wear N95 respirator masks while in the room.
3. For infectious measles or varicella, those without a proven history of infection should not enter the room, or should wear an N95 respirator mask while in the room.

FIGURE 1.1. Recommendations for preventing the spread of airborne pathogens. (From Reference 5).

d. For patients in the infectious stages of rubeola
(measles) and varicella (chickenpox or herpes zoster),
individuals with no prior history of these infections
who are also pregnant, immunocompromised, or
debilitated by disease should not be allowed in the
patient's room. Other susceptible individuals can enter the room, but they must wear an N95 respirator
mask.

III. BLOOD-BORNE INFECTIONS

The greatest infectious risk for ICU personnel is exposure to
blood-borne pathogens like HIV, hepatitis B virus (HBV),
and hepatitis C virus (HCV). This section will describe the
occupational risks and preventive measures for blood-borne
illnesses.

A. Needlestick Injuries

Transmission of blood-borne infections to hospital workers
occurs primarily via needlestick injuries. Each year, about
10% of hospital workers sustain a needlestick injury (13),
and over 50% of housestaff and medical students report a
needlestick injury at some time during their training (14).

1. *Safety-Engineered Needles*

Outside the operating room, most needlestick injuries
occur during recapping and disposal of used needles
(13). To prevent needlestick injuries during recapping,
hollow needles are now equipped with a protective plastic housing that snaps in place over the needle after it is
used. Such "safety-engineered" needles are now mandat-
ed by law in all health care facilities in the United States.

B. Human Immunodeficiency Virus (HIV)

The spread of HIV to hospital workers is universally feared, but is rare. In fact, there are only 56 cases of HIV seroconversion in healthcare workers that can be definitely linked to HIV transmission in the workplace (13).

1. *Percutaneous Exposures*

   Transmission of HIV via needlestick injuries is uncommon.

   a. A single needlestick injury with blood from an HIV-infected patient carries an average 0.3% risk of HIV seroconversion (13,15). Factors that increase the risk of transmission include a deep skin puncture, visible blood on the needle, and injury from a needle that was placed in an artery or vein of the source patient.

2. *Mucous Membrane Exposures*

   The risk of HIV transmission through mucous membranes or nonintact skin is even less than the risk from needlestick injuries.

   a. A single exposure of broken skin or mucous membranes to blood from an HIV-infected patient carries an average 0.09% risk of HIV seroconversion (13,15).

3. *Postexposure Management*

   When a hospital worker sustains a needlestick injury, the HIV status of the source patient is used to determine the need for HIV prophylaxis with antiretroviral drugs. This is outlined in Table 1.4.

   a. If HIV infection is proven or suspected in the source patient, prophylaxis with 2 antiretroviral agents is started immediately. A third drug is added if the source patient has symptomatic HIV infection.

TABLE 1.4 Indications for Antiretroviral Drugs Following Possible HIV Exposure

No Drugs	Two Drugs[1]	Three Drugs[2]
1. When source is HIV-negative	1. When source is HIV-positive but asymptomatic	1. When source is HIV-positive and symptomatic
2. When HIV status of source is not known but HIV is unlikely[3]	2. When HIV status of source is not known but HIV is likely[3]	2. When source is HIV-positive and asymptomatic but exposure is severe[5]
3. When source is not known but HIV is unlikely[4]	3. When source is not known but HIV is likely[4]	

From Reference 15.

[1]The recommended two-drug regimen is zidovudine (200 mg TID) plus lamivudine (150 mg BID) for 4 weeks. The two agents are available together as COMBIVIR™.

[2]Add one of the following drugs to the two-drug regimen: efavirenz (600 mg at bedtime), indinavir (800 mg every 8 hrs, between meals), or nelfinavir (2.5 g daily in 2 or 3 divided doses, with meals).

[3]When the HIV status of the source is unknown, the likelihood of HIV is based on the presence or absence of risk factors.

[4]When the source is unknown, the likelihood of HIV is based on the prevalence of HIV in the population served.

[5]Severe exposure is defined as: deep injury, needle soiled with blood from source patient, and exposure from needle inserted into artery or vein of source patient.

b. If the HIV status of the source patient is unknown and the patient is available, a rapid HIV-antibody test can be performed on the source patient. The results of this bedside test, which are available in minutes, can be used to determine the need for antiretroviral drugs. A negative test not only eliminates the fear of acquiring the illness, it also avoids the use of drugs that tend to be poorly tolerated. A positive test result must be confirmed by standard laboratory tests (e.g., a Western Blot or immunofluorescent antibody assay).

c. The antibody responses to HIV infection can take 4 to 6 weeks to become evident. Therefore, anyone with documented exposure to HIV infection should have serial tests for HIV antibodies at 6 weeks, 3 months, and 6 months post-exposure (5).

C. Hepatitis B Virus (HBV)

Hepatitis B is the most readily transmitted blood-borne illness, but there is a vaccine available that can produce lifelong immunity to HBV.

1. *Hepatitis B Vaccine*

The hepatitis B vaccine confers immunity by stimulating production of an antibody to the hepatitis B surface antigen (anti-HBs). This vaccine is recommended for anyone who has contact with blood, body fluids, and sharp instruments. The only contraindication to the vaccine is a history of anaphylaxis from baker's yeast (15).

a. The vaccine is administered in 3 doses: the first two doses are given 4 weeks apart, and the 3rd dose is administered 5 months later.

b. If the vaccination series is interrupted, it is not necessary to repeat the full sequence. If the second dose is missed, that dose is given as soon as possible, and the 3rd dose is given 2 months later. If the 3rd dose is missed, that dose is given to complete the vaccination series.

Because the initial vaccination sequence does not always confer immunity, the final dose of HBV vaccine should be followed (in 1 to 2 months) by an assay for the antibody to the hepatitis B surface antigen (anti-HBs).

c. Immunity is indicated by an anti-HBs level that is ≥ 10 mIU/mL. If this level is not achieved, the 3-dose vaccination series should be repeated.

Nonresponders have a 30% to 50% chance of responding to the second vaccination series (15). Failure to achieve immunity after the second vaccination series is considered a vaccination failure, and nothing further is done. Responders do not require a booster dose of the vaccine, even though antibody levels wane with time (15).

2. *Risk of HBV Transmission*

The risk of acquiring HBV following an exposure is determined by the immunity of the exposed individual.

a. For individuals who lack HBV immunity (unvaccinated or unresponsive), exposure to HBV-infected blood carries a 60% risk of acquiring HBV, and a 30% risk of developing symptomatic hepatitis (15).

b. For those who are vaccinated and respond appropriately, there is virtually no risk of acquiring HBV infection.

3. *Management Following Possible HBV Exposure*

The management of a subject with possible exposure to HBV is outlined in Table 1.5. The choices are guided by the vaccination status of the exposed individual, and the presence or absence of the hepatitis B surface antigen (HBsAg) in the blood of the source patient.

a. For individuals with vaccine-induced immunity, no treatment is necessary following HBV exposure.

b. For possible exposure in non-immune individuals, proof or suspicion of HBV infection in the source patient should prompt treatment with hepatitis B immune globulin (0.06 mL/kg by intramuscular injection), followed by HBV vaccination.

TABLE 1.5 Management of Possible Exposure to Hepatitis B Virus (HBV)

Immunity of Exposed Person	HBsAg[†] in Source Patient		
	HBsAg (+)	HBsAg (−)	HBsAg (?)
Not vaccinated	HBIG[a] and start HBV vaccination	Start HBV vaccination	Start HBV vaccination
Vaccinated & immune[c]	Do nothing	Do nothing	Do nothing
Vaccinated & not immune[d]	HBIG[a] and start HBV revaccination or HBIG x 2[b]	Do nothing	If source is high risk for HBV, treat as if source is HBsAg (+)
Immunity unknown	Check anti-HBs[††] in exposed person: 1. If immune,[c] no treatment 2. If not immune,[d] HBIG[a] and vaccine booster	Do nothing	Check anti-HBs[††] in exposed person: 1. If immune,[c] no treatment 2. If not immune, vaccine booster & recheck titer in 1–2 months

From Reference 15. [†]HBsAg = hepatitis B surface antigen.
[††]Anti-HBs = antibody to hepatitis B surface antigen.
[a]HBIG = hepatitis B immune globulin, 0.06 mL/kg by intramuscular injection immediately after exposure.
[b]HBIG x 2 = same as (a) above plus second dose one month later.
[c]Immunity defined as postvaccination anti-HBs ≥10 mIU/mL.
[d]Nonimmunity defined as postvaccination anti-HBs <10 mIU/mL.

D. Hepatitis C Virus (HCV)

HCV is a blood-borne pathogen of some concern because infection often leads to chronic hepatitis.

1. *Risk of HCV Transmission*

   a. The prevalence of anti-HCV antibodies in hospital personnel is only 1% to 2% (16), which means that the risk of HCV transmission in the hospital setting is low.

   b. Following a needlestick injury with HCV-infected blood, the average risk of HCV transmission is only 1.8% (15). Transmission from mucous membrane exposure is rare, and there are no documented cases of HCV transmission through breaks in the skin.

2. *Postexposure Management*

   a. There is no effective prophylaxis for HCV following exposure to infected blood.

   b. Following a documented exposure to HCV-infected blood, serial measurements of anti-HCV antibodies is recommended for 6 months (16).

REFERENCES

1. Larson EL, Rackoff WR, Weiman M, et al. APIC guideline for hand antisepsis in health-care settings. Am J Infect Control 1995; 23:251-269.

2. Centers for Disease Control and Prevention. Guidelines for Hand Hygiene in Health-Care Settings: Recommendations of the Healthcare Infection Control Practices Advisory Committee and the HICPAC/SHEA/APIC/IDSA Hand Hygiene Task Force. MMWR 2002; 51 (No.RR-16):1-45.

3. Katz JD. Hand washing and hand disinfection: more than your mother taught you. Anesthesiol Clin North Am 2004; 22:457-471.

4. Laestadius JG, Dimberg L. Hot water for handwashing – where is the proof? J Occup Environ Med 2005; 47:434-435.

5. Garner JS, Hospital Infection Control Practices Advisory Comitee. Guideline for isolation precautions in hospitals. Am J Infect Control 1996; 24:24-52.

6. Centers for Disease Control and Prevention. Guidelines for the prevention of intravascular catheter-related infections. MMWR 2002; 51(No. RR-10): 1-29.

7. Division of Healthcare Quality Promotion, National Center for Infectious Diseases, Centers for Disease Control and Prevention. Standard precautions: excerpted from Guideline for Isolation Precautions in Hospitals. Accessed at www.cdc.gov/ncidod /hip/ISOLAT/std_prec_excerpt.htm

8. Charous L, Charous MA. Is occupational latex allergy causing your patient's asthma? J Respir Dis 2002; 23:250-256.

9. Guin JD. Clinical presentation of patients sensitive to natural rubber latex. Dermatitis 2004; 4:192-196.

10. Hamilton RG, Peterson EL, Ownby DR. Clinical and laboratory-based methods in the diagnosis of natural rubber latex allergy. J Allergy Clin Immunol 2002; 110 (suppl 2): S47-S56.

11. Fennelly KP. Personal respiratory protection against *Mycobacterium tuberculosis*. Clin Chest Med 1997; 18:1-17.

12. Division of Healthcare Quality Promotion, National Center for Infectious Diseases, Centers for Disease Control and Prevention. Airborne precautions: excerpted from Guideline for Isolation Precautions in Hospitals. Accessed at www.cdc.gov/ncidod /hip/ISOLAT/airborne_prec_excerpt.htm

13. National Institute for Occupational Safety and Health. Preventing Needlestick Injuries in Health Care Settings. DHHS (NIOSH) Publication No. 2000-108, 1999.

14. Radechi S, Abbott A, Eloi L. Occupational human immunodeficiency virus exposure among residents and medical students. Arch Intern Med 2000; 160:3107-3100.

15. Centers for Disease Control and Prevention. Updated U.S. Public Health Service Guidelines for the management of occupational exposures to HBV, HCV, and HIV and recommendations for postexposure prophylaxis. MMWR 2001; 50 (No. RR-11):1-52.

16. Centers for Disease Control and Prevention. Immunization of Health-care workers: Recommendations of the Advisory Committee on Immunization Practices (ACIP) and the Hospital Infection Control Practices Advisory Committee (HICPAC). MMWR 1997, 46(RR-18): 1-42.

STRESS-RELATED MUCOSAL INJURY

Stress-related mucosal injury (SRMI) is a term used to describe erosions in the gastric mucosa that occur in patients with acute, life-threatening illness (1,2). This chapter will describe the methods used to prevent troublesome bleeding from these lesions.

I. GENERAL FEATURES

A. Pathogenesis

1. The gastric erosions that appear in acute, life-threatening illness are likely caused by inadequate nutrient blood flow in the gastric mucosa. The erosions are usually superficial and confined to the surface mucosa, but deeper craters that extend into the submucosa can develop. The deeper erosions resemble ulcer craters, and are called *stress ulcers*. (The term "stress ulcer" is often used to represent all types of stress-related gastric erosions. This chapter uses the term in a similar manner.)

2. Stress-related gastric erosions have no protective covering, and the acidity of gastric secretions can aggravate these lesions and promote further mucosal injury. The acidic environment in the stomach can also promote bleeding from the erosions by exerting a thrombolytic effect. The deleterious actions of gastric acidity is the basis for the popularity of gastric acid supression as a prophylactic strategy in this condition (see later).

B. Clinical Manifestations

1. Erosions in the gastric mucosa can be demonstrated in 75% to 100% of patients within 24 hours of admission to the ICU (3). These lesions are often clinically silent, but they can promote mucosal bleeding.

2. Without appropriate preventive measures (see later), gastric erosions can cause clinically apparent bleeding in as many as 25% of ICU patients (3). However, significant bleeding (i.e., causing hypotension or requiring transfusion) occurs in less than 5% of ICU patients (3,4).

TABLE 2.1 Indications for Stress Ulcer Prophylaxis		
Any of the Conditions Listed Below	**OR**	**Two or More of the Conditions Listed Below**

1. Mechanical ventilation > 48 hrs.
 2. Coagulopathy:
   a. Platelets <50,000/mL or
   b. INR > 1.5 or
   c. PTT > 2x control
 3. History of gastritis or peptic ulcer disease, or prior episode of upper GI bleeding.
		1. Hypotension
		 2. Severe sepsis
		 3. Severe head injury
		 4. Multisystem trauma
		 5. Renal failure
		 6. Hepatic failure
		 7. Burns involving >30% of the body surface area

From References 1,4.

C. Predisposing Conditions

The conditions listed in Table 2.1 are associated with an increased risk of troublesome bleeding from gastric erosions.

1. The 3 conditions in the left column (prolonged mechanical ventilation, coagulopathy, and a history of gastritis,

peptic ulcer disease, or upper GI hemorrhage) are independent risk factors, so the presence of any of these conditions represents a risk for significant bleeding.

2. The conditions listed in the right column are not independent risk factors, and at least 2 of these conditions must be present to create a risk for significant bleeding.

3. The predisposing conditions in Table 2.1 should also be used as indications for the preventive measures described next.

II. PREVENTIVE MEASURES

The goal of the preventive measures described here is not to prevent the appearance of gastric erosions (since this may be impossible), but rather to prevent troublesome bleeding from these lesions.

A. Enteral Tube Feedings

1. Enteral tube feedings exert a trophic effect on the bowel mucosa that helps to maintain the structural and functional integrity of the mucosa (see Chapter 37).

2. Clinical studies have shown that enteral tube feedings are effective in preventing overt bleeding from gastric erosions (5,6).

3. Enteral tube feedings should be considered adequate prophylaxis for SRMI-induced bleeding in most patients. Possible exceptions are patients with a coagulopathy, a prior history of bleeding from gastritis or peptic ulcer disease, or active peptic ulcer disease.

B. Reduced Gastric Acidity

The most popular preventive measure for bleeding related to stress ulcers is the use of drugs that can reduce the acidity of gastric secretions (7). The goal of acid suppression therapy is to maintain a pH > 4.0 in gastric secretions.

1. *Histamine Type-2 Receptor Antagonists*

   a. The standard acid-suppressing drugs for stress ulcer prophylaxis are the histamine type-2 receptor antagonists (H_2-blockers). Numerous clinical trials have shown that these drugs reduce the incidence of stress ulcer bleeding to ≤ 3% in high-risk patients (8,9).

   b. The H_2-blockers most often used for stress ulcer prophylaxis are famotidine (Pepcid) and ranitidine (Zantac). Both are given intravenously in the dosing regimens shown in Table 2.2 (10,11). Famotidine is longer-lasting than ranitidine (10–12 hrs. vs. 6–8 hrs.), and is given less frequently. Both drugs are equivalent in their ability to reduce the risk of bleeding from stress ulcers.

   c. Famotidine and ranitidine are excreted unchanged in the urine, and these drugs can accumulate in renal insufficiency and produce a neurotoxic condition characterized by confusion, agitation and seizures (10,11). The dosage of these drugs should be reduced in renal insufficiency (see Table 2.3).

2. *Proton Pump Inhibitors*

   a. Proton pump inhibitors (PPIs) block gastric acid secretion by irreversibly binding to the hydrogen ion pump in gastric parietal cells. These agents have 2 potential advantages over H_2-blockers: they are more effective in reducing gastric acidity (and maintaining gastric pH above 4.0), and their effect is not diminished with repeated use (12).

b. In the ICU setting, PPIs have been used primarily to prevent rebleeding following an episode of acute (non-variceal) upper GI bleeding. There is limited experience with these agents for stress ulcer prophylaxis.

c. There are 2 PPIs available for intravenous use: omeprazole (Prilosec) and pantoprazole (Protonix). The dosage recommendations for each drug are shown in Table 2.2. Note that a continuous infusion is used when the drugs are given to prevent rebleeding.

d. Despite the potential advantage of PPIs over H$_2$-blockers for gastric acid suppression, there is no evidence

TABLE 2.2 Drugs Used to Prevent Bleeding from Stress Ulcers

Agent	Route	Dose Recommendations
1. Histamine H$_2$-Receptor Antagonists		
Famotidine	IV	a. 20 mg every 12 hrs. b. Reduce dose in renal insufficiency (see Table 2.3).
Ranitidine	IV	a. 50 mg every 8 hrs. b. Reduce dose in renal insufficiency (see Table 2.3).
2. Proton Pump Inhibitors		
Omeprazole	IV	a. 80 mg daily as a single dose b. To prevent rebleeding after GI bleed, follow initial dose with a continuous infusion at 8 mg/hr for 1–3 days.
Pantoprazol	IV	a. 40 mg daily as a single dose b. Same as above for omeprazole.
3. Cytoprotective Agent		
Sucralfate	NG Tube	a. 1 g (as a slurry) every 6 hrs. b. Avoid drug interactions.

that PPIs provide more protection against stress ulcer bleeding than H_2-blockers. At the present time, there is no reason to favor PPIs over H_2-blockers for stress ulcer prophylaxis.

TABLE 2.3 Dosage Adjustment of H_2-Blockers in Renal Insufficiency

Creatinine Clearance (mL/min)	Percent of Usual Dose	
	Ranitidine	Famotidine
51 – 75	75%	50%
10 – 50	50%	25%
< 10	25%	10%

From Self TH. Mental confusion induced by H_2-receptor anatgonists: How to avoid. J Crit Illness 2000;15:47.

3. The Hazards of Gastric Acid Suppression

Most microorganisms do not survive in an acid environment, as demonstrated in Figure 2.1. In this case, *Escherichia coli* is completely eradicated in one hour when the pH of the growth medium is reduced from 5 to 3 pH units. The antimicrobial effects of an acid environment were appreciated by Sir Joseph Lister, the father of antiseptic practices in medicine, who used carbolic *acid* as the first antiseptic agent for the skin.

a. In light of the germicidal actions of acidity, it is likely that gastric acid serves as a built-in antiseptic agent that eradicates microorganisms swallowed in saliva and food.

b. Loss of the normal antiseptic actions of gastric acid will result in bacterial overgrowth in the stomach, and this can predispose to certain infections, including infectious gastroenteritis and aspiration pneumonia (13).

c. Several clinical studies have revealed that stress ulcer prophylaxis with H_2-blockers is associated with an increased incidence of pneumonia (9). This is demonstrated in Figure 2.2 (this figure is explained later in the chapter).

d. The loss of antimicrobial defenses with gastric acid suppression is reason to consider preventive measures for stress ulcer bleeding that do not involve gastric acid suppression. One such measure is described next.

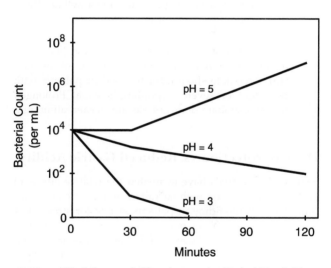

FIGURE 2.1. The influence of pH on the growth of *Escherichia coli*. (From Gianella J et al. Gut 1972;13:251.).

C. Gastric Cytoprotection

1. *Sucralfate*

   a. Sucralfate is an aluminum salt of sucrose sulfate that acts as a *cytoprotective agent* by forming a protective covering on the gastric mucosa (10). The pH of gastric secretions is not altered.

b. The recommended dose of sucralfate to prevent stress ulcer bleeding is shown in Table 2.2. The drug is usually given as a liquid slurry that is instilled through a nasogastric tube.

c. Sucralfate can bind to a number of drugs in the bowel lumen to reduce drug absorption (14). The drug interactions most likely in ICU patients include coumadin, digoxin, fluoroquinolones, phenytoin, quinidine, ranitidine, tetracycline, thyroxine, theophylline. These drugs should be given at least 2 hours before sucralfate to avoid drug interactions.

d. The aluminum in sucralfate can also bind phosphate in the bowel, but hypophosphatemia is uncommon (15). Sucralfate should not be used in patients with persistent or severe hypophosphatemia. Prolonged use of sucralfate does not elevate plasma aluminum levels.

D. Cytoprotection vs. Reduced Gastric Acidity

Several clinical trials have evaluated the relative effects of gastric cytoprotection with sucralfate and gastric acid suppression with ranitidine in patients at risk for stress ulcer bleeding. The results of one of these trials are shown in Figure 2.2 (8). This study involved 1,200 ventilator-dependent patients in 16 ICUs who were randomized to receive sucralfate or ranitidine in the usual doses. The results show the following:

1. Significant bleeding occurs infrequently (< 5%), regardless of the prophylactic drug regimen. This indicates that ranitidine and sucralfate are both effective agents for stress ulcer prophylaxis.

2. Prophylaxis with ranitidine is associated with fewer episodes of bleeding (absolute difference = 2.1%), while

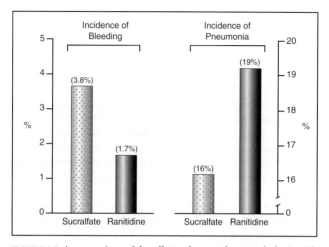

FIGURE 2.2. A comparison of the effects of stress ulcer prophylaxis with sucralfate and ranitidine on the incidence of clinically significant bleeding and hospital-acquired pneumonia in ventilator-dependent patients. (From Reference 8).

prophylaxis with sucralfate is associated with fewer episodes of pneumonia (absolute difference = 2.9%).

3. The increased incidence of pneumonia associated with ranitidine is consistent with the combined results of 8 other clinical trials (9). This association is predicted by the loss of the antibacterial defenses in the upper GI tract as a consequence of reduced gastric acidity, as described earlier.

4. *Reasons to Avoid Gastric Acid Suppression with Ranitidine*

   a. The benefit derived from gastric acid suppression with ranitidine (i.e., fewer episodes of bleeding from stress ulcers) must be weighed against the associated risk (i.e., more frequent episodes of pneumonia). Since nosocomial pneumonia has a higher mortality rate than stress ulcer bleeding (50% vs. 10%), gastric acid suppression with ranitidine can result in more lives lost from pneumonia than lives saved from fewer bleeding episodes. This is one reason to avoid the use of gastric acid suppression with ranitidine (or any other drug) as a preventive strategy for stress-related gastric erosions.

b. Severe sepsis and septic shock are among the leading causes of death in ICU patients, and the gastrointestinal tract is an important reservoir for pathogens in these conditions (16). The suppression of gastric acidity (by any means) will add to this problem by promoting microbial proliferation in the upper GI tract. For this reason, gastric acidity should be preserved whenever possible to preserve the antimicrobial defense system in the bowel and reduce the risk of sepsis from bowel pathogens.

REFERENCES

1. Steinberg KP. Stress-related mucosal disease in the critically ill patient: Risk factors and strategies to prevent stress-related bleeding in the intensive care unit. Crit Care Med 2002; 30 (Suppl):S362-S364.

2. Fennerty MB. Pathophysiology of the upper gastrointestinal tract in the critically ill patient: rationale for the therapeutic benefits of acid suppression. Crit Care Med 2002; 30(Suppl):S351-S355.

3. Muthu GM, Mutlu EA, Factor P. GI complications in patients receiving mechanical ventilation. Chest 2001; 119:1222-1241.

4. Cook DJ, Fuller MB, Guyatt GH. Risk factors for gastrointestinal bleeding in critically ill patients. N Engl J Med 1994; 330:377–381.

5. Raff T, Germann G, Hartmann B. The value of early enteral nutrition in the prophylaxis of stress ulceration in the severely burned patient. Burns 1997; 23:313-318.

6. Pingleton SK, Hadzima SK. Enteral alimentation and gastrointestinal bleeding in mechanically ventilated patients. Crit Care Med 1983; 11:13-16.

7. Daley RJ, Rebuck JA, Welage LS, Rogers FB. Prevention of stress ulceration: current trends in critical care. Crit Care Med 2004; 32: 2008-2013.

8. Cook D, Guyatt G, Marshall J, et al. A comparison of sucralfate and ranitidine for the prevention of upper gastrointestinal bleeding in patients requiring mechanical ventilation. New Engl J Med 1998; 338:791-797.

9. Messori A, Trippoli S, Vaiani M, et al. Bleeding and pneumonia in intensive care patients given ranitidine and sucralfate for prevention of stress ulcer: meta-analysis of randomized controlled trials. Br Med J 2000; 321:1-7.

10. Famotidine. Mosby's Drug Consult. Mosby, Inc., 2006. Accessed at www.mdconsult.com in March, 2007.

11. Ranitidine. Mosby's Drug Consult. Mosby, Inc., 2006. Accessed at www.mdconsult.com. in March, 2007.

12. Morgan D. Intravenous proton pump inhibitors in the critical care setting. Crit Care Med 2002; 30(Suppl): S369-S372.

13. Laheij R, Sturkenboom M, Hassing R-J, et al. Risk of community-acquired pneumonia and use of gastric acid-suppressive drugs. JAMA 2004; 292:1955-1960.

14. McEvoy GK, ed. AHFS Drug Information, 1995. Bethesda, MD: American Society of Health System Pharmacists, 1995:2021–2065.

15. Miller SJ, Simpson J. Medication–nutrient interactions: hypo-phosphatemia associated with sucralfate in the intensive care unit. Nutr Clin Pract 1991; 6:199–201.

16. Marshall JC, Christou NV, Meakins JL, et al. The gastrointestinal tract: the "undrained abscess" of multiple organ failure. Ann Surg 1993; 218:111–119.

Chapter 3

VENOUS THROMBOEMBOLISM

Venous thromboembolism (venous thrombosis and pulmonary embolism) is responsible for an estimated 10% of all hospital deaths (1). This is an alarming estimate considering that venous thromboembolism (VTE) is considered preventable in most cases. This chapter describes the prevention, diagnosis, and treatment of VTE in hospitalized patients, with emphasis on prevention.

I. THE PATIENT AT RISK

The clinical conditions that are most often accompanied by VTE are listed in Table 3.1 (1-3). A patient who has any of these conditions should receive prophylaxis for VTE.

A. Major Surgery

Major surgery (performed under general anesthesia and lasting longer than 30 minutes) is the most common high-risk condition for VTE in hospitalized patients. The major factors promoting VTE after major surgery are vascular injury and thromboplastin release from injured tissues (which produces a hypercoagulable state).

1. *General Surgery*

The risk of VTE after general surgery is determined by 3 factors: the age of the patient, the type of procedure, and the presence or absence of other risk factors for VTE.

Table 3.2 shows how these factors are used in the risk assessment for VTE following general surgery.

a. The lowest risk of VTE occurs after minor procedures performed on young patients (age < 40) who have no other risk factors for VTE .

TABLE 3.1 Risk Assessment for Venous Thromboembolism

If the patient has any of the conditions listed below, place a checkmark in the corresponding box. Check only conditions that are currently present or have occurred within the past week.

Patient Profile

Prior history of thromboembolism	❏
Malignancy	❏
Hypercoagulable state (e.g., estrogen R_x)	❏

Surgery

Major surgery (e.g., abdominal, intracranial)	❏
Orthopedic surgery involving the hip or knee	❏

Trauma

Spinal cord injury or spinal fracture	❏
Fractures involving the pelvis, hip, or leg	❏
Multisystem trauma	❏

Acute Medical Illness

Stroke or acute myocardial infarction	❏
Neuromuscular weakness (e.g., Guillain-Barré)	❏

ICU-Related Conditions

Mechanical ventilation >48 hrs.	❏
Drug-induced neuromuscular paralysis	❏
Central venous or femoral vein catheter	❏

If any of the above boxes is checked, the patient should receive prophylaxis for venous thromboembolism.

From References 1–3

b. The highest risk of VTE occurs after major surgery in older patients (age > 40) who have at least one additional risk factor for VTE.

The incidence of VTE in high-risk general surgery patients is 20% to 40% (1).

2. *Orthopedic Surgery*

The highest incidence of postoperative VTE (40 to 60%) occurs after major surgery involving the hip or knee (1).

3. *Other Surgeries*

a. VTE is a risk after intracranial surgery, open urologic procedures, and gynecologic surgery. The incidence of VTE following these procedures is 20% to 40% (1).

b. Laparoscopy, arterial reconstruction surgery, and closed urologic procedures (e.g., transurethral prostatectomy) have a low risk of VTE, and do not require thromboprophylaxis unless the patient has an inherent risk of VTE (1).

B. Major Trauma

1. Victims of major trauma have a greater than 50% chance of developing VTE while hospitalized, and pulmonary embolism is the leading cause of death in those who survive the first week (1).

2. The trauma conditions with the highest risk of VTE are spinal cord injuries and fractures of the spine and pelvis (1,3).

C. Medical Conditions

1. The acute medical illnesses with a high risk of VTE are stroke, acute myocardial infarction, and neuromuscular

weakness syndromes (e.g., Guillain-Barré). Of these, stroke has the highest incidence of VTE (20% to 50%) (1).

2. ICU patients can have additional risk factors for VTE such as prolonged mechanical ventilation, drug-induced neuromuscular paralysis, and central venous catheterization (4).

TABLE 3.2 Thromboprophylaxis for General Surgery

Risk Categories	Prophylaxis Regimens
I. Low Risk Minor surgery, age <40 yrs. and no other risk factors[a]	I. Early mobilization
II. Moderate Risk Major surgery, age <40 yrs. and no other risk factors	II. $LDUH_1$ or $LMWH_1$, start 2 hr before surgery.
III. High Risk Major surgery, age >40 yrs. or other risk factors	III. $LDUH_2$ or $LMWH_2$, start 2 hr before surgery.
IV. Highest Risk Major surgery, age >40 yrs. and other risk factors	IV. $LDUH_2$ or $LMWH_2$, (start 2 hr before surgery) plus mechanical compression.

Prophylaxis Regimens

Low-Dose Unfractionated Heparin (LDUH):
  $LDUH_1$: 5000 units subcutaneous every 12 hrs.
  $LDUH_2$: 5000 units subcutaneous every 8 hrs.

Low-Molecular-Weight Heparin (LMWH):
  $LMWH_1$: Enoxaparin, 40 mg subcutaneous once daily or
       Dalteparin, 2500 units subcutaneous once daily.

  $LMWH_2$: Enoxaparin, 30 mg subcutaneous every 12 hrs. or
       Dalteparin, 5000 units subcutaneous once daily.

Mechanical Compression:
  Compression stockings or intermittent pneumatic compression.

---

[a]Other risk factors: cancer, obesity, prior history of thromboembolism, hypercoagulable state (e.g., estrogen R_x).

Adapted from Reference 1.

II. THROMBOPROPHYLAXIS

A. Mechanical Compression Devices

The following mechanical compression devices are used as an adjunct to anticoagulant prophylaxis, or as an alternative to anticoagulant prophylaxis in patients who are bleeding or have a high risk of bleeding.

1. *Graded Compression Stockings*

    a. Graded compression stockings are designed to create 18 mm Hg external pressure at the ankles and 8 mm Hg external pressure in the thigh (5). The resulting 10 mm Hg pressure gradient promotes venous outflow from the legs.

    b. Although effective when used alone after abdominal surgery and neurosurgery (6), these stockings are the least effective method of thromboprophylaxis, and are never used alone in patients with a moderate or high risk of VTE.

2. *Pneumatic Compression Devices*

    a. Intermittent pneumatic compression (IPC) devices use an air pump to periodically inflate and deflate distensible bladders that are wrapped around the lower legs. When inflated, the bladders create 35 mm Hg external pressure at the ankle and 20 mm Hg external pressure at the thigh (5).

    b. IPC devices are more effective than graded compression stockings for prophylaxis of VTE (1), and they can be used alone for patients who are not suitable for anticoagulant prophylaxis. These devices are favored after intracranial surgery, spinal cord injury, and multisystem trauma (see Table 3.3).

B. Low-Dose Heparin

Heparin is an indirect-acting anticoagulant that binds to a cofactor (antithrombin III or AT) to produce its effect. The heparin-AT complex is capable of inactivating several coagulation factors, including Factors IIa (thrombin), IXa, Xa, XIa, and XIIa. The inactivation of Factor IIa (antithrombin effect) is a sensitive reaction that occurs at heparin doses far below those needed to inactivate the other coagulation factors (7). This means that small doses of heparin can inhibit thrombus formation without producing full anticoagulation.

1. *Dosing Regimen*
   a. The standard heparin preparation is called unfractionated heparin to distinguish it from low-molecular-weight heparin (see later).
   b. The regimen for low-dose unfractionated heparin (LDUH) is 5,000 units given by subcutaneous injection two or three times daily. The more frequent dosing regimen (three times daily) is recommended for higher risk conditions (see the LDUH$_2$ regimen in Tables 3.2 and 3.3).
   c. When LDUH is used for surgical prophylaxis, the first dose should be given 2 hours before the procedure (because thrombosis can begin during the procedure). Postoperative prophylaxis is continued for 7 to 10 days, or until the patient is fully ambulatory.
   d. Monitoring laboratory tests of coagulation is not necessary with low-dose heparin.

2. *Indications*
   a. LDUH provides effective thromboprophylaxis for high-risk medical conditions and most non-orthopedic surgical procedures (see Tables 3.2 and 3.3).
   b. LDUH is *not* recommended for thromboprophylaxis in major trauma (including spinal cord injury), and for orthopedic surgery involving the hip and knee.

3. *Complications*

a. Bleeding is not considered a complication of low-dose heparin.

b. The heparin-antithrombin III complex binds to platelet Factor 4, and some patients develop a heparin-induced antibody that cross-reacts with this platelet binding site to produce platelet clumping and subsequent thrombocytopenia. This is called *heparin-induced thrombocytopenia*, and it promotes thrombosis rather than bleeding (see Chapter 31).

TABLE 3.3 Thromboprophylaxis for Selected Conditions

Clinical Conditions	Prophylaxis Regimens
1. Major trauma	1. $LMWH_2$ or IPC
2. Spinal cord injury	2. $LMWH_2$ plus IPC
3. Intracranial surgery	3. IPC
4. Gynecologic surgery	
a. Benign disease	4a. $LDUH_1$
b. Malignancy	4b. $LDUH_2$ or $LMWH_2$
5. Urologic surgery	
a. Closed procedures	5a. Early mobilization
b. Open procedures	5b. $LDUH_1$ or IPC
6. High-risk medical condition	6. $LDUH_2$ or $LMWH_1$

Prophylaxis Regimens

Low-Dose Unfractionated Heparin (LDUH):
   $LDUH_1$: 5000 units subcutaneous every 12 hrs.
   $LDUH_2$: 5000 units subcutaneous every 8 hrs.

Low-Molecular-Weight Heparin (LMWH):
   $LMWH_1$: Enoxaparin, 40 mg subcutaneous once daily or
        Dalteparin, 2500 units subcutaneous once daily.
   $LMWH_2$: Enoxaparin, 30 mg subcutaneous every 12 hrs. or
        Dalteparin, 5000 units subcutaneous once daily.

Intermittent Pneumatic Compression (IPC)

Adapted from Reference 1.

C. Low-Molecular-Weight Heparin

1. *Comparison of Heparin Preparations*

   a. Standard (unfractionated) heparin contains molecules that vary widely in size. The anticoagulant activity of heparin is dependent on the size of the molecules (smaller molecules have more activity), so the variable size of the molecules in unfractionated heparin gives it variable anticoagulant activity.

   b. Heparin molecules of variable size can be cleaved enzymatically to produce smaller molecules of more uniform size. Because smaller molecules have more anticoagulant activity, the resultant *low-molecular-weight heparin* (LMWH) is more potent and has more uniform anticoagulant activity than unfractionated heparin.

   c. The advantages of LMWH over unfractionated heparin include less frequent dosing, a lower risk of bleeding and heparin-induced thrombocytopenia, and no need to monitor anticoagulant activity (7,8).

2. *Indications for LMWH*

   LMWH is preferred to unfractionated heparin for thromboprophylaxis in:

   a. Major trauma, including spinal cord injury (see Table 3.3).

   b. Orthopedic procedures involving the hip and knee (see Table 3.4).

   For other conditions where anticoagulant prophylaxis is recommended, LMWH can be used as an alternative to low-dose unfractionated heparin.

3. *Drugs and Dosing Regimens*

   Two LMWH preparations have been studied for thromboprophylaxis: *enoxaparin* (Lovenox) and *dalteparin* (Fragmin). Both drugs are given by subcutaneous injection in the doses shown in Tables 3.2–3.4 (see $LMWH_1$ and $LMWH_2$).

a. Enoxaparin: 40 mg once daily for moderate-risk conditions, and 30 mg twice daily for high-risk conditions.

b. Dalteparin: 2500 units once daily for moderate-risk conditions, and 5000 units once daily for high-risk conditions.

c. For hip and knee surgery, the first dose of LMWH should be given 6 hours after surgery (9). For other surgical procedures, the first dose of LMWH can be given 2 hours before the procedure (1).

d. For patients with renal failure, the prophylactic dose of enoxaparin should be decreased from 30 mg twice daily to 40 mg once daily for high-risk patients (1). No dose adjustment is needed for dalteparin.

TABLE 3.4 Thromboprophylaxis for Hip and Knee Surgery

Drug Regimens
1. Low-molecular-weight heparin (LMWH)
   a. Enoxaparin, 30 mg subcutaneous every 12 hrs. or
   b. Dalteparin, 2500 units subcutaneous initially, then 5000 units subcutaneous once daily.
   c. Give first dose 6 hrs. after surgery.
2. Fondaparinux
   a. 2.5 mg by subcutaneous injection once daily.
   b. Give first dose 6 hrs. after surgery.
   c. Contraindicated when creatinine clearance < 30 mL/min.
3. Adjusted-dose warfarin
   a. 10 mg initially, then 2.5 mg daily. Adjust dose to achieve INR = 2 – 3.
   b. Give first dose the evening before surgery.

Duration of Prophylaxis
1. For elective hip and knee surgery, continue for 10 days after surgery.
2. For hip fracture surgery, continue for 28 to 35 days after surgery.

Adapted from Reference 1.

e. The use of LMWH with spinal anesthesia for hip and knee surgery can result in spinal hematoma and paralysis. When spinal anesthesia is used, the first dose of LMWH should be delayed until 12 to 24 hours after surgery (9), or adjusted-dose warfarin should be used for thromboprophylaxis.

D. Adjusted-Dose Warfarin

Adjusted-dose warfarin is one of three effective regimens for hip and knee surgery (see Table 3.4) It is the most popular prophylactic regimen for hip replacement surgery in North America, despite evidence that LMWH is more effective (1). Warfarin may be preferred in patients who require prolonged prophylaxis after hospital discharge (see later), because of the convenience of oral dosing. For the dosing regimen, see Table 3.4. The target INR of 2 to 3 is not reached for at least 3 days.

E. Fondaparinux

Fondaparinux (Arixtra, GlaxoSmithKline) is a synthetic anticoagulant that selectively inhibits coagulation Factor Xa. The benefits of fondaparinux over heparin include a predictable anticoagulant effect (obviating the need for laboratory monitoring), and lack of an immune-mediated thrombocytopenia (8,10).

1. *Dosing Regimen*
    a. The prophylactic dose of fondaparinux is 2.5 mg given once daily as a subcutaneous injection. When used for surgical prophylaxis, the first dose should be given 6 hours after surgery (if given sooner, there's an increased risk of bleeding) (1).
    b. Fondaparinux is cleared by the kidney, and is contraindicated when the creatinine clearance is <30 mL/min

(11). It is also contraindicated in patients who weigh < 50 kg because of an increased risk of bleeding (11).

2. *Indications*

Fondaparinux is as effective as LMWH for thromboprophylaxis after hip and knee surgery (see Table 3.4) (5).

F. Special Consideration After Hip and Knee Surgery

Following hip and knee surgery, there is an increase in symptomatic VTE after prophylaxis is terminated and patients are discharged from the hospital, and symptomatic VTE is the most common cause of readmission after hip replacement surgery (1). These observations prompted the following recommendations (1):

1. After hip and knee surgery, thromboprophylaxis should be continued for at least 10 days, even after patients are discharged.

2. After hip surgery, patients with additional risk factors for VTE (e.g., malignancy, advanced age, prior history of VTE), should receive prophylaxis for a total of 28 to 35 days.

III. DIAGNOSTIC APPROACH

Thrombosis in the deep veins of the legs is often clinically silent, and becomes apparent only when a portion of the thrombus breaks loose and becomes evident as a pulmonary embolus. Therefore, the diagnostic evaluation of suspected VTE usually involves an evaluation of suspected acute pulmonary embolism.

TABLE 3.5 Clinical and Laboratory Findings in Patients with Suspected Pulmonary Embolism

Findings	Positive Predictive Value	Negative Predictive Value
Dyspnea	37%	75%
Tachycardia	47%	86%
Tachypnea	48%	75%
Pleuritic chest pain	39%	71%
Hemoptysis	32%	67%
Hypoxemia	34%	70%
Elevated plasma D-dimer[a]	27%	92%
Increased dead space ventilation[b]	36%	92%

Positive predictive value is the percentage of patients with the finding who had a pulmonary embolus. It expresses the likelihood that a pulmonary embolus is present when the finding is present.

Negative predictive value is the percentage of patients with the finding who did not have a pulmonary embolus. It expresses the likelihood that a pulmonary embolus is not present when the finding is also not present.

[a]From Reference 14. [b]From Reference 15. Other data from Reference 12.

A. The Clinical Evaluation

The clinical presentation of acute pulmonary embolism is non-specific, and there are no clinical or laboratory findings that will confirm or exclude the presence of pulmonary embolism with certainty (12). The poor predictive value of clinical parameters in the diagnosis of pulmonary embolism is shown in Table 3.5. Two of the parameters in this table deserve mention: plasma D-dimer assays and the alveolar dead space measurement.

1. *Plasma D-Dimer Levels*

   a. Cross-linked fibrin monomers, also called degradation-dimers or *D-dimers*, are products of clot lysis, and plasma levels of these D-dimers are elevated in the presence of active thrombosis.

b. Unfortunately, several conditions other than thrombosis can be associated with elevated plasma D-dimer levels. These include sepsis, malignancy, pregnancy, heart failure, renal failure, and advanced age (13). As a result, up to 80% of ICU patients can have elevated plasma D-dimer levels in the absence of venous thrombosis (14).

c. In the ICU, plasma D-dimer levels may be more valuable for excluding the diagnosis of VTE. As shown in Table 3.5, the negative predictive value of the plasma D-dimer level is 92%, which means that a normal D-dimer level can exclude the presence of VTE with > 90% certainty.

d. The value of the D-dimer assay in excluding VTE is limited by the high prevalence of elevated D-dimer levels in ICU patients.

2. *Alveolar Dead Space*

a. One of the major consequences of a pulmonary embolus is a decrease in pulmonary blood flow and an increase in alveolar dead space ventilation.

b. In patients who present to the emergency room with suspected pulmonary embolism, a normal dead space measurement (i.e., < 15% of total ventilation) can exclude the presence of VTE with > 90% certainty (see the negative predictive value in Table 3.5) (15).

c. The predictive value of the dead space measurement has not been studied in ICU patients.

Because the clinical evaluation of suspected pulmonary embolism has poor predictive value, specialized tests are required. These tests are included in the flow diagram in Figure 3.1.

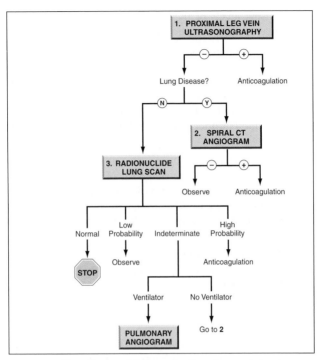

FIGURE 3.1. Flow diagram for the evaluation of suspected pulmonary embolism.

B. Venous Ultrasound

Most pulmonary emboli are believed to originate from thrombi located in large, proximal leg veins (e.g., femoral vein), so the evaluation of suspected pulmonary embolism can begin with an evaluation of the leg veins.

1. *Reliability of Venous Ultrasound*

   a. For the detection of deep vein thrombosis (DVT) in the thigh (proximal DVT), ultrasound has a sensitivity ≥ 95%, a specificity ≥ 97%, a positive predictive value as high as 97%, and a negative predictive value as high as 98% (16). These numbers indicate that ultrasound has a high degree of accuracy for the detection of proximal DVT in the legs.

b. For the detection of venous thrombosis below the knee (calf DVT), ultrasound has a sensitivity of only 33% to 70% (2). Therefore, ultrasound is *not* a reliable method for the diagnosis of DVT below the knee.

2. *When Venous Ultrasound is Unrevealing*

a. As many as 30% of patients with acute pulmonary embolism show no evidence of venous thrombosis in the legs (17). As a result, a negative venous ultrasound evaluation of the legs does not exclude the diagnosis of pulmonary embolus.

b. When venous ultrasound is unrevealing, the next step in the evaluation of pulmonary embolism is either spiral computed tomography (CT) or a radionuclide lung scan (see Figure 3.1)

C. Radionuclide Lung Scan

Ventilation-perfusion lung scans are diagnostic for pulmonary embolism in only 25% to 30% of cases (18). The problem is that the presence of lung disease will produce an abnormal scan in about 90% of cases (18). Lung scans are most helpful in patients with no underlying lung disease (which, unfortunately, excludes most ICU patients). If the decision is made to proceed with a lung scan, the results can be used as follows (18):

1. A normal lung scan excludes the presence of a pulmonary embolus, whereas a high-probability lung scan carries a 90% probability that a pulmonary embolus is present.

2. A low-probability lung scan does not reliably exclude the presence of a pulmonary embolism. However, when

combined with a negative ultrasound evaluation of the legs, a low-probability scan is sufficient reason to stop the diagnostic workup and observe the patient.

3. An intermediate-probability or indeterminate lung scan has no value in predicting the presence or absence of a pulmonary embolus. In this situation, the options include spiral CT angiography (see next) or conventional pulmonary angiography.

D. Spiral CT Angiography

This technique is most valuable in patients with lung disease (where lung scans are often nondiagnostic), but its use in the ICU is limited by the need to breath-hold during the procedure (see below).

1. *Technique*
    a. In conventional computed tomography (CT), the detector is moved in fixed increments to produce a series of images that appear as "slices" of tissue. In spiral CT, the detector is continuously rotated around the patient to produce a volumetric image.
    b. Spiral CT of the thorax takes 30 seconds to complete, and there must be no lung motion during the procedure. This means that *patients must be able to breath-hold for 30 seconds to perform a spiral CT scan*, and this excludes patients who are ventilator-dependent or are unable to follow commands.
    c. When spiral CT is combined with peripheral injection of a contrast agent, the central pulmonary arteries can be visualized. A pulmonary embolus appears as a filling defect.

2. *Performance*
    a. Spiral CT angiography has a sensitivity of 93% and a specificity of 97% for detecting clots in the major pul-

monary arteries (19). The sensitivity is only 30% for detecting clots in smaller, subsegmental arteries (19).

E. Pulmonary Angiography

Pulmonary angiography is the "gold standard" method for detecting pulmonary emboli, but is required in fewer than 15% of cases of suspected pulmonary embolism.

III. ANTITHROMBOTIC THERAPY

A. Anticoagulation

The initial treatment of thromboembolism that is not life-threatening is anticoagulation with heparin.

1. *Unfractionated Heparin*
    a. The standard treatment of VTE is unfractionated heparin given by continuous intravenous infusion using weight-based dosing as shown in Table 3.6 (20).
    b. Unfractionated heparin has unpredictable anticoagulant activity (as described earlier), and anticoagulant activity must be monitored using the partial thromboplastin time (PTT). This test is a reflection of Factor IIa activity, and one of the prominent effects of heparin is inhibition of Factor IIa.

2. *Low-Molecular-Weight Heparin (LMWH)*

    LMWH is as effective as unfractionated heparin (21) and offers some advantages, including simplified dosing and no need to monitor anticoagulant activity (see later).
    a. A standard LMWH treatment for VTE is enoxaparin given in a dose of 1 mg/kg by subcutaneous injection every 12 hours.

   b. Because LMWH is cleared by the kidneys (see earlier), unfractionated heparin is recommended for patients with renal failure (21).

   c. The PTT cannot be used to monitor anticoagulation with LMWH because LMWH acts primarily to inhibit Factor Xa, and the PTT is not a reflection of Factor Xa activity.

   d. Since LMWH produces a predictable level of anticoagulation, monitoring anticoagulant activity is usually not necessary. Factor Xa activity must be measured to determine the anticoagulant response to LMWH (20).

TABLE 3.6 Weight-Based Heparin Dosing Regimen

1. Prepare heparin infusion by adding 20,000 IU heparin to 500 mL diluent (40 IU/mL).
2. Give initial bolus dose of 80 IU/kg and follow with continuous infusion of 18 IU/kg/hr. (Use actual body weight.)
3. Check PTT 6 hrs. after start of infusion, and adjust heparin dose as indicated below.

PTT (sec)	PTT Ratio	Bolus Dose	Continuous Infusion
<35	<1.2	80 IU/kg	Increase by 4 IU/kg/hr
35–45	1.2–1.5	40 IU/kg	Increase by 2 IU/kg/hr
46–70	1.5–2.3	—	—
71–80	2.3–3.0	—	Decrease by 2 IU/kg/hr
>90	>3	—	Stop infusion for 1 hr then decrease by 3 IU/kg/hr

4. Check PTT 6 hrs. after each dose adjustment. When in the desired range (46–70 sec), monitor daily.

From Raschke RA, Reilly BM, Guidry JR, et al. The weight-based heparin dosing nomogram compared with the "standard care" nomogram. Ann Intern Med 1993; 119:874.

3. *Warfarin*

    a. Long-term anticoagulation with warfarin (coumadin) is started on the first day of heparin therapy. The usual starting dose is 5–10 mg once daily. When the prothrombin time reaches an international normalized ratio (INR) of 2 to 3 (which usually takes 3 days or longer), the heparin can be discontinued.

    b. Anticoagulation with coumadin is continued for 3 to 6 months, or longer in patients with cancer-related or recurrent VTE (21).

B. Thrombolytic Therapy

1. Thrombolytic therapy is reserved for life-threatening cases of pulmonary embolism accompanied by hemodynamic instability (21,22). Some recommend lytic therapy for hemodynamically stable patients with right ventricular dysfunction (23), although the benefits in this situation are unproven (21,23).

2. The major problem with lytic therapy is bleeding: there is a 12% incidence of major bleeding (22), and a 1% incidence of intracranial hemorrhage (21,22).

3. All thrombolytic agents are considered equally effective, and systemic drug administration is favored over local infusion into the pulmonary arteries (21). The two drug regimens shown below are designed to achieve rapid clot lysis.

    a. Alteplase: 0.6 mg/kg over 15 minutes (24).

    b. Reteplase: 10 Units by bolus injection and repeat in 30 minutes (25).

4. For more information on the use of thrombolytic agents, see Chapter 14.

IV. INFERIOR VENA CAVA FILTERS

Filter devices can be placed in the inferior vena cava (IVC) to trap thrombi that break loose from leg veins, thus preventing pulmonary embolization.

A. Indications

1. IVC filters are indicated for patients with proximal DVT who have any of the following (26):

   a. A contraindication to anticoagulation

   b. Pulmonary embolization during full anticoagulation

   c. A free-floating thrombus (i.e., the leading edge of the thrombus is unattached).

   d. Poor cardiopulmonary reserve (i.e., unlikely to tolerate a pulmonary embolus).

2. These filters are inserted percutaneously, usually through the internal jugular vein or femoral vein, and are placed below the renal veins, if possible.

B. Efficacy

1. The incidence of post-insertion pulmonary embolism is about 5% (27).

2. Major complications (e.g., migration of the filter) occur in less than 1% of cases (27). Remarkably, septicemia almost never results in seeding of IVC filters, despite their intravascular location.

REFERENCES

1. Geerts WH, Pineo GF, Heit JA, et al. Prevention of venous thromboembolism. The Seventh ACCP Conference on Antithrombotic and Thrombolytic Therapy. Chest 2004; 126(Suppl):338S-400S.

2. Heit JA. Risk factors for venous thromboembolism. Clin Chest Med 2003; 24:1-12.

3. Bick RL, Haas S. Thromboprophylaxis and thrombosis in medical, surgical, trauma, and obstetric/gynecologic patients. Hematol Oncol Clin N Am 2003; 17:217-258.

4. Rocha AT, Tapson VF. Venous thromboembolism in the intensive care unit. Clin Chest Med 2003; 24:103-122.

5. Goldhaber SZ, Marpurgo M, for the WHO/ISFC Task Force on Pulmonary Embolism. Diagnosis, treatment and prevention of pulmonary embolism. JAMA 1992; 268:1727-1733.

6. Wells PS, Lensing AW, Hirsh J. Graduated compression stockings in the prevention of postoperative venous thromboembolism. A meta-analysis. Arch Intern Med 1994; 154:67–72.

7. Hirsch J, Raschke R. Heparin and low-molecular-weight heparin. The Seventh ACCP Conference on Antithrombotic and Thrombolytic Therapy. Chest 2004; 126(Suppl):188S-203S.

8. Bick RL, Frenkel EP, Walenga J, et al. Unfractionated heparin, low molecular weight heparins, and pentasaccharide: Basic mechanism of actions, pharmacology and clinical use. Hematol Oncol Clin N Am 2005; 19:1-51.

9. Raskob G, Hirsch J. Controversies in timing of first dose of anticoagulant prophylaxis against venous thromboembolism after major orthopedic surgery. Chest 2003; 124(Suppl):379S-385S.

10. Bauer KA. New pentasaccharides for prophylaxis of deep vein thrombosis: Pharmacology. Chest 2003; 124(Suppl):364S-370S.

11. Fondaparinux. Mosby's Drug Consult 2005. Accessed at www.mdconsult.com on March 6, 2007.

12. Hoellerich VL, Wigton RS. Diagnosing pulmonary embolism using clinical findings. Arch Intern Med 1986; 146:1699-1704.

13. Kelly J, Rudd A, Lewis RR, Hunt BJ. Plasma D-dimers in the diagnosis of venous thromboembolism. Arch Intern Med 2002; 162:747-756.

14. Kollef MH, Zahid M, Eisenberg PR. Predictive value of a rapid semiquantitative D-dimer assay in critically ill patients with suspected thromboembolism. Crit Care Med 2000; 28:414-420.

15. Kline JA, Israel EG, Michelson EA, et al. Diagnostic accuracy of a bedside D-dimer assay and alveolar dead space measurement for rapid exclusion of pulmonary embolism. JAMA 2001; 285:761-768.

16. Tracey JA, Edlow JA. Ultrasound diagnosis of deep venous thrombosis. Emerg Med Clin N Am 2004; 22:775-796.

17. Hull RD, Hirsh J, Carter CJ, et al. Pulmonary angiography, ventilation lung scanning, and venography for clinically suspected pulmonary embolism with abnormal perfusion scans. Ann Intern Med 1983; 98:891–899.

18. The PIOPED Investigators. Value of the ventilation/perfusion scan in acute pulmonary embolism. Results of the prospective investigation of pulmonary embolism diagnosis (PIOPED). JAMA 1990; 263:2753-2759.

19. Mullins MD, Becker DM, Hagspeil KD, Philbrick JT. The role of spiral volumetric computed tomography in the diagnosis of pulmonary embolism. Arch Intern Med 2000; 160:293-298.

20. Raschke RA, Reilly BM, Guidry JR, et al. The weight-based heparin dosing nomogram compared with a "standard care" nomogram. Ann Intern Med 1993; 119:874–881.

21. Buller HR, Agnelli G, Hull RD, et al. Antithrombotic therapy for venous thromboembolic disease. The Seventh ACCP Conference on Antithrombotic and Thrombolytic Therapy. Chest 2004; 126 (Suppl): 401S-428S.

22. Wood KE. Major pulmonary embolism. Chest 2002; 121:877-905.

23. Comeraota AJ. The role of fibrinolytic therapy in the treatment of venous thromboembolism. Dis Mon 2005; 51:124-134.

24. Goldhaber SZ, Agnelli G, Levine MN. Reduced dose bolus alteplase vs conventional alteplase infusion for pulmonary embolism thrombolysis: an international multicenter randomized trial: the Bolus Alteplase Pulmonary Embolism Group. Chest 1994; 106:718-724.

25. Tebbe U, Graf A, Kamke W, et al. Hemodynamic effects of double bolus reteplase versus alteplase infusion in massive pulmonary embolism. Am Heart J 1999; 138:39-44.

26. Stein PD, Kayali F, Olson RE. Twenty-one year trends in the use of inferior vena cava filters. Arch Intern Med 2004; 164:1541-1545.

27. Athanasoulis CA, Kaufman JA, Halpern EF, et al. Inferior vena cava filters: review of 26-year single-center clinical experience. Radiology 2000; 216:54-66.

VASCULAR CATHETERS

Access to the vascular system is mandatory in the care of critically ill patients. This chapter describes the basic and specialty features of the catheters that provide this access.

I. BASIC FEATURES

A. Composition and Size

1. Vascular catheters are made of polymers impregnated with barium or tungsten salts to enhance radiopacity.

2. Catheters designed for short-term use (days) are made of polyurethane, a polymer known for its strength and durability. Catheters designed for prolonged use are made of a silicone polymer that is more flexible and less thrombogenic than polyurethane.

3. The size of vascular catheters is expressed in terms of their outside diameter. Size can be expressed in a metric-based *French* size or a wire-based *gauge* size.

   a. The French size is a series of whole numbers that increases in increments of roughly 0.33 millimeters (e.g., 1 French = 0.33 mm, 2 French = 0.66 mm).

   b. The gauge size (originally developed for solid wires) has no definable relationship to other units of measurement, and requires a table of reference values like the one in Table 4.1.

TABLE 4.1 Size Chart for Vascular Catheters			
French Size	Gauge	Inner Diameter	Outer Diameter
1	27	0.1 mm	0.4 mm
2	23	0.3 mm	0.6 mm
3	20	0.5 mm	0.9 mm
4	18	0.6 mm	1.2 mm
5	16	0.7 mm	1.7 mm
7	13	1.3 mm	2.4 mm
9	11	1.6 mm	3.2 mm

From www.norfolkaccess.com/Catheters.html. Accessed on 4/7/2007.

B. Determinants of Flow Rate

1. Fluid flow through rigid tubes is defined by the *Hagen-Poisseuille equation:*

$$Q = \Delta P \, (\pi r^4 / 8 \mu L) \qquad (4.1)$$

   Q is the steady-state flow rate.
   ΔP is the pressure gradient along the tube: $(P_{in} - P_{out})$.
   r is the inner radius of the tube.
   L is the length of the tube.
   μ is the viscosity of the fluid.

2. Because flow rate varies directly with the fourth power of the radius, *the radius of a catheter is the principal determinant of flow rate.* For example, if the radius of a catheter is doubled, the flow rate will increase 16-fold: $(2r)^4 = 16r$.

3. Equation 4.1 demonstrates that rapid infusion rates are best achieved with catheters that are short and have a large diameter. The role of catheter size in volume resuscitation is described in Chapter 10.

II. TYPES OF CATHETERS

A. Peripheral Vein Catheters

1. Catheters used to cannulate peripheral veins are short and narrow (length: 5 – 7 cm, diameter: 18 – 22 gauge).

2. These catheters are intended only for short-term use (hours to days) because the plastic polymers in the catheters (e.g., polyethylene) provoke a strong inflammatory reaction upon contact with blood vessels. Because they are short, these catheters also tend to dislodge from blood vessels. The limited life span of these catheters also limits their popularity in the care of ICU patients.

B. Central Venous Catheters

Catheters used to cannulate the large veins entering the thorax (i.e., internal jugular and subclavian veins) are 15 to 25 cm in length, and are available with one, two or three infusion channels. The diameter of central venous catheters (CVCs) varies according to the number and size of the infusion channels.

1. *Multilumen Catheters*

   Multilumen CVCs are popular in the ICU because they allow multiple infusions through a single venipuncture. Table 4.2 shows the variety of multilumen catheter sizes available from one manufacturer (Cook Critical Care). The most popular of these is the 7 French triple-lumen catheter, which is shown in Figure 4.1. This catheter is small enough to pass through introducer catheters (see later), and the channels are large enough to permit adequate flow rates for most patient care needs.

   a. INFECTIOUS RISK. Despite the greater number of infusion channels, multilumen catheters are not associated with a higher incidence of catheter-related infections when compared to single lumen catheters (1).

TABLE 4.2 The Variety of Multilumen Central Venous Catheters

French Size	Cross-Section	Port	Gauge Size	Flow Rate[a]
5.0		Distal	18	52 mL/min
		Mid	23	2 mL/min
		Proximal	23	2 mL/min
7.0		Distal	16	20 mL/min
		Mid	18	22 mL/min
		Proximal	18	24 mL/min
7.5		Distal	14	130 mL/min
		Proximal	21	5 mL/min
9.0		Distal	14	130 mL/min
		Mid	18	29 mL/min
		Proximal	18	31 mL/min
9.5		Distal	13	133 mL/min
		Proximal	18	43 mL/min

[a]The flow rate of purified water flowing from a height of 100 cm.

From Cook Double and Triple Lumen Quick Reference Guide, available at www.cookmedical.com. Accessed on 4/8/2007.

2. Heparin-Bonded Catheters

Thrombus formation has been documented on as many as one-third of indwelling CVCs (2). These thrombi create a risk of vascular occlusion, pulmonary emboli, and catheter-related infection (the infectious risk is due to microorganisms that become trapped and proliferate in the fibrin meshwork of blood clots).

a. CVCs are available with a heparin coating to prevent thrombus formation. However, this heparin coating is washed away by blood flow, and it can be completely lost within a few hours after catheter insertion (2).

b. Heparin bonding is associated with only a small (2%) decrease in the incidence of catheter-related infections (3). Furthermore, the heparin that is washed away from these catheters can cause heparin-induced thrombocytopenia in susceptible individuals (4).

c. Heparin-bonded catheters are now commonplace. However, considering that these catheters provide only limited benefit, yet create a risk of heparin-induced thrombocytopenia, their popularity is undeserved.

3. *Antimicrobial-Impregnated Catheters*

a. CVCs are available that are coated with chlorhexidine and silver sulfadiazine (Arrow International, Reading, PA) or minocycline and rifampin (Cook Critical Care, Bloomington, IN).

b. A single multicenter study comparing both types of antimicrobial catheters showed superior results with the minocycline-rifampin CVCs (5). These catheters show antimicrobial activity for up to 4 weeks, compared to one week for the chlorhexidine-silver sulfadiazine CVCs (6).

c. Antimicrobial-impregnated CVCs should be considered if the rate of catheter-related septicemia in your ICU is higher than the national average (3.8 to 5.3 infections per 1,000 catheter-days in medical-surgical ICUs) (7). They should also be considered in neutropenic patients and burn patients.

C. Introducer Catheters

Large-bore *introducer catheters* like the one shown in Figure 4.1 have a diameter (8 to 9 French) that is large enough to

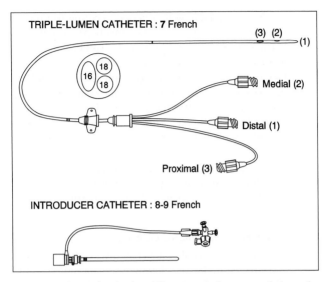

FIGURE 4.1. A popular sized multilumen central venous catheter and a large-bore introducer catheter.

allow passage of central venous catheters (including multilumen catheters) and pulmonary artery catheters. Central venous cannulation usually begins with insertion of an introducer catheter, which is left in place. Narrower catheters can then be inserted and replaced repeatedly without the risks of a new venipuncture. (Figure 7.1 shows a pulmonary artery catheter threaded through an introducer catheter). Introducer catheters can also be used as stand-alone infusion devices. The large diameter of these catheters makes them well suited for rapid infusion rates, which can be advantageous for resuscitation in the bleeding patient (see Chapter 10).

D. Specialty Catheters

1. *Hemodialysis Catheters*

Short-term hemodialysis is performed with specially designed double-lumen catheters like the one shown in Figure 4.2 that are placed in the internal jugular vein or femoral vein. One lumen of the catheter carries blood from the patient to the dialysis membranes, and the other lumen carries blood back to the patient. Each lumen is equivalent in diameter to an introducer catheter (8 French or 12 gauge) to accommodate the rapid flow rates (200 to 300 mL/min) required for effective hemodialysis.

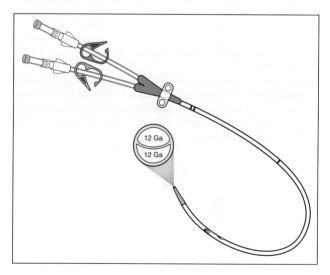

FIGURE 4.2. A large-bore, double-lumen catheter used for short-term hemodialysis.

2. *Pulmonary Artery Catheters*

Pulmonary artery catheters are used for hemodynamic assessments, and can provide as many as 16 measurements of cardiovascular function. These catheters are described in detail in Chapter 7 (see Figure 7.1).

REFERENCES

1. McGee DC, Gould MK. Preventing complications of central venous catheterization. N Engl J Med 2003; 348:1123-1133.

2. Jacobs BR. Central venous catheter occlusion and thrombosis. Crit Care Clin 2003; Vol. 19:489-514.

3. Marin MG, Lee JC, Skurnick JH. Prevention of nosocomial bloodstream infections: effectiveness of antimicrobial-impregnated and heparin-bonded central venous catheters. Crit Care Med 2000; 28:3332-3338.

4. Laster JL, Nichols WK, Silver D. Thrombocytopenia associated with heparin-coated catheters in patients with heparin-associated antiplatelet antibodies. Arch Intern Med 1989; 149:2285-2287.

5. Darouche RO, Raad II, Heard SO, et al. A comparison of antimicrobial-impregnated central venous catheters. N Engl J Med 1999; 340:1-8.

6. Hanna H, Darouche R, Raad I. New approaches for prevention of intravascular catheter-related infections. Infect Med 2001; 18:38-48.

7. Centers for Disease Control and Prevention. Guidelines for the prevention of intravascular catheter-related infections. MMWR 2002; 51(No.RR-10):1-30.

Chapter 5

ESTABLISHING VENOUS ACCESS

This chapter presents some practical guidelines for the insertion of peripheral and central venous catheters, and describes the adverse events that can occur during catheter insertion.

I. PREPARING FOR VASCULAR CANNULATION

A. Hospital Staff

1. Handwashing with an antimicrobial soap or gel is recommended for all vascular catheter insertions (see Table 1.2).

2. Sterile gloves are recommended for insertion of central venous catheters and arterial catheters. Nonsterile disposable gloves can be used for cannulation of peripheral veins as long as the gloved hands do not touch the catheter (see Table 1.3).

3. Masks, gowns, and sterile drapes are recommended for insertion of central venous catheters and peripherally-inserted central catheters (PICCs).

B. Insertion Site

1. The skin around the catheter insertion site should be decontaminated with an antiseptic agent (see Table 1.1).

Chlorhexidine is currently preferred because of its prolonged activity (≥ 6 hrs.).

2. If an iodophor such as povidone-iodine is used, the solution should be left in contact with the skin for a few minutes (see Chapter 1).

II. CATHETER INSERTION TECHNIQUES

A. Catheter-Over-Needle Technique

Short catheters (5 to 7 cm in length) are inserted into small, superficial veins using a catheter-over-needle device like the one shown in Figure 5.1. The entire device (catheter and needle) is advanced toward the target vessel with the bevel of the needle pointed upward. When the tip of the needle enters the blood vessel, blood appears in the transparent flash chamber. When this occurs, the needle is kept stationary and the catheter is advanced over the needle and into the lumen of the blood vessel. The needle is then withdrawn and the catheter is secured to the skin.

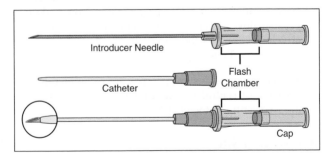

FIGURE 5.1. A catheter-over-needle device used to cannulate peripheral veins. Area of magnification shows needle extending beyond the catheter tip, and the tapered shape of the catheter tip. When the needle enters the vein, blood is visible in the flash chamber.

B. Guidewire Technique

Long catheters (10 to 25 cm in length) are inserted into deeply located veins by threading the catheter over a guidewire. This technique (called the *Seldinger technique* after its founder) is shown in Figure 5.2. A small-bore needle is used to probe for the target blood vessel. When the tip of the needle enters the vessel, a long, flexible wire is passed through the needle and into the lumen of the vessel. The needle is then removed over the guidewire, and the catheter is advanced over the guidewire and into the blood vessel. The guidewire is then removed and the catheter is secured to the skin.

III. VENOUS ACCESS SITES

A. The Upper Extremity

1. *Peripheral Veins*

    The arms are preferred to the legs for peripheral vein cannulation because of ease of access and a lower risk of thrombosis (1). Because the catheters are short and easily dislodged, areas of limited movement (e.g., the forearm of the nondominant hand, away from the wrist and elbow) are most likely to ensure successful cannulation.

2. *Peripherally-Inserted Central Catheters*

    a. Long catheters (50 to 60 cm) are available that can be inserted into the veins of the antecubital fossa and advanced into the superior vena cava. There is no risk of pneumothorax, which is the principal advantage of these *peripherally-inserted central catheters* (PICC).

    b. The basilic vein is preferred to the cephalic vein for PICC placement because it is slightly larger and runs a shorter course up the arm (see Figure 5.3).

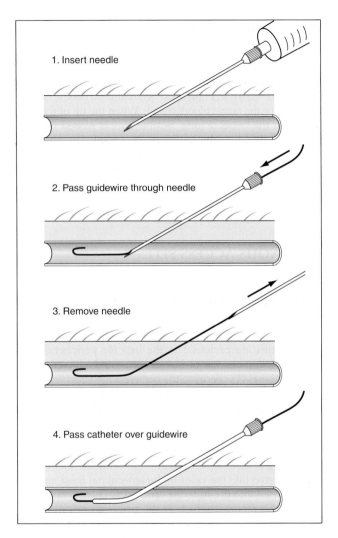

FIGURE 5.2. The steps involved in guidewire-assisted cannulation of blood vessels (the Seldinger technique).

c. PICCs can be placed blindly by adding the length of the vascular segments shown in Figure 5.3. Alternately, the distance from the antecubital fossa to the 3rd anterior intercostal space on the right (where the superior vena cava enters the right atrium) can be measured. However without fluoroscopy, malposition of PICCs is common (2).

d. PICCs offer no advantage over other methods of central venous catheterization. Although there is no risk of pneumothorax with PICCs, the risk of pneumothorax from central venous catheterization is small (see later), at least when performed by trained personnel. PICCs are used primarily for long-term venous access (30 days or longer), and they have no role in the care of critically ill patients.

B. The Subclavian Vein

1. *Anatomy*

a. The subclavian vein is a continuation of the axillary vein as it passes over the first rib. It runs most of its course along the underside of the clavicle and continues to the thoracic inlet, where it joins the internal jugular vein to form the innominate vein. The convergence of the right and left innominate veins then forms the superior vena cava.

b. The average distance from insertion site to the right atrium is 14.5 cm and 18.5 cm for right-sided and left-sided cannulations, respectively. *Subclavian vein catheters should be no longer than 15 cm* to avoid placing the catheter tip in the right side of the heart (3).

2. *Locating the Vessel*

a. Identify the insertion of the sternocleidomastoid muscle on the clavicle. The subclavian vein lies just underneath the clavicle at this point. The vein can be approached from above or below the clavicle, and it should be entered within 2 to 3 cm of the insertion site on the skin.

b. When advancing the probe needle, keep the needle just underneath the clavicle to prevent accidental puncture of the subclavian artery (which runs deep to the subclavian vein).

3. *Benefits and Risks*

a. The subclavian vein is well suited for cannulation because it is a large vessel (diameter of 20 mm) with a predictable anatomic location. Patient tolerance of central venous catheters is highest with subclavian vein catheters.

b. The major concern with subclavian vein cannulation is pneumothorax from puncture of the lung apex. Table 5.1 shows that this is not a common occurrence when the procedure is performed by experienced personnel (4,5).

c. Major bleeding is also uncommon (see Table 5.1), and the presence of a coagulopathy does not increase the risk of bleeding (6,7). The presence of a coagulopathy is not a contraindication to central venous cannulation.

TABLE 5.1 Complications of Large Vein Cannulation

| | Complication Rates | | |
Complication	Subclavian Vein	Internal Jugular Vein	Femoral Vein
Arterial Puncture	1 – 5%	3%	9%*
Major Bleeding	2%	1%	1%
Thrombosis	1%	0	6%*
Pneumothorax	1 – 3%	1%	—
Systemic sepsis	1 – 4%	0 – 8%	2 – 5%

From References 4,5,9,10. Rates are expressed as the nearest whole number.
*Indicates a rate that is significantly different from the others

C. The Internal Jugular Vein

1. *Anatomy*

   a. The internal jugular (IJ) vein is located under the ster-nocleidomastoid muscle in the neck. It runs obliquely along a line drawn from the pinna of the ear to the sterno-clavicular joint. In the lower region of the neck, the vein runs just lateral to the carotid artery, and this proximity creates a risk of carotid artery puncture.

   b. The IJ vein on the right side runs a straight course to the right atrium, and the distance involved is about 15 cm (see Figure 5.3). Therefore, catheters used to cannulate the right IJ vein should be no longer than 15 cm to avoid advancing the catheter into the right side of the heart. (This is the same maximum length recommended for subclavian vein catheters.)

2. *Locating the Vessel*

   Use the right side of the neck when possible (because of the straight course to the heart).

   a. POSTERIOR APPROACH. Identify the point where the external jugular vein crosses over the lateral edge of the sternocleidomastoid muscle. The insertion site is one centimeter superior to this point. The probe needle should be inserted just under the belly of the ster-nocleidomastoid muscle and advanced toward the suprasternal notch. The vein should be entered 5 to 6 cm from the skin.

   b. ANTERIOR APPROACH. At the base of the neck, identify a triangular area where the sternocleidomastoid muscle splits to form the sternal and clavicular heads of the muscle. The probe needle should be inserted at the apex of this triangle and advanced toward the ipsilateral nipple at a 45° angle with the skin. The vein should be entered within 5 cm of the skin. This approach has a higher risk of carotid artery puncture than the posterior approach.

3. *Benefits and Risks*

Cannulation of the IJ vein has few advantages over sub-clavian vein cannulation.

a. The IJ approach was popularized because of the as-sumption that the site of catheter insertion in the neck would eliminate the risk of pneumothorax. However, this is not the case (4,5). In fact, *the incidence of pneu-mothorax is the same with internal jugular vein and subcla-vian vein cannulation* (see Table 5.1). How can the lung be punctured by a catheter inserted in the neck? One possible answer is if the lung apex protrudes into the neck from overinflation during mechanical ventila-tion.

b. The most life-threatening complication of IJ cannula-tion is carotid artery puncture, which occurs during 3% of attempted IJ cannulations (see Table 5.1).

c. The only clear advantage of IJ cannulation is anatom-ic; i.e., the straight course from the right IJ vein to the right atrium. For this reason, the right IJ vein is the preferred site for insertion of pacemaker catheters and hemodialysis catheters.

C. The Femoral Vein

1. *Anatomy*

The femoral vein is the main venous outflow from the legs. In the upper one-third of the thigh, the femoral vein runs adjacent to the femoral artery. Both vessels are locat-ed in the medial portion of the femoral triangle, with the femoral vein situated just medial to the femoral artery (see Figure 5.4). Both vessels are within a few centimeters of the skin at the inguinal crease.

2. *Locating the Vessel*

a. Just below the inguinal crease, palpate the femoral artery pulse in the medial one-third of the leg. The femoral vein is just medial to the palpated pulse.

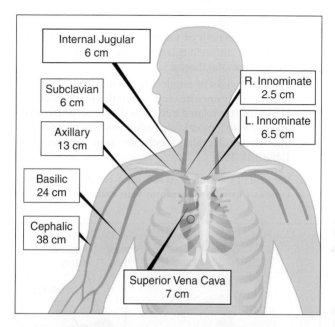

FIGURE 5.3. The length of venous segments involved in the insertion of peripherally inserted central catheters (PICCs) and central venous (subclavian and internal jugular vein) catheters. The circle in the third anterior intercostal space marks the junction of the superior vena cava and right atrium.

> Insert the probe needle within 2 cm of the palpable pulse, and you should enter the femoral vein 2 to 4 cm below the skin.
>
> b. If the femoral artery pulse is not palpable, draw an imaginary line from the anterior superior iliac crest to the pubic tubercle, and divide the line into three equal segments. The femoral artery should be just under the junction between the middle and medial segments of the line, and the femoral vein will be 1 to 2 cm medial to this point. This method has a 90% success rate for locating the femoral vein (8).

3. *Benefits and Risks*

   a. The major benefit of femoral vein cannulation is anatomic: i.e., the vein is large, easily located, and far removed from the thorax.

   b. The major risks of femoral vein cannulation are femoral artery puncture and femoral vein thrombosis (4,9). Catheter-related infections do not occur more frequently with femoral vein catheters when compared to internal jugular and subclavian vein catheters (see Table 5.1) (10).

   c. Because of the enhanced risk for arterial puncture and venous thrombosis, femoral vein catheters should be

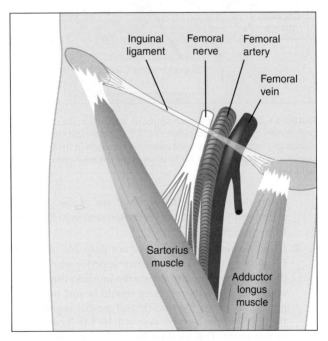

FIGURE 5.4. The anatomy of the femoral triangle.

used only when cannulation of the internal jugular and subclavian veins is not possible. Femoral vein catheters should be removed as soon as possible to limit the risk of venous thrombosis.

IV. IMMEDIATE CONCERNS

A. Venous Air Embolism

When a vascular catheter is advanced into the thorax, the negative intrathoracic pressure generated during spontaneous breathing can draw air into the venous circulation if the catheter is open to the atmosphere. The entrained air can travel to the right side of the heart as a *venous air embolism* and produce life-threatening obstruction in the pulmonary circulation (11).

1. *Preventive Measures*

   Air is prevented from entering the venous circulation when the venous pressure exceeds atmospheric (zero) pressure. The two maneuvers below are designed to increase central venous pressure.

   a. Placing the patient in the Trendelenburg position with the head 15° below the horizontal plane will increase the venous pressure in the head and neck regions, which can be advantageous during cannulation of the subclavian and internal jugular veins. This maneuver is not intended for patients who already have elevated venous pressures from cardiopulmonary disease.

   b. When changing connections in a central venous line, a temporary increase in venous pressure can be achieved by having the patient hum audibly. This not only produces a positive intrathoracic pressure, it also allows you to hear when the desired effect is occurring.

2. *Clinical Presentation*

   a. The earliest clinical manifestation of venous air embolism is acute onset of dyspnea. Hypotension and cardiac arrest can develop rapidly.

   b. Air can pass across a patent foramen ovale and obstruct the cerebral circulation, producing an acute ischemic stroke.

   c. A characteristic "mill wheel" murmur can be heard over the right heart, but it can be fleeting.

3. *Therapeutic Maneuvers*

   a. When air entry is first suspected, the central venous line should be aspirated to remove any residual air, and the patient should be placed with the left side down (so air will collect in the right side of the heart instead of the pulmonary outflow tract).

   b. In dire circumstances, a needle can be inserted through the chest wall and into the right ventricle to aspirate the air. To perform this procedure, insert a long needle in the 4th intercostal space just to the right of the sternum and advance the needle under the sternum at a 45° angle until there is blood return.

   c. In severe cases of venous air embolism, the mortality is high despite the above therapeutic maneuvers.

B. Pneumothorax

Although the risk of pneumothorax from central venous cannulation is small (see Table 5.1), routine chest x-rays are recommended immediately following all cannulations (or attempts) of the subclavian and internal jugular veins.

1. *Radiographic Detection*

   a. Postinsertion chest x-rays should be obtained in the upright position and during expiration, if possible. Expiration decreases the volume of air in the lungs, but not the volume of air in the pleural space, so expiration will facilitate the detection of small pneumothoraces (12).

b. Upright films are not always feasible in ICU patients. If the supine position is used, remember that *pleural air does not collect at the apex of the lung when the patient is in the supine position* (13). In this position, pleural air tends to collect anteriorly and at the base of the lung (see Chapter 20).

2. *Delayed Pneumothorax*

a. Pneumothorax may not be radiographically evident until 24 to 48 hours after catheter insertion (14). Therefore, the absence of a pneumothorax on an immediate postinsertion chest film does not absolutely exclude this complication. However, serial chest x-rays are not justified in asymptomatic patients.

b. Delayed pneumothorax should be a consideration in any patient who develops dyspnea or progressive hypoxemia in the first few days after central venous cannulation.

C. Catheter Position

Chest x-rays are advised after all central venous cannulations to ensure proper catheter placement.

1. *Proper Placement*

A properly placed central venous catheter should run parallel to the shadow of the superior vena cava, and the tip of the catheter should be at or slightly above the third anterior intercostal space (where the superior vena cava meets the right atrium).

2. *Tip in the Right Atrium*

A catheter tip that extends below the third right anterior intercostal space is likely to be in the right side of the heart. If the anterior portion of the third rib cannot be visualized, a catheter tip that extends below the tracheal carina (i.e., the division of the trachea into the right and left mainstem bronchi) can be used as evidence of right heart catheterization. Although cardiac perforation is rare (15), withdrawal of the catheter tip to the appropriate location is advised.

3. *Tip Against the Wall of the Vena Cava*

Catheters inserted from the left side must make an acute turn downward when they enter the superior vena cava from the left innominate vein. Catheters that do not make this turn can end up with the tip pointing directly at the lateral wall of the superior vena cava. These catheters can perforate the superior vena cava, and they should either be withdrawn into the innominate vein or advanced further down the vena cava.

REFERENCES

1. Centers for Disease Control and Prevention. Guidelines for the prevention of intravascular catheter-related infections. MMWR 2002; 51 (No.RR-10):1-30.
2. Heffner JE. A guide to the management of peripherally inserted central catheters. J Crit Illness 2000; 15:165-169.
3. McGee WT, Ackerman BL, Rouben LR, et al. Accurate placement of central venous catheters: a prospective, randomized, multicenter trial. Crit Care Med 1993; 21:1118–1123.
4. Merrer J, DeJonghe B, Golliot F, et al. Complications of femoral and subclavian venous catheterization in critically ill patients. JAMA 2001; 286:700-707.
5. Ruesch S, Walder B, Tramer M. Complications of central venous catheters: internal jugular versus subclavian access – A systematic review. Crit Care Med 2002; 30:454-460.
6. Fisher NC, Mutimer DJ. Central venous cannulation in patients with liver disease and coagulopathy – a prospective audit. Intensive Care Med 1999; 25:481-485.
7. Doerfler M, Kaufman B, Goldenberg A. Central venous catheter

placement in patients with disorders of hemostasis. Chest 1996; 110:185-188.

8. Getzen LC, Pollack EW. Short-term femoral vein catheterization. Am J Surg 1979; 138:875-877.

9. Joynt GM, Kew J, Gomersall CD, et al. Deep venous thrombosis caused by femoral venous catheters in critically ill adult patients. Chest 2000; 117:178-183.

10. Deshpande K, Hatem C, Ulrich H, et al. The incidence of infectious complications of central venous catheters at the subclavian, internal jugular, and femoral sites in an intensive care unit population. Crit Care Med 2005; 33:13-20.

11. Muth CM, Shank ES. Gas embolism. N Engl J Med 2000; 342: 476-482.

12. Marino PL. Delayed pneumothorax: a complication of subclavian vein catheterization. J Parenter Enteral Nutr 1985;9:232.

13. Tocino IM, Miller MH, Fairfax WR. Distribution of pneumothorax in the supine and semirecumbent critically ill adult. Am J Radiol 1985; 144:901–905.

14. Collin GR, Clarke LE. Delayed pneumothorax: a complication of central venous catheterization. Surg Rounds 1994; 17:589–594.

15. McGee WT, Ackerman BL, Rouben LR, et al. Accurate placement of central venous catheters: a prospective, randomized, multicenter trial. Crit Care Med 993; 21:1118–1123.

Chapter 6

THE INDWELLING VASCULAR CATHETER

This chapter describes the routine care and adverse consequences of indwelling vascular catheters, with emphasis on the prevention, diagnosis, and treatment of catheter-related infections.

I. ROUTINE CATHETER CARE

A. Protective Dressings

Catheter insertion sites are covered as a standard antiseptic measure. Sterile gauze pads provide adequate protection in most instances (1).

1. *Adhesive, Semipermeable Dressings*

   Adhesive dressings made of transparent, semipermeable polyurethane membranes are very popular. These dressings partially block the escape of water vapor from the underlying skin, and create a moist environment that is beneficial for wound healing.

   a. Despite their popularity, these dressings do not reduce the incidence of catheter colonization or infection when compared to sterile gauze dressings (1-3). In fact, they can *increase* the risk of infection (2,3) because the moist environment they create favors the growth of microorganisms.

   b. Occlusive dressings can be reserved for skin sites that are close to a source of infectious secretions (e.g., a tracheostomy).

B. Antimicrobial Ointment

The practice of applying antimicrobial gels to the insertion site of central venous catheters does not reduce the incidence of catheter-related infections (4), and it can promote the development of antibiotic-resistant organisms (5). As a result, the routine use of antimicrobial ointments is not recommended (1,4).

C. Flushing Catheters

Vascular catheters are flushed at regular intervals to prevent thrombotic occlusion.

1. *Heparinized Flushes*
   a. The standard flush solution is isotonic saline with heparin (10 to 1000 U/mL).
   b. Catheters that are used intermittently are filled with heparinized saline and capped when idle. (This is called a *heparin lock* because the cap that seals the catheter creates a vacuum that holds the flush solution in place.)
   c. Arterial catheters are flushed continuously (3 mL/hr) using a pressurized bag.

2. *Alternatives to Heparin*

   The small quantities of heparin used in flush solutions can promote heparin-induced thrombocytopenia (see Chapter 31). Alternatives to heparinized flushes are available that eliminate this risk.
   a. For flushing venous catheters, saline alone is as effective as heparinized saline (6).
   b. For flushing arterial catheters, 1.4% sodium citrate is a suitable alternative to heparinized saline (7).

D. Replacing Peripheral Venous Catheters

The concern with prolonged cannulation of peripheral veins is inflammation (phlebitis), not infection. The inflammation is a reaction to the plastic polymers that make up vascular catheters, and is aggravated by mechanical irritation of the blood vessel wall.

1. The incidence of clinically apparent phlebitis increases significantly after peripheral vein catheters are left in place longer than 72 to 96 hours (1).

2. Therefore, replacement of peripheral vein catheters (using a new venipuncture site) is recommended every 72 to 96 hours (1).

E. Replacing Central Venous Catheters

1. *Routine Replacement Not Warranted*

   Septicemia from central venous catheters begins to appear after catheters have been in place for 3 days (1). However, replacing central venous catheters at regular intervals does not reduce the incidence of catheter-related infections (8). In fact, it increases the risk of catheter-related mechanical complications (4), so the overall risk (infectious and mechanical) is increased (9). Therefore, routine replacement of central venous catheters is not advised (1,4).

2. *Indications for Catheter Replacement*

   Catheter replacement is recommended:

   a. When there is purulent drainage from the catheter insertion site. Erythema around the catheter insertion site is not absolute evidence of infection (9), and is not an indication for catheter replacement.

b. When an indwelling vascular catheter is suspected as a source of sepsis and the patient has a prosthetic valve, is immunocompromised, or has severe sepsis or septic shock.

c. When a catheter has been placed emergently, without strict aseptic technique, and it can be replaced safely.

d. When a femoral vein catheter has been in place longer than 48 hours and it can be replaced safely. This will limit the risk of femoral vein thrombosis (see Table 5.1).

II. THE OCCLUDED CATHETER

Catheter occlusion is the most common complication of central venous cannulation (11).

A. Sources of Obstruction

1. Thrombosis is the most common cause of obstruction of central venous catheters (11).

2. Insoluble precipitates in the infusate can accumulate in the catheter lumen and cause obstruction. Possible sources of this type of obstruction include drugs that are insoluble in water (e.g., diazepam, digoxin, phenytoin, and trimethoprim-sulfa), precipitation of inorganic salts (e.g., $CaPO_4$), and lipid residues.

3. The lumen of the catheter can also be compromised by sharp angles and localized indentations. These usually occur during catheter insertion.

B. Restoring Catheter Patency

A protocol for restoring patency in obstructed catheters is shown in Table 6.1. Since thrombosis is the most common cause of catheter occlusion, the initial attempt to restore patency should involve an attempt to lyse the occluding thrombus.

TABLE 6.1 Protocol for Restoring Patency in Occluded Catheters

Drug Preparation

1. Alteplase (tissue plasminogen activator):
   Reconstitute 50 mg vial with 50 mL sterile water (1 mg/mL).

2. Prepare 2 mL aliquots and freeze until needed.

Protocol

1. Thaw two aliquots of drug solution. (Drug must be used within 8 hours after thawing.)

2. Draw 2 mL of drug solution (2mg) into a 5 mL syringe and attach to hub of the occluded catheter.

3. Inject as much volume as possible (up to 2 mL) into the lumen of the catheter and then cap the hub of the catheter.

4. Leave the drug solution in the catheter lumen for 2 hours.

5. Attempt to flush the catheter with a saline solution. Do not use a tuberculin syringe to flush occluded catheters (the high pressure generated by these syringes can fracture the hub of a catheter).

6. If the catheter is still obstructed, repeat steps 1 – 5.

7. If the catheter remains obstructed, consider using 0.1N HCL (2 mL) for drug or $CaPO_4$ precipitates, or 70% ethanol (2 mL) for suspected lipid residue.

8. If the obstruction persists, replace the catheter using a new venipuncture site.

From References 12–15.

---

1. *Thrombotic Occlusion*

Local instillation of the thrombolytic agent alteplase (tissue plasminogen activator), using the regimen in Table 6.1, is 90% effective in restoring patency in catheters with partial or complete occlusion (12,13). The total drug dose in this regimen (up to 4 mg) is too small to cause systemic thrombolysis.

2. *Non-Thrombotic Occlusion*

   a. Catheter occlusion that is refractory to thrombolysis will occasionally respond to instillation of 0.1N hydrochloric acid to promote the solubility of inorganic salts and some medications (14).

   b. If lipid residues are suspected as a cause of catheter occlusion (i.e., in patients receiving lipid emulsions for nutrition), instillation of 70% ethanol (2 mL) can restore catheter patency (15).

3. *Replacing an Occluded Catheter*

   If the obstruction cannot be relieved and the catheter must be replaced, a new venipuncture site is necessary. Catheter replacement over a guidewire is not advised because the guidewire can dislodge the obstructing mass or a thrombus in the surrounding vein (see next) and create a pulmonary embolus.

C. Venous Thrombosis

Thrombotic occlusion of a central venous catheter can be accompanied by thrombosis in the surrounding vein. This is most prominent in the subclavian and femoral veins.

1. *Subclavian Vein Thrombosis*

   a. Clinically apparent thrombosis occurs in about 1% of patients with subclavian vein catheters (see Table 5.1).

   b. The hallmark of subclavian vein thrombosis is unilateral arm swelling (16). The thrombus can extend proximally into the superior vena cava, but complete occlusion of the superior vena cava with the resultant *superior vena cava syndrome* (swelling of neck and face, etc.) is rare (17).

c. Symptomatic pulmonary embolism can occur, but the reported incidence varies from zero to 17% (16,18).

d. Ultrasound has a low sensitivity and specificity (56% and 69%, respectively) for the detection of subclavian vein thrombosis (19), and the diagnosis is often based on the clinical presentation (i.e., unilateral arm swelling). Contrast venography is rarely performed.

e. Treatment involves immediate catheter removal and elevation of the affected arm. Systemic anticoagulation with heparin is popular (16,18), but unproven.

2. *Femoral Vein Thrombosis*

a. Clinically apparent thrombosis is reported in 6% of patients with femoral vein catheters (see Table 5.1).

b. As reported in Chapter 3, venous ultrasound has a high (> 90%) sensitivity and specificity for the detection of proximal deep vein thrombosis in the leg. Treatment includes immediate catheter removal and heparin anticoagulation as described in Chapter 3.

III. CATHETER-RELATED INFECTIONS

Hospital-acquired (nosocomial) bloodstream infections are 2 to 7 times more frequent in ICU patients than in other hospitalized patients (20), and indwelling vascular catheters are responsible for over half of these bloodstream infections (21).

A. Routes of Infection

The routes of infection involving indwelling vascular catheters are described below using the corresponding numbers shown in Figure 6.1.

1. Microbes can gain access to the internal lumen of vascular catheters through break points in the infusion system, such as stopcocks and catheter hubs.

2. Microbes on the skin can migrate along the outer surface of the catheter in the tract created during percutaneous insertion of the catheter. This is considered the major route of catheter-related bloodstream infections.

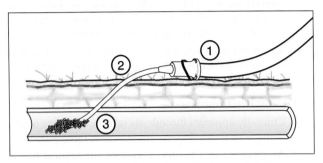

FIGURE 6.1. The routes of catheter-related bloodstream infections.

3. Microbes present in circulating blood can attach to the intravascular portion of an indwelling catheter. Once attached, the microbes can proliferate and become a secondary source of septicemia.

B. Types of Infection

The Centers for Disease Control and Prevention (CDC) has identified the following types of catheter-related infection (1).

1. *Catheter colonization* is characterized by the presence of microbes on the catheter but not in the bloodstream.

2. *Exit-site infection* is characterized by drainage from the catheter insertion site that grows a microorganism on culture. Blood cultures may be positive or negative.

3. *Catheter-related septicemia* is a condition where the same microorganisms are present on the tip of the catheter and in the bloodstream, and the catheter is the primary source of infection.

C. Clinical Features

1. Catheter colonization is asymptomatic, while catheter-related septicemia is usually accompanied by signs of systemic inflammation (i.e., fever, leukocytosis, etc.).

2. There are no specific signs of catheter-related septicemia. The presence of erythema around the insertion site is not predictive of septicemia (10), and the presence of purulent drainage from the insertion site can indicate exit-site infection without septicemia (1,22).

3 . Catheter-related septicemia is usually suspected when a patient with a vascular catheter in place for longer than 48 hours has an unexplained fever. Confirmation is based on the results of appropriate cultures, as described next.

D. Catheter Tip Cultures

The most common approach to suspected catheter-related septicemia is to combine a culture of the catheter tip with a blood culture obtained from a peripheral vein. This method is described below.

1. The catheter is first removed and (using sterile technique) a 2 inch segment is severed from the distal end of the catheter and placed in a sterile culturette tube. There are 2 methods for culturing catheter tips.

2. *Roll-Plate Method*

   a. The catheter tip is rolled directly over the surface of a blood agar plate, and growth is measured as the number of colony-forming units (CFUs) on the plate.

   b. The diagnosis of catheter-related septicemia requires growth of at least 15 CFUs on the culture plate plus isolation of the same organism from the blood culture (22).

   c. This method will detect infection only on the outer surface of the catheter, which explains why it has a sensitivity of only 60% for the detection of catheter-tip infections (see Table 6.2) (22).

3. *Serial Dilution Method*

   a. The catheter tip is placed in culture broth and agitated vigorously to release attached organisms. After serial dilutions, the broth is placed on a blood agar plate, and growth is measured as the number of colony-forming units (CFUs) on the plate.

   b. The diagnosis of catheter-related septicemia requires growth of at least 100 CFUs on the culture plate plus isolation of the same organism from the blood culture.

   c. This method will detect infection on both (outer and inner) surfaces of the catheter, which explains why the sensitivity of this method (80%) is higher than the roll-plate method (see Table 6.2).

TABLE 6.2 Culture Methods for Catheter-Related Septicemia

Method	Catheter Surface Sampled	Sensitivity[†]
Catheter tip culture		
Roll-plate method	Outer surface	60%
Serial dilution method	Outer and inner surfaces	80%
Quantitative blood cultures		
Catheter vs. peripheral blood	Inner surface	50%

[†]From Reference 22.

E. Quantitative Blood Cultures

The disadvantage of catheter tip cultures is the need to remove the catheter. Considering that as many as 70% of catheters that are removed for presumed infection are sterile when cultured (22), an alternative culture method that does not require catheter removal is desirable. The quantitative blood culture technique described below is such a method.

1. This method compares the culture results from 2 blood samples (10 mL each): one sample is drawn through the indwelling catheter, and the other is taken from a peripheral vein. The samples are placed in special culture tubes (e.g., Isolator System, Dupont Co.) for transport to the laboratory.

2. Each blood specimen is processed by first isolating the cells and suspending them in a culture medium. The cells are then lysed to release intracellular organisms, and the supernatant is placed on an agar plate and incubated. Growth is measured as the number of colony-forming units per milliliter (CFU/mL).

3. The diagnosis of catheter-related septicemia requires isolation of the same organism in both blood cultures plus either of the following: growth of at least 100 CFU/mL from the catheter blood or a colony count in catheter blood that is at least 5 times greater than the colony count in peripheral blood (see Figure 6.2).

4. This method will detect infection only on the inner surface of the catheter, and this might explain the low sensitivity of this method (40 to 50%) for the detection of catheter-related infections (see Table 6.2) (22).

F. Which Culture Method is Preferred?

The choice of culture method is dictated largely by the feasibility of removing the catheter. The criteria for catheter removal are listed earlier (See also Figure 6.3).

1. If the catheter should be removed, the catheter tip should be cultured using the serial dilution method (which is more sensitive than the roll-plate method).

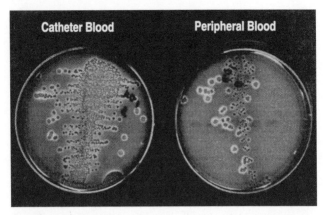

FIGURE 6.2. Comparative growth of quantitative blood cultures from a case of catheter-related septicemia. *Catheter Blood* is blood withdrawn through a central venous catheter. *Peripheral Blood* is blood taken from a peripheral vein. (From Reference 32).

2. If catheter replacement is not necessary (e.g., for patients with isolated fever), or is not easily accomplished (i.e., for tunneled catheters or limited venous access), the comparative blood culture method is appropriate.

G. Empiric Antibiotic Coverage

Empiric antibiotic coverage is indicated in most cases of suspected catheter-related septicemia.

1. *The Microbial Spectrum*

    The selection of empiric antibiotics is dictated by the microbes most likely involved.

    a. A survey of 112 medical ICUs in the United States revealed the following microbial spectrum in primary hospital-acquired bacteremias (most caused by indwelling catheters) (23): *Staphylococcus epidermidis* (36%), enterococci (16%), gram-negative aerobic bacilli (*Pseudomonas aeruginosa, Klebsiella pneumoniae, E. coli,* etc.) (16%), *Staphylococcus aureus* (13%), *Candida* species (11%), and other organisms (8%).

b. About half of the infections involve staphylococci, and half are from organisms usually found in the bowel, including *Candida* organisms.

2. *Recommendations*

The initial management of suspected catheter-related septicemia can be conducted as shown in Figure 6.3.

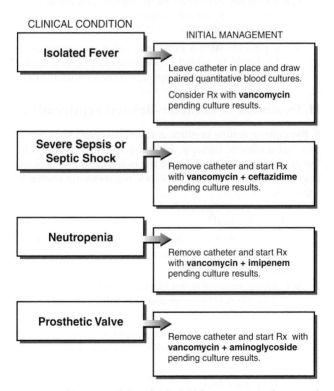

FIGURE 6.3. Recommendations for the initial management of suspected catheter-related septicemia. From References 22 and 24.

a. Despite concern about vancomycin resistance, this antibiotic is well suited for suspected catheter-related infections because it is active against staphylococci (including coagulase-negative and methicillin-resistant strains), and most strains of enterococci, which together account for over 50% of catheter-related infections.

b. Gram-negative coverage with ceftazidime or cefepime (for antipseudomonal activity) can be added for patients with severe sepsis or septic shock.

c. For patients with neutropenia (neutrophil count < 500 /mm³), a carbapenem (imipenem or meropenem) can be added to vancomycin (22,24).

d. For patients with a prosthetic valve, an aminoglycoside should be added to vancomycin (the two agents can be synergistic for *Staph. epidermidis* endocarditis).

H. Treatment of Catheter–Related Septicemia

If the culture results confirm a catheter-related septicemia, directed antibiotic therapy should proceed as dictated by the antibiotic susceptibilities of the isolated microbes. Some popular organism-specific antibiotic regimens are shown in Table 6.3.

1. *Catheter Removal*

a. Catheters that have been left in place should be removed if cultures confirm the presence of catheter-related septicemia. (22).

b. Catheter removal is not always necessary if the patient shows a favorable response to empiric antibiotics and the responsible organism is *Staph. epidermidis* (25).

c. Catheters that are not easily replaced can sometimes be treated successfully with *antibiotic lock therapy* (see next).

2. *Antibiotic Lock Therapy*

a. When a catheter is not used for continuous intravenous infusions, a concentrated antibiotic solution (usually 1 to 5 mg/mL) can be injected into the lumen of an infected catheter and left in place for hours to days (22).

b. This approach is best suited for tunneled catheters that have been in place for longer than 2 weeks because

TABLE 6.3 Popular Antimicrobial Regimens for Catheter-Related Bloodstream Infections

Organism	Antibiotic Regimen
Staphylococci	
Methicillin-sensitive	Nafcillin or oxacillin (2 g every 4 hrs)
Methicillin-resistant (Includes most strains of *S. epidermidis*)	Vancomycin (1 g every 12 hrs)
Enterococci	
Ampicillin-sensitive	Ampicillin (2 g every 4 – 6 hrs)
Ampicillin-resistant	Vancomycin (1 g every 12 hrs)
Vancomycin-resistant	Linezolid (600 mg every 12 hrs)
Gram-negative bacilli	
E. coli *Klebsiella spp* *Enterobacter spp*	Imipenem (500 mg every 6 hrs) or Meropenem (1 g every 8 hrs)
P. aeruginosa	For *P. aeruginosa*, some prefer ceftazidime (2 g every 8 hrs) or an antipseudomonal penicillin
***Candida* organisms**	Fluconazole (6 mg/kg/day) or capsofungin (70 mg load, then 50 mg daily)
	Amphotericin B (0.7 mg/kg/day) for severe infections

Antibiotic regimens are for uncomplicated infections only.

From the guidelines in References 22 and 30.

these catheters are likely to have an intraluminal source of infection (22). The success is limited when *Candida* species are involved (22).

3. *Duration of Therapy*

For uncomplicated cases of catheter-related septicemia, 10 to 14 days of antibiotics is recommended, but only 5 to 7 days is sufficient for most cases of *Staph. epidermidis* septicemia (22).

I. Persistent Sepsis

Continued signs of sepsis after a few days of antibiotic therapy can signal one of the following conditions.

1. *Suppurative Thrombosis*

Thrombosis surrounding the catheter tip is a common finding in catheter-related septicemia (11), and if the thrombus becomes infected, it can transform into an intravascular abscess.

a. Purulent drainage from the catheter insertion site is not always present in this condition (22). Septic emboli in the lungs is an occasional finding.

b. Catheter removal is essential in this condition, and surgical incision and drainage is recommended if peripheral vessels are involved.

c. When this condition involves large central veins, antimicrobial therapy combined with heparin anticoagulation can produce satisfactory results in 50% of cases (26).

2. *Endocarditis*

a. Vascular catheters are the most common cause of nosocomial endocarditis, and *Staph. aureus* is the most common offending organism (22). As such, all cases of catheter-related *Staph. aureus* bacteremia should be evaluated for endocarditis (22).

b. Transesophageal ultrasound is the diagnostic procedure of choice for endocarditis.

c. If endocarditis is documented, catheter removal is mandatory, and antibiotic therapy is continued for 4 to 6 weeks (22).

3. *Disseminated Candidiasis*

a. Vascular catheters are the most common cause of disseminated candidiasis, and the predisposing factors include abdominal surgery, burns, organ transplantation, HIV infection, cancer chemotherapy, long-term steroid therapy, and broad-spectrum antimicrobial therapy (27).

b. The diagnosis can be missed in over 50% of cases because blood cultures are often negative (28). The clinical markers of disseminated candidiasis include isolation of *Candida* organisms in multiple sites, candiduria in the absence of an indwelling urethral catheter, and endophthalmitis.

c. Heavy colonization of the urine in high-risk patients (regardless of the presence or absence of an indwelling urethral catheter) is an indication to initiate empiric antifungal therapy (29).

d. Endophthalmitis can occur in up to one-third of patients with disseminated candidiasis (28), and can lead to permanent blindness. Because the consequences of this condition can be serious, all patients with persistent candidemia should have a detailed eye exam (28).

e. The standard treatment for invasive candidiasis is amphotericin B (0.7 mg/kg/day) (30), which is available in a special lipid formulation (liposomal amphotericin B, 3 mg/kg/day) that produces less nephrotoxicity (see Chapter 44). The antifungal agent capsofungin (70 mg loading dose, followed by 50 mg/day) is equally effective for invasive candidiasis (31), and may become the preferred agent because of its safety profile.

Despite the choice of antimicrobial agent, satisfactory outcomes are achieved in only 60 to 70% of cases of invasive candidiasis (30).

REFERENCES

1. Centers for Disease Control and Prevention. Guidelines for the prevention of intravascular catheter-related infections. MMWR 2002; 51 (No.RR-10):1-30.

2. Hoffman KK, Weber DJ, Samsa GP, et al. Transparent polyurethane film as intravenous catheter dressing. A meta-analysis of infection risks. JAMA 1992; 267:2072–2076.

3. Maki DG, Stolz SS, Wheeler S, Mermi LA. A prospective, randomized trial of gauze and two polyurethane dressings for site care of pulmonary artery catheters: implications for catheter management. Crit Care Med 1994; 22:1729–1737.

4. McGee DC, Gould MK. Preventing complications of central venous catheterization. N Engl J Med 2003; 348:1123-1133.

5. Zakrzewska-Bode A, Muytjens HL, Liem KD, Hoogkamp-Korstanje JA. Muciprocin resistance in coagulase-negative staphylococci after topical prophylaxis for the reduction of colonization of central venous catheters. J Hosp Infect 1995; 31:189-193.

6. Peterson FY, Kirchhoff KT. Analysis of research about heparinized versus non-heparinized intravascular lines. Heart Lung 1991; 20:631–642.

7. Branson PK, McCoy RA, Phillips BA, Clifton GD. Efficacy of 1.4% sodium citrate in maintaining arterial catheter patency in patients in a medical ICU. Chest 1993; 103:882–885.

8. Cook D, Randolph A, Kernerman P, et al. Central venous replacement strategies: a systematic review of the literature. Crit Care Med 1997; 25:1417-1424.

9. Cobb DK, High KP, Sawyer RP, et al. A controlled trial of scheduled replacement of central venous and pulmonary artery catheters. N Engl J Med 1992; 327:1062–1068.

10. Safdar N, Maki D. Inflammation at the insertion site is not predictive of catheter-related bloodstream infection with short-term, noncuffed central venous catheters. Crit Care Med 2002; 30:2632-2635.

11. Jacobs BR. Central venous catheter occlusion and thrombosis. Crit Care Clin 2003; 19:489-514.

12. Davis SN, Vermeulen L, Banton J, et al. Activity and dosage of alteplase dilution for clearing occlusions of vascular-access devices. Am J Health Syst Pharm 2000; 57:1039-1045.

13. Zacharias JM. Alteplase versus urokinase for occluded hemodialysis catheters. Ann Pharmacother 2003; 37:27-33.

14. Shulman RJ, Reed T, Pitre D, Laine L. Use of hydrochloric acid to clear obstructed central venous catheters. J Parenter Enteral Nutr 1988; 12:509–510.

15. Calis KA ed. Pharmacy Update. Drug Information Service, National Institutes of Health, Bethesda MD, Nov-Dec, 1999 (Accessed at www.cc.nih.gov/phar/updates/99nov-dec.html)

16. Mustafa S, Stein P, Patel K, et al. Upper extremity deep venous thrombosis. Chest 2003; 123:1953-1956.

17. Otten TR, Stein PD, Patel KC, et al. Thromboembolic disease involving the superior vena cava and brachiocephalic veins. Chest 2003; 123:809-812.

18. Hingorani A, Ascher E, Hanson J, et al. Upper extremity versus lower extremity deep venous thrombosis. Am J Surg 1997; 174:214-217.

19. Mustafa BO, Rathbun SW, Whitsett TL, Raskob GE. Sensitivity and specificity of ultrasonography in the diagnosis of upper extremity deep venous thrombosis. A systematic review. Arch Intern Med 2002; 162:401-404.

20. Pittet D, Tarara D, Wenzel RP. Nosocomial bloodstream infection in critically ill patients. JAMA 1994; 271:1598–1601.

21. EdgeworthJ, Treacher D, Eykyn S. A 25-year study of nosocomial bacteremia in an adult intensive care unit. Crit Care Med 1999; 27:1421-1428.

22. Mermel LA, Farr BM, Sherertz RJ, et al. Guidelines for the management of intravascular catheter-related infections. Clin Infect Dis 2001; 32:1249-1272.

23. Richards M, Edwards J, Culver D, Gaynes R. Nosocomial infections in medical intensive care units in the United States. Crit Care Med 1999; 27:887-892.

24. Hughes WT, Armstrong D, Bodey GP, Bow EJ, et al. 2002 guidelines for the use of antimicrobial agents in neutropenic patients with cancer. Clin Infect Dis 2002; 34:730-751.

25. Raad I, Davis S, Khan A, et al. Impact of central venous catheter removal on the recurrence of catheter-related coagulase-negative staphylococcal bacteremia. Infect Control Hosp Epidemiol 1992; 154:808-816.

26. Verghese A, Widrich WC, Arbeit RD. Central venous septic thrombophlebitis: the role of antimicrobial therapy. Medicine 1985; 64:394–400.

27. Ostrosky-Zeichner L, Rex JH, Bennett J, Kullberg B-J. Deeply invasive candidiasis. Infect Dis Clin North Amer 2002; 16:821-835.

28. Calandra T. *Candida* infections in the intensive care unit. Curr Opin Crit Care 1997; 3:335-341.

29. British Society for Antimicrobial Chemotherapy Working Party. Management of deep *Candida* infection in surgical and intensive care unit patients. Intensive Care Med 1994; 20:522–528.

30. Pappas PG, Rex JH, Sobel JD, et al. Guidelines for the treatment of candidiasis. Clin Infect Dis 2004; 38:161-189.

31. Mora-Duarte J, Betts R, Rotstein C, et al. Comparison of capsofungin and amphotericin B for invasive candidiasis. N Engl J Med 2002; 347:2020-2029.

32. Curtas S, Tramposch K. Culture methods to evaluate central venous catheter sepsis. Nutr Clin Pract 1991; 6:43.

Chapter 7

THE PULMONARY ARTERY CATHETER

The emergence of critical care medicine as a specialty is largely the result of two innovations: positive-pressure mechanical ventilation and the pulmonary artery catheter. This chapter will introduce you to the pulmonary artery catheter and the information it provides (1-3).

I. THE CATHETER

A. The Principle

The pulmonary artery (PA) catheter is equipped with an inflatable balloon that acts like a rubber raft and allows the flow of venous blood to carry the catheter tip through the right side of the heart and out into the pulmonary circulation. This *balloon flotation* method makes it possible to perform a right heart catheterization at the bedside without fluoroscopic guidance.

B. Catheter Design

The basic features of a PA catheter are illustrated in Figure 7.1.

1. The catheter is 110 cm long and has an outside diameter of 2.3 mm (about 7 French). There are two internal channels: One runs the entire length of the catheter and opens at the tip (the distal or PA lumen), and the other ends 30 cm from the catheter tip and is usually in the right atrium (the proximal or RA lumen).

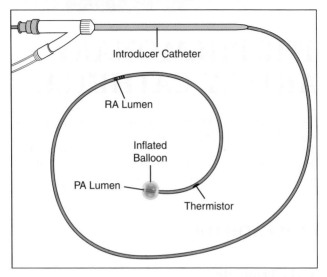

FIGURE 7.1. The basic features of the balloon-flotation pulmonary artery catheter. Note that the catheter is threaded through a large-bore introducer catheter (see Chapter 4 for a description of introducer catheters).

2. The tip of the catheter has a small balloon (1.5 mL capacity) that is used as just described. When inflated, the balloon creates a recess for the tip of the catheter that prevents the tip from scraping along the vessel wall as the catheter is advanced.

3. The catheter also has a small thermistor (i.e., a transducer that senses changes in temperature) located 4 cm from the catheter tip. This device can measure the cardiac output using the *thermodilution* method, which is described later in the chapter.

II. CATHETER PLACEMENT

The PA catheter is usually inserted through a large-bore

(9 French) introducer catheter that has been placed in the subclavian or internal jugular vein (see Figure 7.1). Just prior to insertion, the distal lumen is attached to a pressure transducer. When the tip of the PA catheter emerges from the introducer catheter, a venous pressure waveform appears. The balloon is then inflated and the catheter is advanced. The location of the catheter tip is determined by the pressure tracings recorded from the distal lumen, as shown in Figure 7.2.

1. The superior vena cava pressure is a nonpulsatile pressure with small amplitude oscillations. The pressure waveform is unchanged after the catheter tip is advanced into the right atrium. The normal pressure in the superior vena cava and right atrium is 2 to 8 mm Hg.

2. When the catheter tip moves across the tricuspid valve and into the right ventricle, a pulsatile waveform appears. The peak (systolic) pressure is a function of the strength of right ventricular contraction, and the lowest (diastolic) pressure is equivalent to the right-atrial pressure. The systolic pressure in the right ventricle is normally 15 to 30 mm Hg.

3. When the catheter moves across the pulmonic valve and into a main pulmonary artery, the pressure wave shows a sudden rise in diastolic pressure caused by flow resistance in the pulmonary circulation. This diastolic pressure is normally 6 to 12 mm Hg.

4. As the catheter is advanced further into the pulmonary circulation, the pulsatile waveform eventually disappears, leaving a venous-type waveform at the same pressure level as the pulmonary artery diastolic pressure (6 to 12 mm Hg). This is the pulmonary artery occlusion pressure, also called the *pulmonary capillary wedge pressure* (PCWP), or simply the *wedge pressure*. This pressure is a reflection of the diastolic filling pressure of the left ventricle (as explained in the next chapter).

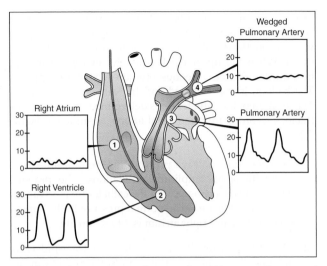

FIGURE 7.2. The pressure waveforms used to guide proper placement of pulmonary artery catheters.

5. When the wedge pressure first becomes evident, the balloon at the tip of the catheter should be deflated. This should result in a return of the pulsatile pressure tracing. If this occurs, the PA catheter should be left in place with the balloon deflated.

6. In about 25% of PA catheter placements, the pulsatile PA pressure never disappears as the catheter is advanced the maximum distance along the pulmonary artery (1,2). If this occurs, the pulmonary artery diastolic pressure can be used as a reflection of the wedge pressure (in the absence of pulmonary hypertension, the two pressures should be equivalent).

A. The Balloon

1. The balloon should remain deflated while the PA catheter

is left in place (sustained balloon inflation can result in pulmonary artery rupture or pulmonary infarction). Balloon inflation is permitted only when measuring the wedge pressure.

2. When measuring the wedge pressure, DO NOT fully inflate the balloon with 1.5 mL air all at once (catheters often migrate into smaller pulmonary arteries, and a fully inflated balloon could result in vessel rupture). The balloon should be slowly inflated until a wedge pressure tracing is obtained.

3. Once the wedge pressure is recorded, the balloon should be fully deflated. Detaching the syringe from the balloon injection port will help prevent inadvertent balloon inflation while the catheter is in place.

III. THERMODILUTION

A. The Method

The thermodilution method is illustrated in Figure 7.3. A dextrose or saline solution that is colder than blood is injected through the proximal port of the catheter in the right atrium. The cold fluid mixes with blood in the right heart chambers, and the cooled blood is ejected into the pulmonary artery and flows past the thermistor on the distal end of the catheter. The thermistor records the change in blood temperature with time and sends this information to an electronic instrument that records and displays a temperature–time curve. The area under this curve is inversely proportional to the rate of blood flow in the pulmonary artery. In the absence of intracardiac shunts, this flow rate is equivalent to the (average) cardiac output.

B. Technical Considerations

1. Although the indicator solution is usually cooled before injection (to optimize the temperature difference between blood and injectate), room temperature injectates produce reliable measurements in most patients (4,5).

2. Serial measurements are recommended for each cardiac output determination. Three measurements are sufficient if they differ by 10% or less, and the cardiac output is taken as the average of all measurements. Serial measurements that differ by more than 10% are considered unreliable (6).

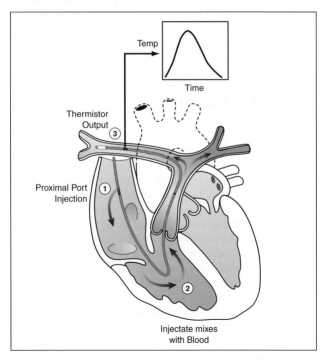

FIGURE 7.3. The thermodilution method of measuring cardiac output.

C. Variability

Thermodilution cardiac output can vary by as much as 10% without any apparent change in the clinical condition of the patient (7). *A change in thermodilution cardiac output must exceed 10% to be considered clinically significant.*

D. Confounding Conditions

The following clinical conditions can affect the accuracy of cardiac output measurements.

1. *Tricuspid Regurgitation*

   This condition may be common during positive-pressure mechanical ventilation. The regurgitant flow causes the indicator fluid to be recycled, producing a prolonged, low-amplitude thermodilution curve characteristic of a low cardiac output. Therefore, this condition results in falsely low cardiac output measurements (8).

2. *Intracardiac Shunts*

   Intracardiac shunts produce falsely elevated cardiac output measurements.

   a. In right-to-left shunts, a portion of the injectate fluid passes through the shunt, creating an abbreviated thermodilution curve similar to the one seen in high output states.

   b. In left-to-right shunts, the shunted blood increases the blood volume in the right side of the heart, and this dilutes the injectate fluid and produces an abbreviated thermodilution curve similar to the one seen in high output states.

E. Continuous Cardiac Output Measurements

A specialized PA catheter is available (from Baxter Edwards Critical Care) that can provided frequent and automatic measurements of cardiac output (9). A thermal filament wrapped around a distal portion of the catheter is used to generate low-energy heat pulses that warm the surrounding blood. The change in blood temperature is then sensed by a thermistor on the catheter, and the average cardiac output over successive 3-minute time intervals is recorded and displayed.

1. This "continuous" thermodilution method produces more accurate cardiac output measurements (10) than the intermittent bolus-injection method, and it does not require the time or expertise of an operator.

IV. HEMODYNAMIC PARAMETERS

The PA catheter can provide a wealth of information about cardiovascular function and systemic oxygen transport. This section provides a brief description of the hemodynamic parameters that can be measured or derived with PA catheters. These parameters are listed in Table 7.1.

A. Cardiovascular Parameters

1. *Central Venous Pressure*

   The proximal port of the PA catheter measures the pressure in the superior vena cava, which is equivalent to the pressure in the right atrium. This pressure is commonly called the *central venous pressure* (CVP). In the absence of a tricuspid valve abnormality, the CVP or right-atrial pressure (RAP) is equivalent to the right ventricular end-diastolic pressure (RVEDP):

   CVP = RAP = RVEDP

   Because the CVP is equivalent to the RVEDP, it is used as a measure of right-ventricular filling. (See Chapter 8 for more information on the CVP).

TABLE 7.1 Hemodynamic & Oxygen Transport Parameters

Parameter	Abbreviation	Normal Range
Central Venous Pressure	CVP	2 – 8 mm Hg
Pulmonary Capillary Wedge Pressure	PCWP	6 – 12 mm Hg
Cardiac Index	CI	2.4 – 4.0 L/min/m^2
Stroke Index	SI	40 – 70 L/m^2
Systemic Vascular Resistance Index	SVRI	25 – 30 Wood units[†]
Pulmonary Vascular Resistance Index	PVRI	1 – 2 Wood units[†]
Oxygen Delivery	DO$_2$	520 – 570 mL/min/m^2
Oxygen Uptake	VO$_2$	110 – 160 mL/min/m^2
Oxygen Extraction Ratio	O$_2$ER	0.2 – 0.3

[†]mm Hg per liter per minute per square meter.

2. *Pulmonary Capillary Wedge Pressure*

When the inflated balloon on a PA catheter creates a complete obstruction in the involved artery, the pressure at the tip of the PA catheter (which is called the *pulmonary capillary wedge pressure* or PCWP) is equivalent to the pressure in the left atrium. In the absence of a mitral valve abnormality, the PCWP or left-atrial pressure (LAP) is equivalent to the left-ventricular end-diastolic pressure (LVEDP):

PCWP = LAP = LVEDP

Because the PCWP is equivalent to the LVEDP, it is used as a measure of left-ventricular filling. (See Chapter 8 for a detailed description of the wedge pressure).

3. *Cardiac Index*

Cardiac output varies with body size, so the conventional practice is to adjust the measured cardiac output for the size of the patient. The size-dependent changes in cardiac output show a closer correlation with changes in body surface area (BSA) than with changes in body weight, so BSA is used as the measure of body size. A simple method for determining the BSA based on height (Ht) and weight (Wt) is shown below (11).

$$\textbf{BSA (m}^2\textbf{) = Ht (cm) + Wt (kg) − 60 /100} \qquad (7.1)$$

To adjust for body size, the BSA is divided into the cardiac output (CO). The size-adjusted parameter is called the *cardiac index* (CI), and is expressed as L/min/m².

$$\textbf{CI = CO /BSA} \qquad (7.2)$$

The average-sized adult has a BSA of 1.6 to 1.9 m², so the cardiac index is normally about 50 to 60% of the measured cardiac output. The normal range for CI in adults is shown in Table 7.1.

4. *Stroke Index*

The stroke volume (the volume of blood ejected by the ventricles during systole) is a reflection of the systolic performance of the heart, and is superior to the cardiac output in this regard because it is not influenced by heart rate. The stroke volume should be adjusted for body size, as in Equation 7.3, by dividing the heart rate (HR) into the cardiac index (CI), not cardiac output. The size-adjusted stroke volume, or *stroke index* (SI), is expressed as mL/m².

$$\textbf{SI = CI /HR} \qquad (7.3)$$

The normal range of SI in adults is shown in Table 7.1. An abnormally low SI can be the result of reduced ventricular filling (e.g., hypovolemia), impaired contractility (systolic heart failure), or increased impedance to ventricular emptying (e.g., aortic stenosis).

5. *Systemic Vascular Resistance Index*

The systemic vascular resistance (SVR) is traditionally calculated as the pressure drop across the systemic circulation, or the mean arterial pressure minus the central venous pressure (MAP – CVP) divided by the cardiac output (CO). These relationships are shown in Equation 7.4 using the cardiac index (CI) to derive the size-adjusted SVR or *systemic vascular resistance index* (SVRI).

$$\textbf{SVRI = (MAP – CVP) / CI} \qquad (7.4)$$

The SVRI is expressed as Wood units (mm Hg/L/min /m^2), and the normal range is shown in Table 7.1. A common practice is to multiply Wood units by 80 to express vascular resistance in more conventional units (dynes•sec^{-1}•cm^{-5}/m^2), but this practice offers no advantage (12).

   a. CAVEAT. The hydraulic resistance in the systemic circulation is not a measurable entity for a number of reasons (e.g., resistance varies in different tissues, resistance is flow-dependent, the vessels are compressible and not rigid, etc.). *The SVRI is not a true measure of hydraulic resistance;* it merely describes the global relationship between blood pressure and blood flow in the systemic circulation.

6. *Pulmonary Vascular Resistance Index*

The pulmonary vascular resistance (PVR) is derived as the pressure gradient across the lungs, or the mean pulmonary artery pressure minus the left-atrial or wedge pressure (PAP – PCWP) divided by the cardiac output (CO). These relationships are shown below using the cardiac index (CI) to derive the size-adjusted PVR, or *pulmonary vascular resistance index* (PVRI).

$$PVRI = (PAP - PCWP)/CI \qquad (7.5)$$

The PVRI is expressed as Wood units (mm Hg/L/min /m^2), and the normal range is shown in Table 7.1. Note that the PVRI is only a small fraction of the SVRI, which is a reflection of the low pressures in the pulmonary circulation. The PVRI suffers from the same shortcoming as the SVRI as a measure of hydraulic resistance.

B. Oxygen Transport Parameters

There are 3 parameters used to define systemic oxygen transport. These are described in detail in Chapter 9, and are presented only briefly here.

1. *Oxygen Delivery*

The rate of oxygen transport in arterial blood, or *oxygen delivery* (DO$_2$), is determined by the cardiac output and the O$_2$ content in arterial blood (CaO$_2$). The equation below shows the determinants of the size-adjusted DO$_2$, which is expressed as mL/min/m^2.

$$DO_2 = CI \times (1.34 \times Hb \times SaO_2) \times 10 \qquad (7.6)$$

The term (1.3 x Hb x SaO$_2$) represents the arterial O$_2$ content (CaO$_2$), and is described in more detail in Chapter 9. The normal range for the size-adjusted DO$_2$ is shown in Table 7.1

2. *Oxygen Uptake*

Oxygen uptake (VO$_2$) is the rate at which oxygen is taken up from the systemic capillaries into the tissues. Since oxygen is not stored in tissues, the VO$_2$ is equivalent to the O$_2$ consumption in the tissues. The equation below shows the determinants of the size-adjusted VO$_2$, which is expressed as mL/min/m^2.

$$VO_2 = CI \times 1.34 \times Hb \times (SaO_2 - SvO_2) \times 10 \qquad (7.7)$$

(The components of this equation are described in Chapter 9). The normal range for the size-adjusted VO_2 is shown in Table 7.1.

3. *Oxygen Extraction Ratio*

The oxygen extraction ratio (O_2ER) is the fractional uptake of oxygen from the systemic microcirculation, and is equivalent to the ratio of O_2 uptake to O_2 delivery.

$$\textbf{O}_2\textbf{ER} = \textbf{VO}_2 / \textbf{DO}_2 \qquad (7.8)$$

The normal O_2ER is 0.2 to 0.3 (see Table 7.1), which means that only 20% to 30% of the oxygen that is delivered to the tissues is consumed.

V. APPLICATIONS

A. Hemodynamic Profiles

Most hemodynamic problems are identified by noting the pattern of changes in three hemodynamic parameters: ventricular filling pressure (CVP or PCWP), cardiac output, and systemic or pulmonary vascular resistance. This is demonstrated in Table 7.2 using the 3 classic forms of shock: hypovolemic, cardiogenic, and vasogenic. Each of these conditions produces a distinct pattern or *profile* of hemodynamic changes. Since there are 3 parameters and 3 possible conditions (low, normal, or high), there are 3^3 or 27 possible profiles, each representing a distinct hemodynamic condition.

B. Oxygen Uptake (VO_2)

Hemodynamic profiles can identify a hemodynamic problem, but they provide no information about the impact of the problem on tissue oxygenation. The addition of the oxygen uptake (VO_2) to hemodynamic profiles can help in this regard. An abnormally low VO_2, in the absence of hypometabolism, is evidence of impaired tissue oxygenation. Therefore, if a hemodynamic problem is associated with a low VO_2 (less than 100 ml/min/m²), the condition is potentially life-threatening and deserves immediate attention. (See Chapter 9 for more information on the VO_2).

TABLE 7.2 Hemodynamic Patterns in Different Types of Shock

Parameter	Hypovolemic Shock	Cardiogenic Shock	Vasogenic Shock
CVP or PCWP	Low	High	Low
Cardiac Output	Low	Low	High
Systemic Vascular Resistance	Low	High	Low

REFERENCES

1. Swan HJ. The pulmonary artery catheter. Dis Mon 1991; 37: 473–543.
2. Pinsky MR. Hemodynamic monitoring in the intensive care unit. Clin Chest Med 2003; 24:549-560.
3. American Society of Anesthesiologists Task Force on Pulmonary Artery Catheterization. Practice guidelines for pulmonary artery catheterization: an updated report by the American Society of Anesthesiologists Task Force on Pulmonary Artery Catheterization. Anesthesiology 2003; 99:988-1014.
4. Nelson LD, Anderson HB. Patient selection for iced versus room temperature injectate for thermodilution cardiac output determinations. Crit Care Med 1985; 13:182–184.
5. Pearl RG, Rosenthal MH, Nielson L, et al. Effect of injectate volume and temperature on thermodilution cardiac output determi-

nations. Anesthesiology 1986; 64:798–801.

6. Nadeau S, Noble WH. Limitations of cardiac output measurement by thermodilution. Can J Anesth 1986; 33:780–784.

7. Sasse SA, Chen PA, Berry RB, et al. Variability of cardiac output over time in medical intensive care unit patients. Chest 1994; 22:225–232.

8. Konishi T, Nakamura Y, Morii I, et al. Comparison of thermodilution and Fick methods for measurement of cardiac output in tricuspid regurgitation. Am J Cardiol 1992; 70:538–540.

9. Yelderman M, Ramsay MA, Quinn MD, et al. Continuous thermodilution cardiac output measurement in intensive care unit patients. J Cardiothorac Vasc Anesth 1992; 6:270–274.

10. Mihaljevic T, vonSegesser LK, Tonz M, et al. Continuous versus bolus thermodilution cardiac output measurements – A comparative study. Crit Care Med 1995; 23:944-949.

11. Mattar JA. A simple calculation to estimate body surface area in adults and its correlation with the Dubois formula. Crit Care Med 1989; 17:846–847.

12. Bartlett RH. Critical Care Physiology. New York: Little Brown & Co., 1996: 36.

Chapter 8

CARDIAC FILLING PRESSURES

As mentioned in the last chapter, the central venous pressure and the pulmonary artery occlusion (wedge) pressure are the diastolic filling pressures of the right and left ventricles, respectively (see Table 8.1). This chapter describes how these pressures are measured, and highlights the limitations and misinterpretations that haunt these pressures (1-3).

I. VENOUS PRESSURES IN THE THORAX

A. Intravascular vs. Transmural Pressure

1. The pressure recorded from an indwelling vascular catheter is the *intravascular pressure*, which is measured relative to atmospheric (zero reference point) pressure.

2. The pressure that distends the ventricles and drives edema fluid into the tissues is the *transmural pressure*, or the difference between intravascular and extravascular pressures. This is the physiologically important pressure.

3. The intravascular and transmural pressures are equivalent only when the extravascular pressure is zero. In the thorax, this normally occurs at the end of expiration (see next section).

B. Influence of Thoracic Pressure

Respiratory changes in intrathoracic pressure can be transmitted across the wall of blood vessels in the thorax. This creates phasic changes in intravascular pressure similar to the central venous pressure (CVP) tracing in Figure 8.1. Despite these changes in intravascular pressure, there is little or no change in the transmural pressure (because the changes in thoracic pressure are transmitted across the wall of the blood vessels). This means that respiratory variations in the CVP and wedge pressures do not reflect changes in the cardiac filling pressure (i.e., the transmural pressure).

TABLE 8.1 The Cardiac Filling Pressures

	Right Heart	**Left Heart**
Measurement	Superior vena cava pressure	Pulmonary artery occlusion pressure
Common Term	Central venous pressure	Wedge pressure
Equivalent Pressures	Right atrial pressure, Right ventricular end-diastolic pressure	Left atrial pressure, Left ventricular end-diastolic pressure*
Normal Range	2 – 8 mm Hg	6 –12 mm Hg

*Is NOT a measure of pulmonary capillary hydrostatic pressure.

1. The End of Expiration

   a. In the thorax, intravascular pressures should be equivalent to transmural pressures at the end of expiration, when the intrathoracic (extravascular) pressure is at atmospheric or zero reference level. Therefore, when respiratory variations are apparent in the CVP or wedge pressure tracing, the pressure should be measured at the end of expiration.

   b. The mean pressure (which is often displayed by bedside monitors) should never be used as the CVP or wedge pressure when respiratory variations are present.

2. *Positive End-Expiratory Pressure*

   a. Cardiac filling pressures recorded at the end of expiration will be falsely elevated in the presence of positive end-expiratory pressure (PEEP).

   b. When PEEP is applied during mechanical ventilation, the patient should be disconnected from the ventilator to measure the CVP and wedge pressure (4).

   c. In the presence of intrinsic PEEP (caused by incomplete emptying of the lungs during exhalation), accurate recordings of the CVP and wedge pressures can be difficult (5). See Chapter 20 for a method of correcting the CVP and wedge pressure measurements in patients with intrinsic PEEP.

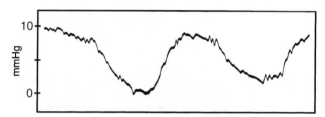

FIGURE 8.1. Respiratory variations in the central venous pressure (CVP). The true cardiac filling pressure (the transmural pressure) is at end-expiration, which corresponds to the peak pressures during spontaneous breathing, and trough pressures during mechanical ventilation.

C. Spontaneous Variations

In addition to respiratory variations, the CVP and wedge pressures can vary spontaneously, without apparent cause. The spontaneous variation in wedge pressure is 4 mm Hg or less in 60% of patients, but it can be as high as 7 mm Hg (6). In general, *a change in the CVP or wedge pressure should exceed 4 mm Hg to be considered a clinically significant change.*

II. THE WEDGE PRESSURE

The pulmonary artery occlusion pressure (known as the *wedge pressure*) is the measurement that prompted the introduction of the pulmonary artery catheter in 1970. Despite years of enormous popularity (which is waning), the wedge pressure is often misinterpreted (3,7-9).

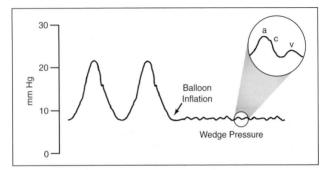

FIGURE 8.2. The transition from a pulsatile pulmonary artery pressure to a balloon-occlusion (wedge) pressure. The magnified area shows 3 components that identify the wedge pressure as a venous pressure.

A. The Wedge Pressure Tracing

1. When the pulmonary artery (PA) catheter is properly positioned, inflation of the balloon at the distal end of the catheter will obstruct flow in the involved artery, and the pulsatile pressure recorded from the tip of the catheter will disappear (see Figure 8.2).

2. The nonpulsatile or "wedged" pressure has 3 component waves: the a wave is produced by left atrial contraction, the c wave is produced by closure of the mitral valve during isometric contraction of the left ventricle, and the v wave is produced by contraction of the left ventricle

against a closed mitral valve. These waves identify the wedge pressure as a venous (cardiac filling) pressure.

B. The Principle of the Wedge Pressure

1. The principle of the wedge pressure is easily explained using the hydraulic relationships in the following equation (see Figure 8.3):

$$\mathbf{P_c} - \mathbf{P_{LA}} = \mathbf{Q} \times \mathbf{R_v} \qquad (8.1)$$

Where: P_c is the pressure at the tip of the PA catheter
P_{LA} is the pressure in the left atrium
Q is the rate of blood flow (cardiac output)
R_v is the resistance to flow in the pulmonary veins

2. If the balloon at the distal end of the PA catheter is inflated to obstruct flow, the following is predicted by Equation 8.1:

When: $Q = 0$
Then: $P_c - P_{LA} = 0$
And: $P_c = P_{LA}$

Thus, the absence of flow eliminates the pressure gradient between the tip of the PA catheter and the left atrium, and this allows the pressure at the tip of the PA catheter (the wedge pressure) to be used as a measure of the left atrial pressure.

3. The left atrial pressure (the wedge pressure) will be equivalent to the end-diastolic pressure (the filling pressure) of the left ventricle as long as there is no obstruction at the mitral valve orifice.

4. Thus, the principle of the wedge pressure measurement is to create an obstruction to flow so that the pressure at

the tip of the PA catheter can be used as a surrogate measure of the left ventricular filling pressure.

C. Checking for Accuracy

The following factors can be used to determine if the wedge pressure is an accurate reflection of the pressure in the left atrium.

1. *Catheter Tip Position*

   a. The tip of the PA catheter must be in a lung region where capillary (venous) pressure exceeds alveolar pressure (if not, the pressure at the tip of the PA catheter will reflect the alveolar pressure). This corresponds to the most dependent lung region (see Figure 8.3).

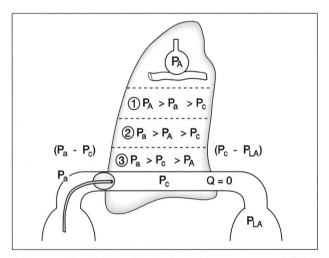

FIGURE 8.3. The principle of the wedge pressure measurement. When flow ceases because of balloon inflation ($Q = 0$), the pulsatile arterial pressure (P_a) is lost, and the pressure at the catheter tip (P_c) is the same as the pressure in the left atrium (P_{LA}). This occurs only in the most dependent lung zone, where the capillary pressure (P_c) exceeds the alveolar pressure (P_A).

b. The lung regions where capillary pressure exceeds alveolar pressure are usually below the level of the left atrium. Therefore, the tip of the PA catheter should be located below the level of the left atrium (3). Confirming this location requires a lateral chest x-ray (which is not a common practice).

2. *Respiratory Variations*

Prominent respiratory variations in the wedge pressure tracing indicates that the wedge pressure is a reflection of alveolar pressure more than left atrial pressure. In this situation, the wedge pressure should be measured at the end of expiration, when the alveolar pressure is normally zero.

3. *Wedged Blood PO_2*

As many as 50% of the non-pulsatile pressures produced by balloon inflation are damped pulmonary artery pressures and not true wedge (i.e., venous) pressures (10). Aspiration of blood from the catheter tip during balloon inflation can help to identify a true wedge pressure.

a. A true wedge pressure will have a "wedged blood" PO_2 that is at least 20 mm Hg higher than the arterial PO_2 (10). This indicates that the blood sampled is from the pulmonary capillaries.

D. Wedge vs. Capillary Hydrostatic Pressure

1. The pressure at the tip of the PA catheter measured during balloon inflation is often used as a measure of the hydrostatic pressure in the pulmonary capillaries. The problem here is that the wedge pressure is measured in the absence of flow. *When the balloon is deflated and blood flow resumes, the pressure at the tip of the PA catheter (the capillary hydrostatic pressure) will increase relative to the left-atrial (wedge) pressure* (this is the pressure gradient that drives blood flow from the pulmonary capillaries to the

left atrium) (11). This is expressed below using Equation 8.1 and substituting the pulmonary capillary wedge pressure (PCWP) for the left atrial pressure (P_{LA}).

$$P_c - PCWP = Q \times R_v \qquad (8.2)$$

$$\text{If:} \quad Q \times R_v > 0$$
$$\text{Then:} \quad P_c - PCWP > 0$$
$$\text{And:} \quad P_c > PCWP$$

2. The discrepancy between the capillary hydrostatic pressure and the wedge pressure is partly determined by the resistance to flow in the pulmonary veins. This may be exaggerated in critically ill patients because conditions that promote venoconstriction (e.g., hypoxia, endotoxemia, ARDS) are common in these patients (12). Therefore, the capillary hydrostatic pressure may be significantly higher than the wedge pressure in critically ill patients.

3. Because the capillary hydrostatic pressure is higher than the wedge pressure, *a normal wedge pressure does not exclude the diagnosis of cardiogenic pulmonary edema.*

III. RELIABILITY

A. Pressure vs. Volume

1. According to the *Frank Starling Law of the Heart,* the volume in the ventricles at the end of diastole is the principal factor that governs the strength of cardiac contraction (13). Therefore, the important measure of cardiac filling is ventricular end-diastolic volume.

2. End-diastolic volume is not easy to measure, so the ventricular end-diastolic pressure (as measured by the CVP

and wedge pressure) is used as the clinical measure of cardiac filling.

3. Unfortunately, the CVP and wedge pressures show an inconsistent relationship to the end-diastolic volume (14,15), as demonstrated in Figure 8.4. Note that only half of the wedge pressure measurements are within the normal range (the shaded area) even though the study included only healthy subjects.

4. Observations like those in Figure 8.4 indicate that *isolated measurements of cardiac filling pressures are unreliable as measures of cardiac filling.* Trends in cardiac filling pressures may be more reliable than single measurements.

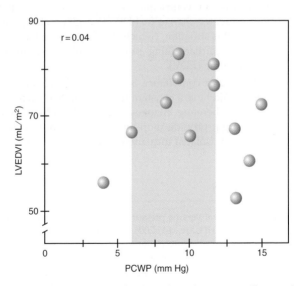

FIGURE 8.4 The relationship between the pulmonary capillary wedge pressure (PCWP) and the left-ventricular end-diastolic volume index (LVEDVI) in 12 normal subjects. The shaded area represents the normal range for PCWP, and the r value is the correlation coefficient. From Reference 15.

B. Ventricular Compliance

1. Cardiac filling pressures are determined not only by end-diastolic volume, but also by the distensibility (compliance) of the ventricles. Therefore, the poor correlation between the cardiac filling pressures and end-diastolic volume may be due to variations in ventricular compliance.

2. Ventricular compliance describes the relationship between changes in end-diastolic volume (EDV) and end-diastolic pressure (EDP):

$$\textbf{Compliance} = \Delta\ \textbf{EDV}\ /\ \Delta\ \textbf{EDP} \qquad (8.3)$$

   a. A decrease in ventricular compliance is associated with a greater change in EDP for a given change in EDV. In this situation, (which may be common in ICU patients), cardiac filling pressures will overestimate cardiac filling (EDV).

   b. If ventricular compliance is constant, changes in the EDP should have a constant relationship to changes in the EDV. Therefore, changes in the cardiac filling pressures might provide more information about cardiac filling than isolated measurements.

REFERENCES

1. Magder S. Central venous pressure: A useful but not so simple measurement. Crit Care Med 2006; 34:2224-2227.
2. Pinsky MR. Hemodynamic monitoring in the intensive care unit. Clin Chest Med 2003; 24:549-560.
3. O'Quin R, Marini JJ. Pulmonary artery occlusion pressure: clinical physiology, measurement, and interpretation. Am Rev Respir Dis 1983; 128:319–326.
4. Pinsky M, Vincent J-L, De Smet J-M. Estimating left ventricular filling pressure during positive end-expiratory pressure in humans. Am Rev Respir Dis 1991; 143:25–31.

5. Teboul J-L, Pinsky MR, Mercat A, et al. Estimating cardiac filling pressure in mechanically ventilated patients with hyperinflation. Crit Care Med 2000; 28:3631-3636.

6. Nemens EJ, Woods SL. Normal fluctuations in pulmonary artery and pulmonary capillary wedge pressures in acutely ill patients. Heart Lung 1982; 11:393–398.

7. Jacka MJ, Cohen MM, To T, et al. Pulmonary artery occlusion pressure estimation: How confident are anesthesiologists. Crit Care Med 2002; 30:1197-1203.

8. Nadeau S, Noble WH. Misinterpretation of pressure measurements from the pulmonary artery catheter. Can Anesth Soc J 1986; 33:352–363.

9. Komandina KH, Schenk DA, LaVeau P, et al. Interobserver variability in the interpretation of pulmonary artery catheter pressure tracings. Chest 1991; 100:1647–1654.

10. Morris AH, Chapman RH. Wedge pressure confirmation by aspiration of pulmonary capillary blood. Crit Care Med 1985; 13:756–759.

11. Cope DK, Grimbert F, Downey JM, et al. Pulmonary capillary pressure: a review. Crit Care Med 1992; 20:1043–1056.

12. Kloess T, Birkenhauer U, Kottler B. Pulmonary pressure–flow relationship and peripheral oxygen supply in ARDS due to bacterial sepsis. Second Vienna Shock Forum, 1989:175–180.

13. Opie LH. Mechanisms of cardiac contraction and relaxation. In Braunwald E, Zipes DP, Libby P (eds). Heart disease: A textbook of cardiovascular medicine. 6th ed., Philadelphia: W.B. Saunders, 2001:443-478.

14. Diebel LN, Wilson RF, Tagett MG, Kline RA. End-diastolic volume. A better indicator of preload in the critically ill. Arch Surg 1992; 127:817–822.

15. Kumar A, Anel R, Bunnell E, et al. Pulmonary artery occlusion pressure and central venous pressure fail to predict ventricular filling volume, cardiac performance, or the response to volume infusion in normal subjects. Crit Care Med 2004; 32:691-699.

Chapter 9

SYSTEMIC OXYGENATION

One of the seminal goals of patient care in the ICU is to maintain adequate tissue oxygenation. This chapter describes the parameters used to monitor systemic oxygen transport and how they are used to evaluate tissue oxygenation.

I. SYSTEMIC OXYGEN TRANSPORT

There are four parameters used to evaluate systemic O_2 transport: the concentration of O_2 in blood, the rate of O_2 transport in arterial blood, the rate of O_2 uptake into tissues, and the extent of hemoglobin desaturation in capillary blood.

A. Oxygen Content of Blood

The concentration of O_2 in blood (called the O_2 content) is the summed contribution of the O_2 that is bound to hemoglobin and the O_2 that is dissolved in plasma.

1. *Hemoglobin-Bound O_2*

$$HbO_2 = 1.34 \times Hb \times SO_2 \qquad (9.1)$$

   a. HbO_2 is the concentration of hemoglobin-bound O_2 (mL O_2 per 100 mL whole blood).
   b. Hb is the hemoglobin concentration in blood (grams per 100 mL blood).

    c. 1.34 is the O_2 binding capacity of hemoglobin (1.34 mL O_2 per gram Hb).

    d. SO_2 is the O_2 saturation of hemoglobin, which is expressed as the ratio of oxygenated Hb to total Hb ($SO_2 = HbO_2$/total Hb). SO_2 should be expressed as a decimal rather than a percentage (e.g., 0.9 instead of 90%).

Equation 9.1 states that, when Hb is fully saturated with oxygen ($SO_2 = 1$), each gram of Hb binds 1.34 mL O_2.

2. *Dissolved O_2* (mL O_2/100 mL blood)

$$\textbf{Dissolved O}_2 = \textbf{0.003} \times \textbf{PO}_2 \qquad (9.2)$$

    a. PO_2 is the partial pressure of O_2 in blood (mm Hg).

    b. 0.003 is the solubility coefficient of O_2 in plasma at normal body temperature This number represents the volume of oxygen (mL) that will dissolve in 100 mL plasma for each 1 mm Hg increment in the PO_2 (mL O_2/100 mL blood/mm Hg).

Equation 9.2 demonstrates that *oxygen is relatively insoluble in plasma*. For example, if the arterial PO_2 of blood is 100 mm Hg, each 100 mL of blood contains only 0.3 mL of dissolved O_2 (or one liter of blood will contain only 3 mL of dissolved O_2).

3. *Total O_2 Content* (mL O_2/100 mL blood)

$$\textbf{O}_2 \textbf{ Content} = \textbf{(1.34} \times \textbf{Hb} \times \textbf{SO}_2\textbf{)} + \textbf{(0.003} \times \textbf{PO}_2\textbf{)} \qquad (9.3)$$

Table 9.1 shows the normal concentrations of O_2 (bound, dissolved, and total O_2) in arterial and venous blood. Note that the contribution of dissolved O_2 is very small. Because dissolved O_2 is such a small fraction of total O_2 in blood, the *O_2 content of blood is considered equivalent to the Hb-bound fraction*.

$$\textbf{O}_2 \textbf{ Content} = \textbf{1.34} \times \textbf{Hb} \times \textbf{SO}_2 \qquad (9.4)$$

TABLE 9.1 Normal Levels of Oxygen in Arterial and Venous Blood[1]

Parameter	Arterial Blood	Venous Blood
PO_2	90 mm Hg	40 mm Hg
O_2 Saturation of Hb	0.98	0.73
HbO_2	19.7 mL/dL	14.7 mL/dL
Dissolved O_2	0.3 mL/dL	0.1 mL/L
Total O_2 content	20 mL/dL	14.8 mL/dL
Blood volume[2]	1.25 L	3.75 L
Volume of O_2	250 mL	555 mL

[1]Values shown are for a body temperature of 37°C and a hemoglobin concentration of 15 g/dL (150 g/L) in blood.

[2]Volume estimates are based on a total blood volume (TBV) of 5 liters, an arterial blood volume that is 25% of TBV, and a venous blood volume that is 75% of TBV.

Abbreviations: Hb = hemoglobin, HbO_2 = hemoglobin-bound O_2, PO_2 = partial pressure of O_2, dL = deciliter (100 mL).

B. Oxygen Delivery (DO_2)

The rate of O_2 transport in arterial blood is known as O_2 *delivery* (DO_2).

$$DO_2 = Q \times CaO_2 \times 10 \qquad (9.5)$$

a. DO_2 is the delivery rate of O_2 in arterial blood (mL/min).

b. Q is cardiac output (L/min).

c. CaO_2 is the O_2 content of arterial blood (mL/100mL).

d. The multiplier of 10 is used to convert the CaO_2 from mL/100 mL to mL/L, which allows the DO_2 to be expressed as mL/min.

If the CaO_2 is broken down into its components (1.34 x Hb x SaO_2), where SaO_2 is the oxyhemoglobin saturation in arterial blood, the DO_2 equation can be rewritten as:

$$DO_2 = Q \times (1.34 \times Hb \times SaO_2) \times 10 \qquad (9.6)$$

Table 9.2 shows the normal range of DO_2 in adults. The size-adjusted values are determined using the body surface area in meters squared, as described in Chapter 7 (see Equation 7.1).

TABLE 9.2 Normal Ranges for Oxygen Transport Parameters

Parameter	Absolute Range	Size-Adjusted Range[1]
Cardiac Output	5–6 L/min	2.4–4.0 L/min/m²
O_2 Delivery	900–1100 mL/min	520–570 mL/min/m²
O_2 Uptake	200–270 mL/min	110–160 mL/min/m²
O_2 Extraction Ratio	0.20–0.30	

[1]Size-adjusted values represent the absolute values divided by the patient's body surface area (BSA) in square meters (m²).

C. Oxygen Uptake (VO_2)

The rate at which O_2 moves out of the capillaries and into the tissues is called the O_2 *uptake* (VO_2). Because O_2 is not stored in tissues in significant quantities, the VO_2 is also a measure of the O_2 *consumption* of the tissues. The VO_2 can be calculated or measured directly.

1. *Calculated VO_2*

The uptake of any substance into a tissue bed is a reflection of 2 variables: the rate of blood flow through the tissue bed, and the decrease in concentration of the substance from arterial to venous blood. When O_2 is the substance, this relationship can be stated as follows:

$$VO_2 = Q \times (CaO_2 - CvO_2) \times 10 \qquad (9.7)$$

a. VO_2 is the rate of O_2 uptake into tissues (mL/min).

b. Q is the cardiac output (L/min).

c. $CaO_2 - CvO_2$ is the difference in oxygen content between arterial and venous blood.

d. The multiplier of 10 is needed for the same reason as explained for the DO_2.

CaO_2 and CvO_2 share a common term (1.34 x Hb), so Equation 9.7 can be rewritten as:

$$VO_2 = Q \times (1.34 \times Hb) \times (SaO_2 - SvO_2) \times 10 \qquad (9.8)$$

where $SaO_2 - SvO_2$ is the difference in oxyhemoglobin saturation between arterial and mixed venous (pulmonary artery) blood. The determinants of VO_2 in this equation are all measurable quantities (a pulmonary artery catheter is needed to measure cardiac output and SvO_2, as described in Chapter 7).

2. *Measured VO_2*

   The VO_2 can be measured as the rate of O_2 uptake from the lungs.

$$VO_2 = V_E \times (FiO_2 - FeO_2) \qquad (9.9)$$

a. VO_2 is the rate of O_2 uptake from the lungs (mL/min).

b. V_E is the volume of gas that is exhaled per minute (L/min).

c. FiO_2 and FeO_2 represent the fractional concentration of O_2 in inhaled and exhaled gas, respectively.

The VO_2 can be measured at the bedside with a specialized device that is equipped with an oxygen sensor.

3. *Calculated vs. Measured VO_2*

   The measured VO_2 is superior to the calculated VO_2 for the following reasons:

   a. The calculated VO_2 has a greater variability because it involves four measurements (Q, Hb, SaO_2, SvO_2), and each of these measurements has its own variability (see Table 9.3) (1–4).

b. The calculated VO_2 is less accurate as a measure of whole-body VO_2 because it does not include the VO_2 of the lungs. Although the lungs normally contribute only 5% or less to the whole-body VO_2, this contribution can increase to 20% or more when there is inflammation in the lungs (e.g., pneumonia or ARDS). (5).

The normal VO_2 in a resting adult is shown in Table 9.2. Note that the VO_2 is only a small fraction of the DO_2. This is explained in the next section.

TABLE 9.3 Variability of Calculated and Measured VO_2

Parameter	Variability
Thermodilution Cardiac Output	± 10%
Hemoglobin Concentration	± 2%
Arterial O_2 Saturation (SaO_2)	± 2%
Mixed Venous O_2 Saturation (SvO_2)	± 5%
Calculated VO_2	± 19%
Measured VO_2	± 5%

From References 1–4.

D. Oxygen Extraction

The ratio of O_2 uptake to O_2 delivery is called the *oxygen extraction ratio* (O_2ER).

$$O_2ER = VO_2 / DO_2 \qquad (9.10)$$

(This ratio can be multiplied by 100 and expressed as a percentage.) Since the VO_2 and DO_2 share common terms ($Q \times 1.34 \times Hb \times 10$), Equation 9.10 can be expressed as follows:

$$O_2ER = (SaO_2 - SvO_2) / SaO_2 \qquad (9.11)$$

When the SaO_2 is close to 1.0 (which is usually the case), the O_2ER is roughly equivalent to $SaO_2 - SvO_2$:

$$O_2ER \approx SaO_2 - SvO_2 \qquad (9.12)$$

The O_2ER is normally about 0.25 (range = 0.2 – 0.3), as shown in Table 9.2. This means that *only 25% of the oxygen delivered to the systemic capillaries is taken up into the tissues.* Although O_2 extraction is normally low, it can increase when O_2 delivery is impaired, as explained in the next section.

II. CONTROL OF OXYGEN UPTAKE

A. The Role of O_2 Extraction

The oxygen transport system operates to maintain a constant flow of oxygen into the tissues (a constant VO_2) in the face of changes in oxygen supply (varying DO_2). This behavior is made possible by the ability of O_2 extraction to adjust to changes in O_2 delivery (6). The control system for VO_2 can be described by rearranging Equation 9.10 to make VO_2 the dependent variable:

$$VO_2 = DO_2 \times O_2ER \qquad (9.13)$$

Thus, the VO_2 will remain constant if changes in O_2 delivery are accompanied by equivalent and reciprocal changes in O_2 extraction. However, if the O_2 extraction remains fixed, changes in DO_2 will be accompanied by equivalent changes in VO_2. The ability of O_2 extraction to adjust to changes in DO_2 therefore determines the tendency of VO_2 to remain constant in the face of changes in DO_2.

A. The $DO_2 - VO_2$ Relationship

The response to a progressive decrease in O_2 delivery is illustrated in the graph in Figure 9.1 (The equation at the top of the figure is similar to Equation 9.13, but the $SaO_2 - SvO_2$ difference is used as the O_2ER.) At the point indicating a normal DO_2, the arterial O_2 saturation (SaO_2) is 98%, the mixed venous O_2 saturation (SvO_2) is 73%, and the O_2 extraction ($SaO_2 - SvO_2$) is 25%. As the DO_2 decreases (moving left along the horizontal axis of the graph), the VO_2 remains constant until a point is reached where the SvO_2 has decreased to 50% and the corresponding O_2 extraction ($SaO_2 - SvO_2$) has increased to 48%. This is the maximum O_2 extraction that can be achieved in response to decreases in O_2 delivery. When O_2 extraction is maximal, further decreases in DO_2 will result in equivalent decreases in VO_2. When this occurs, the VO_2 is referred to as being *supply-dependent*, which means that the rate of aerobic metabolism is limited by the supply of oxygen. This condition is known as *dysoxia*, and it is accompanied by lactate accumulation (from anaerobic glycolysis) and impaired cell function.

1. ***Critical DO_2***

   The DO_2 at which the VO_2 becomes supply-dependent is called the *critical oxygen delivery* (critical DO_2). It is the lowest DO_2 that is capable of fully supporting aerobic metabolism. Although important conceptually, the critical DO_2 has little clinical value for the following reasons:

   a. The critical DO_2 has varied widely in studies of critically ill patients (6–8), and thus it is not possible to predict the critical DO_2 in any individual patient.

   b. The $DO_2 - VO_2$ curve does not always have a distinct point that marks the transition to a supply-dependent VO_2 (9).

   Although it is not possible to identify the critical DO_2 in each patient, you can avoid the critical DO_2 in most patients by maintaining the DO_2 at a rate that is at least four times higher than the VO_2.

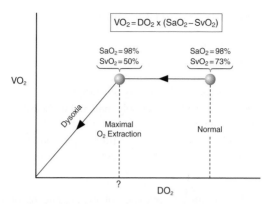

FIGURE 9.1. Graph showing the effects of a progressive decrease in systemic O_2 delivery (DO_2) on whole-body O_2 uptake (VO_2), and the O_2 saturation of hemoglobin in arterial blood (SaO_2) and mixed venous blood (SvO_2).

III. TISSUE OXYGENATION

It is not possible to measure tissue PO_2 directly. Instead, the oxygen transport variables and blood lactate levels are used to evaluate tissue oxygenation. Table 9.4 shows the markers of threatened or impaired tissue oxygenation.

TABLE 9.4 Clinical Markers of Threatened or Impaired Tissue Oxygenation

I. Oxygen Transport Variables
  1. VO_2 < 100 mL/min/m^2 (when not due to hypometabolism).
  2. (SaO_2 – SvO_2) ≥ 50%
  3. SvO_2 ≤ 50%

II. Lactate Concentration in Blood
  1. > 2 mEq/L is abnormal.
  2. > 4 mEq/L has prognostic implications.

A. Oxygen Transport Parameters

1. *Oxygen Uptake (VO_2)*

   a. The adequacy of tissue oxygenation is determined by the balance between the metabolic requirement for O_2 (MRO_2) and the tissue oxygen supply (VO_2).

   b. Normally, the VO_2 is closely matched to the MRO_2, and aerobic metabolism continues unimpeded.

   c. If the VO_2 falls below the MRO_2, a portion of metabolism will be carried out anaerobically. Therefore, an abnormally low VO_2 (< 100 mL/min/m²), in the absence of hypometabolism (which is not common in ICU patients), is evidence of inadequate tissue oxygenation.

2. *Oxygen Extraction ($SaO_2 - SvO_2$)*

   a. The graph in Figure 9.1 shows that in conditions where oxygen delivery is reduced (e.g., anemia, hypoxemia, or low cardiac output), an increase in O_2 extraction to 50% is the maximum adjustment possible to maintain tissue oxygenation.

   b. Therefore, an O_2 extraction ($SaO_2 - SvO_2$) that is at or near 50% indicates that tissue oxygenation is either impaired or is on the verge of impairment.

   c. Consistent with this reasoning, an O_2 extraction of 50% has been suggested as a "transfusion trigger" to prompt the transfusion of erythrocytes to correct anemia (10).

3. *Venous O_2 Saturation (SvO_2)*

   a. As mentioned earlier, the SvO_2 can be used as a surrogate measure of O_2 extraction if the SaO_2 is close to 100%.

   b. According to the graph in Figure 9.1, a decrease in SvO_2 to 50% occurs when O_2 extraction is maximal.

   c. Therefore, an SvO_2 of 50% can be used as a surrogate marker of maximum O_2 extraction.

d. The SvO_2 is traditionally measured in "mixed venous" (pulmonary artery) blood, but superior vena cava blood (from a central venous catheter) can be a suitable alternative (10). However, multiple measurements of the central venous SvO_2 must be averaged to gain close agreement with the SvO_2 in mixed venous blood (11).

B. Blood Lactate

The accumulation of lactate in blood is the most widely used marker of inadequate tissue oxygenation. Lactate can be measured in whole blood or plasma (12), and concentrations above 2 mEq/L are considered abnormal. Increasing the threshold to 4 mEq/L may be more appropriate for predicting survival (12).

1. *Other Sources of Lactate*

   a. Unfortunately, lactate accumulation in blood is not specific for impaired tissue oxygenation.
   b. Other sources of hyperlactatemia in ICU patients include hepatic insufficiency (which impairs lactate clearance), thiamine deficiency (which inhibits pyruvate entry into mitochondria), severe sepsis (same mechanism as thiamine deficiency), and intracellular alkalosis (which stimulates glycolysis) (13,14).

2. *Severe Sepsis*

   a. The predominant cause of lactate accumulation in severe sepsis appears to be cytokine-mediated inhibition of pyruvate dehydrogenase, an enzyme involved in pyruvate transport into mitochondria (15). The result is pyruvate accumulation in the cell cytoplasm and subsequent conversion to lactate.
   b. The absence of anaerobic conditions in sepsis is supported by a study showing that PO_2 levels in muscle are *elevated* in patients with severe sepsis (16).
   c. Thus, elevation of blood lactate does not appear to be

a useful marker of impaired tissue oxygenation in severe sepsis.

d. There is a strong correlation between hyperlactatemia and mortality in severe sepsis (12,17), particularly when 4 mEq/L is used as the threshold for lactate elevation (12). Therefore, elevated blood lactate levels have prognostic implications in severe sepsis.

See Chapter 23 for more information on lactate accumulation in blood.

REFERENCES

1. Sasse SA, Chen PA, Berry RB, et al. Variability of cardiac output over time in medical intensive care unit patients. Chest 1994; 22:225-232.

2. Noll ML, Fountain RL, Duncan CA, et al. Fluctuations in mixed venous oxygen saturation in critically ill medical patients: a pilot study. Am J Crit Care 1992; 3:102-106.

3. Bartlett RH, Dechert RE. Oxygen kinetics: Pitfalls in clinical research. J Crit Care 1990; 5:77-80.

4. Schneeweiss B, Druml W, Graninger W, et al. Assessment of oxygen-consumption by use of reverse Fick-principle and indirect calorimetry in critically ill patients. Clin Nutr 1989; 8:89–93.

5. Jolliet P, Thorens JB, Nicod L, et al. Relationship between pulmonary oxygen consumption, lung inflammation, and calculated venous admixture in patients with acute lung injury. Intensive Care Med 1996; 22:277-285.

6. Leach RM, Treacher DF. The relationship between oxygen delivery and consumption. Dis Mon 1994; 30:301-368.

7. Shoemaker WC. Oxygen transport and oxygen metabolism in shock and critical illness. Crit Care Clin 1996; 12:939-969.

8. Ronco J, Fenwick J, Tweedale M, et al. Identification of the critical oxygen delivery for anaerobic metabolism in critically ill septic and nonseptic humans. JAMA 1993; 270:1724-1730.

9. Lebarsky DA, Smith LR, Sladen RN, et al. Defining the relationship of oxygen delivery and consumption: use of biological system models. J Surg Res 1995; 58:503-508.

10. Levy PS, Chavez RP, Crystal GJ, et al. Oxygen extraction ratio: a valid indicator of transfusion need in limited coronary vascular reserve? J Trauma 1992; 32:769–774.

11. Dueck MH, Kilmek M, Appenrodt S, et al. Trends but not individual values of central venous oxygen saturation agree with mixed venous oxygen saturation during varying hemodynamic conditions. Anesthesiology 2005; 103:249-257.

12. Aduen J, Bernstein WK, Khastgir T, et al. The use and clinical importance of a substrate-specific electrode for rapid determination of blood lactate concentrations. JAMA 1994; 272:1678–1685.

13. Duke T. Dysoxia and lactate. Arch Dis Child 1999; 81:343-350.

14. Mizock BA, Falk JL. Lactic acidosis in critical illness. Crit Care Med 1992; 20:80–93.

15. Curtis SE, Cain SM. Regional and systemic oxygen delivery/uptake relations and lactate flux in hyperdynamic, endotoxin-treated dogs. Am Rev Respir Dis 1992; 145:348–354.

16. Sair M, Etherington PJ, Winlove CP, et al. Tissue oxygenation and perfusion in patients with systemic sepsis. Crit Care Med 2001; 29:1343.

17. Bakker J, Coffernils M, Leon M, et al. Blood lactate levels are superior to oxygen-derived variables in predicting outcome in septic shock. Chest 1991; 99:956–962.

Chapter 10

HEMORRHAGE AND HYPOVOLEMIA

The circulatory system operates with a relatively small volume and a volume-sensitive pump. This is an energy efficient design, but it suffers from a limited tolerance to acute blood loss. Loss of less than 50% of the blood volume can be fatal, whereas major organs like the lungs, liver, and kidneys can lose as much as 75% of their functional mass without a fatal outcome. Because of the limited tolerance to blood loss, successful management of the bleeding patient requires prompt intervention to halt bleeding and replace volume deficits.

I. BODY FLUIDS AND BLOOD LOSS

A. Distribution of Body Fluids

Table 10.1 shows the volume of body fluids for adult men and women expressed in relation to lean body weight in kilograms. Note the following:

1. Total body water in liters is equivalent to 60% of the lean body weight (600 mL/kg) in males, and 50% of the lean body weight (500 mL/kg) in females.

2. Blood volume (66 mL/kg in males, and 60 mL/kg in females) is only a small fraction (11 to 12%) of the total body water. The meager distribution of body fluids in the vascular compartment is an important factor in the limited tolerance to blood loss.

3. Plasma volume represents about about one quarter of the volume of extracellular fluid (interstitial fluid plus plasma). This relationship is important for understanding the effects of colloid and crystalloid resuscitation fluids (described later in the chapter).

TABLE 10.1 Body Fluid Volumes in Adult Men & Women

Fluid	Men		Women	
	mL/kg	75 kg†	mL/kg	60 kg†
Total Body Water	600	45 L	500	30 L
Interstitial Fluid	120	9 L	100	6 L
Whole Blood	66	5 L	60	3.6 L
Plasma	40	3 L	36	2.2 L

All weights are lean body weight.

†Average body weight (lean) for an adult male and female.

From American Association of Blood Banks Technical Manual. 10th ed. Arlington, VA, American Association of Blood Banks, 1990: 650.

B. Severity of Blood Loss

The following classification system is based the severity of acute blood loss (1).

1. *Class I*
   a. Loss of 15% or less of the blood volume (or ≤10 mL/kg).
   b. The volume loss in this instance is fully replaced by interstitial fluid shifts (transcapillary refill) so that blood volume is maintained, and clinical findings are minimal or absent.

2. *Class II*
   a. Loss of 15–30% of the blood volume (or 10–20 mL/kg).
   b. This represents the compensated phase of hypovo-

lemia. Blood volume is reduced, but blood pressure is maintained by systemic vasoconstriction. Postural changes in pulse and blood pressure may be evident, but not consistently (see later). Urine output can fall to 20 or 30 mL/hr, and splanchnic flow may be compromised.

3. *Class III*

   a. Loss of 30–45% of the blood volume (or 20–30 mL/kg).

   b. This marks the onset of decompensated hypovolemia or *hypovolemic shock*, with hypotension, oliguria (urine output <15 mL/hr), depressed mentation, and lactate accumulation in the blood (>2 mEq/L).

4. *Class IV*

   a. Loss of more than 45% of the blood volume (or >30 mL/kg).

   b. This condition can be irreversible and fatal. Hypotension and oliguria can be profound (e.g., urine output <5 mL/hr) and refractory to volume replacement. Blood lactate levels are typically greater than 4 to 6 mEq/L.

   This classification system can be used to determine the replacement volume in individual patients with acute blood loss (see later).

II. CLINICAL EVALUATION

The clinical evaluation of acute blood loss is limited in accuracy, as described next.

A. Vital Signs

The sensitivity of vital signs for detecting blood loss is poor, as shown in Table 10.2 (2).

1. Contrary to popular belief, supine tachycardia (>90 bpm) is absent in a majority of patients with acute blood loss, regardless of severity.

2. Supine hypotension (systolic pressure <90 mm Hg) appears only in advanced stages of blood loss, when volume deficits exceed 30% of blood volume (about 1.5 liters or more in an average-sized adult).

3. *Postural Changes*

   a. To record postural changes in pulse and blood pressure, the position should change from supine to standing (not sitting), and at least one minute should elapse before measurements are obtained (2).

   b. A significant postural change is defined as an increase in pulse rate of at least 30 bpm or a decrease in systolic pressure of at least 20 mm Hg (2).

   c. The most sensitive test is the postural pulse increment, which can become evident after 15–20% loss of blood volume (about 750–1,000 mL in an average-sized adult).

   d. In general, orthostatic vital signs add little to the evaluation of hypovolemia.

B. Hemoglobin and Hematocrit

1. Acute hemorrhage involves loss of whole blood, which is not expected to alter the blood hemoglobin concentration or hematocrit. This explains why there is a poor correlation between blood volume deficits and hemoglobin or hematocrit in acute hemorrhage (3).

2. A drop in hemoglobin and hematocrit in the early hours after acute hemorrhage is a reflection of volume resuscitation with crystalloid or colloid fluids, (which expands the plasma volume and causes a dilutional decrease in the hemoglobin and hematocrit) (4).

3. For the reasons stated above, the hemoglobin and hematocrit should NEVER be used to evaluate acute blood loss.

TABLE 10.2 Sensitivity of Vital Signs in Detecting Acute Blood Loss

	Reported Sensitivities[†]	
	Moderate Loss (450 – 630 mL)	**Severe Loss (630 – 1150 mL)**
Supine Tachycardia	0 – 42%	5 – 24%
Supine Hypotension	0 – 50%	21 – 47%
Postural Pulse Increment[a]	6 – 48%	91 – 100%
Postural Hypotension[b]		
Age <65 yrs	6 – 12%	——
Age ≥65 yrs	14 – 40%	——

[a]Increase in pulse rate ≥30 beats/min on standing.
[b]Decrease in systolic pressure >20 mm Hg on standing.
[†]Combined results of 9 clinical studies. From Reference 2.

C. Invasive Hemodynamics

1. *Cardiac Filling Pressures*

   a. Cardiac filling pressures show a poor correlation with ventricular end-diastolic volume (see Chapter 8, Figure 8.4), and they do not predict responsiveness to volume infusion (5).

   b. Hypovolemia is associated with a decrease in ventricular distensibility (compliance) (6), which means that cardiac filling pressures will overestimate the intravascular volume in hypovolemic patients.

   c. *Changes* in cardiac filling pressures in response to volume infusion are considered more meaningful than single measurements. It is believed that rapid infusion of 500 mL isotonic saline will not raise the cardiac filling pressures more than 2 mm Hg in hypovolemic patients (7), but the validity of this belief is unproven.

2. *Systemic Oxygen Transport*

(See Chapter 9 for a description of the O_2 transport parameters). Hypovolemia is accompanied by a decreased cardiac output and an associated decrease in systemic O_2 delivery (DO_2). The effect of this decline in DO_2 on the systemic O_2 uptake (VO_2) can help to distinguish compensated hypovolemia from hypovolemic shock.

a. In compensated hypovolemia, the VO_2 will remain normal ($110-160$ mL/min/m^2) because O_2 extraction has increased to compensate for the decrease in DO_2.

b. In hypovolemic shock, the VO_2 falls below normal (<100 mL/min/m^2) because O_2 extraction has reached its maximum level (approximately 50%) and cannot increase further in response to the declining DO_2. These DO_2-VO_2 relationships are demonstrated in Figure 9.1.

D. Acid-Base Parameters

The arterial base deficit and blood lactate level can provide information about the effects of hypovolemia on tissue oxygenation.

1. *Arterial Base Deficit*

a. The base deficit is the amount (in millimoles) of base needed to titrate one liter of whole blood to a pH of 7.40 (at a temperature of 37°C and a PCO_2 of 40 mm Hg). Because base deficit is measured when the PCO_2 is normal, it is a measure of non-respiratory acid-base disturbances. In the hypovolemic patient, an elevated base deficit is a marker of global tissue acidosis from impaired oxygenation (8).

b. Most blood gas analyzers detemine the base deficit routinely (using a PCO_2/HCO_3 nomogram), and the results are included in the blood gas report. The base deficit can also be calculated using Equation 10.1 (9), where BD is base deficit in mmol/L, Hb is the hemoglobin concentration in blood, and HCO_3 is the serum bicarbonate concentration.

$$\textbf{BD} = [(1 - 0.014\ \textbf{Hb}) \times \textbf{HCO}_3] - 24$$
$$+ [(9.5 + 1.63\ \textbf{Hb}) \times (\textbf{pH} - 7.4)] \qquad (10.1)$$

c. The normal range for base deficit is +2 to -2 mmol/L. Increases in base deficit are classified as mild (-2 to -5 mmol/L), moderate (-6 to -14 mmol/L), and severe ($\geq$ -15 mmol/L).

d. In the bleeding patient, there is a direct correlation between the magnitude of increase in base deficit and the extent of blood loss (10). Correction of the base deficit within hours after volume resuscitation is associated with a favorable outcome, while persistent elevations in base deficit can be a sign of impending multiorgan failure (10).

2. *Blood Lactate*

a. As described in Chapter 9, hyperlactatemia (blood lactate > 2 mEq/L) can be a sign of a global shift to anaerobic metabolism.

b. When compared with the base deficit, elevations in blood lactate show a closer correlation with both the magnitude of blood loss (11), and the likelihood of a fatal outcome (11,12).

III. VOLUME INFUSION

The mortality in hypovolemic shock is directly related to the magnitude and duration of hypoperfusion of the vital organs (1). This means that the rate of volume replacement can have an impact on outcome in hypovolemic shock. This section describes the factors that influence the infusion rate of resuscitation fluids.

A. Catheter Size

1. There is a tendency to cannulate the large central veins to achieve more rapid infusion rates. However, *the rate of volume infusion is determined by the dimensions of the vascular catheter, not the size of the vein.*

2. The influence of catheter size on infusion rate is defined by the Hagen-Poisseuille equation, which is described in Chapter 4 (see Equation 4.1) and is shown below.

$$\mathbf{Q} = \Delta \mathbf{P} \ (\pi \mathbf{r}^4 / 8 \mu \mathbf{L}) \tag{10.2}$$

According to this equation, steady flow (Q) through a catheter is directly related to the driving pressure (ΔP) for flow and the fourth power of the radius (r) of the catheter, and is inversely related to the length (L) of the catheter and the viscosity (μ) of the infusate.

3. Equation 10.2 predicts that flow through central venous catheters (which are at 6–8 inches in length) will be much slower than flow through peripheral vein catheters (which are 2 inches in length) if the diameter of the infusion channels is equivalent.

4. The influence of catheter length on infusion rate is demonstrated in Figure 10.1 (13). Using catheters of equal diameter (16 gauge), flow in the 2-inch catheter is about 50% higher than flow in the 5.5-inch catheter, and is more than twice the flow rate in the 12-inch catheter. Therefore, *for rapid volume resuscitation, cannulation of peripheral veins with short catheters is preferred to cannulation of large central veins with long catheters.*

5. *Introducer Catheters*

Volume resuscitation of trauma victims may require flow
rates in excess of 5 L/min (14). Because flow increases
with the fourth power of the radius of a catheter, very
rapid flow rates are best achieved with large-bore catheters like the *introducer catheters* described in Chapter 4
(see Figure 4.1). These catheters are normally used as
conduits for pulmonary artery catheters, but they can be
used as stand-alone infusion devices.

a. Gravity-driven flow through introducer catheters can
   reach 15 mL/sec, which is only slightly less than the
   gravity-driven flow rate (18 mL/sec) through standard (3 mm diameter) intravenous tubing (15).
b. The side infusion port on the hub of introducer catheters (see Figure 4.1) has a flow capacity that is only
   25% of the flow capacity of the catheter (15). Therefore, the side port on these catheters should not be
   used for rapid volume infusion.

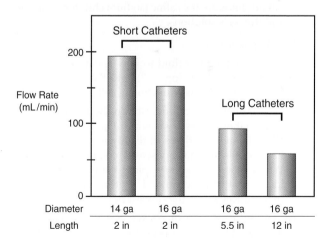

FIGURE 10.1. The influence of catheter size on the gravity-driven flow
rate of water. Catheter dimensions are indicated below the horizontal
axis of the graph. (From Reference 13).

B. Type of Resuscitation Fluid

1. *Types of Fluid*

   There are three types of resuscitation fluid:

   a. Fluids that contain red blood cells; i.e., whole blood and erythrocyte concentrates or "packed cells". Whole blood is rarely available for resuscitation, and packed cells are used to increase the oxygen carrying capacity of blood.

   b. Fluids that contain large molecules with limited movement out of the bloodstream. These are called *colloid* fluids, and they are designed to expand the plasma volume. Common colloid fluids include albumin solutions, hetastarch, and the dextrans.

   c. Fluids that contain electrolytes and other small molecules that move freely out of the bloodstream. These are called *crystalloid* fluids, and they are used to expand the extracellular volume. The most notable crystalloid fluids are the saline (sodium chloride) solutions and Ringer's solutions.

2. *Flow Characteristics*

   a. The tendency for a fluid to flow is determined by its viscosity (see Equation 10.2), and the viscosity of resuscitation fluids is a function of cell density.

   b. The influence of cell density on the infusion rate of resuscitation fluids is shown in Figure 10.2 (16). The albumin solution flows as readily as water because it has no cells and has a viscosity comparable to water. Whole blood flows less rapidly than the cell-free fluids, and the concentrated erythrocyte preparation (packed RBCs) has the slowest flow rate.

   c. The infusion rate of packed RBCs is enhanced by increasing the driving pressure with an inflatable cuff wrapped around the blood bag, and also by adding an equal volume of isotonic saline to reduce the viscosity of the infusate.

IV. RESUSCITATION STRATEGIES

The ultimate goal of volume resuscitation for acute blood loss is to maintain oxygen uptake (VO_2) into tissues and sustain aerobic metabolism. The strategies used to maintain VO_2 are identified by the determinants of VO_2 in Equation 10.3. (This equation is described in detail in Chapter 9.)

$$VO_2 = Q \times Hb \times 1.34 \times (SaO_2 - SvO_2) \times 10 \qquad (10.3)$$

Acute blood loss affects two components of this equation: cardiac output (Q) and hemoglobin concentration in blood (Hb). Therefore, promoting cardiac output and correcting hemoglobin deficits are the two goals of resuscitation for acute blood loss.

A. Promoting Cardiac Output

The consequences of a low cardiac output are far more

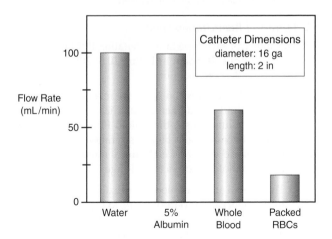

FIGURE 10.2. Comparative infusion rates of erythrocyte-containing and cell-free resuscitation fluids. Catheter size and driving pressure are the same for all infusions. (From Reference 16).

threatening than the consequences of anemia, so t*he first priority in the bleeding patient is to support cardiac output.*

1. *The Trendelenburg Position*

   a. The Trendelenburg position (legs elevated 45° above the horizontal plane and head down 15° below the horizontal plane) is a popular "autotransfusion maneuver" that is believed to promote cardiac output by shifting blood from the legs to more central veins to augment venous return. However, *these presumed effects have not been demonstrated in experimental studies.*

   b. Studies have shown that the Trendelenburg position does not increase central blood volume (17,18), and does not increase cardiac output in hypovolemic patients (19).

   c. Because there is no proof of efficacy, the Trendelenburg position is not advised for the management of hypovolemia. It is axiomatic that *the appropriate treatment of hypovolemia is volume replacement.*

2. *Efficacy of Resuscitation Fluids*

   The ability of each type of resuscitation fluid to augment cardiac output is shown in Figure 10.3 (20). The following results deserve mention:

   a. A colloid fluid (dextran-40) is the most effective resuscitation fluid for augmenting cardiac output. On a volume-to-volume basis, the colloid fluid is about twice as effective as whole blood, six times more effective than packed cells, and eight times more effective than the crystalloid fluid (lactated Ringer's).

   b. The limited ability of blood (particularly packed RBCs) to augment cardiac output is due to the viscosity effects of erythrocytes. Some studies have shown that packed RBCs can actually *decrease* cardiac output (21).

   If augmenting cardiac output is the first priority in acute hemorrhage, the results in Figure 10.3 indicate that *blood is not the fluid of choice for early volume resuscitation in acute blood loss.*

3. *Colloid vs. Crystalloid Resuscitation*

   a. The marked difference in the ability of colloid and crystalloid fluids to augment cardiac output, as demonstrated in Figure 10.3, is due to differences in volume distribution.

   b. Crystalloid fluids are distributed evenly in the extracellular fluid and, because plasma represents only 25% of the extracellular fluid, *only 25% of the infused volume of crystalloid fluids will remain in the vascular space and expand the plasma volume* (22).

   c. Colloid fluids are primarily restricted to the plasma

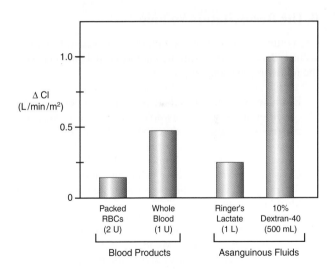

FIGURE 10.3. Graph showing the change in cardiac index (ΔCI) following a one-hour infusion of the specified resuscitation fluids. The volume of whole blood (1 unit = 450 mL) packed RBCs (2 units = 500 mL) and dextran-40 (500 mL) is equivalent, while the volume of Ringers lactate (1 Liter) is twice that of the other fluids. (From Reference 20).

because these fluids contain large molecules that do not readily move into the interstitial fluid. *At least 75% of the infused volume of colloid fluids will remain in the vascular space and expand the plasma volume* in the first few hours after infusion (22).

d. Thus, colloid fluids are more effective for augmenting cardiac output because they are more effective for augmenting plasma volume.

e. Crystalloid fluids can achieve the same augmentation of plasma volume and cardiac output as seen with colloid fluids, but the infusion volume must be at least three times greater than that of colloid fluids.

Colloid and crystalloid resuscitation is described in detail in the next chapter.

B. The Resuscitation Volume

The volume of colloid or crystalloid fluid needed to replace volume deficits can be estimated in individual patients using the following two-step approach.

1. Estimate the volume deficit by matching the patient's condition as closely as possible to one the four stages of progressive blood loss described earlier in the chapter. The corresponding volume deficits are as follows: Class I = 5 mL/kg, Class II = 15 mL/kg, Class III = 25 mL/kg, Class IV = 35 mL/kg (these values are midway between the range of values shown earlier). Remember to use ideal body weight.

2. The resuscitation volume (V_{Infuse}) is then determined as the volume deficit (V_{Lost}) divided by the fraction of the infused volume that is retained in the plasma. The latter variable is the ratio of the increment in plasma volume to the infused volume ($\Delta V_{plasma}/V_{Infuse}$), and can be called the *plasma retention ratio*.

$$V_{Infuse} = V_{Lost} \text{ / Plasma Retention Ratio} \qquad (10.4)$$

For colloid fluids, at least 75% of the infused volume will remain in the plasma, so the plasma retention ratio is ≥ 0.75. For crystalloid fluids, only 25% of the infused volume is retained in plasma, so the plasma retention ratio is 0.25.

3. *Example*

   Assume that an adult male with an ideal body weight of 70 kg presents with acute GI hemorrhage, and the physical exam shows only a postural increase in pulse rate of 35 bpm. The latter finding makes this a Class II hemorrhage with an estimated volume loss of 15 mL/kg, so the volume loss in this patient is 15 x 70 =1,050 mL. If a crystalloid fluid is used for volume resuscitation, the resuscitation volume is 1,050/0.25 =4,200 mL. If a colloid fluid is used, the minimum resuscitation volume is 1,050/0.75 =1,400 mL. Therefore, resuscitation with a crystalloid fluid requires at least 3 times more volume than resuscitation with a colloid fluid.

C. Correcting Anemia

After volume deficits are replaced and cardiac output is restored, attention can be directed to correcting hemoglobin deficits. The use of RBC transfusions to correct anemia is described in Chapter 30.

D. End-Points of Resuscitation

1. *Traditional End-Points*

   a. The traditional end-points of volume resuscitation are normalization of blood pressure and urine output.

   b. As many as 85% of patients with hypovolemic shock will have continued evidence of impaired tissue oxygenation after the blood pressure and urine output return to normal (23).

   c. Therefore, normalization of blood pressure and urine output should not mark the end of resuscitation, but should be followed by an evaluation of systemic oxygenation.

2. *Systemic Oxygenation*

   a. The clinical measures listed below are used as indirect evidence of adequate tissue oxygenation (see Chapter 9), and thus they can also be used as end-points of volume resuscitation in hypovolemic shock.

> Oxygen uptake (VO_2) > 100 mL/min/m^2
> Arterial base deficit > 2 mmol
> Serum lactate < 2 mEq/L

   b. The goal is to reach these end-points within 24 hours of the onset of hypovolemic shock (23). Unfortunately, this is not always possible, and the more prolonged the circulatory shock, the greater the risk of a fatal outcome. In one study of trauma victims (24), there were no mortalities when blood lactate levels returned to normal within 24 hours, but the mortality rate rose to 85% when hyperlactatemia persisted for longer than 48 hours.

REFERENCES

1. Falk JL, O'Brien JF, Kerr R. Fluid resuscitation in traumatic hemorrhagic shock. Crit Care Clin 1992; 8:323-340.
2. McGee S, Abernathy WB, Simel DL. Is this patient hypovolemic. JAMA 1999; 281:1022-1029.
3. Cordts PR, LaMorte WW, Fisher JB, et al. Poor predictive value of hematocrit and hemodynamic parameters for erythrocyte deficits after extensive vascular operations. Surg Gynecol Obstet 1992; 175:243–248.
4. Stamler KD. Effect of crystalloid infusion on hematocrit in nonbleeding patients, with applications to clinical traumatology. Ann Emerg Med 1989; 18:747–749.

5. Kumar A, Anel R, Bunnell E, et al. Pulmonary artery occlusion pressure and central venous pressure fail to predict ventricular filling volumes, cardiac performance, or the response to volume infusion in normal subjects. Crit Care Med 2004; 32:691-699.

6. Walley KR, Cooper DJ. Diastolic stiffness impairs left ventricular function during hypovolemic shock in pigs. Am J Physiol 1991; 260:H702–712.

7. Barbeito A, Mark JB. Arterial and central venous pressure monitoring. Anesthesiol Clin 2006; 24:717-735.

8. Kincaid EH, Miller PR, Meredith JW, et al. Elevated arterial base deficit in trauma patients: a marker of impaired oxygen utilization. J Am Coll Surg 1998; 187:384-392.

9. Landow L. Letter to the editor. J Trauma 1994; 37:870-871.

10. Davis JW, Shackford SR, Mackersie RC, Hoyt DB. Base deficit as a guide to volume resuscitation. J Trauma 1998; 28:1464-1467.

11. Moomey CB Jr, Melton SM, Croce MA, et al. Prognostic value of blood lactate, base deficit, and oxygen-derived variables in an LD_{50} model of penetrating trauma. Crit Care Med 1999; 27:154-161.

12. Husain FA, Martin MJ, Mullenix PS, et al. Serum lactate and base deficit as predictors of mortality and morbidity. Am J Surg 2003; 185:485-491.

13. Mateer JR, Thompson BM, Aprahamian C, Darin JC. Rapid fluid resuscitation with central venous catheters. Ann Emerg Med 1983; 12:149–152.

14. Buchman TG, Menker JB, Lipsett PA. Strategies for trauma resuscitation. Surg Gynecol Obstet 1991; 172:8–12.

15. Hyman SA, Smith DW, England R, et al. Pulmonary artery catheter introducers: Do the component parts affect flow rate? Anesth Analg 1991; 73:573–575.

16. Dula DJ, Muller A, Donovan JW. Flow rate variance of commonly used IV infusion techniques. J Trauma 1981; 21:480–482.

17. Bivins HG, Knopp R, dos Santos PAL. Blood volume distribution in the Trendelenburg position. Ann Emerg Med 1985; 14:641–643.

18. Gaffney FA, Bastian BC, Thal ER, Atkins JM. Passive leg raising does not produce a significant autotransfusion effect. J Trauma 1982; 22:190–193.

19. Sing R, O'Hara D, Sawyer MJ, Marino PL. Trendelenburg position and oxygen transport in hypovolemic adults. Ann Emerg Med 1994; 23:564–568.

20. Shoemaker WC. Relationship of oxygen transport patterns to the pathophysiology and therapy of shock states. Intensive Care Med 1987; 213:230–243.
21. Marik PE, Sibbald WJ. Effect of stored-blood transfusion on oxygen delivery in patients with sepsis. JAMA 1993; 269:3024–3029.
22. Imm A, Carlson RW. Fluid resuscitation in circulatory shock. Crit Care Clin 1993; 9:313–333. .
23. Tisherman SA, Barie P, Bokhari F, et al. Clinical practice guideline: Endpoints of resuscitation. Winston-Salem (NC): Eastern Association for Surgery of Trauma, 2003. Available at www.east.org/tpg/endpoints.pdf (accessed 6/18/07)
24. Abramson D, Scalea TM, Hitchcock R, et al. Lactate clearance and survival following injury. J Trauma 1993; 35:584-589.

Chapter 11

COLLOID AND CRYSTALLOID RESUSCITATION

Intravenous fluids are classified as crystalloid or colloid fluids. This chapter describes the comparative features of each type of fluid, and the individual fluids available for clinical use. A brief description of hypertonic fluid resuscitation is included at the end of the chapter.

I. CRYSTALLOID FLUIDS

Crystalloid fluids are electrolyte solutions that contain only small molecules capable of unrestricted movement between plasma and interstitial fluid. The principal ingredient in crystalloid fluids is the inorganic salt sodium chloride (which takes advantage of sodium's role as the principal solute in extracellular fluid).

A. Crystalloid Distribution

1. Crystalloid fluids are distributed uniformly in the extracellular fluid. Since the interstitial fluid represents about 75% of the extracellular fluid (excluding bone), then 75% of infused crystalloid fluids will be distributed in the interstitial fluid.

2. The tendency for crystalloid fluids to distribute more in the interstitial fluid than in plasma is demonstrated in Figure 11.1. In this case, infusion of one liter of 0.9% sodi-

um chloride (isotonic saline) adds of 275 mL to the plasma, and 825 mL to the interstitial fluid (1). The total volume increment (1,100 mL) is more than the volume infused because isotonic saline is slightly hypertonic to interstitial fluid, and will draw water out of cells.

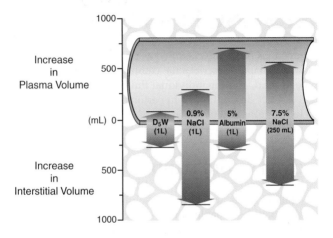

FIGURE 11.1. The effects of selected colloid and crystalloid fluids on the plasma volume and interstitial fluid volume. The infusion volume for each fluid is shown in parentheses. (From Reference 1).

B. Isotonic Saline

The classic crystalloid fluid is 0.9% sodium chloride (0.9% NaCL), which is also called *isotonic saline* (even though it is not isotonic to plasma) or normal saline (even though it is not a one-normal solution) .

1. *Composition*

When compared to plasma (see Table 11.1) isotonic saline has a higher sodium concentration (154 vs. 140 mEq/L), a much higher chloride concentration (154 vs. 103 mEq /L), a much lower pH (5.7 vs. 7.4) and a slightly higher osmolality (308 vs. 290 mOsm/L). The chloride difference has significance, as described next.

2. *Adverse Effects*

Large volume infusions of isotonic saline can produce a *hyperchloremic metabolic acidosis* (2). The culprit is the excess chloride in isotonic saline, which will promote renal bicarbonate excretion. This condition has no adverse consequences, but it can create confusion in the resuscitation of diabetic ketoacidosis, as explained in Chapter 23.

C. Lactated Ringer's Solution

Ringer's solution was introduced in 1880 as a calcium-containing fluid that could promote cardiac contraction in frog heart preparations. It was later adopted for clinical use, and lactate was added as a buffer in 1930.

1. *Composition*

a. Ringer's solutions contain potassium and calcium in concentrations that approximate the free (ionized) concentrations in plasma. The addition of these cations requires a reduction in sodium concentration for electrical neutrality, and the resultant sodium concentration is lower than in isotonic saline or plasma (see Table 11.1).

b. The addition of lactate (28 mEq/L) requires a drop in chloride concentration, and the resultant chloride concentration (109 mEq/L) is close to that of plasma (103 mEq/L). This eliminates the risk of hyperchloremic metabolic acidosis observed after large-volume infusions of isotonic saline.

2. *Adverse Effects*

a. The calcium in Ringer's solutions can bind to drugs (e.g., amphotericin, ampicillin, thiopental) and reduce

TABLE 11.1 Comparative Features of Crystalloid Fluids and Plasma

| Fluid | mEq/L | | | | | | | Osmolality (mOsm/L) |
	Na	Cl	K	Ca	Mg	Buffers	pH	
Plasma	140	103	4	5	2	HCO_3	7.4	290
0.9% NaCl	154	154	—	—	—	—	5.7	308
Ringer's Lactate	130	109	4	3	—	Lactate	6.4	273
7.5% NaCl*	1283	1283	—	—	—	—	5.7	2567
Normosol Plasma-Lyte Isolyte†	140	98	5	—	3	Acetate & Gluconate	7.4	295

*From Stapczynski JS et al. Emerg Med Rep 1994; 15:245.
†Isolyte also contains phosphate (1 mEq/L).

efficacy (3). These drugs should not be mixed with Ringer's solutions.

b. The calcium in Ringer's can also bind to the citrated anticoagulant in blood products. This inactivates the anticoagulant and promotes clot formation in donor blood. According to the American Association of Blood Banks, *Ringer's solutions are contraindicated as a diluent for red blood cell transfusions* (4).

D. Normal pH Fluids

1. Three crystalloid fluids (Normosol, Isolyte, and Plasma-Lyte) contain both acetate and gluconate buffers to a-chieve a pH of 7.4 (see Table 11.1). All three fluids con-tain potassium (5 mEq/L) and magnesium (3 mEq/L), while Isolyte also contains phosphate (1 mEq/L).

2. These fluids are not popular, but they have been recommended as preferable to isotonic saline for washing or diluting salvaged red blood cells (5).

II. DEXTROSE SOLUTIONS

A. Protein-Sparing Effect

1. Dextrose was originally added to intravenous fluids as a nutrient. One gram of dextrose provides 3.4 kilocalories (kcal) when fully metabolized, so a 5% dextrose solution (50 grams per liter) provides 170 kcal per liter.

2. Daily infusion of 3 liters of a 5% dextrose (D_5) solution provides about 500 kcal per day, which is enough non-protein calories to limit the breakdown of endogenous proteins to meet daily caloric requirements. This *protein-sparing effect* is responsible for the early popularity of dextrose-containing fluids.

3. The current availability of enteral and parenteral nutrition regimens obviates the need for 5% dextrose solutions as a source of calories.

B. Volume Effects

1. The addition of dextrose to an intravenous fluid does not enhance the performance of the fluid for volume resuscitation because the dextrose is taken up by cells and metabolized.

2. The poor performance of 5% dextrose-in-water (D_5W) as a resuscitation fluid is shown in Figure 11.1. In this case, infusion of one liter of D_5W is associated with a minimal (about 100 mL) increment in plasma volume.

3. Note in Figure 11.1 that the combined increments in plasma volume (100 mL) and interstitial fluid volume (250 mL) are far less than the volume infused. The volume difference (650 mL) is the result of fluid movement into cells, which means that D$_5$W *expands the intracellular volume* (which is not a desirable effect).

C. Adverse Effects

1. *Enhanced Lactate Production*

   In healthy subjects, only 5% of glucose metabolism leads to lactate production, but in critically ill patients with tissue hypoperfusion, as much as 85% of glucose metabolism is diverted to lactate production (6). Thus when tissue oxygenation is impaired, glucose is a source of metabolic acid production more than metabolic energy production.

2. *Hyperglycemia*

   a. Hyperglycemia has several undesirable effects in critically ill patients, including immunosuppression (7), aggravation of ischemic brain injury (8), and increased mortality (9,10).

   b. Clinical studies have shown improved survival in ICU patients when there is a protocol for strict glycemic control with insulin infusions (9,10). The mechanism for this effect is not known.

   Because 5% dextrose solutions offer no benefit, and can be harmful, the routine use of these solutions should be abandoned.

III. COLLOID FLUIDS

The behavior of colloid fluids is determined by an osmotic force that is described briefly in the next section.

A. Colloid Osmotic Pressure

1. Colloid fluids contain large molecules that do not readily move out of the vascular compartment. These molecules create an osmotic pressure called the *colloid osmotic pressure* that favors the retention of water in the vascular compartment.

2. The following relationship identifies the role of the colloid osmotic pressure in capillary fluid exchange.

$$Q \propto (P_c - COP) \qquad (11.1)$$

   a. Q is the flow rate across the capillaries.
   b. P_c is the hydrostatic pressure in the capillaries.
   c. COP is the colloid osmotic pressure of plasma. This pressure is created by plasma proteins (mostly albumin), and the normal range is 20–25 mm Hg.

3. The two pressures (P_c and COP) act in opposition: P_c favors the movement of fluid out of the capillaries, and COP favors movement into the capillaries.

4. Colloid fluids that are used to replace volume losses have a COP that is equivalent to the COP of plasma. This helps to retain most of the infused volume in the plasma.

5. Some colloid fluids have a COP that is much higher than the COP of plasma: these fluids are used to draw interstitial fluid into the plasma.

B. Volume Effects

1. The effect of colloid fluid resuscitation on plasma and interstitial fluid volumes is shown in Figure 11.1 The colloid fluid in this case is a 5% albumin solution, which has a COP (20 mm Hg) that is equivalent to the COP of plasma. Infusion of one liter of this solution adds 700 mL to the plasma and 300 mL to the interstitial fluid.

2. Comparing the effects of the colloid and crystalloid fluid on plasma volume in Figure 11.1 reveals that *the colloid fluid is about three times more effective than the crystalloid fluid for increasing the plasma volume* (1,11–13).

3. Colloid fluids differ in their ability to increase the plasma volume, and this difference is a function of the COP of each fluid. This is demonstrated in Table 11.2, which shows that fluids with a higher COP produce greater increments in plasma volume.

TABLE 11.2 Comparative Features of Colloid Fluids

Fluid	Colloid Osmotic Pressure	Δ Plasma Volume Infused Volume	Duration of Effect
25% Albumin	70 mm Hg	4.0 – 5.0	12 h
10% Dextran-40	40 mm Hg	1.0 – 1.5	6 h
6% Hetastarch	30 mm Hg	1.0 – 1.3	24 h
5% Albumin	20 mm Hg	0.7 – 1.3	12 h

From References 1,11–13,17.

C. Albumin Solutions

Albumin solutions are heat-treated preparations of human serum albumin that are available as a 5% solution (50 g/L) and a 25% solution (250 g/L) in isotonic saline.

1. *Volume Effects*

   a. The 5% albumin solution has an albumin concentration (5 g/dL) and a COP (20 mm Hg) that are equivalent to plasma. This solution is given in aliquots of 250 mL, and the acute volume effect (70% retention in plasma, as shown in Figure 11.1) is lost after 12 hours (1,11).

b. The 25% albumin solution has a COP (70 mm Hg) that is about three times higher than the COP of plasma. As a result, 25% albumin draws fluid from the interstitial space, and the increment in plasma volume can be four to five times greater than the volume infused (see Table 11.2). This colloid fluid is given in small aliquots (50 mL) to shift interstitial fluid into the plasma in conditions where hypovolemia is associated with edema (e.g., hypoalbuminemia). It is not appropriate for replacing volume losses.

2. *Safety*

Early claims of increased mortality attributed to albumin infusions (14) have not been corroborated in more recent studies (15). In addition, there is evidence of reduced morbidity when albumin is used instead of crystalloid fluids (16).

D. Hydroxyethyl Starch

Hydroxyethyl starch (hetastarch) is a synthetic starch polymer that is available as a 6% solution in isotonic saline. There are 3 preparations based on molecular weight (high MW, medium MW, and low MW), but only the high MW preparation is available in the United States (17).

1. *Volume Effects*

Overall, 6% hetastarch is considered equivalent to 5% albumin as a plasma volume expander (even though the COP is higher, and the increment in plasma volume is slightly greater, as shown in Table 11.2).

2. *Side Effects*

a. High MW hetastarch can cause a bleeding tendency due to decreased levels of Factor VIII and von Willebrand factor, and impaired platelet adhesiveness (17, 18). This effect becomes pronounced when more than 1.5 L hetastarch is infused within a 24 hr period (17).

Overt bleeding is inconsistent. This side effect is not seen with low MW hetastarch (18).

b. Serum amylase levels are elevated (2 to 3 times normal) for one week after hetastarch infusion (the amylase cleaves hetastarch prior to clearance by the kidneys) (17), and this could be misinterpreted as indicating pancreatitis.

3. *Clinical Role*

Hetastarch is a less costly alternative to 5% albumin (see Table 11.3), but the resuscitation volume should be less than 1,500 mL daily to avoid a troublesome coagulopathy.

E. The Dextrans

The dextrans are glucose polymers prepared as 10% dextran-40 and 6% dextran-70, each with a different molecular weight. Both preparations use isotonic saline as the diluent.

1. *Volume Effects*

Both dextran preparations have a COP of 40 mm Hg, and cause a greater increase in plasma volume than 5% albumin or 6% hetastarch (see Table 11.2). Dextran-70 may be preferred because the duration of action (12 hours) is longer than that of dextran-40 (6 hours) (11).

2. *Side Effects*

a. Dextrans produce a dose-related bleeding tendency that involves impaired platelet aggregation, decreased levels of Factor VIII and von Willebrand factor, and enhanced fibrinolysis (18). These effects are minimal when the dextran dose is limited to 20 mL/kg daily.

b. Dextrans coat the surface of red blood cells and can interfere with the ability to cross-match blood. Red cell preparations must be washed to eliminate this problem. Dextrans also increase the erythrocyte sedimentation rate as a result of their interactions with red blood cells (19).

c. Dextrans have been implicated as a cause of acute renal failure (19), but a causal link is unproven.

3. *Clinical Role*

The dextrans have fallen out of favor because of their side effects.

TABLE 11.3 Cost Comparison for Resuscitation Fluids

Fluid	Manufacturer	Unit Size	AWP[†]
Crystalloid Fluids			
Isotonic Saline	Hospira	1,000 mL	$1.46
Lactated Ringer's	Hospira	1,000 mL	$1.48
Colloid Fluids			
5% Albumin	Bayer	250 mL	$30.63
25% Albumin	Bayer	50 mL	$30.63
6% Hetastarch	Abbott	500 mL	$27.63
6% Dextran-70	Hospira	500 mL	$14.96

[†]Average wholesale price listed in 2005 Redbook. Montvale, NJ, Thomson PDR, 2005.

IV. COLLOIDS vs. CRYSTALLOIDS

There is a longstanding debate concerning the type of fluid (crystalloid or colloid) that is most appropriate for volume resuscitation.

A. Colloid Fluids

1. *Pros*

The major point in favor of colloid fluids is their effectiveness in expanding the plasma volume. Colloid fluids will achieve a given increment in plasma volume with only one-quarter to one-third the volume required of crystalloid fluids. Since the goal of volume resuscitation is to support the intravascular volume, colloid fluids are the logical choice over crystalloid fluids

2. *Cons*

The major argument against colloid fluids is the expense (see Table 11.3) and the lack of a documented survival benefit to justify the expense. The bulk of evidence shows no difference in mortality in patients who are resuscitated with colloid or crystalloid fluids (15,20).

B. Crystalloid Fluids

1. *Pros*

The proponents of crystalloid resuscitation claim that crystalloid fluids can achieve the same increment in plasma volume as colloid fluids (if enough crystalloid fluid is infused) but at a much lower cost.

2. *Cons*

The major argument against crystalloid fluids is their poor performance as plasma volume expanders. *The principal effect of crystalloid infusions is to expand the interstitial fluid volume, not the plasma volume.*

C. Preferences

Instead of selecting one type of fluid for all occasions, it seems more reasonable to select the most appropriate fluid for the clinical condition. For example, a crystalloid fluid is more appropriate for a patient with hypovolemia due to dehydration (where there is a uniform loss of extracellular fluid), whereas a colloid fluid is more appropriate for a patient with life-threatening hypovolemia due to hemorrhage.

V. HYPERTONIC RESUSCITATION

Volume resuscitation with 7.5% NaCL (hypertonic saline), which has an osmolality about 8.5 times greater than that of plasma (see Table 11.1), is being investigated as a method of small-volume resuscitation.

A. Volume Effects

1. As shown in Figure 11.1, the increment in plasma volume following infusion of 250 mL of 7.5% NaCL is about twice the infused volume. The same increment in plasma volume would require infusion of 2 liters of isotonic saline (or eight times the volume of hypertonic saline).

2. Figure 11.1 also shows 7.5% NaCL produces an increase in extracellular fluid volume (1,235 mL) that is 4 to 5 times greater than the infused volume (250 mL). The additional volume comes from intracellular fluid that moves out of cells and into the extracellular space. This highlights one of the feared consequences of hypertonic resuscitation: i.e., cell dehydration.

B. Clinical Role?

1. Small-volume resuscitation with hypertonic saline has potential benefits in the following clinical situations:
   a. In trauma victims with hypotension and closed head injuries (to limit the severity of cerebral edema) .
   b. In cases of acute hemorrhage from a vascular injury (to limit blood loss through the injured vessel until the injury can be surgically repaired).
   c. In patients with subarachnoid hemorrhage, a combination of hypertonic saline in 6% hetastarch has been successful in reducing intracranial pressure (21).

2. At the present time, there are no firm indications for hypertonic saline over more traditional resuscitation fluids.

REFERENCES

1. Imm A, Carlson RW. Fluid resuscitation in circulatory shock. Crit Care Clin 1993; 9:313-333.
2. Scheingraber S, Rehm M, Schmisch C, Finsterer U. Rapid saline infusion produces hyperchloremic acidosis in patients undergoing gynecologic surgery. Anesthesiology 1999; 90:1265-1270.
3. Griffith CA. The family of Ringer's solutions. J Natl Intravenous Ther Assoc 1986; 9:480–483.
4. American Association of Blood Banks Technical Manual. 10th ed. Arlington, VA: American Association of Blood Banks, 1990:368.
5. Halpern NA, Alicea M, Seabrook B, et al. Isolyte S, a physiologic multielectrolyte solution, is preferable to normal saline to wash cell saver salvaged blood: conclusions from a prospective, randomized study in a canine model. Crit Care Med 1997; 12:2031-2038.
6. Gunther B, Jauch W, Hartl W, et al. Low-dose glucose infusion in patients who have undergone surgery. Arch Surg 1987; 122:765–771.
7. Turina M, Fry D, Polk HC, Jr. Acute hyperglycemia and the innate immune system: Clinical, cellular, and molecular aspects. Crit Care Med 2005; 33:1624-1633.
8. Sieber FE, Traystman RJ. Special issues: glucose and the brain. Crit Care Med 1992; 20:104–114.
9. Van Den Berghe G, Wouters P, Weekers F, et al. Intensive insulin therapy in critically ill patients. N Engl J Med 2001; 345:1359-1367.
10. Finney SJ, Zekveld C, Elia A, Evans TW. Glucose control and mortality in critically ill patients. JAMA 2003; 290: 2041-2047.
11. Griffel MI, Kaufman BS. Pharmacology of colloids and crystalloids. Crit Care Clin 1992; 8:235–254.
12. Kaminski MV, Haase TJ. Albumin and colloid osmotic pressure: implications for fluid resuscitation. Crit Care Clin 1992; 8:311–322.
13. Sutin KM, Ruskin KJ, Kaufman BS. Intravenous fluid therapy in neurologic injury. Crit Care Clin 1992; 8:367–408.

14. Cochrane Injuries Group Albumin Reviewers. Human albumin administration in critically ill patients: Systematic review of randomized, controlled trials. Br Med J 1998; 317:235-240.

15. SAFE Study Investigators. A comparison of albumin and saline for fluid resuscitation in the Intensive Care Unit. N Engl J Med 2004; 350:2247-2256.

16. Vincent J-L, Navickis RJ, Wilkes MM. Morbidity in hospitalized patients receiving human serum albumin: A meta-analysis of randomized, controlled trials. Crit Care Med 2004; 32:2029-2038.

17. Treib J, Baron JF, Grauer MT, Strauss RG. An international view of hydroxyethyl starches. Intensive Care Med 1999; 25:258-268.

18. de Jonge E, Levi M. Effects of different plasma substitutes on blood coagulation: A comparative review. Crit Care Med 2001; 29:1261-1267.

19. Nearman HS, Herman ML. Toxic effects of colloids in the intensive care unit. Crit Care Clin 1991; 7:713–723.

20. Choi PT, Yip G, Quinonez LG, et al. Crystalloids vs. colloids in fluid resuscitation: A systematic review. Crit Care Med 1999; 27: 200-210.

21. Bentsen G, Breivik H, Lundar T, Stubhaug A. Hypertonic saline (7.2%) in 6% hydroxyethyl starch reduces intracranial pressure and improves hemodynamics in a placebo-controlled study involving stable patients with subarachnoid hemorrhage. Crit Care Med 2006; 34:2912-2917.

Chapter 12

ACUTE HEART FAILURE(S)

Acute, decompensated heart failure is the leading cause of hospital admissions for adults over the age of 65 (1). Heart failure is not a single entity, but can be classified according to the side of the heart that is involved (right-sided and left-sided heart failure) and the portion of the cardiac cycle that is affected (diastolic and systolic heart failure). This chapter describes the diagnosis and management of these heart failure(s) in the ICU.

I. HEMODYNAMIC ALTERATIONS

A. Progressive Heart Failure

The influence of progressive heart failure on cardiac performance is shown in Figure 12.1. Changes in cardiac performance occur in 3 distinct stages (as indicated by the circled numbers in Figure 12.1):

1. The earliest stage of heart failure is characterized by an isolated increase in ventricular end-diastolic pressure (the wedge pressure in Figure 12.1). The stroke volume and cardiac output are maintained, but at the expense of venous congestion.

2. The next stage is characterized by a decrease in stroke volume and a corresponding increase in heart rate. The tachycardia offsets the reduction in stroke volume, so the cardiac output remains unchanged.

3. The final stage is characterized by a steady decline in cardiac output and an accelerated rise in the wedge pressure. (Note the blunted heart rate response, which is responsible for the drop in cardiac output). These changes mark the onset of *decompensated heart failure*. If left unchecked, the steady decline in cardiac output will eventually lead to hypoperfusion of the vital organs and ischemic tissue injury: a condition known as *cardiogenic shock*.

4. The changes in cardiac performance in progressive heart failure are summarized in Table 12.1. The following points deserve mention:

   a. Because the cardiac output does not decline until the later stages of heart failure, cardiac output monitoring is not a sensitive method of detecting heart failure

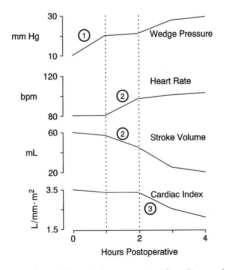

FIGURE 12.1. Serial changes in measures of cardiac performance in a patent who developed rapidly progressive heart failure in the immediate postoperative period.

b. The optimal measure of cardiac performance for the detection of cardiac pump failure is the relationship between end-diastolic pressure and stroke volume. An increase in end-diastolic pressure without a corresponding rise in stroke volume is the earliest sign of pump failure (see Table 12.1).

TABLE 12.1 Cardiac Performance in Progressive Heart Failure

Performance Measure	Cardiac Pump Failure		
	Mild	**Moderate**	**Advanced**
End-Diastolic Pressure	High	High	High
Stroke Volume	Normal	Low	Low
Cardiac Output	Normal	Normal	Low

B. Systolic vs. Diastolic Heart Failure

1. *The Entities*

   a. Heart failure is classically described as failure of cardiac contraction during systole. This condition is now known as *systolic heart failure*.

   b. Systolic function is normal in 40 to 50% of newly-diagnosed cases of heart failure (1). In these cases, the heart failure is due to a decrease in ventricular distensibility during diastole. This condition is known as *diastolic heart failure* (2). Common causes of diastolic heart failure in ICU patients include ventricular hypertrophy, myocardial ischemia (stunned myocardium), and positive-pressure mechanical ventilation.

2. *Pressure-Volume Curves*

   The pressure volume relationships in Figure 12.2 will be used to point out the similarities and differences between systolic and diastolic heart failure.

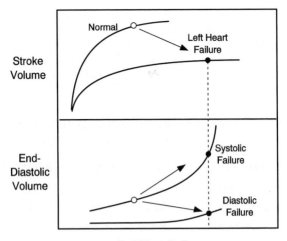

End-Diastolic Pressure

FIGURE 12.2. Graphs showing the effects of heart failure on pressure-volume relationships during systole (upper curves) and diastole (lower curves). Left heart failure is associated with an increase in end-diastolic pressure, and this is associated with an *increased* end-diastolic volume in systolic failure and a *decreased* end-diastolic volume in diastolic failure.

a. The curves at the top of Figure 12.2 demonstrate that heart failure is associated with an increased end-diastolic pressure (EDP) and a decreased stroke volume. These changes occur in both types of heart failure, as indicated in Table 12.2.

b. The lower set of curves in Figure 12.2 show the pressure–volume relationships during diastole in both types of heart failure. Note that in systolic heart failure, the increased EDP is associated with an increase in end-diastolic volume (EDV), while in diastolic heart failure, the increased EDP is associated with a decrease in EDV. Therefore, *end-diastolic volume, not end-diastolic pressure, is the parameter that distinguishes diastolic from systolic heart failure* (see Table 12.2).

c. Unfortunately, end-diastolic volume is not easily measured at the bedside, but there is another measure that has discriminatory value (see next).

TABLE 12.2 Features of Diastolic & Systolic Heart Failure

Parameter	Diastolic Failure	Systolic Failure
End-Diastolic Pressure	High	High
Stroke Volume	Low	Low
End-Diastolic Volume	Low	High
Ejection Fraction	Normal	Low

Note that only the parameters below the dotted line can distinguish between the two types of heart failure.

3. *Ventricular Ejection Fraction*

a. The ventricular *ejection fraction* (EF) expresses the stroke volume (SV) as a fraction of the end-diastolic volume (EDV):

$$EF = SV/EDV \qquad (12.1)$$

The EF provides a measure of cardiac contractile strength during diastole.

b. The EF is normal in patients with diastolic heart failure, and reduced in patients with systolic heart failure. The normal ejection fraction of each ventricle is shown below:

Ejection Fraction (EF)	Normal Range
Right Ventricle	0.50-0.55
Left Ventricle	0.40-0.50

c. Cardiac ultrasound can be used to measure EF at the bedside. Transthoracic ultrasound can be used to measure the EF of the left ventricle (2,3), and transesophageal ultrasound can be used to measure the EF of the right ventricle (4). A specialized pulmonary artery catheter is also available that can monitor the EF of the right ventricle (see next section).

C. Right Heart Failure

1. Right heart failure is more common than suspected in the ICU (5), but it may be clinically apparent only in the later stages of illness.

2. Right heart failure is usually systolic failure, and thus is associated with an increased end-diastolic volume and a decreased ejection fraction.

3. The central venous pressure (CVP) is normal in about one-third of cases of right heart failure (6). The CVP begins to rise only when right ventricular dilatation has reached a point where it is impeded by the pericardium (6). This differs from left heart failure, where the pulmonary capillary wedge pressure (PCWP) rises early in the course of illness (see Figure 12.1).

4. A specialized pulmonary artery catheter is available that can measure the end-diastolic volume and ejection fraction of the right ventricle (see Reference 7 for a description of this catheter). Transesophageal ultrasound can also be used to measure right ventricular EF, as mentioned earlier.

II. B-TYPE NATRIURETIC PEPTIDE

Brain-type (B-type) natriuretic peptide (BNP) is a hormone that is released by the ventricular myocardium in response to volume and pressure overload. Plasma levels of BNP increase in direct relation to increases in ventricular end-diastolic volume and end-diastolic pressure (both right-sided and left-sided), and the rise in BNP produces both vasodilation and an increase in renal sodium excretion (8).

A. Diagnostic Value

1. In patients who present to the emergency room with dyspnea of unknown etiology, a plasma BNP > 100 picograms/milliliter (pg/mL) will identify heart failure almost 90% of the time (9).

2. Plasma BNP levels also show a direct correlation with the severity of heart failure (8), which means that plasma BNP levels may be useful for evaluating treatment responses and selecting end-points of management.

3. Plasma BNP levels are also influenced by gender, age, and renal function. The levels are 50% higher in females than in males, and levels in both sexes can triple in advanced age (>75 years) (8). However, these factors do not raise the BNP levels above the 100 pg/mL threshold for the diagnosis of heart failure.

4. Renal insufficiency increases plasma BNP levels because BNP is cleared by the kidneys, and plasma levels can exceed the 100 pg/mL threshold if there is associated volume overload (10).

B. Any Role in the ICU?

1. Plasma BNP has been studied primarily in the emergency room setting. Few studies have been performed in the ICU.

2. It is unlikely that plasma BNP will replace more traditional methods of evaluating heart failure in the ICU, but BNP levels could prove useful for monitoring the response to treatment.

III. MANAGEMENT STRATEGIES

The management of heart failure described here is intended only for the ICU environment because the treatments are based on invasive hemodynamic measurements rather than symptoms, and the drugs that are used are given by continuous intravenous infusion. Table 12.3 contains a list of the drugs and the recommended dose rates. (These drugs are presented in much more detail in Chapter 45.)

TABLE 12.3 Drugs Used to Manage Acute Heart Failure

Drug	Dose Range	Principal Actions
Dobutamine	3–15 µg/kg/min	Positive inotropic effect and systemic vasodilatation
Dopamine	1–3 µg/kg/min	Renal vasodilatation and natriuresis
	3–10 µg/kg/min	Positive inotropic effect and systemic vasodilatation
	>10 µg/kg/min	Systemic vasoconstriction
Milrinone	50 µg/kg bolus, then 0.25–1 µg/kg/min	Positive inotropic effect and lusitropic effect, and systemic vasodilatation
Nitroglycerin	1–50 µg/min	Venous vasodilatation
	>50 µg/min	Arterial vasodilatation
Nitroprusside	0.3–2 µg/kg/min	Systemic vasodilatation

A. Left-Sided Systolic Heart Failure

Contractile failure involving the left ventricle is the prototype model of heart failure, and the one for which most treatments are designed. The treatments described here are for decompensated heart failure, which corresponds to the point on the lower curve in Figure 12.3. The goal of therapy is to move the point to the left and upward (as indicated by the arrow). The treatments are organized according to the condition of the patient's blood pressure (i.e., high, normal, or low).

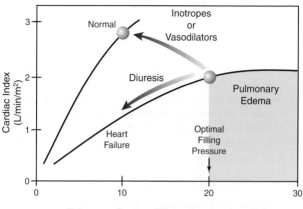

FIGURE 12.3. Cardiac performance curves for the normal and failing left ventricle. The point on the lower curve represents decompensated heart failure.

1. *High Blood Pressure*

   Decompensated heart failure with elevated blood pressure is a familiar condition in the early period after cardiopulmonary bypass surgery.

   Profile: High PCWP/Low CO/High BP

   Treatment: Vasodilator therapy with nitroprusside or nitroglycerin. If the PCWP remains above 20 mm Hg, add diuretic therapy with furosemide.

   a. Vasodilator drugs like nitroprusside and nitroglycerin will dilate both arteries and veins, and the overall effect will be a reduction in blood pressure, an increase in cardiac output, and a decrease in the wedge pressure (11).

   b. Nitroprusside is a more effective vasodilator than nitroglycerin, but drug safety is a concern. The major problem with nitroprusside is *cyanide toxicity*, which is described in Chapter 45. Nitroprusside is also not advised in patients with ischemic heart disease because the drug can produce a "coronary steal syndrome" (12).

c. Nitroglycerin is a safer alternative to nitroprusside. Low infusion rates (<50 μg/min) will dilate veins selectively (which can reduce cardiac output further), and dose rates in excess of 50 μg/min are usually required to produce effective arterial vasodilation. The major drawback with nitroglycerin infusions is the development of tolerance, which can appear after 16 to 24 hours (12).

d. Diuretic therapy with furosemide is indicated only if vasodilator therapy does not reduce the wedge pressure below 20 mm Hg. (The effects of diuretic therapy are described later in the chapter).

e. The wedge pressure should be kept just under 20 mm Hg because this is the highest pressure that will augment cardiac output without producing pulmonary edema. This is shown in Figure 12.3 as the highest point on the lower curve that does not enter the hatched (pulmonary edema) region.

2. *Normal Blood Pressure*

This is the usual presentation of heart failure caused by non-hypertensive heart disease (e.g., ischemic heart disease).

Profile: High PCWP/Low CO/Normal BP

Treatment: Inodilator therapy with dobutamine or milrinone, or vasodilator therapy with nitroglycerin. If the PCWP does not drop below <20 mm Hg, add diuretic therapy with furosemide.

a. Dobutamine and milrinone are called *inodilators* because they have both positive inotropic and vasodilator actions (13,14). Dobutamine is a β-receptor agonist, while milrinone is a phosphodiesterase inhibitor. Both drugs augment cardiac output and reduce ventricular filling pressures. Blood pressure is usually unaffected in the usual doses, but dobutamine can increase blood pressure, and milrinone can promote hypotension.

b. Because dobutamine can increase myocardial oxygen (because of its positive inotropic actions), vasodilator therapy (e.g., nitroglycerin) has been recommended as a safer alternative to dobutamine in patients with ischemic heart disease (13,14).

c. Milrinone is preferred to dobutamine in patients receiving β-blocker drugs because its efficacy is independent of β-receptors.

d. Diuretic therapy has the same role in this situation as it did for hypertensive heart failure: i.e., it is reserved for cases where the wedge pressure remains above 20 mm Hg despite inodilator or vasodilator therapy.

3. *Low Blood Pressure*

Decompensated heart failure accompanied by hypotension is the *sine qua non* of cardiogenic shock., and requires prompt intervention.

Profile: High PCWP/Low CO/Low BP

Treatment: Dopamine in vasoconstrictor doses. Consider a mechanical assist device in patients with coronary artery disease and a correctable lesion.

a. Hemodynamic drugs are notoriously unsuccessful in cardiogenic shock, and the mortality rate continues to be is as high as 80% (15).

b. Increasing blood pressure (to a mean pressure of 60 mm Hg) is a priority, and dopamine is a popular choice because it acts as a vasopressor in high doses (>10 µg/kg/min) and retains some positive inotropic actions associated with lower doses (5 to 10 µg/kg /min) (12-14). However, low cardiac output states are accompanied by systemic vasoconstriction, and vasopressor drugs can further aggravate tissue hypoperfusion.

c. Mechanical cardiac support is indicated if myocardial function is expected to improve spontaneously (as occurs in the early period following cardiopulmonary bypass surgery), or when a corrective procedure (e.g., angioplasty) is planned. A description of the support devices is beyond the scope of this text.

4. *Limited Role for Diuretics*

a. Diuretics should be used cautiously in acute heart failure because *intravenous furosemide can cause a 15 to 20% drop in cardiac output in this situation* (16,17). The expected effect of diuresis in decompensated heart failure is shown by the arrow in Figure 12.3.

b. Drugs that augment cardiac output should always be given priority over diuretics in acute heart failure. In fact, if cardiac output can be restored, the stimulus to retain salt and water will be eliminated, and diuretics will not be necessary.

5. *Furosemide by Continuous Infusion*

a. Critically ill patients can have an attenuated response to furosemide (18), possibly as a result of reduced transport proteins and chloride depletion (furosemide acts by inhibiting chloride reabsorption in the Loop of Henle).

b. Because the diuretic effect of furosemide is closely related to its urinary excretion rate (19), continuous infusion of the drug will produce a more vigorous diuresis than bolus injection.

c. INDICATION. Continuous furosemide infusion should be considered when an 80 mg IV bolus dose of furosemide fails to produce more than 2 liters of urine output in the ensuing four hours.

d. DOSAGE. Start with 100 mg furosemide as an IV bolus, and immediately follow with a continuous infusion of furosemide at 40 mg/hr. Double the dose rate every 12 hours if needed to achieve a urine output of at least 100 mL/h. The dose rate should not exceed 170 mg/hr (20).

6. *Nesiritide*

   a. Nesiritide (Natrecor) is a recombinant human B-type natriuretic peptide that acts as a systemic vasodilator to augment cardiac output.

   b. DOSAGE. Give initial bolus of 2 µg/kg and follow with a continuous infusion at 0.01 µg/kg/min. This dose rate can be increased 0.01 µg/kg/min every 3 hours to a maximum dose of 0.03 µg/kg/min (21).

   c. Clinical studies show that nesiritide offers no advantage over traditional vasodilators such as nitroglycerin (21). In fact, there is a report of increased short-term (30 day) mortality attributed to nesiritide (22), which prompted an FDA safety alert about the drug.

B. Left–Sided Diastolic Heart Failure

The prevalence of diastolic dysfunction in acute heart failure is not known, but heart failure associated with left ventricular hypertrophy or acute myocardial ischemia is probably diastolic failure. There is no general agreement about the optimal treatment of diastolic heart failure (3), but the following recommendations seem valid.

1. Because systolic function is normal or only mildly impaired in diastolic heart failure, *positive inotropic agents have no role in the treatment of diastolic heart failure*.

2. Because ventricular filling is impaired in diastolic heart failure, *diuretic therapy is counterproductive in diastolic heart failure*.

3. Vasodilator therapy is appropriate for diastolic failure resulting from hypertension-induced left ventricular hy-

pertrophy. Some vasodilator agents, such as nitroglycerin and milrinone, can promote ventricular relaxation during diastole (3,14), and these *lusitropic effects* are well-suited for diastolic heart failure.

C. Right Heart Failure

The therapeutic strategies below are meant for cases of primary right heart failure and not for patients with right heart failure secondary to lung disease. The pulmonary capillary wedge pressure (PCWP) and right ventricular end-diastolic volume (RVEDV) are used as the focal points of management. (The RVEDV can be measured with a specialized PA catheter as described previously).

1. If PCWP is below 15 mm Hg, infuse volume until the PCWP or CVP increases by 5 mm Hg or either one reaches 20 mm Hg (6).

2. If the RVEDV is less than 140 mL/m², infuse volume until the RVEDV reaches 140 mL/m² (23).

3. If PCWP is above 15 mm Hg or the RVEDV is 140 mL/m² or higher, infuse dobutamine, beginning at a rate of 5 µg/kg/minute (24,25).

4. In the presence of AV dissociation or complete heart block, institute sequential A-V pacing and avoid ventricular pacing (3).

The response to volume infusion must be carefully monitored in right heart failure because excessive volume can overdistend the right ventricle, causing the interventricular septum to bulge into the left ventricular cavity and impair left ventricular filling. This process whereby the right ventricle can influence the function of the left ventricle is called interventricular interdependence.

REFERENCES

1. Nieminen MS, Harjola V-P. Definition and etiology of acute heart failure syndromes. Am J Cardiol 2005; 96(Suppl):5G-10G.

2. Zile MR, Baicu CF, Gaasch WH. Diastolic heart failure. Abnormalities in active relaxation and passive stiffness of the left ventricle. N Engl J Med 2004; 350:1953-1959.

3. Aurigemma GP, Gaasch WH. Diastolic heart failure. N Engl J Med 2004; 351:1097-1015.

4. Numi Y, Haki M, Ishiguro Y, et al. Determination of right ventricular function by transesophageal echocardiography: Impact of proximal right coronary artery stenosis. J Clin Anesthesia 2004; 16:104-110.

5. Hurford WE, Zapol WM. The right ventricle and critical illness: a review of anatomy, physiology, and clinical evaluation of its function. Intensive Care Med 1988; 14:448-457.

6. Isner JM. Right ventricular myocardial infarction. JAMA 1988; 259:712-718.

7. Vincent JL, Thirion M, Brimioulle S, et al. Thermodilution measurement of right ventricular ejection fraction with a modified pulmonary artery catheter. Intensive Care Med 1986; 12:33-38.

8. Maisel AS, Wanner EC. Measuring BNP levels in the diagnosis and treatment of CHF. J Crit Illness 2002; 17:434-442.

9. Maisel AS, Krishnaswamy P, Nomak RM, et al. Rapid measurement of B-type natriuretic peptide in the emergency diagnosis of heart failure. N Engl J Med 2002; 347:161-167.

10. Takami Y, Horio T, Iwashima Y, et al. Diagnostic and prognostic value of plasma bran natriuretic peptide in non-dialysis-dependent CRF. Am J Kidney Dis 2004; 44:420-428.

11. Stough WG, O'Connor CM, Gheorghiade M. Overview of current noninodilator therapies for acute heart failure syndromes. Am J Cardiol 2005; 96(Suppl):41G-46G.

12. The Task Force on Acute Heart failure of the European Society of Cardiology. Guidelines on the diagnosis and treatment of heart failure. European Society of Cardiology Web Site. Available at www.escardio.org.

13. Bayram M, De Luca L, Massie B, Gheorghiade M. Reassessment of dobutamine, dopamine, and milrinone in the management of acute heart failure syndromes. Am J Cardiol 2005; 96(Suppl): 47G-58G.

14. Chatterjee K, De Marco T. Role of nonglycosidic inotropic agents: indications, ethics, and limitations. Med Clin N Am 2003; 87:391-418.

15. Samuels LE, Darze ES. Management of acute cardiogenic shock. Cardiol Clin 2003; 21:43-49.

16. Kiely J, Kelly DT, Taylor DR, Pitt B. The role of furosemide in the treatment of left ventricular dysfunction associated with acute myocardial infarction. Circulation 1973; 58:581–587.

17. Mond H, Hunt D, Sloman G. Haemodynamic effects of frusemide in patients suspected of having acute myocardial infarction. Br Heart J 1974; 36:44–53.

18. Brater DC. Resistance to loop diuretics: why it happens and what to do about it. Drugs 1985; 30:427-443.

19. van Meyel JJM, Smits P, Russell FGM, et al. Diuretic efficiency of furosemide during continuous administration versus bolus injection in healthy volunteers. Clin Pharmacol Ther 1992; 51:440–444.

20. Howard PA, Dunn MI. Aggressive diuresis for severe heart failure in the elderly. Chest 2001; 119:807-810.

21. Vasodilation in the Management of Acute CHF (VMAC) Investigators. Intravenous nesiritide vs nitroglycerin for treatment of decompensated congestive heart failure. JAMA 2002; 287:1531-1540.

22. Sackner-Bernstein JD, Kowalski M, Fox M, Aaronson K. Short-term risk of death after treatment with nesiritide for decompensated heart Failure. JAMA 2005; 293:1900-1905.

23. Reuse C, Vincent JL, Pinsky MR. Measurement of right ventricular volumes during fluid challenge. Chest 1990; 98:1450-1454.

24. Vincent RL, Reuse C, Kahn RJ. Effects on right ventricular function of a change from dopamine to dobutamine in critically ill patients. Crit Care Med 1988; 16:659–662.

25. Dell'Italia LJ, Starling MR, Blumhardt R, et al. Comparative effects of volume loading, dobutamine and nitroprusside in patients with predominant right ventricular infarction. Circulation 1986; 72:1327–1335.

Chapter 13

CARDIAC ARREST

Cardiac arrest is managed with a variety of interventions known in total as *cardiopulmonary resuscitation* or CPR. Since fewer than 10% of cardiac arrest victims survive the experience (1), CPR can hardly be called effective, yet it is universally embraced as a standard of care. This chapter presents the essential features of CPR as described in the most recent guidelines on the subject (2).

I. BASIC LIFE SUPPORT

Basic life support involves 3 directives: establish and maintain patency of the upper airways, provide ventilation through periodic lung inflations, and promote circulation with chest compressions (3).

A. Airway Patency

1. Airway patency is a concern for all unconscious patients.

2. The oropharyngeal airway, an S-shaped device that is passed over the tongue and into the pharynx, is easily placed and can prevent a flaccid tongue from occluding the oropharynx.

3. Translaryngeal intubation should be the preferred method for maintaining airway patency in the hospital setting, where trained personnel are available.

B. Ventilation

1. Ventilation in BLS means periodic lung inflations with self-inflating "ventilating bags" that are attached to a face mask or endotracheal tube.

2. The recommended rate of lung inflations is 8 to 10 per minute, and it is not necessary to deliver the inflations between chest compressions.

3. The inflation volumes should be just enough to produce a rise in the chest wall, and the inflation time should not exceed one second to allow time for the lungs to empty.

4. *Excessive Ventilation*

   a. There is a tendency to overventilate patients during CPR, which can be counterproductive. In one survey of CPR techniques, the rate of lung inflations was 20/min (double the recommended rate) in 60% of the resuscitations (4).

   b. The problem with rapid breathing and large inflation volumes is the inability of the lungs to fully empty during exhalation. The retained air creates a positive end-expiratory pressure (called *intrinsic PEEP*), and this pressure can reduce cardiac output by impeding venous return and restricting ventricular distension during diastole. This will only add to the high mortality in this situation (5).

   c. To avoid excessive ventilation during CPR, it is imperative to keep the rate of lung inflations at 8–10/minute. Inflation volumes can be reduced by using one hand to compress the ventilating bag. The capacity of these bags is about 1,600 mL, which is about three times greater than the tidal volume of an average-sized adult (about 7 mL/kg, or 500 mL in a 70 kg subject). One-handed compression will expel a volume of about 800 mL, which is closer to the normal tidal volume than completely emptying the bag with two-handed compression.

C. Chest Compressions

1. Chest compressions should be delivered over the mid-

sternum with the elbows locked and the arms straight. Each compression is a thrust delivered through the heel of the hands (one on top of the other) to depress the sternum 1.5 to 2 inches. When the compression is released, the sternum should be allowed to recoil completely before the next compression.

2. The rate of chest compressions should be at least 100 per minute, and a compression-ventilation ratio of 30:2 is recommended (3).

3. It is important to avoid unnecessary interruptions in chest compressions. One survey of CPR revealed that interruptions in chest compressions accounted for one-quarter of the total resuscitation time (4).

II. ADVANCED LIFE SUPPORT

Advanced life support (also called advanced cardiac life support or ACLS) includes measures for ventilatory support (intubation and mechanical ventilation), hemodynamic support (drugs) and cardiac rhythm support (defibrillation). This section describes the use of these support measures in the management of pulseless cardiac arrest. This information is included in the flow diagrams in Figure 13.1 and 13.2.

A. Defibrillation

Direct-current (DC) cardioversion is the treatment of choice for ventricular tachycardia (V-Tach) and ventricular fibrillation (V-Fib), and it is the only treatment modality that has had an impact on survival from cardiac arrest.

1. *Timing*
   a. The survival benefit of electrical cardioversion is a function of the time elapsed from onset of cardiac ar-

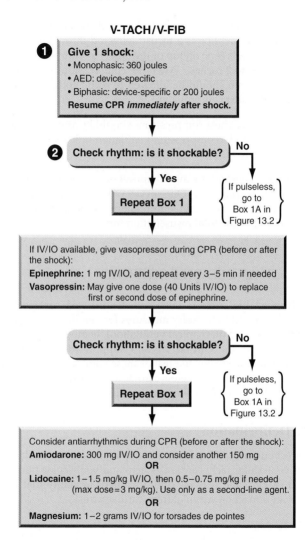

FIGURE 13.1. Flow diagram for the management of pulseless cardiac arrest due to ventricular tachycardia (*V-Tach*) and ventricular fibrillation (*V-Fib*). Adapted from Reference 8.

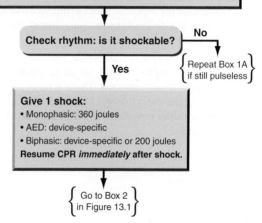

FIGURE 13.2. Flow diagram for the management of cardiac arrest due to asystole or pulseless electrical activity (*PEA*). Adapted from Reference 8.

rest to the first electric shock (6,7). This is demonstrated in Figure 13.3. Note that 40% of patients survived when the first shock was delivered 5 minutes after the arrest, while only 10% of patients survived if defibrillation was delayed for 20 minutes.

b. For out-of-hospital cardiac arrests when the response time exceeds 5 minutes, a brief period of CPR (1.5 to 3 minutes) is recommended prior to the initial countershock. This recommendation is based on evidence that chest compressions can enhance the response to electrical cardioversion (1).

2. *Technical Considerations*

The effectiveness of electric countershocks depends on the type of waveform delivered. Newer defibrillators deliver biphasic shocks, which are effective at lower energy levels than the monophasic shocks used by older defibrillators.

a. The recommended energy level for the first shock is 200 joules for biphasic shocks (unless otherwise specified by the defibrillator manufacturer) and 360 joules for monophasic shocks (11).

b. If the first shock is ineffective, two additional shocks can be attempted (don't forget to perform CPR between successive shocks). There is no evidence that increasing the energy levels in successive shocks is more effective than maintaining the energy level of the initial shock.

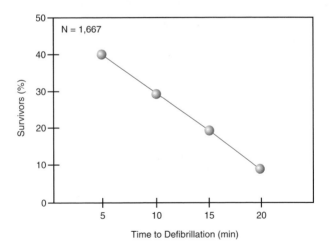

FIGURE 13.3. The relationship between survival rate and time to defibrillation in patients with ventricular fibrillation. N = number of subjects studied. (From Reference 7).

3. *Automated External Defibrillators*

Automated external defibrillators (AEDs) are designed to operate with minimal human input (6).

a. The AED has 2 electrode pads: one is placed on the right anterior chest wall, and the other is placed on the left lateral chest wall.

b. Sensors in the pads act like precordial leads to record the cardiac rhythm. The AED analyzes the rhythm and then displays a prompt indicating if defibrillation is appropriate. The operator does not see the cardiac rhythm. If defibrillation is indicated, the operator simply presses a button to deliver the shock. The machine automatically selects the strength of the pulse.

c. After the shock is delivered, the machine will again analyze the cardiac rhythm and determine if a second shock is necessary. This sequence can continue until three shocks are delivered.

d. AEDs have been used primarily for cardiac arrests that occur outside the hospital, but they are also available in most hospitals as well. The ability to deliver rapid DC cardioversion without introducing human error should make AEDs popular in all settings.

B. Routes of Drug Administration

1. *Intravenous Route*

a. The intravenous route is preferred for drug delivery during CPR, and *peripheral veins are preferred to central veins* because cannulation of peripheral veins does not require interruption of CPR (8).

b. Drugs given via peripheral veins should always be injected as a bolus, followed by a 20 mL bolus of an intravenous fluid (8). The extremity should be elevated for 10 to 20 seconds to facilitate drug delivery to the heart.

c. If the initial drug injection is unsuccessful, central venous cannulation can be performed for subsequent drug administration. This latter maneuver reduces the transit time for drugs to reach the heart by 1 to 2 minutes (8).

2. *Alternate Routes*

a. When venous access is not readily available, drugs can be delivered by puncturing a marrow cavity (usually in the sternum) or injecting the drug into the upper airways.

b. The *intraosseous (IO) route is preferred to the airway route* because drug absorption from the airways is erratic (8). However, the airways route continues to be a popular alternative in adults.

3. *The Endotracheal Route*

a. The drugs that can be given via the endotracheal route are atropine, epinephrine, vasopressin, and lidocaine.

b. The endotracheal dose of each drug should be 2 to 2.5 times the recommended intravenous dose (8).

c. All drugs injected into the airways should be diluted in 5 to 10 mL of water or isotonic saline. Water may be the preferred diluent because of enhanced drug absorption (8).

C. Vasopressor Drugs

Vasopressor drugs are recommended for most cases of pulseless cardiac arrest (see Figures 13.1 and 13.2).

1. *Epinephrine*

a. Epinephrine, which is a β-receptor agonist in low doses and an α-receptor agonist in high doses, is the traditional vasopressor used in cardiac arrest.

b. The recommended dose is 1 mg (10 mL of a 1:10,000 solution) as a bolus injection (IV/IO), repeated every 3 to 5 minutes if necessary (see Table 13.1).

c. Endotracheal epinephrine (usual dose is 2 to 2.5 mg) is not advised because poor absorption can result in prominent β-receptor stimulation and unwanted cardiac stimulation (8).

2. *Vasopressin*

a. Vasopressin is a nonadrenergic vasoconstrictor that can be used in a single bolus dose of 40 Units (IV/IO) to replace the first or second dose of epinephrine.

TABLE 13.1 Cardiopulmonary Resuscitation Drugs

Drug	Dosage (IV or IO)	Indications
Vasopressors		
Epinephrine	1 mg first dose and repeat every 3−5 min if needed	Asystole, PEA, and shock-resistant V-Fib or V-Tach
Vasopressin	40 U as a single dose	Can replace the first or 2nd dose of epinephrine
Antiarrhythmic Agents		
Amiodarone	300 mg first dose, then 150 mg once if needed	V-Fib or V-Tach that is refractory to defibrillation and vasopressors
Lidocaine	1−1.5 mg/kg first dose, then 0.5−0.75 mg/kg to a total of 3 doses or 3 mg/kg	Alternative to amiodarone
Magnesium	1−2 g over 5 minutes	Torsades de pointes associated with a prolonged QT interval
Atropine	1 mg first dose and repeat every 3−5 min if needed to a total of 3 doses	Bradyarrhythmias, or as an adjunct to vasopressors for asystole and slow-rate PEA

From Reference 8.

Abbreviations: IV = intravenous, V-Fib = ventricular fibrillation, V-Tach = ventricular tachycardia, PEA = pulseless electrical activity.

b. The use of vasopressin has two potential benefits: (1) vasopressin acts as a cerebral vasodilator, and (2) there is no risk of unwanted cardiac stimulation from epinephrine. The disadvantage of vasopressin is its actions as a coronary artery vasoconstrictor (8).

c. Several clinical trials have shown *no survival benefit when vasopressin is substituted for epinephrine* (9).

D. Antiarrhythmic Agents

1. *Amiodarone*

   a. Amiodarone is recommended for cases of V-Fib and pulseless V-Tach that are refractory to defibrillation and vasopressor drugs (8,10).

   b. The initial dose is 300 mg (IV/IO), followed by a second dose of 150 mg if needed.

   c. Amiodarone can produce hypotension and bradycardia (10), but these effects have been minimized by a new aqueous formulation that does not contain vasoactive solvents (8).

2. *Lidocaine*

   a. Lidocaine has been the traditional antiarrhythmic agent used for shock-resistant V-Fib and V-Tach. However, because amiodarone seems to produce better results for short-term survival (11), lidocaine is now recommended only as a second-line agent (8).

   b. The recommended dosage of lidocaine is 1–1.5 mg/kg (IV/IO) initially, then 0.5–0.75 mg/kg every 5 to 10 minutes if needed to a maximum of 3 doses or 3 mg/kg.

3. *Magnesium*

   a. Intravenous magnesium is effective in terminating polymorphic V-Tach (also called "torsades de pointes") associated with a prolonged QT interval (see Chapter 15).

b. The recommended dose of magnesium is 1–2 grams (IV/IO) infused over 5 minutes (8).

4. *Atropine*

a. Atropine is an anticholinergic agent that is recommended as an adjunct to vasopressor therapy for cardiac arrest associated with asystole or slow-rate pulseless electrical activity (see Figure 13.2). The recommended dose is 1 mg (IV/IO), which can be repeated every 3 to 5 minutes to a total dose of 3 mg (the dose that produces complete vagal blockade) (8).

III. MONITORING DURING CPR

The goal of the resuscitation effort is to restore circulatory flow. Since it is not possible to directly measure blood flow (global or regional) during CPR, indirect or surrogate measures of blood flow are used. These measurements, which are described below, are limited and sometimes misleading.

A. Arterial Pulse and Pressure

Despite their popularity, the arterial pulse and pressure are not reliable markers of circulatory blood flow. This is demonstrated in Figure 13.4, which shows the effect of chest compressions on the arterial pressure and central venous pressure in a patient with asystole. If the arterial blood pressure is considered in isolation, the size of the pressure pulse (50 mm Hg) would be interpreted as indicating that the chest compressions are successful in promoting systemic blood flow. However, the central venous pressure is roughly the same magnitude as the arterial pressure, indicating that *there is no pressure gradient for systemic blood flow*. Therefore, the arterial pressure in this case is unlikely to be associated with a significant rate of blood flow.

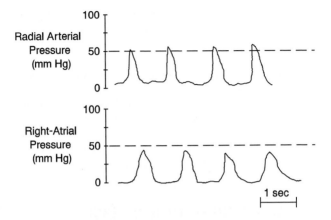

FIGURE 13.4. The influence of chest compressions on arterial and central venous pressure tracings in a patient with asystolic cardiac arrest. Although there is a systolic pressure of 50 mm Hg, the central venous pressure is equivalent, so there is no pressure gradient to drive systemic blood flow.

1. *Mean Arterial Pressure*

   Despite the fact that blood pressure is an unreliable marker of blood flow during CPR, a popular goal of resuscitation is a mean arterial pressure of 60 mm Hg, which is considered the minimum pressure needed for adequate cerebral blood flow.

2. *Coronary Perfusion Pressure*

   a. The pressure gradient that drives coronary blood flow, which is called the *coronary perfusion pressure* (CPP) is the difference between the aortic diastolic pressure and the right-atrial pressure.

   b. Clinical studies have shown that a CPP ≥15 mm Hg during CPR is associated with a successful outcome (12,13).

   c. When CPR is performed on a patient with indwelling arterial and central venous catheters, the CPP can be estimated by using the peripheral arterial diastolic pressure as a substitute for the aortic diastolic pressure.

B. End-Tidal PCO$_2$

The excretion of carbon dioxide in exhaled gas is a direct function of pulmonary blood flow, and the partial pressure of CO_2 in end-expiratory gas (the end-tidal PCO$_2$) can be used as an indirect indicator of cardiac output during CPR (16,18–20). The end-tidal PCO$_2$ is easily measured at the bedside with infrared sensing devices called capnometers that are connected to an artificial airway (i.e., a tracheal tube).

   a. An increase in end-tidal PCO$_2$ during CPR is an indication that the resuscitation effort is successful in promoting cardiac output.

   b. Clinical studies have shown that an increase in end-tidal PCO$_2$ during CPR is predictive of a successful

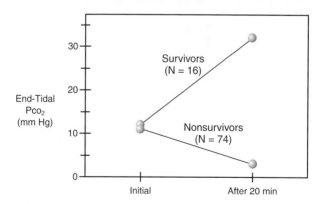

FIGURE 13.5. Changes in end-tidal PCO$_2$ during CPR in survivors and nonsurvivors of cardiac arrest due to pulseless electrical activity. Data points represent the mean end-tidal PCO$_2$ for each group. (From Reference 15).

outcome (12,14,15). This is demonstrated in Figure 13.5. Note that the end-tidal PCO_2 increased (from 12 to 31 mm Hg) after 20 minutes of CPR in the survivors, while the end-tidal PCO_2 decreased during CPR in nonsurvivors.

  c. A threshold of 10 mm Hg for end-tidal PCO_2 can be used to predict outcome: i.e., *when end-tidal PCO_2 does not rise above 10 mm Hg during CPR, the resuscitative effort is unlikely to be successful.*

C. Venous Blood Gases

During CPR, arterial blood gas analysis often reveals a respiratory alkalosis (indicating operator-induced hyperventilation), while venous blood gas analysis often reveals a metabolic acidosis (indicating systemic hypoperfusion) (16,17). Therefore, venous blood gas analysis is more appropriate for evaluating tissue perfusion during CPR.

IV. POST-RESUSCITATION CONCERNS

The immediate goal of CPR is to restore spontaneous circulation, but this does not ensure a satisfactory recovery. This section describes some concerns in the post-resuscitation management that will help to optimize the recovery from cardiac arrest.

A. Fever Suppression

1. Animal studies show that ischemic brain injury is aggravated by increased body temperature (18), and clinical studies show that increased body temperature after CPR is associated with an unfavorable neurologic outcome (19). These studies suggest that it is wise to avoid increased body temperature following cardiac arrest.

2. Acetaminophen (10–15 mg/kg per dose, 3 to 4 times a day) can be used for antipyresis. This drug must be given

enterally, and should not be given to patients with hepatic dysfunction.

3. Cooling blankets are problematic because they can induce shivering (which increases body temperature) and can provoke vasospasm in diseased coronary arteries (20).

TABLE 13.2 Induced Hypothermia after Cardiac Arrest

Eligible Patients

Patients with out-of-hospital cardiac arrest due to V-Fib or V-Tach who remain comatose after return of spontaneous circulation

Inclusion Criteria

All of the following criteria must be satisfied:
   a. Cardiac arrest is cardiac in origin
   b. Body temperature is not reduced
   c. Patient is hemodynamically stable
   d. Patient is intubated and on a ventilator

Methodology
1. Cooling should begin within 1 to 2 hours after CPR.
2. Use cooling blamket to achieve a body temperature of 32°C to 34°C (89.6°F to 93.2°F).
3. Use sedation and neuromuscular blockade to avoid shivering.
4. Watch for hyperkalemia and hyperglycemia during hypothermia
5. Maintain hypothermia for 12–24 hours, and then allow passive rewarming.

From References 21 and 22.

B. Therapeutic Hypothermia

1. Induced hypothermia has been shown to improve neurologic outcome in patients who remain comatose after out-of-hospital cardiac arrest due to V-Fib or V-Tach (21,22).

2. The eligibility criteria for post-CPR hypothermia are listed in Table 13.2, along with important aspects of the methodology.

a. The target body temperature is 32°C to 34°C (89.6°F to 93.2°F), and this should be maintained for no less than 12 hours and no longer than 24 hours (21).

b. External cooling can provoke shivering, which is counterproductive for the reasons stated earlier. Therefore, shivering should be suppressed by administering a neuromuscular blocker (e.g., atracurium).

c. Hypothermia is associated with hyperkalemia (usually mild) and hyperglycemia (27), so vigilance for these changes is warranted.

C. Glycemic Control

1. Hyperglycemia following cardiac arrest is associated with a poor neurologic outcome (23).

2. There are no studies to show that aggressive management of hyperglycemia improves neurologic outcome after cardiac arrest, but this practice has been shown to reduce morbidity and mortality in ICU patients (24).

3. Based on these observations, the recent American Heart Association Guidelines for CPR recommend avoiding hyperglycemia in the post-resuscitation period (25). This goal is accomplished by using insulin infusions when necessary, and avoiding dextrose-containing intravenous solutions when possible. Careful monitoring of blood glucose is necessary during insulin infusions because hypoglycemia can also be injurious to the central nervous system.

D. Predicting Neurologic Outcome

In patients who do not awaken immediately after CPR, the single most important concern is the likelihood of neurologic recovery. The following clinical factors will help to predict the likelihood of a satisfactory neurologic recovery.

1. *Duration of Coma*

   a. Failure to regain consciousness after CPR has prognostic significance if the coma persists for longer than 4 to 6 hours.

   b. Fewer than 15% of patients will recover fully if their coma persists for longer than 4 to 6 hours after cardiac arrest (26).

   c. If a patient is not awake 24 hours after a cardiac arrest, there is only a 10% chance of satisfactory neurologic recovery (26).

   d. A Glasgow Coma Score less than 5 points (see Chapter 40) on the third day following cardiac arrest will identify patients with little or no chance of neurologic recovery (27).

2. *Other Prognostic Signs*

   A review of 11 studies involving patients who did not awaken immediately after CPR identified four clinical signs that act as independent predictors of death or poor neurologic recovery after cardiac arrest (28).

   a. No corneal reflex.

   b. No pupillary light reflex.

   c. No withdrawal to pain.

   d. No motor response.

   The presence of any of these signs 24 hours after cardiac arrest carries a poor prognosis for neurologic recovery.

REFERENCES

1. Ristagno G, Gullo A, Tang W, Weil MH. New cardiopulmonary resuscitation guidelines 2005: Importance of uninterrupted chest compressions. Crit Care Clin 2006; 22:531-538.

2. 2005 American Heart Association Guidelines for Cardiopulmonary Resuscitation and Emergency Cardiovascular Care. Circu-

lation, 2005; 112(Suppl).

3. 2005 American Heart Association Guidelines for Cardiopulmonary Resuscitation and Emergency Cardiovascular Care. Part 4: Adult basic life support. Circulation 2005; 112 (Suppl):IV-19–IV-34.

4. Abella BS, Alvarado JP, Mykelbust H, et al. Quality of cardiopulmonary resuscitation during in-hospital cardiac arrest. JAMA 2005; 293:305-310.

5. Aufderheide TP, Lurie KG. Death by hyperventilation: A common and life-threatening problem during cardiopulmonary resuscitation. Crit Care Med 2004; 32(Suppl):S345-S351.

6. 2005 American Heart Association Guidelines for Cardiopulmonary Resuscitation and Emergency Cardiovascular Care. Part 5: Electrical therapies: Automated external defibrillators, defibrillation, cardioversion, and pacing. Circulation 2005; 112(Suppl):IV-35–IV-46.

7. Larsen MP, Eisenberg M, Cummins RO, Hallstrom AP. Predicting survival from out-of-hospital cardiac arrest: a graphic model. Ann Emerg Med 1993; 22:1652–1658.

8. 2005 American Heart Association Guidelines for Cardiopulmonary Resuscitation and Emergency Cardiovascular Care. Part 7.2: Management of cardiac arrest. Circulation 2005; 112(Suppl):IV-58–IV-66.

9. Aung K, Htay T. Vasopressin for cardiac arrest: a systematic review and meta-analysis. Arch Intern Med 2005; 165:17–24.

10. Kudenchuk PJ, Cobb LA, Copass MK, et al. Amiodarone for out-of-hospital cardiac arrest due to ventricular fibrillation. N Engl J Med 1999; 341:871–878.

11. Dorian P, Cass D, Schwartz B, et al. Amiodarone as compared to lidocaine for shock-resistant ventricular fibrillation. N Engl J Med 2002; 346:884–890.

12. 2005 American Heart Association Guidelines for Cardiopulmonary Resuscitation and Emergency Cardiovascular Care. Part 7.4: Monitoring and medications. Circulation 2005; 112 (Suppl):IV-78–IV-83.

13. Paradis NA, Martin GB, Rivers EP, et al. Coronary perfusion pressure and the return of spontaneous circulation in human cardiopulmonary resuscitation. JAMA 1990; 263:1106–1113.

14. Falk JL, Rackow EC, Weil MH. End-tidal carbon dioxide concentration during cardiopulmonary resuscitation. N Engl J Med 1988; 318:607–611.

15. Wayne MA, Levine RL, Miller CC. Use of end-tidal carbon dioxide to predict outcome in prehospital cardiac arrest. Ann Emerg Med 1995; 25:762–767.

16. Weil MH, Rackow EC, Trevino R. Difference in acid–base state between venous and arterial blood during cardiopulmonary resuscitation. N Engl J Med 1986; 315:153–156.

17. Steedman DJ, Robertson CE. Acid–base changes in arterial and central venous blood during cardiopulmonary resuscitation. Arch Emerg Med 1992; 9:169–176.

18. Hickey RW, Kochanek PM, Ferimer H, et al. Induced hyperthermia exacerbates neurologic neuronal histologic damage after asphyxial cardiac arrest in rats. Crit Care Med 2003; 31:531–535.

19. Zeiner A, Holzer M, Sterz F, et al. Hyperthermia after cardiac arrest is associated with an unfavorable neurologic outcome. Arch Intern Med 2001; 161:2007–2012.

20. Nobel EG, Gang P, Gordon JB, et al. Dilation of normal and constriction of atherosclerotic coronary arteries cause by the cold pressor test. Circulation 1987; 77:43–52.

21. The Hypothermia After Cardiac Arrest Study group. Mild therapeutic hypothermia to improve the neurologic outcome after cardiac arrest. N Engl J Med 2002; 346:549–556.

22. Bernard SA, Gray TW, Buist MD, et al. Treatment of comatose survivors of out-of-hospital cardiac arrest with induced hypothermia. N Engl J Med 2002; 346:557–563.

23. Calle PA, Buylaert WA, Vanhaute OA. Glycemia in the postresuscitation period. The Cerebral Resuscitation Study group. Resuscitation 1989; 17(Suppl):S181–S188.

24. van der Berghe G, Wouters P, Weekers F, et al. Intensive insulin therapy in critically ill patients. N Engl J Med 2001; 345: 1359–1367.

25. 2005 American Heart Association Guidelines for Cardiopulmonary Resuscitation and Emergency Cardiovascular Care. Part 7.5: Postresuscitation support. Circulation 2005; 112(Suppl I): IV-84–IV-88.

26. Levy DE, Caronna JJ, Singer BH, et al. Predicting outcome from hypoxic-ischemic coma. JAMA 1985; 253:1420–1426.

27. Edgren E, Hedstrand U, Kelsey S, et al. Assessment of neurologic prognosis in comatose survivors of cardiac arrest. Lancet 1994; 343:1055–1059.

28. Booth CM, Boone RH, Tomlinson G, Detsky AS. Is this patient dead, vegetative, or severely neurologically impaired? Assessing outcome for comatose survivors of cardiac arrest. JAMA 2004; 291:870–879.

Chapter 14

ACUTE CORONARY SYNDROMES

The management of patients with acute coronary syndromes requires timely interventions (often within hours after the onset of symptoms). These interventions are described here using information from guidelines listed in the bibliography at the end of the chapter (1-3).

I. THE CORONARY SYNDROMES

A. Definitions

Acute coronary syndromes (ACS) are characterized by the sudden onset of coronary insufficiency as a result of thrombotic occlusion of one or more coronary arteries. The following conditions are identified:

1. ST-segment elevation myocardial infarction (STEMI), caused by complete and sustained coronary occlusion.

2. Non-ST-segment elevation myocardial infarction (non-STEMI) and unstable angina (UA), which are caused by partial coronary occlusion or transient occlusion with spontaneous revascularization.

B. Pathogenesis

The seminal event in all these conditions is thrombus formation in one or more coronary arteries. The inciting event is rupture of an atherosclerotic plaque, which exposes the blood to thrombogenic lipids and leads to activation of platelets and clotting factors. The trigger for plaque disruption is not known, but liquefaction caused by local inflammation and inflammatory mediators is believed to be involved.

II. ROUTINE MEASURES

The routine measures used for all patients with ACS are shown in Figure 14.1. These measures should be initiated immediately after ACS is suspected.

A. Relieving Chest Pain

1. *Nitroglycerin*
   a. Nitroglycerin (0.4 mg sublingual tablets or aerosol spray) is given for up to three doses (each 5 minutes apart) to relieve chest pain. If the chest pain persists after 3 doses of nitroglycerin, immediate administration of morphine is indicated.
   b. Intravenous infusion of nitroglycerin is recommended for patients with recurrent chest pain due to unstable angina. The initial dose rate is 5–10 µg/min, and this can be increased by 5–10 µg/min every 5 minutes until pain relief is achieved. (See Chapter 45 for a nitroglycerin dose chart.)
   c. Nitroglycerin is NOT advised in patients who have taken a nitric oxide synthetase inhibitor or phosphodiesterase inhibitor for erectile dysfunction within the past 24 hours (because of the risk for hypotension).

2. *Morphine*

   Morphine is the drug of choice for chest pain that is refractory to nitroglycerin.
   a. The initial dose is 5 mg given by slow intravenous

push (e.g., 1 mg/minute), and this can be repeated every 5 to 10 minutes if necessary. Pain relief can be sustained with a morphine infusion (1–5 mg/hr).

b. Morphine may cause a decrease in blood pressure, which is primarily due to reduced sympathetic nervous system activity. This usually requires no interven-

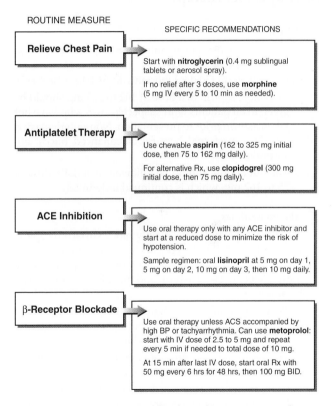

ROUTINE MEASURE

SPECIFIC RECOMMENDATIONS

Relieve Chest Pain

Start with **nitroglycerin** (0.4 mg sublingual tablets or aerosol spray).

If no relief after 3 doses, use **morphine** (5 mg IV every 5 to 10 min as needed).

Antiplatelet Therapy

Use chewable **aspirin** (162 to 325 mg initial dose, then 75 to 162 mg daily).

For alternative Rx, use **clopidogrel** (300 mg initial dose, then 75 mg daily).

ACE Inhibition

Use oral therapy only with any ACE inhibitor and start at a reduced dose to minimize the risk of hypotension.

Sample regimen: oral **lisinopril** at 5 mg on day 1, 5 mg on day 2, 10 mg on day 3, then 10 mg daily.

β-Receptor Blockade

Use oral therapy unless ACS accompanied by high BP or tachyarrhythmia. Can use **metoprolol**: start with IV dose of 2.5 to 5 mg and repeat every 5 min if needed to total dose of 10 mg.

At 15 min after last IV dose, start oral Rx with 50 mg every 6 hrs for 48 hrs, then 100 mg BID.

FIGURE 14.1 Routine measures for the early management of acute coronary syndromes. Abbreviation: ACE = angiotensin-converting-enzyme.

tion. A drop in blood pressure to hypotensive levels usually indicates hypovolemia, and can be corrected by volume infusion (2). Pressor agents should NEVER be used to correct morphine-induced decreases in blood pressure.

B. Antiplatelet Therapy

1. *Aspirin*

   Aspirin causes irreversible inhibition of platelet aggregation by inhibiting thromboxane production (4), and reduces short-term (30 day) mortality in ACS by 2 to 3% (5).

   a. Chewable aspirin in a dose of 162 to 325 mg should be given to all patients with suspected ACS who have not taken aspirin prior to presentation. Non-enteric-coated aspirin is preferred because of enhanced buccal absorption.

   b. The initial dose should be followed by a daily dose of 75 to 162 mg, which is continued indefinitely.

2. *Thienopyridines*

   The thienopyridines irreversibly block surface receptors involved in ADP-induced platelet aggregation (4). This mechanism of action differs from that of aspirin, so the antiplatelet effects of aspirin and the thienopyridines can be additive.

   a. There are 2 drugs in this class: **clopidogrel** (Plavix) and **ticlodipine** (Ticlid). Clopidogrel seems to be preferred because of fewer side effects (4).

   b. The recommended dose of clopidogrel in ACS is 300 mg initially, followed by 75 mg daily (2).

   c. Clopidogrel has been used as a substitute for aspirin. However, combined therapy with clopidogrel and aspirin in ACS is associated with a lower mortality than that seen with aspirin therapy alone (6).

C. β-Receptor Blockade

Beta-receptor blockade is recommended for all patients with ACS except those with contraindications (e.g., bradycardia) and those with cocaine-induced myocardial infarction (because of the risk of coronary vasospasm from unopposed α-receptor activity) (7).

    a. Oral therapy is suitable for most cases of ACS. Intravenous therapy is more appropriate for patients with hypertension or tachyarrhythmias.

    b. The agents used most often are **atenolol** (Tenormin) and **metoprolol** (Lopressor), which are selective β_1-receptor antagonists. The oral and intravenous dosing regimens for metoprolol are shown below (8).

    Oral regimen: Start with intravenous metoprolol dose of 2.5 to 5 mg and repeat every 5 minutes if needed to a total dose of 10 mg. Fifteen minutes after the last IV dose, start oral therapy with 50 mg every 6 hours for 48 hours, then 100 mg BID.

    IV regimen: Add 5 mg metoprolol to 50 mL D_5W and infuse over 15 to 30 minutes. Repeat every 6 hours.

D. Angiotensin-Converting-Enzyme Inhibition

Angiotensin-converting-enzyme (ACE) inhibitors reduce cardiac work, and may also have an inhibitory effect on the cardiac remodeling that contributes to post-MI heart failure.

    1. ACE inhibitors are recommended for all patients with acute MI, but they provide the most benefit in the following conditions (9):

      a. Anterior MI

      b. Acute MI with left ventricular dysfunction (LV ejection fraction <0.40) or symptomatic left heart failure.

      c. Acute MI with tachycardia.

2. Contraindications to ACE inhibitors include hypotension, serum creatinine >2.5 mg/dL, and bilateral renal artery stenosis.

3. Any ACE inhibitor can be used, and the first dose should be given within 24 hours after symptom onset (2). One effective ACE inhibitor regimen is shown in Figure 14.1 (10). Oral therapy only is recommended, to minimize the risk of hypotension.

4. Angiotensin-receptor blockers (ARBs) are considered as a suitable alternative to ACE inhibitors in patients with acute MI complicated by LV dysfunction or heart failure (2). One successful ARB regimen is oral **valsartan** given in a dose of 20 mg initially, followed by a gradual increase to 160 mg twice daily by the end of the hospitalization (11).

III. REPERFUSION THERAPY

Reperfusion therapy is designed to alleviate thrombotic obstruction and restore patency in occluded coronary arteries. There are two approaches to reperfusion: pharmacologic (using thrombolytic agents) and mechanical (using balloon angioplasty).

A. Thrombolytic Therapy

1. *Indications*

Patients are candidates for thrombolytic therapy when all of the following conditions are satisfied.

a. Onset of chest pain between 30 minutes and 12 hours prior to presentation.

b. 12-lead ECG shows ST elevation of at least 0.1 mV (1 mm) in two contiguous leads, or a new left bundle branch block.

c. Coronary angioplasty not immediately available.

d. No hypotension or evidence of heart failure.

e. No contraindication to thrombolytic therapy (see Table 14.1).

Recent guidelines (2) include true posterior MI as an indication for thrombolytic therapy if treatment is started within 12 hours of symptom onset. This condition should be suspected when the ECG shows ST-segment depression with upright T waves in leads V_1 through V_4 (12).

TABLE 14.1 Contraindications to Thrombolytic Therapy

Absolute Contraindications

Active bleeding other than menses

Malignant intracranial neoplasm (primary or metastatic)

Cerebrovascular anomaly (e.g., AV malformation)

Suspected aortic dissection

Ischemic stroke within 3 months (but not within 3 hours)

Prior history of intracranial hemorrhage

Significant closed-head or facial trauma within 3 months

Relative Contraindications

Systolic BP >180 mm Hg or diastolic BP >110 mm Hg

Active bleeding within the past 4 weeks

Noncompressible vascular punctures

Major surgery within the past 3 weeks

Traumatic or prolonged (>10 min) CPR

Ischemic stroke over 3 months ago

Dementia

Active peptic ulcer disease

Pregnancy

Ongoing therapy with anticoagulants

From Reference 2.

---

2. *Timing*

The survival benefit of thrombolytic therapy is greatest

when therapy is initiated in the first few hours after the onset of chest pain. Thereafter, the survival benefit declines steadily with time and is eventually lost 12 hours after symptom onset. To ensure timely initiation of thrombolytic therapy, emergency rooms in the United States have adopted the following guidelines (2):

a. When a patient with sudden onset of chest pain enters the emergency room, a 12-lead ECG should be performed and interpreted within 10 minutes (door-to-ECG time <10 minutes).

b. Thrombolytic therapy, if indicated, should be started within 30 minutes after the patient enters the emergency room (door-to-needle time <30 minutes).

TABLE 14.2 Thrombolytic Agents

Agent	Dose	Comments
Streptokinase (SK)	1.5 million Units IV over 60 min	Less effective and more frequent side effects than alteplase
Alteplase (tPA)	15 mg IV bolus, +0.75 mg/kg over 30 min +0.5 mg/kg over 60 min (90 min total)	Most frequently used lytic agent
Reteplase (rPA)	10 Units as IV bolus and and repeat in 30 min	Bolus doses are easier to give and produce more rapid clot lysis than tPA
Tenecteplase (TNK)	IV bolus of: 30 mg for BW<60 kg 35 mg for BW=60–69 kg 40 mg for BW=70–79 kg 45 mg for BW=80–89 kg 50 mg for BW≥90 kg	Most clot-specific and rapidly acting lytic agent Easiest to use because of single bolus dose

3. *Fibrinolytic Agents*

The available fibrinolytic agents and recommended dosing regimens for acute MI are shown in Table 14.2. All of these agents act by converting plasminogen to plasmin, which then breaks fibrin strands into smaller subunits. Streptokinase acts on circulating plasminogen and produces a systemic lytic state, while the other agents act only on fibrin-bound plasminogen and produce clot-specific lysis. This distinction (clot-specific versus systemic lysis), however, has little clinical relevance.

a. **Streptokinase** was the first thrombolytic agent that showed a survival benefit in acute MI. The popularity of this agent has waned over the years, in part because of troublesome side effects. Streptokinase is a bacterial protein and acts as an antigen to promote fever (20 to 40% of cases), allergic reactions (5% of cases), and accumulation of neutralizing antibodies (with repeated use) (13).

b. **Alteplase** (tissue plasminogen activator or tPA) provides a greater survival benefit than streptokinase (14) and has fewer side effects. It is currently the favored lytic agent for reperfusion therapy, but its popularity is being challenged by newer lytic agents capable of more rapid clot lysis.

c. **Reteplase** (rPA) is a molecular variant of tPA that is given as two bolus doses 30 minutes apart (see Table 14.3). Despite more rapid clot lysis (15), reteplase does not produce better outcomes than alteplase (16).

d. **Tenecteplase** (TNK-tPA) is another variant of tPA that is given as a single bolus. Clot lysis occurs in less time than with the other lytic agents (17), but the mortality rate is no different than with other lytic agents (18).

Excluding streptokinase, there is no clear favorite among the thrombolytic agents in terms of promoting survival in STEMI. However, *bolus therapy with reteplase or tenecte-*

plase should probably be favored because of the more rapid clot lysis (which is desirable even if survival is unaffected) and the simplified dosing regimens.

4. *Bleeding*

   a. The bleeding tendency that haunts thrombolytic therapy is the result of systemic fibrinolysis with depletion of circulating fibrinogen levels.

   b. Intracerebral hemorrhage is the most feared complication of thrombolytic therapy, and occurs in 0.5 to 1% of cases (17). Alteplase, reteplase, and tenecteplase share the same risk for this serious complication.

   c. Troublesome bleeding elsewhere (i.e., that requires blood replacement) occurs in 5 to 15% of patients, regardless of the lytic agent used (19).

   d. The hemostatic defect produced by fibrinolytic agents can be partially corrected by cryoprecipitate administration (10 to 15 bags) to raise the serum fibrinogen level to 1 g/L (19). If bleeding persists, fresh frozen plasma (up to 6 units) will elevate fibrinogen levels further, and will provide volume replacement as well.

   e. Antifibrinolytic agents such as epsilon-aminocaproic acid (5 grams infused over 15 to 30 minutes) should be reserved only for the most serious and refractory cases of bleeding because these agents can promote widespread thrombosis (19).

5. *Reocclusion*

   Reocclusion (occurring within days) is reported in about one of every four patients who receive thrombolytic therapy (2,17). Thrombin released during clot dissolution is believed to be the culprit. This risk of reocclusion has prompted the use of antithrombotic therapy with heparin and antiplatelet agents after successful clot lysis. This adjunctive therapy is described later in the chapter.

B. Coronary Angioplasty

The use of balloon-tipped catheters to open occluded arteries was adapted for use in the coronary arteries in 1977, and this method of *percutaneous coronary angioplasty is now the preferred method of reperfusion in acute coronary syndromes.*

1. *Angioplasty vs. Lytic Therapy*

   Several clinical trials have compared coronary angioplasty and thrombolytic therapy in patients with STEMI who present within 12 hours of symptom onset. The pooled results show a significant reduction in both mortality rate and reinfarction rate when angioplasty is used instead of thrombolytic therapy. *For every 100 patients treated with angioplasty instead of thrombolytic therapy, there are 2 fewer deaths and 4 fewer (non-fatal) reinfarctions* (20).

2. *Timing*

   Clinical trials in patients with STEMI have shown that the survival benefit of angioplasty falls significantly when the procedure is delayed for more than 2 hours after the patient arrives at the hospital (21). This observation has prompted the recommendation that *no more than 90 minutes should elapse from the time the patient arrives in the emergency room and the time the angioplasty is performed* (2).

3. *Interhospital Transfer*

   Less than 25% of hospitals in the United States (and less than 10% of the hospitals in Europe) have the capability to perform coronary angioplasty. One potential remedy for this situation is timely interhospital transfer of patients. Clinical studies have shown that interhospital transfer for coronary angioplasty, if completed in one to two hours, can retain the survival benefit of angioplasty (2,22). The following recommendations have been proposed for hospitals without angioplasty capability (2):

a. If the symptom duration is less than 3 hours, thrombolytic therapy is recommended (because lytic therapy is most effective in this time period) unless interhospital transfer will not delay reperfusion therapy by more than one hour.

b. If the symptom duration is longer than 3 hours, interhospital transfer for angioplasty is recommended. The total door-to-balloon time, including the transfer time, should be close to 90 minutes to achieve the optimal benefit of angioplasty.

IV. ADJUNCTS TO REPERFUSION THERAPY

Antithrombotic therapy with antiplatelet agents and heparin has a proven benefit when used alone or in combination with reperfusion therapy. When used in combination, antithrombotic therapy reduces the risk of reocclusion and reinfarction.

A. Heparin

1. *Which Heparin for Which Condition*

   The following is a summary of the ACC/AHA recommendations for the use of unfractionated heparin (UFH) and low-molecular-weight heparin (LMWH) in acute coronary syndromes (2,3). (See Chapter 3 for a description of the different heparin preparations).

   a. LMWH is preferred to UFH for patients with unstable angina (UA) and non-ST-segment elevation myocardial infarction (non-STEMI) (3,23).

   b. UFH and LMWH are considered equivalent in patients with ST-segment elevation myocardial infarction (STEMI) who do not receive reperfusion therapy (2).

   c. Despite promising results with LMWH (24), UFH is recommended for patients with STEMI who undergo angioplasty or thrombolytic therapy (2).

2. *Dosing Regimens*

The ACC/AHA recommendations for heparin dosing in acute coronary syndromes are shown below (1-3). Enoxaparin is used as the LMWH because this agent has been studied most in clinical trials.

Enoxaparin: Start with an intravenous bolus of 40 mg and follow with subcutaneous injections of 1 mg/kg twice daily for 5 days (3). Reduce the dose in patients with renal insufficiency using the guidelines in Table 14.3.

UFH: Start with an intravenous bolus of 60–70 Units/kg, and follow with an infusion of 12–15 Units/kg/hr. Use the lowest doses (bolus dose of 60 Units/kg and infusion rate of 12 Units/kg/hr) when UFH is combined with thrombolytic therapy and use a larger bolus dose (70 to 100 Units/kg) when UFH is combined with angioplasty. Measure the activated partial thromboplastin time (aPTT) 3 hours after starting the infusion, and adjust the infusion rate to maintain the aPTT at 1.5 to 2 times control (3).

TABLE 14.3 Enoxaparin Dosage Based on Renal Function

GFR[†] (mL/min)	SC Dose (mg/kg q 12h)	GFR[†] (mL/min)	SC Dose (mg/kg q 12h)
≥ 80	1.0	40 – 49	0.6
70 – 79	0.9	30 – 39	0.5
60 – 69	0.8	20 – 29	0.4
50 – 59	0.7	10 – 19	0.3

[†]GFR (mL/min) = (140 – age) × wt (kg)/ 72 × serum creatinine (mg/dL)
For females, multiply GFR by 0.5.

From Green B. et al. Dosing Strategy for enoxaparin in patients with renal impairment presenting with acute coronary syndromes. Br J Clin Pharmacol 2004; 59:281.

B. Aspirin

When used in combination with fibrinolytic agents, aspirin reduces the rate of reinfarction. The dosing regimen for aspirin is described earlier in the chapter.

C. Platelet Glycoprotein Inhibitors

When platelets are activated, specialized glycoproteins on the platelet surface (called IIb/IIIa receptors) change configuration and begin to bind fibrinogen. Fibrinogen binding to adjacent platelets then promotes platelet aggregation. A class of drugs known as *platelet glycoprotein (IIb/IIIa) inhibitors* can bind to the IIb/IIIa receptors on platelets and prevent the binding of fibrinogen. The final result is inhibition of platelet aggregation. Because the IIb/IIIa receptors are the final common pathway for platelet aggregation, the IIb/IIIa inhibitors are the most powerful antiplatelet agents available.

1. *Drug Preparations*

   The platelet glycoprotein inhibitors available for clinical use are included in Table 14.4, along with the dosing regimen for each.

   a. **Abciximab** (try to pronounce it!) is a monoclonal antibody and is the most expensive. most potent, and longest-acting drug in the group. The bleeding time can take 12 hours to normalize after discontinuing this drug (4). This prolonged activity is a disadvantage when emergency coronary bypass surgery is required.

   b. **Eptifibatide** (a synthetic peptide) and **tirofiban** (a tyrosine derivative) are short-acting agents that are cleared by the kidneys. After discontinuing these drugs, bleeding times return to normal in 15 minutes (for eptifibatide) to 4 hours (for tirofiban) (4).

   c. Dose adjustments are recommended for the short-acting agents in patients with renal insufficiency (see Table 14.4). Abciximab is cleared by the reticuloendothelial system and does not require dose adjustments in renal failure.

TABLE 14.4 Platelet Glycoprotein (IIb/IIIa) Inhibitors

Agent	Commercial Preparation	Dosing Regimen
Abciximab	ReoPro	0.25 mg/kg as IV bolus followed by infusion of 0.125 µg/kg/min (maximum 10 µg/min)
Eptifibatide	Integrilin	180 µg/kg as IV bolus followed by infusion of 2 µg/kg/min for up to 96 hours
		For serum creatinine of 2–4 mg/dL, first reduce dose to 130 µg/kg and reduce infusion rate to 0.5 µg/kg/min[†]
Tirofiban	Aggrastat	0.4 µg/kg/min for 30 minutes followed by infusion of 0.1 µg/kg/min
		For creatinine clearance <30 mL/min, reduce both dose rates by 50%.[†]

[†]Manufacturer's recommendation.

2. *Indications*

Platelet glycoprotein inhibitors are primarily used in patients with unstable angina (UA) and non-ST-elevation myocardial infarction (non-STEMI) when the following conditions are present (3):

a. When coronary angioplasty is planned in the next 24 to 48 hours.

b. When there is evidence of continuing myocardial ischemia.

c. When there are risk factors for recurrent ischemic

events, such as age >75 years, heart failure, new or worsening mitral regurgitation, markedly elevated cardiac troponin levels, and cardiogenic shock (3).

The greatest benefit occurs when these agents are used in conjunction with angioplasty (1-3,23), and abciximab is used only when angioplasty is performed. These drugs are also gaining popularity in patients with STEMI, and are usually given in combination with angioplasty or thrombolytic therapy (2,3).

3. *Adverse Effects*

Abnormal bleeding is, of course, the major concern with platelet glycoprotein inhibitors.

   a. Mucocutaneous bleeding is the most common side effect, but the true incidence is difficult to ascertain because these drugs are often given in combination with aspirin and heparin. Intracranial hemorrhage has not been reported in association with these drugs.

   b. Thrombocytopenia is reported in 2% of patients who receive abciximab, and is more common with repeated use of the drug (23).

4. *Contraindications*

   a. Active bleeding is an absolute contraindication to platelet glycoprotein inhibitors.

   b. Relative contraindications include major surgery within the past 3 months, stroke in the past 6 months, systolic pressure >180 mm Hg or diastolic pressure >110 mm Hg, and severe thrombocytopenia (23).

V. EARLY COMPLICATIONS

A. Mechanical Complications

Mechanical complications are usually the result of transmural MI. All are serious, and all require prompt action.

1. *Acute mitral regurgitation* is the result of papillary muscle rupture, and presents with the sudden onset of pulmonary edema and the characteristic holosystolic murmur radiating to the axilla. The pulmonary artery occlusion pressure may reveal prominent V waves, but this can be a nonspecific finding. The diagnosis is confirmed by echocardiography, and arterial vasodilators (e.g., hydralazine) are often needed to relieve pulmonary edema pending surgery. The mortality rate is 70% without surgery and 40% with surgery (24).

2. *Ventricular septal rupture* can develop at any time in the first 5 days after an acute MI. The diagnosis can be elusive without cardiac ultrasound. There is a step-up in O_2 saturation from the right atrium to the pulmonary artery, but this is rarely measured. The initial management involves vasodilator (e.g., nitroglycerin) infusions combined with mechanical support (the intraaortic balloon pump) if needed. The mortality rate is 90% without surgery and 20 to 50% with surgery (2).

3. *Ventricular free wall rupture* occurs in up to 6% of cases of STEMI, and is more common with anterior MI, fibrinolytic or steroid therapy, and advanced age (2). Early manifestations include recurrence of chest pains and new ST-segment abnormalities on the ECG. Accumulation of blood in the pericardium often leads to rapid deterioration and cardiovascular collapse from pericardial tamponade. Diagnosis is made by cardiac ultrasound (if time permits), and prompt pericardiocentesis combined with aggressive volume resuscitation is required for hemodynamic support. Immediate surgery is the only course of action, but fewer than half of the patients survive despite surgery (2).

B. Arrhythmias

Cardiac rhythm disturbances are common after acute MI, and this topic is covered in detail in the next chapter.

C. Cardiac Pump Failure

About 15% of cases of acute MI are accompanied by cardiac pump failure and cardiogenic shock (24). The management involves hemodynamic support (usually with intraaortic balloon counterpulsation) followed by reperfusion using coronary angioplasty or coronary bypass surgery. The mortality rate in cardiogenic shock is high (60 to 80%) (25), despite our best efforts.

1. *Hemodynamic Support*

The goal of hemodynamic support in this situation is to augment cardiac output without increasing myocardial oxygen consumption. Table 14.5 shows the effects of different types of hemodynamic support on the determinants of myocardial O_2 consumption (preload, contractility, afterload, and heart rate) in decompensated heart failure and cardiogenic shock. As indicated by the net effect on myocardial O_2 consumption, vasodilator therapy is superior to dobutamine in heart failure, and the

TABLE 14.5 Hemodynamic Support and Myocardial Oxygen Consumption

Parameter	Heart Failure		Cardiogenic Shock	
	Vasodilators	Dobutamine	IABP	Dopamine
Preload	↓	↓	↓	↑
Contractility	—	↑↑	—	↑↑
Afterload	↓↓	↓	↓	↑
Heart Rate	—	↑	—	↑
Net effect on myocardial VO_2	↓↓↓	↑	↓↓	↑↑↑↑↑

IABP = Intraaortic balloon pump; VO_2 = oxygen consumption.

intraaortic balloon pump (IABP) is superior to dopamine in cardiogenic shock. (See Chapter 12 for more information on the treatment of cardiac pump failure).

2. *Reperfusion Therapy*

   a. The ACC/AHA guidelines recommend coronary angioplasty when cardiogenic shock appears within 36 hours of acute MI and when the angioplasty can be performed within 18 hours of the onset of shock (2).

   b. Coronary artery bypass surgery is considered if the cardiac catheterization reveals multivessel disease that is not suitable for angioplasty, or the obstruction involves the left main coronary artery (2).

VI. ACUTE AORTIC DISSECTION

Aortic dissection is included in this chapter because the clinical presentation can be mistaken as an acute coronary syndrome, and a missed diagnosis can be fatal.

A. Chest Pain

1. Chest pain is the most common complaint in acute aortic dissection. The pain is often sharp, and is described as "ripping or tearing" in about 50% of cases (26). Radiation to the jaws and arms is uncommon.

2. The chest pain in aortic dissection *can subside spontaneously* for hours to days (26,27), and this is a source of missed diagnoses. The recurrence of pain after a pain-free interval is often a sign of impending aortic rupture.

B. Clinical Findings

1. Hypertension and aortic insufficiency are each present in about 50% of cases, and hypotension is reported in 25% of cases (26,27).

2. Dissection can cause obstruction of the left subclavian artery leading to blood pressure differences in the arms. However, this finding is absent in up to 85% of cases (27).

3. Mediastinal widening is evident on routine chest x-rays in 60% of patients with aortic dissection. This finding neither confirms nor excludes the presence of aortic dissection.

C. Diagnosis

1. The diagnosis requires one of four imaging modalities (28):

   a. Magnetic resonance imaging (MRI): sensitivity and specificity 98%.

   b. Contrast-enhanced computed tomography: sensitivity 94%, specificity 87%.

   c. Transesophageal echocardiography: sensitivity 98%, specificity 77%.

   d. Aortography: sensitivity 88%, specificity 94%.

2. MRI is the diagnostic modality of choice for aortic dissection. CT angiography and transesophageal ultrasound are high-yield alternatives to MRI.

D. Management

1. Acute dissection in the ascending thoracic aorta is a surgical emergency.

2. Prompt control of hypertension is warranted prior to surgery to reduce the risk of aortic rupture. The blood pressure reduction should not be accompanied by an increase in cardiac output because increased flow rates in the aorta will create shear forces that promote further dissection.

3. The drug regimens shown in Table 14.6 will reduce blood pressure without increasing cardiac output (26,27). One regimen uses a vasodilator (nitroprusside) infusion com-

bined with a β-blocker (esmolol) infusion. The β-blocker is given first to prevent the vasodilator-induced increase in cardiac output. Esmolol is used as the β-blocker because it has a short duration of action (9 minutes) and thus is easy to titrate. Single-drug therapy with labetalol, a combined α- and β-receptor antagonist, will produce the same result.

TABLE 14.6 Treating Hypertension in Aortic Dissection

Combined therapy with β-blocker and vasodilator:

Start with esmolol:	500 µg/kg bolus and follow with 50 µg/kg/min.
	Increase infusion by 25 µg/kg/min every 5 min until heart rate 60–80 bpm.
	Maximum dose rate is 200 µg/kg/min.
Add nitroprusside:	Start infusion at 0.2 µg/kg/min and titrate upward to desired effect.
	See the nitroprusside dosage chart in Chapter 45.

Monotherapy with combined α-β receptor antagonist:

Labetalol:	20 mg IV over 2 min, then infuse 1–2 mg/min to desired effect and stop infusion.
	Maximum cumulative dose is 300 mg.

REFERENCES

1. 2005 American Heart Association Guidelines for Cardiopulmonary Resuscitation and Emergency Cardiovascular Care. Part 8: Stabilization of the patient with acute coronary syndromes. Circulation 2005; 112(Suppl I):IV89-IV110.

2. Antman EM, Anbe DT, Armstrong PW, et al. ACC/AHA guidelines for the management of patients with ST-elevation myocardial infarction – executive summary: a report of the American College of Cardiology/American Heart Association Task Force

on Practice Guidelines (Writing Committee to Revise the 1999 Guidelines for the Management of Patients with Acute Myocardial Infarction). Circulation 2004; 110:588-636.

3. Braunwald E, Antman EM, Beasley JW, et al. ACC/AHA 2002 guideline update for the management of patients with unstable angina and non-ST-segment myocardial infarction – summary article: a report of the American College of Cardiology/American Heart Association Task Force on Practice Guidelines (Committee on the Management of Patients with Unstable Angina). J Am Coll Cardiol 2002; 40:1366-1374.

4. Patrono C, Coller B, Fitzgerald G, et al. Platelet-active drugs: The relationships among dose, effectiveness, and side effects. Chest 2004; 126:234S-264S.

5. ISIS-2 (Second International Study of Infarct Survival) Collaborative Group. Randomized trial of intravenous streptokinase, oral aspirin, both, or neither among 17,187 cases of suspected acute myocardial infarction: ISIS-2. Lancet 1988; 2:349-360.

6. Clopidogrel in Unstable Angina to Prevent Recurrent Events Trial Investigators. Effects of clopidogrel in addition to aspirin in patients with acute coronary syndromes without ST-segment elevation. N Engl J Med 2001; 345:494-502.

7. Kloner RA, Hale S. Unraveling the complex effects of cocaine on the heart. Circulation 1993; 87:1046-47.

8. Metoprolol succinate and metoprolol tartrate. In: McEvoy GK, ed. AHFS drug information, 2001. Bethesda, MD: American Society for Health System Pharmacists, 2001:1622-1629.

9. ACE Inhibitor Myocardial Infarction Collaborative Group. Indications for ACE inhibitors in the early treatment of acute myocardial infarction: systematic overview of individual data from 100,000 patients in randomized trials. Circulation 1998; 97:2202-2212.

10. Gruppo Italiano per lo Studio della Sopravvivenza nell'infarto Miocardico (GISSI). GISSI-3: effects of lisinopril and transdermal glyceryl trinitrate singly and together on 6-week mortality and ventricular function after acute myocardial infarction. Lancet 1994; 343:1115-1122.

11. Pfeffer MA, McMurray JJ, Velazquez EJ, et al, for the Valsartan in Acute Myocardial Infarction Trial Investigators. Valsartan, captopril, or both in myocardial infarction complicated by heart failure, left ventricular dysfunction, or both. N Engl J Med 2003; 349:1893-1906.

12. Boden WE, Kleiger RE, Gibson RS, et al. Electrocardiographic evolution of posterior acute myocardial infarction: importance of early precordial ST-segment depression. Am J Cardiol 1987; 59: 782-787.

13. Guidry JR, Raschke R, Morkunas AR. Anticoagulants and thrombolytics. In: Blumer JL, Bond GR, eds. Toxic effects of drugs in the ICU. Critical care clinics. Vol. 7. Philadelphia: WB Saunders, 1991; 533–554.

14. GUSTO Investigators. An international randomized trial comparing four thrombolytic strategies for acute myocardial infarction. N Engl J Med 1993; 329:673–682.

15. Smalling RW, Bode C, Kalbfleisch J, et al. More rapid, complete, and stable coronary thrombolysis with bolus administration of reteplase compared with alteplase infusion in acute myocardial infarction. Circulation 1995; 91:2725-2732.

16. GUSTO-III Investigators. An international, multicenter, randomized comparison of reteplase with alteplase for acute myocardial infarction. N Engl J Med 1997; 337:1118-1123.

17. Llevadot J, Giugliano RP, Antman EM. Bolus fibrinolytic therapy in acute myocardial infarction. JAMA 2001; 286:442-449.

18. Assessment of the Safety and Efficacy of a New Thrombolytic (ASSENT-2) Investigators. Single-bolus tenecteplase compared with front-loaded alteplase in acute myocardial infarction. Lancet 1999; 354:716-722.

19. Young GP, Hoffman JR. Thrombolytic therapy. Emerg Med Clin 1995; 13:735–759.

20. Keeley EC, Boura JA, Grines CL. Primary angioplasty versus intravenous thrombolytic therapy for acute myocardial infarction: a quantitative review of 23 randomized trials. Lancet 2003; 361:13-20.

21. Cannon CP, Gibson CM, Lambrew CT, et al. Relationship of symptom onset to balloon time and door-to-balloon time with mortality in patients undergoing angioplasty for acute myocardial infarction. JAMA 2000; 283:2941-2947.

22. Andersen HR, Nielsen TT, Rasmussen K, et al. for the DANAMI-2 Investigators. A comparison of coronary angioplasty with fibrinolytic therapy in acute myocardial infarction. N Engl J Med 2003; 349:733-742.

23. Bhatt DL, Topol EJ. Current role of platelet glycoprotein IIb/IIIa inhibitors in acute coronary syndromes. JAMA 2000; 284:1549-1558.

24. Thompson CR, Buller CE, Sleeper LA, et al. Cardiogenic shock due to acute severe mitral regurgitation complicating acute myocardial infarction: a report from the SHOCK trial registry. J Am Coll Cardiol 2000; 36:1104-1109.

25. Samuels LF, Darze ES. Management of acute cardiogenic shock. Cardiol Clin 2003; 21:43-49.

26. Khan IA, Nair CK. Clinical, diagnostic, and management perspectives of aortic dissection. Chest 2002; 122:311-328.

27. Knaut AL, Cleveland JC. Aortic emergencies. Emerg Med Clin N Am 2003; 21:817-845.

28. Zegel HG, Chmielewski S, Freiman DB. The imaging evaluation of thoracic aortic dissection. Appl Radiol 1995; (June):15–25.

Chapter 15

TACHYCARDIAS

This chapter describes the diagnosis and management of rapid rhythm disturbances using clinical practice guidelines developed by consensus groups in the United States and Europe (see References 1–3).

I. DIAGNOSTIC APPROACH

The diagnostic approach to tachycardias (heart rate >100 beats/minute) can be organized as shown in Figure 15.1. This approach is based on selected components of the electrocardiogram, including 1) the duration of the QRS complex, 2) the uniformity of the R-R intervals, and 3) the pattern of atrial activity.

A. QRS Duration

1. A normal QRS duration (≤ 0.12 second) identifies tachycardias that originate above the AV conduction system. These *narrow QRS complex tachycardias* (also called supraventricular tachycardias) include sinus tachycardia, atrial tachycardias, AV nodal re-entrant tachycardia (a type of paroxysmal supraventricular tachycardia), atrial flutter and atrial fibrillation (see Figure 15.1).

2. A prolonged QRS duration (> 0.12 seconds) is most often the result of a tachycardia that originates below the AV conduction system; i.e., ventricular tachycardia (VT). Occasionally, a wide QRS complex tachycardia is the result of a supraventricular tachycardia (SVT) with prolonged conduction through the AV node.

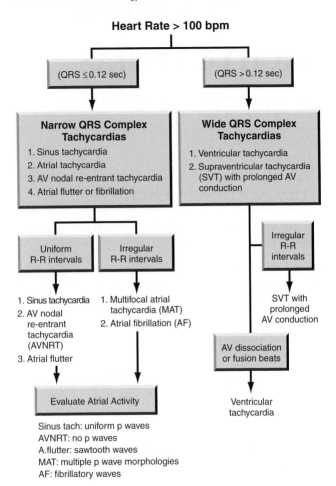

FIGURE 15.1. Flow diagram for the evaluation of tachycardias using selected criteria from the electrocardiogram.

B. Uniformity of the R-R intervals

The regularity of the cardiac rhythm is determined by the

distance between R waves (the R-R interval) in a series of consecutive heart beats. (A regular rhythm will produce R-R intervals that are uniform in length from beat to beat). The diagnostic implications of uniform and non-uniform R-R intervals is shown in Figure 15.1, and is summarized below.

1. *Narrow QRS Complex Tachycardias*

   a. If the R-R interval is uniform (indicating a regular rhythm), the possible rhythms include sinus tachycardia, AV nodal re-entrant tachycardia, and atrial flutter.

   b. If the R-R interval is non-uniform (indicating an irregular rhythm), the most likely rhythms are multifocal atrial tachycardia and atrial fibrillation.

2. *Wide QRS Complex Tachycardias*

   a. A uniform R-R interval does not help to distinguish ventricular tachycardia from an SVT with prolonged AV conduction. In this situation, look for AV dissociation or fusion beats, which are evidence of ventricular tachycardia (these ECG findings are described later in the chapter)

   b. An irregular R-R interval is evidence of an SVT with prolonged AV conduction.

C. Atrial Activity

The pattern of atrial activity can be very useful in identifying the cause of a narrow QRS complex tachycardia, as indicated at the bottom of Figure 15.1.

1. For a narrow QRS complex tachycardia with a regular rhythm:

   a. The presence of uniform p waves and a fixed PR interval is evidence of a sinus tachycardia.

   b. The absence of p waves is evidence of an AV nodal re-entrant tachycardia (see Figure 15.2).

   c. The presence of sawtooth waves is evidence of atrial flutter.

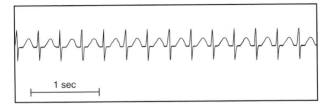

FIGURE 15.2 AV nodal re-entrant tachycardia, a type of paroxysmal supraventricular tachycardia (PSVT). Note the absence of p waves, which are hidden in the QRS complexes.

2. For a narrow QRS complex tachycardia with an irregular rhythm (see Figure 15.3):

a. The presence of multiple p wave morphologies is evidence of multifocal atrial tachycardia.

b. The presence of fibrillatory waves is evidence of atrial fibrillation.

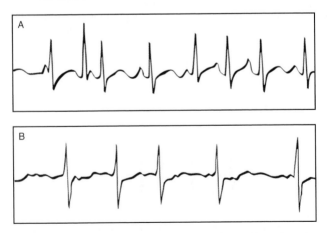

FIGURE 15.3. Narrow QRS complex tachycardias with an irregular rhythm. Panel A is a multifocal atrial tachycardia (note the multiple p wave morphologies and variable PR intervals) and panel B is atrial fibrillation. (From the CD ROM provided with Critical care nursing: A holistic approach. Philadelphia: Lippincott Williams & Wilkins, 2005.)

II. ATRIAL FIBRILLATION

Atrial fibrillation (AF) is the most prevalent cardiac arrhythmia, affecting about 1% of the adult population (3).

A. Predisposing Factors

1. Most patients with AF are elderly (median age 75 years) and have underlying heart disease. About 15% are younger (<60 yrs) and have no comorbid conditions (3). This latter condition is known as *lone atrial fibrillation.*

2. Hyperthyroidism is considered the major extracardiac source of AF, but the importance of this condition may be overestimated. In one survey of nursing home residents with AF, not a single case of hyperthyroidism was discovered (4).

3. AF is very common in the first 3 to 4 days after cardiac surgery. The incidence is 30% following coronary artery bypass surgery and 60% following valve surgery (5). The etiology is unclear, but 90% of cases convert spontaneously to sinus rhythm within 2 months (3).

B. Adverse Consequences

1. *Cardiac Performance*
   a. The principal threat from AF is impaired ventricular filling. The contributing factors are loss of atrial contractions (which normally contribute 25% of the ventricular end-diastolic volume) and a rapid heart rate (which reduces diastolic filling time). Diastolic dysfunction (e.g., from left ventricular hypertrophy) magnifies the deleterious effects of AF on ventricular filling.
   b. Cardiac stroke output will decrease in response to the change in ventricular filling, but the magnitude of change will depend on several factors (e.g., the presence and severity of systolic dysfunction).

2. *Atrial Thrombosis*

Thrombus formation in the left atrium can be apparent 72 hours after the onset of AF (7). These thrombi can (and do) break loose and enter the cerebral circulation to produce embolic stroke. The management issues related to atrial thrombosis in AF are described later in the chapter.

C. DC Cardioversion

Direct-current (DC) cardioversion, which is a painful and anxiety-provoking experience for awake patients, should be reserved only for cases of AF with severe hemodynamic compromise (hypotension or acute pulmonary edema). The following protocol has proven successful in 90% of cardioversion attempts (3):

1. Premedication with an opiate (morphine or fentanyl) is advised, and will provide both analgesia and sedation.

2. The DC shocks should be synchronized to the R wave of the QRS complex to avoid electrical stimulation during the vulnerable period of ventricular repolarization, which usually coincides with the peak of the T wave (3).

3. If the defibrillator is an older model that delivers monophasic shocks, begin with 200 joules (J) for atrial fibrillation and 50 J for atrial flutter. If additional shocks are needed, increase the energy level by 100 J for each shock until a maximum strength of 400 J is reached.

4. For biphasic shocks (the waveform used by newer model defibrillators), follow the protocol for monophasic shocks but decrease the energy of each shock by 50%.

D. Pharmacologic Cardioversion

1. *Indications*

Acute cardioversion with an antiarrhythmic agent is

appropriate for *first episodes of AF that are less than 48 hours in duration and are not associated with hemodynamic compromise*. Successful cardioversion in this situation will avoid the need for long-term anticoagulation. The decision to attempt cardioversion must be weighed against the fact that 50% of cases of new-onset AF convert spontaneously to sinus rhythm in the first 72 hours (6).

2. **Drug Regimen**

The most successful antiarrhythmic agent for acute termination of AF is **ibutilide** (see dose recommendation in Table 15.1). Successful cardioversion is achieved in over 50% of cases, and 80% of the responses occur within 30 minutes of drug administration (7). The only risk associated with ibutilide is torsades de pointes (described later), which is reported in 4% of cases (7).

E. Acute Rate Control

When there is no immediate threat to life, the management of AF is directed at slowing the heart rate to a target level of 60 to 80 bpm (3). This is accomplished with the drug regimens shown in Table 15.1. The drugs in this table share the ability to slow impulse transmission through the AV node.

1. *Diltiazem*

   a. Diltiazem is a calcium-channel blocker that *achieves satisfactory rate control in 85% of patients with AF* (8). The acute response dissipates in 1–3 hours, so a continuous infusion (5 to 15 mg/hr) is recommended to maintain rate control.

   b. Diltiazem has negative inotropic actions, but is generally safe to use in patients with systolic heart failure (3).

2. β-*Blocker*s

   a. β-Blockers are preferred for rate control when AF is associated with hyperadrenergic states (e.g., after cardiac surgery).

TABLE 15.1 Acute Pharmacotherapy of Atrial Fibrillation

Drug	Dose Regimen	Comments
Cardioversion		
Ibutilide	1 mg IV over 10 min and repeat once if needed.	Successful cardioversion in 50% of cases, usually within 30 min.
Acute Rate Control		
Diltiazem	0.25 mg/kg IV over 2 min, then 0.35 mg/kg 15 min later if needed. Follow with infusion of 5–15 mg/hr for 24 hr.	Effective rate control in 85% of patients. Safe to use in patients with heart failure.
Esmolol	500 µg/kg IV over 1 min, then infuse at 50 µg/kg/min. Increase dose rate by 25 µg/kg/min every 5 min if needed to maximum of 200 µg/kg/min.	Ultra-short-acting ß-blocker that permits rapid dose titration.
Metoprolol	2.5–5 mg IV over 2 min. Repeat every 10–15 min if needed to total of 3 doses.	Bolus dosing regimen not optimal for precise rate control.
Amiodarone	300 mg IV over 15 min, then 45 mg/hr for 24 hr.	A suitable alternative for patients who do not tolerate more effective rate-reducing drugs.

From Reference 3. Amiodarone dose regimen from Reference 17.

b. The β-blockers with proven efficacy in AF include **esmolol** and **metoprolol**. Esmolol is preferred for acute rate control because it is ultra–short-acting (serum half-life of 9 minutes) and the dose rate can be titrated rapidly to maintain the desired heart rate (9).

3. *Amiodarone*

 a. When given as recommended in Table 15.1, amiodarone will produce satisfactory rate reduction in 75% of patients with AF (10).

 b. Amiodarone is less effective than diltiazem, but it produces less cardiac depression and hypotension than diltiazem (10). This creates a possible niche for amiodarone in patients who do not tolerate diltiazem.

 c. The adverse effects of intravenous amiodarone include hypotension (15%), infusion phlebitis (15%), bradycardia (5%), and elevated liver enzymes (3%) (7,11).

 d. There are several potential drug interactions because amiodarone is metabolized by the cytochrome P450 enzyme system in the liver. The interactions with digoxin and warfarin (blood levels increased by amiodarone) are most relevant in the ICU (11).

F. Antithrombotic Therapy

The risk of atrial thrombosis and subsequent embolic stroke is one of the major concerns in patients with AF.

1. *Risk Categories*

 There are 3 risk categories for embolic stroke (high, moderate, and low risk), and Table 15.2 shows the clinical characteristics for each category, along with the therapeutic recommendations.

 a. For patients in the high risk category, the incidence of embolic stroke is 6% per year without treatment, and 3% per year with coumadin anticoagulation to achieve an INR of 2 to 3. (12)

 b. Patients in the moderate-risk category have a 2% annual incidence of embolic stroke (which is lower than the incidence reported during anticoagulation therapy with coumadin). Antiplatelet therapy with aspirin (325 mg daily) is recommended for these patients.

c. Patients with lone atrial fibrillation (i.e., AF without comorbid conditions in a patient younger than 60 yrs of age) have the same risk of embolic stroke as the general population, so antithrombotic therapy is not required in these patients.

2. *Cardioversion*

For cardioversion of AF that is less than 48 hours in duration, the risk of embolism with cardioversion is low (<1%), so anticoagulation is not needed prior to cardioversion (3). When the duration of AF exceeds 48 hours, the risk of embolization with cardioversion is about 6%, and anticoagulation is recommended for 3 weeks before cardioversion is attempted.

TABLE 15.2 Antithrombotic Therapy & Risk of Embolic Stroke

High Risk

  I. Oral Anticoagulation (INR = 2 – 3)

    Age > 75 yrs

    Age ≥ 60 yrs plus diabetes or coronary artery disease

    Heart failure with LV ejection fraction < 0.35

    Heart failure with hypertension or thyrotoxicosis

    Prosthetic heart valves (mechanical or tissue)

    Rheumatic mitral valve disease

    Prior thromboembolism

Moderate Risk

  II. Antiplatelet Therapy (Aspirin, 325 mg daily)

    Age < 60 yrs with heart disease, but no risk factors[†]

    Age ≥ 60 yrs with no risk factors[†]

Low Risk

  III. No Therapy Required

    Age < 60 yrs and no heart disease *(Lone AF)*

[†]Risk factors include heart failure, LV ejection fraction <0.35. and a history of hypertension.

G. Wolff–Parkinson–White (WPW) Syndrome

1. The WPW syndrome (short P–R interval and delta waves before the QRS) is characterized by recurrent supraventricular tachycardias that originate from an accessory (re-entrant) pathway in the AV conduction system (2). One of these tachycardias is atrial fibrillation.

2. *In cases of AF associated with WPW syndrome, calcium-channel blockers and digoxin are contraindicated* because these drugs can paradoxically accelerate the ventricular rate (by blocking the wrong pathway).

3. The treatment of choice for this type of tachycardia is electrical cardioversion or cardioversion with procainamide. (The procainamide dosing regimen is: 100 mg IV over 2 minutes, then up to 25 mg/min IV to a maximum of one gram in the first hour, then 2 to 6 mg/min.)

III. MULTIFOCAL ATRIAL TACHYCARDIA

A. Features

Multifocal atrial tachycardia (MAT) is a narrow QRS tachycardia with an irregular rhythm, and is characterized by multiple p wave morphologies and a variable P–R interval (see Figure 15.3). It is seen most often in the elderly (average age = 70), and over half of the cases occur in patients with chronic lung disease (13).

B. Acute Management

MAT can be difficult to manage, but the following measures can be effective.

1. Start with intravenous **magnesium**: mix 2 grams $MgSO_4$ in 50 mL saline and infuse over 15 minutes, then mix 6

grams $MgSO_4$ in 500 mL saline and infuse over 6 hours (14). This regimen has been successful in converting MAT to sinus rhythm in 88% of attempts, even when serum magnesium levels are normal. The mechanism is unclear, but the actions of magnesium as a calcium-channel blocker may be responsible.

2. Correct hypomagnesemia and hypokalemia if present. If these electrolyte disorders co-exist, the magnesium deficiency must be corrected before potassium replacement is started. (The reason for this is explained in Chapter 28). Use the following replacement protocol: 2 mg $MgSO_4$ (in 50 mL saline) IV over 15 minutes, then 40 mg potassium IV over 1 hour.

3. If the above measures are ineffective, give IV **metoprolol** (a β-blocker) as directed in Table 15.1. This regimen has been successful in converting MAT to sinus rhythm in as many as 80% of attempts (13).

   a. If metoprolol cannot be given safely (e.g., patient has reactive airways disease), give **verapamil** (a calcium-channel blocker) in a dose of 7–150 mg/kg IV over 2 minutes (3). Verapamil converts MAT to sinus rhythm in less than 50% of cases, but it can also slow the ventricular rate. Watch for hypotension, which is a common side effect of verapamil.

IV. PAROXYSMAL SUPRAVENTRICULAR TACHYCARDIA

A. Features

1. Paroxysmal supraventricular tachycardia (PSVT) is a narrow QRS complex tachycardia with a regular rhythm and an abrupt onset.

2. The source of these arrhythmias is an *accessory pathway* that conducts impulses at a different speed than the normal conduction pathways. The difference in conduction velocities allows an impulse traveling down one pathway (antegrade transmission) to travel up the other pathway (retrograde transmission). This circuitous transmission of impulses creates a self-sustaining *re-entrant tachycardia*. The trigger is an ectopic impulse that travels through one of the pathways.

3. There are 5 different types of PSVT, each with a different location for the accessory pathway. The most common is *AV nodal re-entrant tachycardia*, where the accessory pathway is in the AV node.

B. AV Nodal Re-entrant Tachycardia

1. *Features*

   a. AV nodal re-entrant tachycardia (AVNRT) is a narrow QRS complex tachycardia with a regular rhythm and a rate between 140 and 220 bpm. It differs from sinus tachycardia in that the onset is abrupt and there are no discernible p waves on the ECG (see Figure 15.2).

   b. This arrhythmia is typically seen in relatively young adults with no comorbid conditions who complain of the sudden onset of palpitations, dyspnea, and chest pains.

2. *Adenosine*

   a. Adenosine is an endogenous purine nucleotide that briefly depresses activity in the sinus and AV nodes. When given by rapid intravenous injection, adenosine terminates AV re-entrant tachycardias in over 90% of cases (15). The effect is usually apparent within 30 seconds, and the AV block lasts only 1–2 minutes.

   b. A summary of the clinical use of adenosine is presented in Table 15.3

c. Note that peripheral veins are preferred for adenosine injection. This is based on reports showing that adenosine injection (in standard doses) through central venous catheters can provoke brief periods of cardiac standstill (16). If a central venous catheter is used for adenosine injection, the dose must be reduced by 50%.

d. Side effects are common after adenosine injection, but most disappear rapidly because of adenosine's ultra-short duration of action. One of the troublesome side effects is bronchoconstriction in asthmatic subjects (17), which is why adenosine should NOT be used in patients with asthma.

TABLE 15.3 Adenosine for AV Nodal Re-entrant Tachycardia

I. Injection site:
   Use a peripheral vein for drug injection if possible.
   If a central vein is used, reduce adenosine dose by 50%.

II. Dosing Regimen:
   1. Give 6 mg by rapid injection and follow with 20 mL saline flush.
   2. If no response after 2 min, give a second dose of 12 mg.
   3. The 12 mg dose can be repeated once if necessary.

III. Transient Reactions:
   • Facial flushing (50%)
   • Sinus bradycardia, AV block (50%)
   • Dyspnea (35%)
   • Chest pain (20%)
   • Nausea, headache, dizziness (5–10%)

IV. Drug Interactions:
   • Theophylline antagonizes the actions of adenosine.
   • Adenosine effect is enhanced by ß-blockers, calcium-channel blockers, and dipyridamole. (Reduce adenosine dose 50%).

V. Contraindications: Asthma, AV block, sick sinus syndrome

AV = atrioventricular. From References 15–17.

3. *Calcium-Channel Blockers*

In uncommon cases where adenosine is ineffective or not tolerated, calcium-channel blockers can be used to terminate AVNRT. One recommended drug regimen is shown below (18):

Diltiazem: 0.25 mg/kg IV over 2 minutes. If no response, give 0.35 mg/kg over 2 minutes. After conversion to sinus rhythm, infuse at 5–15 mg/hr for 24 hours.

It is very important to rule out Wolff-Parkinson-White (WPW) syndrome as a cause of the PSVT before giving calcium-channel blockers because of the potential for these drugs to increase the ventricular rate in tachycardias associated with WPW (see earlier in the chapter).

V. VENTRICULAR TACHYCARDIA

Ventricular tachycardia (VT) is a wide QRS complex tachycardia that has an abrupt onset, a regular rhythm, and a rate above 100 bpm. VT that lasts longer than 30 seconds (sustained VT) is a potentially life-threatening arrhythmia that requires prompt attention.

A. VT versus SVT

VT can be difficult to distinguish from an SVT with prolonged conduction through the AV node. This is demonstrated in Figure 15.4 The tracing in the upper panel shows a wide QRS complex tachycardia that looks like VT. The tracing in the lower panel shows spontaneous conversion to sinus rhythm. Note that the QRS complex remains unchanged after the arrhythmia is terminated, revealing an underlying bundle branch block. Thus, the apparent VT in the upper panel is actually a paroxysmal SVT with a pre-existing bundle branch block.

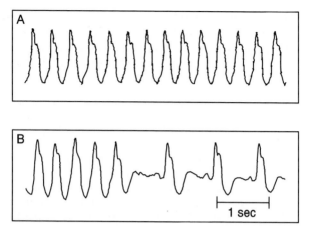

FIGURE 15.4. An apparent VT (upper panel) that is actually an SVT with aberrant (prolonged) AV conduction. The correct diagnosis is evident only when spontaneous conversion to sinus rhythm (in the lower panel) reveals a pre-existing bundle branch block. (Tracings courtesy of Dr. Richard M. Greenberg, M.D.).

1. *Evidence of VT*

   The presence of either of the following ECG abnormalities is evidence that the rhythm disturbance is VT.

   a. AV DISSOCIATION. The atria and ventricles beat independently in VT, so the lack of a fixed relationship between P waves and QRS complexes is evidence of VT.

   b. FUSION BEATS. A fusion beat is an irregularly-shaped QRS complex that just precedes the onset of VT. These complexes are the result of retrograde transmission of a ventricular ectopic impulse that merges (fuses) with a normal QRS complex. The presence of a fusion beat is therefore evidence of ventricular ectopic activity.

2. *Primary Heart Disease*

   A simplified approach to distinguishing VT from SVT with aberrant conduction is to consider the presence or absence of heart disease.

   a. VT is the cause of 95% of wide complex tachycardias
      in patients with primary heart disease (19).

   b. Therefore, *a wide QRS complex tachycardia in any patient*
      with primary heart disease should be treated as VT.

B. Acute Management

The management of patients with a wide QRS complex
tachycardia can proceed as follows. This approach is organized in a flow diagram in Figure 15.5.

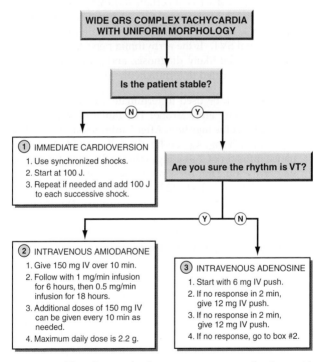

FIGURE 15.5. Flow diagram for the acute management of patients with
wide QRS complex tachycardias. (From Reference 1).

1. If there is evidence of hemodynamic compromise, initiate DC cardioversion immediately with an initial shock of 100 J, followed by repetitive shocks of 200, 300, and 360 J, if necessary. This is necessary regardless of whether the rhythm is VT or SVT with aberrant conduction.

2. If there is no evidence of hemodynamic compromise and the diagnosis of VT is certain, start intravenous **amiodarone** to terminate the arrhythmia (see Figure 15.5 for the amiodarone dosing regimen) (1).

3. If there is no evidence of hemodynamic compromise and the diagnosis of VT is uncertain, *intravenous adenosine can help to unmask a paroxysmal SVT*. Adenosine will not terminate VT, but it will abruptly terminate most cases of paroxysmal SVT. If the arrhythmia persists after adenosine, VT is the likely diagnosis, and intravenous amiodarone is indicated to terminate the rhythm.

4. **Lidocaine** can be used to terminate VT in patients who do not tolerate amiodarone. The initial dose is 1 to 1.5 mg/kg by bolus injection. After 5 minutes, a second dose of 0.5 to 0.75 mg/kg can be given if needed. A maintenance infusion of 2 to 4 mg/min can be used for continued arrhythmia suppression. Lidocaine infusions should not extend beyond 6 to 12 hours because prolonged infusions can produce an excitatory neurotoxic syndrome.

VI. TORSADES DE POINTES

A. General Features

1. Torsades de pointes ("twisting around the points") is a polymorphic VT that is associated with a prolonged QT interval (20). The name derives from the appearance of the QRS complexes as twisting around the isoelectric line of the ECG (see Figure 15.6).

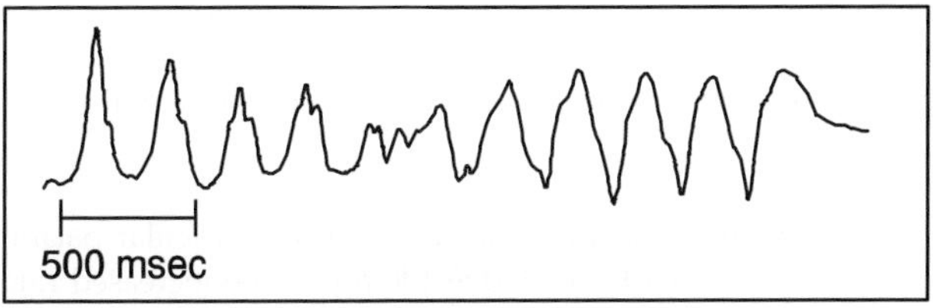

FIGURE 15.6. Torsades de pointes, a polymorphic ventricular tachycardia that appears to be twisting around the isoelectric line of the ECG. (Tracing courtesy of Dr. Richard M. Greenberg, M.D.).

2. Polymorphic VT with a normal QT interval is not torsades de pointes, and is simply called polymorphic VT.

3. *Measuring the QT Interval*

   The QT interval is usually measured in limb lead II, and must be corrected for the heart rate. The rate-corrected QT interval (QTc) is equivalent to the measured QT interval divided by the square root of the R-R interval (21).

   $$\textbf{QTc = QT/}\sqrt{\textbf{RR}} \qquad (15.1)$$

   A prolonged QT interval is defined as a QTc > 0.44 seconds.

B. Etiologies

Torsades de pointes can be congenital (idiopathic) or acquired. The acquired form is caused by a variety of drugs and electrolyte disorders that prolong the QT interval.

1. The drugs that can trigger this arrhythmia are listed in Table 15.4 (22,23).

2. The electrolyte disorders that may be responsible are hypokalemia, hypomagnesemia, or hypocalcemia (20).

C. Management

The management of polymorphic VT with a normal QT

interval is the same as described for monomorphic VT (i.e., amiodarone). The management of torsades de pointes depends on whether the QT prolongation is congenital or acquired.

1. The congenital form is managed with ventricular pacing to raise the heart rate above 100 bpm. The increased rate shortens the QT interval and reduces the tendency for VT.

2. The acquired form is treated as follows:

   a. Use intravenous magnesium (Mg^{++}) for acute management: Start with 2 grams Mg^{++} (as $MgSO_4$) injected over one minute, and repeat 10 minutes later if needed. Follow with a continuous infusion of 1 gram Mg^{++} per hour for the next 6 hours.

   b. Identify and discontinue any drugs that prolong the QT interval.

   c. Identify and correct any relevant electrolyte abnormalities. Mg^{++} deficiency is the principal concern here, particularly since hypokalemia and hypocalcemia can be the result of an underlying Mg^{++} deficiency. (For more information on Mg^{++} deficiency, see Chapter 28).

TABLE 15.4 Drugs That Can Trigger Torsades de Pointes

Antiarrhythmics	Anti-microbials	Anti-psychotics	Others
IA { Quinidine	Clarithromycin	Chlorpromazine	Cisapride
IA { Procainamide	Erythromycin	Haloperidol	Droperidol
Flecainide	Gatifloxacin	Thioridazine	Methadone
III { Ibutilide	Levofloxacin		
III { Sotalol	Pentamidine		

From References 22,23.

REFERENCES

1. 2005 American Heart Association Guidelines for Cardiopulmonary Resuscitation and Emergency Cardiovascular Care. Part 7.3: Management of symptomatic bradycardia and tachycardia. Circulation 2005; 112 (Suppl I):IV67–IV77.

2. Blomstrom-Lunqvist C, Scheinmann MM, Haliot EM, et al. ACC /AHA/ESC guidelines for the management of patients with supraventricular arrhythmias: a report of the American College of Cardiology/American Heart Association Task Force on Practice Guidelines and the European Society of Cardiology Committee on Practice Guidelines. J Am Coll Cardiol 2003; 42:1493–1531.

3. Fuster V, Ryden LE, Asinger RW, et al. ACC/AHA/ESC guidelines for the management of patients with atrial fibrillation: a report of the American College of Cardiology/American Heart Association Task Force on Practice Guidelines and the European Society of Cardiology Committee on Practice Guidelines and Policy Conferences. J Am Coll Cardiol 2001; 38:1266i–lxx.

4. Siebers MJ, Drinka PJ, Vergauwen C. Hyperthyroidism as a cause of atrial fibrillation in long-term care. Arch Intern Med 1992; 152:2063–2064.

5. Hogue CW, Creswell LL, Gutterman DD, Fleisher LA. American College of Chest Physicians guidelines for the prevention and management of postoperative atrial fibrillation after cardiac surgery. Epidemiology, mechanisms, and risks. Chest 2005; 128 (Suppl):9S–16S.

6. Danias PG, Caulfield TA, Weigner MJ, et al. Likelihood of spontaneous conversion of atrial fibrillation to sinus rhythm. J Am Coll Cardiol 1998; 31:588–592.

7. VerNooy RA, Mounsey P. Antiarrhythmic drug therapy in atrial fibrillation. Cardiol Clin 2004; 22:21–34.

8. Ellenbogen KA, Dias VC, Plumb VJ, et al. A placebo-controlled trial of continuous intravenous diltiazem infusion for 24-hour heart rate control during atrial fibrillation and atrial flutter: a multicenter study. J Am Coll Cardiol 1991; 18:891–897.

9. Gray RJ. Managing critically ill patients with esmolol. An ultra-short-acting β-adrenergic blocker. Chest 1988; 93:398–404.

10. Karth GD, Geppert A, Neunteufl T, et al. Amiodarone versus diltiazem for rate control in critically ill patients with atrial tachyarrhythmias. Crit Care Med 2001; 29:1149–1153.

11. Chow MSS. Intravenous amiodarone: pharmacology, pharmaco-kinetics, and clinical use. Ann Pharmacother 1996; 30:637–643.

12. Ezekowitz MD, Falk RH. The increasing need for anticoagulant therapy to prevent stroke in patients with atrial fibrillation. Mayo Clin Proc 2004; 79:904–913.

13. Kastor J. Multifocal atrial tachycardia. N Engl J Med 1990; 322: 1713–1720.

14. Iseri LT, Fairshter RD, Hardeman JL, Brodsky MA. Magnesium and potassium therapy in multifocal atrial tachycardia. Am Heart J 1985; 312:21–26.

15. Chronister C. Clinical management of supraventricular tachycardia with adenosine. Am J Crit Care 1993; 2:41–47.

16. McCollam PL, Uber W, Van Bakel AB. Adenosine-related ventricular asystole. Ann Intern Med 1993;118:315–316.

17. Cushley MJ, Tattersfield AE, Holgate ST. Adenosine-induced bronchoconstriction in asthma. Am Rev Respir Dis 1984; 129:380–384.

18. Opie LH. Calcium channel blockers. In: Opie LH, Gersh BJ, eds. Drugs for the Heart, 5th ed. Philadelphia: WB Saunders, 2001:53–83.

19. Akhtar M, Shenasa M, Jazayeri M, et al. Wide QRS complex tachycardia. Ann Intern Med 1988; 109:905–912.

20. Vukmir RB. Torsades de pointes: a review. Am J Emerg Med 1991; 9:250–262.

21. Garson A Jr. How to measure the QT interval: what is normal? Am J Cardiol 1993; 72:14B–16B.

22. Frothingham R. Rates of torsades de pointes associated with ciprofloxacin, oflaxacin, levofloxacin, gatifloxacin, and moxifloxacin. Pharmacotherapy 2001; 21:1468–1472.

23. Roden DM. Drug-induced prolongation of the QT interval. N Engl J Med 2004; 350:1013–1022.

Chapter 16

ACUTE RESPIRATORY DISTRESS SYNDROME

The condition described in this chapter, which has the non-descript name *acute respiratory distress syndrome* (ARDS), is the leading cause of acute respiratory failure, and is characterized by widespread inflammation in the lungs, often accompanied by inflammatory injury in other organs (1–3).

I. FEATURES

A. Pathogenesis

1. ARDS is a diffuse inflammatory process that involves both lungs.

2. The process usually begins with activation of circulating neutrophils, which adhere to the endothelium of the pulmonary capillaries. The neutrophils then release the contents of their cytoplasmic granules, which damages the endothelium and produces a leaky-capillary type of exudation into the lung parenchyma.

3. Neutrophils cross the capillary endothelium and produce an inflammatory injury of the lung parenchyma, and this tissue damage promotes further inflammation, creating a vicious cycle that leads to progressive respiratory insufficiency.

B. Predisposing Conditions

A variety of conditions predispose to ARDS, and the most notable are listed in Table 16.1.

1. The most common predisposing conditions are those that trigger a systemic inflammatory response (i.e., fever and leukocytosis). The most common of these is the *sepsis syndrome*, which is a local or bloodstream infection associated with a systemic inflammatory response. The incidence of ARDS in the sepsis syndrome is as high as 40% (4).

TABLE 16.1 Predisposing Conditions for ARDS

1. Conditions associated with a systemic inflammatory response (fever, leukocytosis):
   a. Sepsis syndrome
   b. Endotoxemia
   c. Extensive tissue injury
   d. Cardiopulmonary bypass

2. Local conditions in the lungs:
   a. Gastric acid aspiration
   b. Pneumonia
   c. Pulmonary contusion
   d. Ventilator-induced lung injury

3. Embolism syndromes:
   a. Fat embolism syndrome
   b. Amniotic fluid embolism

4. Miscellaneous conditions:
   a. Blood transfusions
   b. Drugs
   c. Pancreatitis
   d. Intracranial hypertension.

---

2. If the predisposing conditions are combined, the incidence of ARDS is about 25%, and the presence of ARDS increases the mortality rate threefold (4).

C. Clinical Manifestations

1. The earliest signs of ARDS include tachypnea and progressive hypoxemia, which is often refractory to supplemental oxygen. Fever is common and may be present from a predisposing condition.

2. The chest x-ray can be unrevealing in the first few hours of the illness. However by 24 hours after symptom onset, the chest x-ray reveals bilateral pulmonary infiltrates (see Figure 16.1).

3. Progressive hypoxemia leading to dependence on mechanical ventilation often occurs in the first 48 hours of the illness.

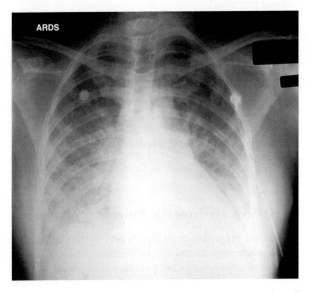

FIGURE 16.1. Portable chest x-ray from a patient with ARDS. The infiltrates appear to be distributed uniformly throughout both lower lung fields. The actual location of the infiltrates in ARDS is shown in Figure 16.2.

II. DIAGNOSIS

A. Diagnostic Criteria

1 The diagnosis of ARDS requires all of the conditions listed in Table 16.2 (5). Note the term *acute lung injury* (ALI), which is a less severe form of ARDS.

2. The conditions most often confused with ARDS are *multilobar pneumonia* and *cardiogenic pulmonary edema*. Multilobar pneumonia can be indistinguishable from ARDS based on the diagnostic criteria in Table 16.2, and cardiogenic pulmonary edema can be mistaken as ARDS because of the limitations of the wedge pressure measurement (see next).

TABLE 16.2 Diagnostic Criteria for ARDS and ALI

1. Acute onset
2. Presence of a predisposing condition
3. Bilateral infiltrates on chest x-ray
4. $PaO_2/FiO_2 < 200$ mm Hg for ARDS
   $PaO_2/FiO_2 = 200 - 300$ mm Hg for ALI
5. Pulmonary artery occlusion pressure ≤ 18 mm Hg or no clinical evidence of left heart failure.

B. ARDS vs. Hydrostatic Pulmonary Edema

The clinical presentation of ARDS and hydrostatic (cardiogenic) pulmonary edema can be indistinguishable, and the pulmonary artery occlusion pressure (known as the *wedge pressure* and described in Chapter 8) is considered a valuable measurement for differentiating between the 2 conditions. As indicated in Table 16.2, a wedge pressure ≤ 18 mm Hg is considered evidence of ARDS, and a wedge pressure above

18 mm Hg is considered evidence of hydrostatic pulmonary edema. The problem here is that the wedge pressure is not a measure of capillary hydrostatic pressure (see next).

1. *Pitfalls of the Wedge Pressure*

   a. As described in Chapter 8, the wedge pressure is a measure of left atrial pressure, and the pulmonary capillary hydrostatic pressure is higher than the left atrial pressure (if the 2 pressures were equivalent, there would be no pressure gradient for flow in the pulmonary veins).

   b. The wedge pressure will therefore underestimate the actual capillary hydrostatic pressure. In conditions where the pulmonary venous resistance is elevated (e.g., during mechanical ventilation), the wedge pressure may be considerably lower than the capillary hydrostatic pressure. This means that *a wedge pressure ≤18 mm Hg does not exclude the possibility of hydrostatic pulmonary edema.*

2. *Bronchoalveolar Lavage*

   Although rarely used, bronchoalveolar lavage is a reliable test for distinguishing ARDS from hydrostatic pulmonary edema. This procedure is performed at the bedside using a flexible bronchoscope that is advanced into one of the involved lung segments. Once in place, the lung segment is lavaged with isotonic saline. The lavage fluid is then analyzed for neutrophil density and protein concentration.

   a. In pulmonary edema, neutrophils will make up less than 5% of the cells recovered in lung lavage fluid, whereas in ARDS, as many as 80% of the recovered cells are neutrophils (6).

   b. Inflammatory exudates are rich in proteinaceous material, and lung lavage fluid in ARDS is similarly rich in protein. When the protein concentration in lung lavage fluid is expressed as a fraction of the plasma protein concentration, the following criteria can be applied (7):

lavage protein/plasma protein < 0.5 = hydrostatic edema

lavage protein/plasma protein > 0.7 = ARDS

III. MANAGEMENT

Since ARDS was first described in 1967, only one therapeutic manipulation has proven effective in improving survival in ARDS: i.e., the use of reduced inflation volumes during mechanical ventilation. This is not really a specific therapy for ARDS, but is a lessening of the harmful effects of mechanical ventilation on the lungs.

A. Ventilator-Induced Lung Injury

Since the introduction of positive-pressure mechanical ventilation, large inflation volumes (tidal volumes) have been used to reduce the tendency for atelectasis during mechanical ventilation.

1. The standard tidal volumes during mechanical ventilation are 10 to 15 mL per kg body weight, which are about twice the size of normal tidal volumes recorded during quiet breathing (6 to 7 mL/kg).

2. In patients with ARDS, the large inflation volumes are delivered into lungs that have a marked reduction in functional volume. The decreased functional volume in ARDS is evident in Figure 16.2. Note that the lung consolidation is confined to the posterior or dependent lung regions. The relatively small region of uninvolved lung in the anterior portion of the thorax is the region where the inflation volumes from the ventilator are distributed.

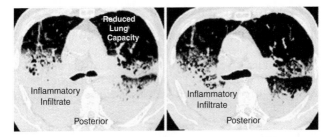

FIGURE 16.2 CT images of lung slices in a patient with ARDS. Lung capacity is reduced by the consolidation in the posterior lung regions, and the bulk of mechanical ventilation is delivered to the uninvolved lung regions in the anterior thorax. (CT images digitally retouched. From Rouby J-J, et al. Crit Care Med 2003; 31(Suppl):S285-S295.)

3. Because the functional lung volume in ARDS is markedly reduced, the large inflation volumes delivered by mechanical ventilation cause overdistension and rupture of the distal airspaces. This volume-related injury is known as *volutrauma*. (Pressure-related lung injury is called *barotrauma*).

4. Volutrauma produces stress-fractures in the alveolar capillary interface, and this leads to infiltration of the distal airspaces with an inflammatory cells and proteinaceous material. The resulting clinical condition is called *ventilator-induced lung injury*, and the pathologic changes look strikingly similar to ARDS (8).

5. The damaging effects of mechanical ventilation may not be confined to the lungs; i.e., inflammatory mediators that accumulate in the lungs in response to volutrauma could enter the systemic circulation and travel to distant organs to produce widespread inflammatory injury and multiorgan dysfunction (9).

B. Low-Volume Ventilation

To reduce the risk of ventilator-induced lung injury, a new strategy has been adopted for mechanical ventilation in ARDS that uses reduced tidal volumes (6 mL/kg instead of the usual 10 to 15 mL/kg). Some clinical trials have shown a survival benefit associated with low-volume ventilation in ARDS (10,11).

1. *Protocol*

   a. A protocol for low-volume ventilation in ARDS is shown in Table 16.3. This protocol has 3 objectives: (1) maintain a tidal volume no higher than 6 mL/kg, (2) keep the end-inspiratory plateau pressure below 30 cm H_2O (this pressure is described in Chapter 18), and (3) avoid severe respiratory acidosis.

   b. Note that the tidal volumes in this protocol are based on *predicted body weight* (which is the weight that best corresponds to normal lung volumes).

2. *Permissive Hypercapnia*

   One of the consequences of low-volume ventilation is reduced CO_2 elimination, which can lead to hypercapnia and respiratory acidosis. Allowing hypercapnia to persist in favor of maintaining low-volume ventilation is known as *permissive hypercapnia* (12).

   a. Clinical trials of permissive hypercapnia have shown that arterial PCO_2 levels of 60 to 70 mm Hg and arterial pH levels of 7.2 to 7.25 are safe for most patients (13). The protocol in Table 16.3 is designed to keep the arterial pH above 7.15, but the preferred arterial pH is 7.30 to 7.45.

   b. Carbon dioxide is a powerful respiratory stimulant, and even mild degrees of hypercapnia can lead to increases in respiratory rate that interfere with effective mechanical ventilation. If this occurs, neuromuscular paralysis may be necessary.

TABLE 16.3 Protocol for Low-Volume Ventilation in ARDS

I. First Stage:

1. Calculate patient's predicted body weight (PBW).

   Males: PBW = 50 + [2.3 x (height in inches − 60)]
   Females: PBW = 45.5 + [2.3 x (height in inches − 60)]

2. Set initial tidal volume (V_T) at 8 mL/kg PBW.

3. Add positive end-expiratory pressure (PEEP) of 5−7 cm H_2O.

4. Reduce V_T by 1 mL/kg every 2 hours until V_T = 6 mL/kg.

5. Adjust FiO_2 to achieve $SaO_2 \geq 90\%$.

II. Second Stage:

1. When V_T = 6 mL/kg, measure plateau pressure (Ppl).

2. If Ppl >30 cm H_2O, decrease V_T in 1 mL/kg increments until Ppl <30 cm H_2O or V_T = 4 mL/kg.

III. Third Stage:

1. Monitor arterial blood gases for respiratory acidosis.

2. If pH = 7.15−7.30, increase respiratory rate (RR) until pH >7.30 or RR = 35 bpm.

3. If pH <7.15, increase RR to 35 bpm. If pH still <7.15, increase V_T in 1 mL/kg increments until pH >7.15.

IV. Optimal Goals:

V_T = 6 mL/kg, Ppl <30 cm H_2O, pH = 7.30−7.45

Adapted from the protocol developed by ARDS Network, available at www.ardsnet.org/studies/arma.

3. *Positive End-Expiratory Pressure (PEEP)*

Low-volume ventilation is often accompanied by collapse of terminal airways at the end of expiration and reopening of the airways during lung inflation. This repetitive opening and closing of terminal airways can itself be a source of lung injury (possibly by creating shear forces that damage the airway epithelium) (14). This problem can be corrected (at least partially) by using positive end-expiratory pressure (PEEP) to reduce the tendency for airway collapse at end-expiration. (PEEP is described in Chapter 20.)

a. The use of low-level PEEP (5–7 cm H_2O) is a standard practice during low-volume ventilation. There is no added benefit from higher levels of PEEP (for preventing airways collapse) (15).

b. Higher levels of PEEP can be used, if necessary, to reduce the fractional concentration of inhaled oxygen (FiO_2) to safe levels. PEEP opens distal airspaces (alveolar recruitment), and this effect improves arterial oxygenation and allows a reduction in the FiO_2. When an $FiO_2 > 60\%$ is needed to maintain an $SaO_2 \geq 90\%$ (or $\geq 88\%$ if a pulse oximeter is used to measure SaO_2), PEEP is added in increments of 2–4 cm H_2O until the FiO_2 can be reduced below 60%. (The risk of pulmonary oxygen toxicity is considered minimal when the FiO_2 is below 60%).

C. Fluid Management

Fluid management in ARDS is usually aimed at reducing extravascular lung water with diuretics. While this approach has shown modest benefits in clinical measures like lung compliance, gas exchange, and length of time on the ventilator, there is little evidence of a consistent survival benefit (16,17). The following are some problems with diuretic therapy in ARDS that deserve mention.

1. *Problems with Diuretic Therapy in ARDS*

a. The first problem with diuretic therapy in ARDS is the nature of the lung infiltration. Diuretics are used to reduce watery edema fluid. However, *the lung infiltration in ARDS is an inflammatory process, and diuretics don't reduce inflammation.*

b. The second problem with diuretic therapy in ARDS is the risk for hemodynamic compromise. Most patients with ARDS are receiving positive-pressure mechanical ventilation, and venous pressures must be higher than normal to exceed the positive intrathoracic pressures and maintain venous return to the heart. Diuretic therapy can compromise venous return to the heart, and the resulting decrease in cardiac output will adversely affect systemic oxygen transport. Hemodynamic monitoring with a pulmonary artery catheter can provide valuable information if aggressive diuretic therapy is planned.

B. Blood Transfusions

1. The traditional practice of transfusing RBCs to maintain a hemoglobin of 10 gm/dL has no documented benefit in ICU patients, including ventilator-dependent patients (18). A lower transfusion threshold of 7 gm/dL has proven safe in ICU patients, except possibly patients with active coronary artery disease (19).

2. Considering that blood transfusions can *cause* ARDS, and that this complication may be much more common than recognized (20), it is wise to avoid RBC transfusions whenever possible in patients with ARDS.

3. See Chapter 30 for more information on anemia and blood transfusions in the ICU.

C. Pharmacotherapy

1. *Steroids*

High-dose steroid therapy has no effect on ARDS when given within 24 hours of the onset of illness (21). However when steroids are given later in the course of illness, during the fibrinoproliferative phase that begins 7–14 days after the onset of illness, there is a definite survival benefit (22). One of the successful regimens involves methylprednisolone in a dose of 2 to 3 mg/kg/day.

2. *Failed Therapies*

Several attempted therapies for ARDS have failed to show a survival benefit. The failed therapies include surfactant (in adults), nitric oxide, pentoxyphylline, lisophylline, ibuprofen, prostaglandin E_1, ketoconazole, and N-acetylcysteine (16,17).

D. Misdirected Therapy?

Attempts at treating ARDS have been directed primarily at the lungs, but a majority of deaths in patients with ARDS are the result of multiorgan failure rather than respiratory (23–25). The relationship between mortality and multiorgan failure in ARDS is shown in Figure 16.3 (24,25). Note the steady rise in mortality rate as the number of organ failures increases. This relationship suggests that the therapeutic

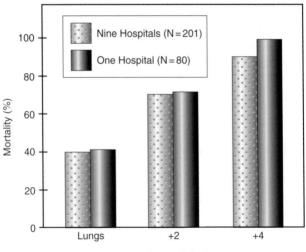

FIGURE 16.3. Mortality rate in ARDS as a function of number of organs failed. Data from References 24 and 25.

approach to ARDS should be directed away from the lungs and toward a more systemic inflammatory disorder if there is to be a survival benefit.

REFERENCES

1 Ware LB, Matthay MA. The acute respiratory distress syndrome. N Engl J Med 2000; 342:1334-1349.

2. Abraham E, Matthay MA, Dinarello C, et al. Consensus conference definitions for sepsis, septic shock, acute lung injury and acute respiratory distress syndrome: Time for a reevaluation. Crit Care Med 2000; 28:232–235.

3. The Fourth Margaux Conference on Critical Illness. Acute lung injury—understanding mechanisms of injury and repair. Crit Care Med 2003; 31(Suppl):S183–S337.

4. Hudson LD, Milberg JA, Anardi D, Maunder RJ. Clinical risks for development of the acute respiratory distress syndrome. Am Rev Respir Crit Care Med 1995; 151:293–301.

5 Bernard GR, Artigas A, Brigham KL, et al. The American–European Consensus Conference on ARDS: definitions, mechanisms, relevant outcomes, and clinical trial coordination. Am Rev Respir Crit Care Med 1994; 149:818–824.

6. Idell S, Cohen AB. Bronchoalveolar lavage in patients with the adult respiratory distress syndrome. Clin Chest Med 1985; 6:459–471.

7. Sprung CL, Long WM, Marcial EH, et al. Distribution of proteins in pulmonary edema. The value of fractional concentrations. Am Rev Respir Dis 1987;136:957–963.

8. Dreyfuss D, Saumon G. Ventilator-induced lung injury. Am J Respir Crit Care Med 1998; 157:294–323.

9. Ranieri VM, Giunta F, Suter P, Slutsky AS. Mechanical ventilation as a mediator of multisystem organ failure in acute respiratory distress syndrome. JAMA 2000; 284:43–44.

10. Fan E, Needham DM, Stewart TE. Ventilator management of acute lung injury and acute respiratory distress syndrome. JAMA 2005; 294:2889–2896.

11. The Acute Respiratory Distress Syndrome Network. Ventilation with lower tidal volumes as compared with traditional tidal volumes for acute lung injury and the acute respiratory distress syndrome. N Engl J Med 2000; 342:1301–1308.

12. BidaniA, Tzouanakis AE, Cardenas VJ, Zwischenberger JB. Permissive hypercapnia in acute respiratory failure. JAMA 1994; 272:957–962.

13. Hickling KG, Walsh J, Henderson S, et al. Low mortality rate in adult respiratory distress syndrome using low-volume, pressure-limited ventilation with permissive hypercapnia: A prospective study. Crit Care Med 1994; 22:1568–1578.

14. Muscedere JG, Mullen JBM, Gan K, et al. Tidal ventilation at low airway pressures can augment lung injury. Am J Respir Crit Care Med 1994; 149:1327–1334.

15. The National Heart, Lung, and Blood Institute ARDS Clinical Network. Higher versus lower positive end-expiratory pressures in patients with acute respiratory distress syndrome, N Engl J Med 2004; 351:327–336.

16. Brower RG, Ware LB, Berthiaume Y, Matthay MA. Treatment of ARDS. Chest 2001; 120:1347–1367.

17. McIntyre RC Jr, Pulido EJ, Bensard DD, et al. Thirty years of clinical trials in acute respiratory distress syndrome. Crit Care Med 2000; 28:3314–3331.

18. Hebert PC, Blajchman MA, Cook DJ, et al. Do blood transfusions improve outcomes related to mechanical ventilation? Chest 2001; 119:1850–1857.

19. Hebert PC, Yetisir E, Martin C, et al. Is a low transfusion threshold safe in critically ill patients with cardiovascular disease. Crit Care Med 2001; 29:227–234.

20. Goodnough LT. Risks of blood transfusion. Crit Care Med 2003; 31(Suppl):S678–S686.

21. Bernard GR, Luce JM, Sprung CL, et al. High-dose corticosteroids in patients with adult respiratory distress syndrome. N Engl J Med 1987; 317:1565–1570.

22. Meduri GU, Chinn A. Fibrinoproliferation in late adult respiratory distress syndrome. Chest 1994; 105(Suppl):127S–129S.

23. Montgomery AB, Stager MA, Carrico J, Hudson LD. Causes of mortality in patients with the adult respiratory distress syndrome. Am Rev Respir Dis 1985; 132:485–489.

24. Bartlett RH, Morris AH, Fairley B, et al. A prospective study of acute hypoxic respiratory failure. Chest 1986; 89:684–689.

25. Gillespie DJ, Marsh HMM, Divertie MB, Meadows JA III. Clinical outcome of respiratory failure in patients requiring prolonged (> 24 hours) mechanical ventilation. Chest 1986; 90:364–369.

Chapter 17

ASTHMA AND COPD IN THE ICU

This chapter describes the management of patients with acute exacerbations of asthma and chronic obstructive pulmonary disease (COPD). The focus here is on the use of pharmacologic agents to relieve airways obstruction. The principles of mechanical ventilation are described in the next section of the book.

I. ACUTE EXACERBATION OF ASTHMA

A. Peak Expiratory Flow Rate

The management of acute asthma requires an assessment of the severity of airflow obstruction, but the physical examination is unreliable in this regard (1). The *peak expiratory flow rate* (PEFR) is an objective measure of airflow obstruction that is easily obtained at the bedside.

1. The PEFR is the greatest flow velocity that can be generated during a forced exhalation from total lung capacity (i.e., when the lungs are fully inflated). The measurement is obtained with a hand-held device (called a *peak flow meter*) that the patient exhales into. A series of 3 measurements should be obtained, if possible, and the highest value is taken as the PEFR.

2 The PEFR is an effort-dependent measurement, and is reliable only when the patient gives a maximum expiratory effort. Patients who are in respiratory distress may be unable to perform this maneuver.

269

3. Figure 17.1 shows the normal PEFR for adult men and women (2). As indicated, the PEFR varies with age, gender, and height. For men, PEFR readings up to 100 L/min below predicted are considered within normal limits. For women, the equivalent figure is 85 L/min.

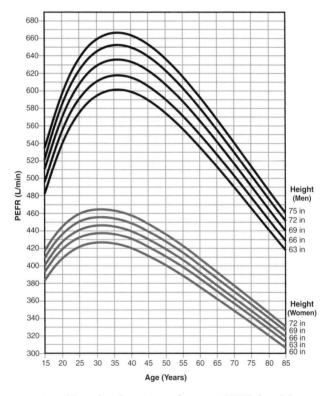

FIGURE 17.1 Normal peak expiratory flow rates (PEFR) for adult men and women. Adapted from Reference 2 for the Mini-Wright Peak Flow Meter™.

4. The PEFR can be used in acute asthma as shown in Figure 17.2 (3,4).

   a. PEFR >70% of normal values indicates minimal or no airflow obstruction.
   b. PEFR = 50–70% of normal values indicates moderate airflow obstruction.
   c. PEFR <50% of normal values indicates severe airflow obstruction.

B. Aerosol Drug Therapy

The drugs used to relieve airflow obstruction (i.e., bronchodilators) are delivered as inhaled aerosols. This mode of delivery is more effective than oral or intravenous therapy (5,6), and has fewer side effects. Two devices are used to generate bronchodilator aerosols: nebulizers and metered-dose inhalers.

1. *Nebulizers*

   Small-volume nebulizers use a reservoir volume of 3 to 6 mL (drug plus saline diluent). A narrow capillary tube is submerged in the solution and a rapidly flowing stream of gas is passed over the open end of the tube. This gas jet creates a viscous drag that draws the drug solution up the capillary tube. When the solution reaches the gas jet, it is pulverized to form an aerosol spray, which is then inhaled by the patient. The reservoir volume is completely aerosolized in less than 10 minutes.

2. *Metered-Dose Inhalers*

   The metered-dose inhaler (MDI) operates like a can of hair spray. The device has a pressurized canister that contains a drug solution with a boiling point below room temperature. When the canister is squeezed between the thumb and fingers, a valve opens that releases a fixed volume of the drug solution. The liquid immediately vaporizes when it emerges from the canister, and a liquid propellant in the solution creates a high-velocity spray.

a. The high velocity of MDI sprays is problematic because most of the aerosol spray impacts on the posterior wall of the oropharynx and is not inhaled. The velocity of the spray can be reduced by using a spacer device to increase the distance between the MDI and

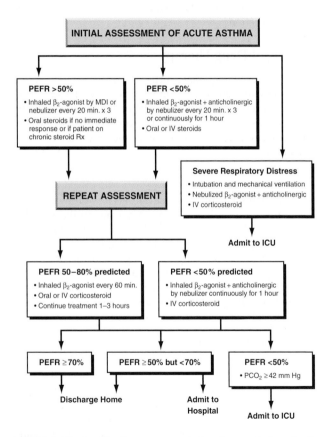

FIGURE 17.2 Protocol for the management of acute exacerbation of asthma. Adapted from Reference 3. $PEFR$ = peak expiratory flow rate.

mouth. Spacer devices (which are usually chambers that hold several sprays from an MDI) should be used routinely to improve lung deposition of MDI sprays.

3. *Nebulizer vs. MDI*

The dose of bronchodilators delivered by nebulizers is far greater than the dose delivered by MDIs, but the bronchodilator response is the same. This is demonstrated in Figure 17.3 (7). Because MDIs are equivalent to nebulizer treatments but are less labor intensive (i.e., do not require a respiratory therapist to administer), *MDIs are favored over nebulizers for bronchodilator therapy* (don't forget to use a spacer with the MDI).

C. β-Receptor Agonists

The favored bronchodilators in asthma are drugs that stimulate β-adrenergic receptors in bronchial smooth muscle (β_2 subtype) to promote smooth muscle relaxation (8). Short-acting agents are preferred for acute therapy because they can be given more frequently. The most popular short-acting β_2-agonist is **albuterol**. When inhaled as an aerosol, albuterol produces an effect within 5 minutes, and it lasts 2–5 hours (8). The dose of aerosolized albuterol in acute asthma is shown in Table 17.1.

1. *Intermittent vs. Continuous Aerosol Therapy*

For acute exacerbation of asthma, albuterol can be given as a series of intermittent aerosol treatments (using a nebulizer or MDI) every 20 minutes, or as a single continuous nebulizer treatment (see Table 17.1 for the doses). Most studies show no difference in efficacy between the two regimens (9). Continuous aerosol therapy is favored by many because it is easier to administer.

2. *Parenteral Therapy*

For the rare asthmatic patient who does not tolerate bronchodilator aerosols (usually because of excessive

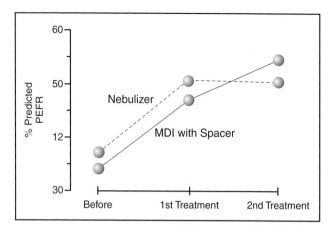

FIGURE 17.3 Bronchodilator response to albuterol delivered by nebulizer (2.5 mg per treatment) and metered-dose inhaler (*MDI*) (0.4 mg per treatment) in patients with acute exacerbation of asthma. *PEFR* = peak expiratory flow rate. Adapted from Reference 7.

coughing), the following regimens are effective (1):

  a. **Epinephrine:** 0.3–0.5 mg by subcutaneous injection every 20 minutes x 3, or

  b. **Terbutaline:** 0.25 mg by subcutaneous injection every 20 minutes x 3.

3. *Side Effects*

High-dose aerosol therapy with β_2-agonists can produce a number of side effects, including tachycardia, tremors, hyperglycemia, hypokalemia, hypomagnesemia, and hypophosphatemia (8,10,11). Cardiac ischemia is rare (11).

C. Anticholinergic Agents

1.Anticholinergic agents are less effective than β_2-agonists in asthma, and are used only in in combination with β_2-agonists (see Figure 17.2) (3,4,12).

2. The only anticholinergic agent approved for clinical use is **ipatropium bromide**, a derivative of atropine that blocks muscarinic receptors in the airways. The aerosol dose of ipatropium in acute asthma is shown in Table 17.1.

TABLE 17.1 Drug Therapy for Acute Exacerbation of Asthma

Drug Preparation	Dose	Comments
Short-Acting β_2-Receptor Agonist		
Albuterol nebulizer solution (5 mg/mL)	2.5–5 mg every 20 min x 3 doses, or 10–15 mg/hr continuously, then 2.5–10 mg every 1–4 hrs as needed.	Dilute albuterol solution to final volume of 5 mL and deliver at gas flows of 6–8 L/min.
Albuterol by MDI (90 µg/puff)	4–8 puffs every 20 min up to 4 hrs, then every 1–4 hrs as needed.	As effective as nebulizer R_x. MDI should be used with spacer device.
Anticholinergic Agent		
Ipatropium bromide nebulizer solution (0.25 mg/mL)	0.5 mg every 20 min for 3 doses, then every 2–4 hrs as needed.	Can mix in same nebulizer as albuterol. Should not be used alone as first-line therapy.
Ipatropium bromide by MDI (18 µg/puff)	4–8 puffs as needed.	MDI delivery has not been studied in acute asthma.
Corticosteroids		
Methylprednisolone (IV), or prednisone (oral)	120–180 mg/day in 3 or 4 divided doses for 48 hrs, then 60–80 mg/day until PEFR ≥70% of predicted.	No difference in efficacy between IV and oral R_x. Onset of effect takes several hours.

From Reference 3. Drug doses are for adults only.

3. Systemic absorption of aerosolized ipatropium is minimal, so there is little risk of anticholinergic side effects; i.e., tachycardia, dry mouth, blurred vision, and urinary retention.

D. Corticosteroids

Steroids are recommended for all patients with acute asthma (see Figure 17.2). The steroid preparations used most often are **methylprednisolone** (for intravenous therapy) and **prednisone** (for oral therapy), and the recommended doses are shown in Table 17.1. The following points about steroid therapy deserve mention.

1. There is no difference in efficacy between oral and intravenous steroids (13).

2. The beneficial effects of steroids may not be apparent until 12 hours after therapy is started (13).

3. There is no clearly defined dose-response curve for steroids, which means that higher doses of steroids are not superior to lower doses (13).

4. A 10-day course of steroids can be stopped abruptly without a tapering dose (14).

5. A *myopathy* has been reported in ventilator-dependent asthmatic patients treated with high-dose steroids and neuromuscular blocking agents (15).

   a. Unlike the traditional steroid myopathy, which is characterized by proximal muscle weakness, this myopathy involves both proximal and distal muscles, and is often associated with rhabdomyolysis. The muscle weakness can hamper weaning from mechanical ventilation.

   b. Once the disorder is suspected, rapid taper of the paralyzing agents and steroids is advised.

   c. The muscle weakness can be prolonged, but the disorder is usually reversible.

E. Other Considerations

The following are some important considerations for the management of acute asthma in the emergency department:

1. Supplemental oxygen is not necessary if the arterial O_2 saturation measured by pulse oximetry is 92% or higher.

2. Chest x-rays are not necessary unless there is suspicion of a condition other than asthma (e.g., pneumonia).

3. Arterial blood gases are not necessary unless the patient is *in extremis*, is cyanotic, or is refractory to initial bronchodilator therapy.

4. Antibiotics are not necessary unless there is evidence of a *treatable* infection.

II. ACUTE EXACERBATIONS OF COPD

Acute exacerbations of COPD (i.e., chronic bronchitis and emphysema) are responsible for about half a million hospital admissions yearly in the United States, and half of these are ICU admissions (16).

A. Bronchodilator Therapy

1. Short-acting β_2-agonists like albuterol are used routinely in acute exacerbation of COPD. The usual dose is 2.5–5 mg via nebulizer or 2 puffs by MDI every 4 to 6 hours.

2. Unlike the case in asthma, aerosolized ipatropium bromide can be used alone as a bronchodilator in acute exac-

erbations of COPD (17,18). The usual dose is 0.5 mg by nebulizer or 2 to 4 puffs by MDI every 4 to 6 hours. The common practice is to combine ipatropium with β_2-agonist therapy, but some studies do not support this practice (18).

B. Corticosteroids

A short course (2 weeks) of corticosteroid therapy is recommended for all patients with acute exacerbation of COPD (16-18). One example of an effective 2-week steroid regimen is shown below (19).

Methylprednisolone: 125 mg IV every 6 hrs on days 1–3,
Prednisone: 60 mg once daily on days 4–7,
40 mg once daily on days 8–11,
20 mg once daily on days 12–15.

C. Antibiotic Therapy

1. Infection in the airways is believed to be the inciting event in 80% of cases of acute exacerbation of COPD, and bacteria are isolated in at least half of the cases (20). The infections are usually polymicrobial, and the most frequent treatable isolates are *Chlamydia pneumoniae, Hemophilus influenza,* and *Streptococcus pneumoniae.*

2. Despite the prevalence of airway infection, the benefit of antimicrobial therapy in acute exacerbation of COPD has been difficult to prove. The most recent evidence using pooled data from 11 clinical trials indicates that antimicrobial therapy is beneficial in patients who are at risk for a poor outcome (18).

3. Antibiotic therapy in acute exacerbation of COPD is not based on sputum cultures, but rather on the risk for a poor outcome. Recommendations for antibiotic therapy based on risk assessment are shown in Table 17.2.

4. The optimal duration of antimicrobial therapy is not known: the common practice is to continue therapy for at least 7 days.

TABLE 17.2 Antibiotic Therapy for Acute Exacerbation of COPD Based on Risk Assessment

I. Risk Assessment

Answer the following questions:

	Yes	No
1. Is the FEV_1 less than 50% of predicted?	☐	☐
2. Does the patient have cardiac disease or other significant comorbid conditions?	☐	☐
3. Has the patient had 3 or more exacerbations in the previous 12 months?	☐	☐

If the answer is **YES** to at least one of these questions, the patient is considered to be high-risk for an unfavorable outcome.

II. Antibiotic Selection

High Risk Patients: Amoxicillin-clavulanate or a newer fluoroquinolone (gatifloxacin, levofloxacin, or moxifloxacin)

Low Risk Patients: Doxycycline, a second-generation cephalosporin (e.g., cefuroxime) or a newer macrolide (azithromycin or clarithromycin)

From Reference 20. FEV_1 = Forced expiratory volume in 1 second.

D. Oxygen Therapy

In patients with COPD and chronic hypercapnia, inhalation of high concentrations of oxygen can aggravate the hypercapnia (21). To minimize this risk, the concentration of inhaled O_2 should be just enough to keep the arterial oxyhemoglobin saturation (SaO_2) at 88–90%. There is no evidence that raising the SaO_2 above this level will further enhance tissue oxygenation.

REFERENCES

1. Shim CS, Williams MH. Evaluation of the severity of asthma: patients versus physicians. Am J Med 1980; 68:11–13.

2. Nunn AJ, Gregg I. New regression equations for predicting peak expiratory flow in adults. Br Med J 1989; 298:1068–1070.

3. National Asthma Education and Prevention Program Expert Panel Report 2. Guidelines for the diagnosis and management of asthma. NIH Publication No. 97-4051, July, 1997.

4. National Asthma Education and Prevention Program Expert Panel Report: Guidelines for the diagnosis and management of asthma. Update on selected topics, 2002. NIH Publication No. 02-5074, June, 2003.

5. Shim C, Williams MH. Bronchial response to oral versus aerosol metaproterenol in asthma. Ann Intern Med 1980; 93:428–431.

6. Salmeron S, Brochard L. Mal H, et al. Nebulized versus intravenous albuterol in hypercapnic acute asthma. Am J Respir Crit Care Med 1994; 149:1466–1470.

7. Idris AH, McDermott MF, Raucci JC, et al. Emergency department treatment of severe asthma: Metered-dose inhaler plus holding chamber is equivalent in effectiveness to nebulizer. Chest 1993; 103:665–672.

8. Dutta EJ, Li JTC. β-agonists. Med Clin N Am 2002; 86:991–1008.

9. Rodrigo GJ, Rodrigo C. Continuous vs. intermittent beta-agonists in the treatment of acute adult asthma: A systematic review with meta-analyses. Chest 2002; 122:1982–1987.

10. Truwit JD. Toxic effect of bronchodilators. Crit Care Clin 1991; 7:639–657.

11. Bodenhamer J, Bergstrom R, Brown D, et al. Frequently nebulized beta-agonists for asthma: Effects on serum electrolytes. Ann Emerg Med 1992; 21:1337–1342.

12. Rodrigo G, Rodrigo C. The role of anticholinergics in acute asthma treatment. An evidence-based evaluation. Chest 2002; 121:1977–1987.

13. Rodrigo G, Rodrigo C. Corticosteroids in the emergency department therapy of acute adult asthma. An evidence-based evaluation. Chest 1999; 116:285–295.

14. Cydulka RK, Emerman CL. A pilot study of steroid therapy after emergency department treatment of acute asthma: Is a taper needed? J Emerg Med 1998; 16:15–19.

15. Griffin D, Fairman N, Coursin D, et al. Acute myopathy during treatment of status asthmaticus with corticosteroids and steroidal muscle relaxants. Chest 1992; 102:510–514.

16. Stoller JK. Acute exacerbations of chronic obstructive pulmonary disease. N Engl J Med 2002; 346:988–994.

17. Snow V, Lascher S, Mottur-Pilson C, for the Joint Expert Panel on COPD of the American College of Chest Physicians and the American College of Physicians-American Society of Internal Medicine. The evidence base for management of acute exacerbations of COPD. Chest 2001; 119:1185–1189.

18. McCrory DC, Brown C, Gelfand SE, Bach PB. Management of acute exacerbations of COPD. A summary and appraisal of published evidence. Chest 2001; 119:1190–1209.

19. Niewoehner DE, Erbland ML, Deupree RH, et al. Effect of systemic glucocorticoids on exacerbations of chronic obstructive pulmonary disease. N Engl J Med 1999; 340:1941–1947.

20. Sethi S. Acute exacerbations of COPD: A "multipronged" approach. J Respir Dis 2002; 23:217–225.

21. Campbell EJM. The J. Burns Amberson Lecture. The management of acute respiratory failure in chronic bronchitis and emphysema. Am Rev Respir Dis 1967; 96:626–639.

Chapter 18

BASICS OF MECHANICAL VENTILATION

Patient care in any ICU requires a working knowledge of mechanical ventilation. Much of this is learned by repeated exposure to ventilators at the bedside, but the information in the next few chapters can serve as a starting point.

I. POSITIVE-PRESSURE VENTILATION

A. Pressure-Volume Relationships

1. During mechanical ventilation, the ventilator creates a positive pressure that pushes air into the lungs. This inflation pressure is transmitted into the thorax to create a positive intrathoracic pressure.

2. The inflation pressure is influenced by the volume that is delivered (the inflation volume) and the mechanical properties of the lungs. This is demonstrated in Figure 18.1. Note the following:

   a. The inflation pressure increases as the inflation volume increases.

   b. In conditions of increased airways resistance and reduced lung compliance, the inflation pressure is higher at any given inflation volume (i.e., the curve is shifted to the left).

3. The inflation pressure is roughly equivalent to the intra-

thoracic pressure. Therefore, Figure 18.1 shows that *the influence of mechanical ventilation on intrathoracic pressure is determined by the volume delivered and the mechanical properties of the lungs.*

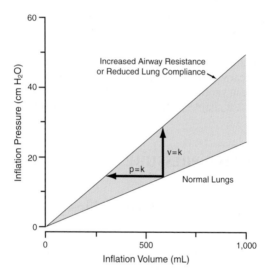

FIGURE 18.1 Pressure-volume relationships during positive-pressure mechanical ventilation. The vertical arrow ($v = k$) represents volume-cycled ventilation, and the horizontal arrow ($p = k$) represents pressure-cycled ventilation.

B. Pressure vs. Volume Control

1. A mechanical breath can be terminated at a preset pressure (pressure-cycled ventilation) or a preset volume (volume-cycled ventilation).

2. During pressure-cycled ventilation, the inflation volume varies with changes in the mechanical properties of the lungs. This is shown by the horizontal arrow in Figure

18.1; i.e., when lung mechanics are abnormal, the inflation volume decreases.

3. During volume-cycled ventilation, the inflation volume
is constant regardless of the mechanical properties of the
lungs. This is shown by the vertical arrow in Figure 18.1;
i.e., when lung mechanics are abnormal, the ventilator
develops higher inflation pressures to deliver the preset
volume.

4. Volume-cycled ventilation is favored because of the ability
to maintain a constant inflation volume despite changes in
the mechanical properties of the lungs (which can occur
frequently in ventilator-dependent patients). However,
intrathoracic pressures can reach very high levels during
volume-cycled ventilation (particularly when the lungs
are noncompliant), and this can adversely affect the cardiac output (see next).

C. Cardiac Performance

Positive-pressure ventilation can influence both ventricular
filling and ventricular emptying (1).

1. *Ventricular Filling*

   Positive-pressure lung inflation can reduce ventricular
   filling by the following mechanisms:

   a. Positive intrathoracic pressure impedes venous return
   by reducing the pressure gradient for venous inflow
   into the thorax.

   b. Positive pressure exerted on the outer surface of the
   heart reduces cardiac distensibility, and this can reduce ventricular filling during diastole.

2. *Ventricular Emptying*

   Positive intrathoracic pressure can facilitate ventricular
   emptying by reducing the transmural pressure that must
   be developed by the ventricle to eject the stroke volume.

(The positive intrathoracic pressure acts like a hand that squeezes the ventricles during systole).

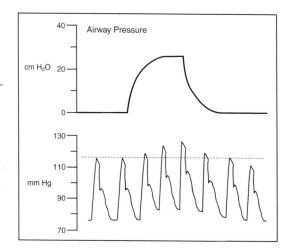

FIGURE 18.2 Respiratory variation in blood pressure. The positive-pressure lung inflation (depicted in the upper graph) is associated with a transient rise in blood pressure, reflecting an increase in cardiac stroke output.

3. *Cardiac Output*

The effect of mechanical ventilation on cardiac stroke output will depend on which of the two effects on cardiac performance (a decrease in ventricular filling or an increase in ventricular emptying) is predominant.

a. In conditions where the intrathoracic pressure exceeds the central venous pressure (e.g., hypovolemia), the predominant effect of mechanical ventilation is to reduce ventricular filling and thereby decrease cardiac stroke output.

b. When ventricular filling is adequate, the predominant effect of mechanical ventilation is to enhance ventricular emptying and thereby increase cardiac stroke output.

c. The effect of mechanical ventilation on cardiac output can be inferred from the respiratory variations in blood pressure. When cardiac stroke output is increased, there is an increase in blood pressure associated with each lung inflation, as demonstrated in Figure 18.2. When cardiac stroke output is decreased, each lung inflation produces a decrease in blood pressure.

II. INITIATING MECHANICAL VENTILATION

A. Tracheal Intubation

Positive-pressure ventilation requires tracheal intubation with specialized *endotracheal tubes* that have an inflatable balloon (called a cuff) at the distal end to prevent air from escaping around the tube during lung inflation.

1. Endotracheal tubes are sized according to their internal diameter, which varies from 5 to 10 mm (in adults). Tube sizes of 7 or 8 (i.e., internal diameters of 7 or 8 mm) are recommended for adults. Smaller sized (narrower) tubes create an obstruction to air flow, while larger-sized (wider) tubes increase the risk of laryngeal damage.

2. Intubation of the trachea is accomplished by inserting the endotracheal tube through the nose or mouth and advancing the tube through the larynx and into the trachea. The nasal route is reserved for elective intubations in awake patients.

3. Once the endotracheal tube is in place, the balloon at the distal end of the tube is inflated (with an air-filled syringe) until there is no evidence of an air leak (i.e., no audible sounds of air escaping out through the mouth when the lungs are manually inflated).

4. To verify tube placement in the trachea, exhaled CO_2 is measured with a disposable, colorimetric CO_2 detector (Easy Cap II, Nellcor, Pleasantville, CA). If the exhaled CO_2 is above 0.5% (which produces a tan or yellow color on the CO_2 detector), the tube is in the trachea (2). A lower concentration of exhaled CO_2 indicates that the tube is in the esophagus, and should be removed immediately.

5. Listening for breath sounds when air is forced through the endotracheal tube is an unreliable method for distinguishing between tracheal and esophageal intubation (3).

6. Once tracheal intubation is verified, a portable chest x-ray should be obtained to determine the location of the tip of the tube. The tube is properly placed when the tip is located 3 to 5 cm above the tracheal carina (with the head in a neutral position) (4).

B. Low-Volume Ventilation

Following successful tracheal intubation, mechanical ventilation can proceed according to the protocol shown in Table 18.1. This protocol was developed for patients with acute respiratory distress syndrome (ARDS), and it is described in detail in Chapter 16 (see Table 16.3).

1. Low-volume ventilation is designed to reduce the risk of *ventilator-induced lung injury* (5), a condition characterized by overdistension and rupture of alveoli in nondiseased lung segments. This condition is caused by inflation volumes that are too large for the volume of nondiseased lung, where most of the inflation volume is distributed. This condition is described in Chapter 16 (section III-A).

2. The inflation volume (also called *tidal volume*) in low-volume ventilation is 6 mL/kg, which is about half the traditional inflation volume (10 to 12 mL/kg). Note that the *predicted body weight* is used to determine the tidal volume. Predicted body weight is the preferred measure of

TABLE 18.1 Protocol for Initiating Low-Volume Ventilation

Step 1: Initial Ventilator Settings

1. Select assist-control mode of ventilation with NO ventilator sighs
2. Set initial tidal volume (V_T) at 8 mL/kg using the patient's predicted body weight (PBW).

    Males: PBW = 50 + [2.3 x (height in inches − 60)]
    Females: PBW = 45.5 + [2.3 x (height in inches − 60)]

3. Set respiratory rate (RR) at 12−14 breaths.
4. Add positive end-expiratory pressure (PEEP) of 5−7 cm H_2O.
5. Set inspired O_2 concentration (FiO_2) at 100%.

Step 2: Volume Reduction

1. Reduce V_T by 1 mL/kg every 2 hrs until V_T is 6 mL/kg.
2. When V_T is 6 mL/kg, measure end-inspiratory plateau pressure (Ppl).
3. If Ppl > 30 cm H_2O, decrease V_T in 1 mL/kg increments until Ppl < 30 cm H_2O or V_T = 4 mL/kg.

Step 3: Adjustments for Respiratory Acidosis

1. Measure arterial blood gases for evidence of acute respiratory acidosis. If present, proceed as follows.
2. If arterial pH is 7.15−7.30, increase RR until pH > 7.30 or RR = 35 bpm.
3. If arterial pH < 7.15, increase RR to 35 bpm. If pH still < 7.15, increase V_T in 1 mL/kg increments until pH > 7.15.

Step 4: Achieving a Non-Toxic FiO_2

1. Decrease FiO_2 in 10–20% increments until the FiO_2 < 60% or the SaO_2 = 80% (by pulse oximetry).
2. If the FiO_2 remains > 60%, add PEEP in increments of 2–3 cm H_2O until the FiO_2 < 60% and the SaO_2 ≥88%.

Adapted from the protocol for low volume ventilation in ARDS (see Table 16.3).

body size because it is closely associated with normal lung volumes.

3. The use of low-level positive end-expiratory pressure (PEEP) is a standard practice during low-volume ventilation, and is used to counteract the tendency for small airways to collapse at end-expiration when inflation volumes are reduced (6).

4. The end-inspiratory plateau pressure (described later in the chapter), which is the elastic recoil pressure of the lungs and thorax, is kept below 30 cm H_2O because a large clinical study showed that this condition was associated with improved outcomes during low-volume ventilation (7).

5. The CO_2 is allowed to rise during low-volume ventilation (a condition known as *permissive hypercapnia*), but the arterial pH is not allowed to drop below 7.15.

6. To reduce the risk of pulmonary oxygen toxicity, the fractional concentration of inspired oxygen (FIO_2) should be kept below 60% in all patients who breathe supplemental oxygen for more than 48 hours. Additional PEEP can be used to achieve this goal if necessary (The actions of PEEP to improve arterial oxygenation are described in Chapter 19).

III. MONITORING LUNG MECHANICS

A. Mechanical Properties of the Lungs

1. The mechanical properties of the lungs include the resistance to flow in the airways and the elastic recoil force of the lung parenchyma.

2. The elastic recoil of the lungs is measured as *compliance*, which is a measure of the distensibility of the lungs (i.e., a decrease in lung compliance indicates a decrease in lung distensibility).

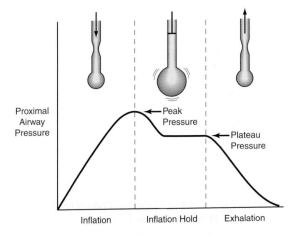

FIGURE 18.3 Airway pressure profile during an inflation-hold maneuver.

A. Proximal Airway Pressures

The proximal airway pressures depicted in Figure 18.3 can be used to evaluate the mechanical properties of the lungs during mechanical ventilation (8,9).

1. *Peak Pressure*

   The peak pressure at the end of inspiration (P_{peak}) varies in the same direction as changes in airways resistance, and varies in the opposite direction to changes in lung compliance (see Table 18.2).

   a. When the inflation volume is constant, an increase in P_{peak} indicates either an increase in airway resistance, a decrease in lung compliance, or both.

2. *Plateau Pressure*

   If the inflation volume is held in the lungs by occluding the expiratory limb of the ventilator tubing, the proximal airway pressure decreases initially and then reaches a steady level (see Figure 18.3). This inflation-hold pressure is called the *plateau pressure*.

a. The plateau pressure ($P_{plateau}$) varies in the opposite direction to changes in lung compliance; i.e., an increase in $P_{plateau}$ indicates a decrease in lung compliance.

b. Because $P_{plateau}$ is obtained in the absence of airflow, it is not influenced by changes in airway resistance (see Table 18.2).

c. Because airways resistance influences only peak pressure, the pressure difference ($P_{peak} - P_{plateau}$) is a measure of changes in airway resistance (see Table 18.2).

TABLE 18.2 Influence of Abnormal Lung Mechanics on Proximal Airway Pressures

Abnormal Condition	Changes in Proximal Airway Pressures		
	P_{peak}	$P_{plateau}$	($P_{peak} - P_{plateau}$)
Decreased lung compliance	Increased	Increased	No Change
Increased airway resistance	Increased	No Change	Increased

3. *Summary*

a. Changes in lung compliance are detected by changes in $P_{plateau}$.

b. Changes in airway resistance are detected by changes in ($P_{peak} - P_{plateau}$).

CAVEAT. Since airways pressures are measured relative to atmospheric pressure, they are *transthoracic pressures*, and are influenced by conditions in the chest wall as well as the lungs. This can be an important consideration for the evaluation of compliance; i.e., contraction of the chest wall muscles can reduce the compliance of the chest wall, and this can be misinterpreted as a decrease in lung compliance. Thus, the term *thoracic compliance* is a more accurate description of this parameter.

B. Practical Applications

The following are two situations where interpretation of proximal airway pressures can be useful.

1. *Bedside Evaluation of Respiratory Distress*

   The flow diagram in Figure 18.4 demonstrates how the proximal airway pressures can be used to evaluate a ventilator-dependent patient who develops sudden onset of respiratory deterioration.

   a. If the peak pressure is increased but the plateau pressure is unchanged, the problem is an increase in airways resistance. In this situation, the major concerns are obstruction of the tracheal tube, airway obstruction from secretions, and acute bronchospasm. Therefore, immediate interventions should include airways suctioning to clear secretions and an aerosolized bronchodilator treatment.

   b. If the peak and plateau pressures are both increased, the problem is a decrease in thoracic compliance. In this situation, the major concerns in the lungs are pneumothorax, lobar atelectasis, acute pulmonary edema, worsening pneumonia, and progression of ARDS. The appropriate interventions in this situation include auscultation of the lungs (diminished breath sounds can be a sign of pneumothorax or lobar atelectasis) and a STAT chest x-ray (all of the conditions just mentioned should be apparent on a chest x-ray).

   c. If the peak pressure is decreased, the problem may be a cuff leak that allows part of the inflation volume to escape from the lungs. A sudden drop in peak pressure can also be the result of a hyperventilating patient who is generating enough negative intrathoracic pressure to decrease the peak airway pressure.

2. *Bronchodilator Responsiveness*

The proximal airway pressures can be used to evaluate responsiveness to aerosolized bronchodilators during mechanical ventilation.

a. A favorable bronchodilator response should be accompanied by a decrease in P_{peak} with no change in $P_{plateau}$; i.e., a decrease in ($P_{peak} - P_{plateau}$).

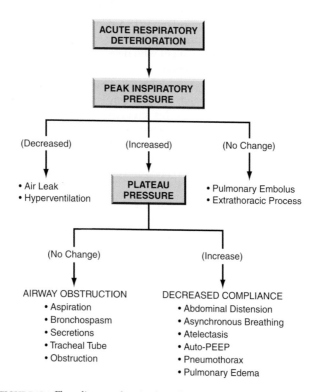

FIGURE 18.4. Flow diagram showing how the peak and plateau pressures can be used to identify the likely cause(s) of acute respiratory problems.

C. Thoracic Compliance

The compliance of the lungs and chest wall (thoracic compliance) can be determined as the ratio of the tidal volume (V_T) to the elastic recoil pressure measured at end-inspiration (i.e., $P_{plateau}$).

$$C_{stat} = V_T/P_{plateau} \qquad (18.1)$$

Since the plateau pressure is measured in the absence of airflow, the resulting compliance is referred to as "static" compliance (C_{stat}).

1. *Expected Range of Values*

   In an intubated patient without lung disease (e.g., a drug overdose), a tidal volume (V_T) of 500 mL should be associated with a plateau pressure no higher than 10 cm H_2O. The thoracic compliance in this situation is: 500 mL ÷ 10 cm H_2O = 50 mL/cm H_2O.

   a. Thoracic compliance is normally 50–80 mL/cm H_2O (8).

   b. In patients with stiff lungs due to severe infiltrative lung disease, thoracic compliance is reduced to 10–20 mL/cm H_2O (10).

D. Inspiratory Resistance

The pressure difference ($P_{peak} - P_{plateau}$) is the pressure gradient needed to overcome resistance to airflow during lung inflation. Therefore, the resistance to flow during inspiration (R_{insp}) can be determined using the ($P_{peak} - P_{plateau}$) and the inspiratory flow rate (Q_{insp}) generated by the ventilator.

$$R_{insp} = (P_{peak} - P_{plateau})/Q_{insp} \qquad (18.2)$$

The R_{insp} is a measure of the summed resistances of the connector tubing, the endotracheal tube, and the airways, and is often called the *total inspiratory resistance*.

1. *Expected Range of Values*

   For ventilator-dependent patients who have no cardio-pulmonary disease, the following measurements are typical: inspiratory flow rate=60 L/min (1 L/sec), peak pressure=20 cm H_2O, plateau pressure=10 cm H_2O. The resulting R_{insp} is $(20 - 10) \div 1 = 10$ cm H_2O /L/sec.

   a. Total inspiratory resistance is normally 10–15 cm H_2O/L/sec.

   b. The minimal flow resistance in large-bore endotracheal tubes is 3–7 cm H_2O/L/sec (11), so nonpulmonary resistive elements can account for a considerable portion of the total inspiratory resistance. This is a major shortcoming of the inspiratory resistance measurement.

REFERENCES

1. Pinsky MR. Cardiovascular issues in respiratory care. Chest 2005; 128:592S–597S.

2. Ornato JP, Shipley JB, Racht EM, et al. Multicenter study of a portable, hand-size, colorimetric end-tidal carbon dioxide detection device. Ann Emerg Med 1992; 21:518–523.

3. Mizutani AR, Ozake G, Benumoff JL, et al. Auscultation cannot distinguish esophageal from tracheal passage of tube. J Clin Monit 1991; 7:232–236.

4. Goodman LR, Putman CE. Critical Care Imaging. 3rd ed, Philadelphia: WB Saunders, 1992:35–56.

5. Dreyfuss D, Saumon G. Ventilator-induced lung injury. Am J Respir Crit Care Med 1998; 157:294–323.

6. Fan E, Needham DM, Stewart TE. Ventilator management of acute lung injury and acute respiratory distress syndrome. JAMA 2005; 294:2889–2896.

7. The Acute Respiratory Distress Syndrome Network. Ventilation with lower tidal volumes as compared with traditional tidal volumes for acute lung injury and the acute respiratory distress syndrome. N Engl J Med 2000; 342:1301–1308.

8. Tobin MJ. Respiratory monitoring. JAMA 1990; 264:244–251.

9. Marini JJ. Lung mechanics determinations at the bedside: instrumentation and clinical application. Respir Care 1990; 35:669–696.

10. Katz JA, Zinn SE, Ozanne GM, Fairley BB. Pulmonary, chest wall, and lung-thorax elastances in acute respiratory failure. Chest 1981; 80:304–311.

11. Marini JJ. Strategies to minimize breathing effort during mechanical ventilation. Crit Care Clin 1990; 6:635–662.

Chapter 19

MODES OF POSITIVE-PRESSURE BREATHING

Positive airway pressure can be used to inflate the lungs, prevent the lungs from deflating, provide full ventilatory support, or support spontaneous breathing. This chapter presents these different forms of positive-pressure breathing.

I. THE VENTILATOR BREATH

The cornerstone of positive-pressure breathing is the positive-pressure lung inflation (i.e., the *ventilator breath*) like the one shown in Figure 19.1. These lung inflations can be volume-cycled (where inflation continues to a preset volume), pressure-cycled (where inflation continues to a preset pressure), or time-cycled (where inflation continues for a preset period of time). The description that follows is for volume-cycled ventilation, which is the most common method of positive-pressure breathing.

A. Basic Features

The components of a ventilator breath are described below using the corresponding numbers in Figure 19.1.

1. *Initiating the Breath*

The initial portion of the tracing has a negative pressure deflection, which represents a spontaneous inspiratory effort by the patient. If the negative pressure reaches a

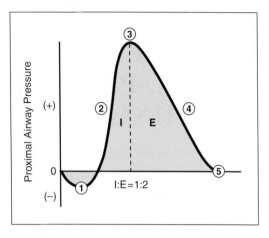

FIGURE 19.1 Changes in airway pressure during a ventilator breath. The components of the ventilator breath are marked by the circled numbers (see text for explanation).

threshold level (which is usually set 2 cm H_2O below the baseline pressure), a pressure-activated valve in the ventilator is opened, and the ventilator delivers the breath. Patients who are able to initiate or "trigger" ventilator breaths will be ventilated at their own intrinsic rate.

2. *Lung Inflation*

The lungs are usually inflated at a constant flow rate, which produces a steady rise in airway pressure and lung volume. Inspiratory flow rates are usually set at 60 L/min (1 L/sec), which ensures rapid lung inflation (i.e., a typical inflation volume of 500 mL will be delivered in less than one second) and allows enough time for the lungs to empty.

3. *Peak Airway Pressure*

The peak pressure at the end of the lung inflation is determined by three factors: the inflation volume, the resistance to flow in the airways and ventilator tubing, and the compliance (distensibility) of the lungs and chest wall. This pressure can be used to evaluate the mechanical properties of the lungs, as described in Chapter 18.

4. *Exhalation*

Exhalation is a passive process (at least during quiet breathing), and is driven by the elastic recoil pressure of the lungs. Exhalation is faster in patients with noncompliant lungs (e.g., ARDS), and slower in patients with obstructive airway disease (e.g., asthma). The time allowed for exhalation should be at least twice the time of lung inflation: this is expressed as an I:E ratio of 1:2, as shown.

5. *End-Expiratory Pressure*

Under normal circumstances, the lungs empty the tidal volume before the next breath begins, and the pressure in the airways and distal airspaces returns to zero (atmospheric) pressure at the end of expiration. Positive pressure can be applied to the airways at the end of expiration as described later in the chapter.

II. COMMON PATTERNS OF VENTILATION

This section describes two common methods of delivering ventilator breaths: *assist-control ventilation* and *intermittent mandatory ventilation.*

A. Assist-Control Ventilation

Assist-control ventilation is the traditional method of delivering positive-pressure lung inflations. As the name implies, this method allows patients to initiate ventilator breaths (assisted ventilation), but can also provide ventilator breaths for patients unable to interact with the ventilator (controlled ventilation).

1. *Ventilatory Pattern*

   The upper panel of Figure 19.2 shows two ventilator breaths delivered during assist-control ventilation (ACV). The first is a patient-initiated or "triggered" breath similar to the one in Figure 19.1. The second breath is not preceded by an inspiratory effort, and is not initiated by the patient. The first breath is an example of *assisted ventilation*, and the second breath is an example of *controlled ventilation*.

2. *Rate of Ventilation*

   During assisted (triggered) ventilation, the patient's intrinsic breathing rate determines the number of ventilator breaths delivered each minute. During controlled (nontriggered) ventilation, the number of ventilator breaths delivered each minute is selected on the ventilator control panel. This rate is usually set at 10 to 12 breaths/minute.

3. *Rapid Breathing*

   A ventilator breath is delivered for each inspiratory effort during assisted ventilation, and this can create problems for patients who are breathing rapidly; i.e., the shorter time to exhale during rapid breathing can hamper the ability to fully exhale the tidal volume. Incomplete emptying of the lungs leads to air trapping and progressive hyperinflation, and can culminate in alveolar rupture with pneumothorax and pneumomediastinum. The following measures will reduce the risk of air trapping:

   a. Use low tidal volumes (6 mL/kg) instead of traditional tidal volumes (12 mL/kg).

   b. Increase the inspiratory flow rate: this prolongs expiration and allows more time to exhale the tidal volume.

   c. Sedation is advised but may not be effective for slowing respirations. Neuromuscular paralysis may be needed for patients in respiratory distress, but this should only be used as a short-term measure.

d. Change to a mode of ventilation that allows spontaneous breathing (e.g., IMV, CPAP). This helps because
rapid breathing is usually accompanied by reduced
tidal volumes (except in anxiety states), which compensates for the shorter exhalation times.

B. Intermittent Mandatory Ventilation

Intermittent mandatory ventilation (IMV) allows patients to
breathe spontaneously in the interval between ventilator
breaths. This design is more suitable than assisted (triggered) ventilation for rapidly breathing patients because
only a fraction of the patient's inspiratory efforts will trigger
a ventilator breath.

1. *Ventilatory Pattern*

The pattern of breathing during IMV is shown in the
lower panel of Figure 19.2. The first breath (dotted line)

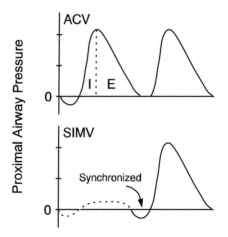

FIGURE 19.2 Ventilatory patterns during assist-control ventilation (*ACV*)
and "synchronized" intermittent mandatory ventilation (*SIMV*). The
dotted line in the SIMV panel represents a spontaneous breath.

is a spontaneous breath, and the second breath is a positive-pressure lung inflation that is synchronized to the patient's own breathing pattern (hence the term "synchronized" IMV). IMV thus combines spontaneous breathing with periods of assist-control ventilation.

2. *IMV Rate*

The number of positive-pressure lung inflations during IMV is selected on the control panel of the ventilator. This rate is usually set at 10 to 12 bpm initially, and can be adjusted upward or downward as dictated by the patient's spontaneous breathing (fewer breaths are required as the patient's spontaneous breathing approaches normal or premorbid levels).

3. *Spontaneous Breathing*

The work of breathing is increased during the period of spontaneous breathing (because of the high resistance imposed by tracheal tubes and ventilator tubing), and this is often a source of patient distress during IMV. Adding pressure-support ventilation (described later in the chapter) at 10 cm H_2O decreases the work of spontaneous breathing (1), and improves patient tolerance of IMV.

4. *Cardiac Performance*

IMV has an adverse effect on cardiac output in patients with left-ventricular dysfunction (2). This effect is the result of the negative intrathoracic pressures generated during the spontaneous breathing period. (Negative pressure in the thorax holds the ventricles open during systole, which impedes ventricular emptying).

5. *When to Use IMV*

The principal role of IMV is for patients who are breathing rapidly and are at risk for air trapping during ACV. IMV should NOT be used to wean patients from mechanical ventilation, as explained in Chapter 21.

III. PRESSURE-MODULATED VENTILATION

A. Pressure-Controlled Ventilation

1. Pressure-controlled ventilation (PCV) uses a constant, preselected pressure to inflate the lungs.

2. The ventilatory pattern during PCV is shown in the top panel in Figure 19.3 Note the absence of an inspiratory effort (i.e., a negative pressure deflection) at the beginning of the ventilator breaths. This highlights the fact that ventilation during PCV is completely controlled by the ventilator, with no patient interaction (similar to controlled ventilation in ACV).

3. The proposed advantage of PCV over ACV is a decreased risk of ventilator-induced lung injury (described in Chapter 16) because of the lower airway pressures. However, this is unproven.

4. There is one major disadvantage with PCV; i.e., *the inflation volume varies with changes in the mechanical properties of the lungs*. This is demonstrated in Figure 18.1. Note that when the inflation pressure is constant ($p = k$), the inflation volume decreases when there is an increase in airway resistance or a decrease in lung compliance (distensibility). This behavior is a major concern in patients with acute respiratory failure because the mechanical properties of the lungs are likely to change frequently in these patients.

B. Inverse Ratio Ventilation

1. When PCV is combined with a prolonged inflation time, the result is *inverse ratio ventilation* (IRV) (3).

2. The ventilatory pattern during IRV is shown in the middle panel of Figure 19.3. A decrease in inspiratory flow rate is used to prolong the time for lung inflation, and the usual I:E ratio of 1:2 is reversed to a ratio of 2:1.

3. The prolonged inflation time during IRV prevents alveolar collapse and improves gas exchange. However, prolonged inflation times also hamper exhalation and favor progressive hyperinflation and alveolar rupture.

4. The only indication for IRV at present is for patients with ARDS who have refractory hypoxemia or hypercapnia during ACV (4).

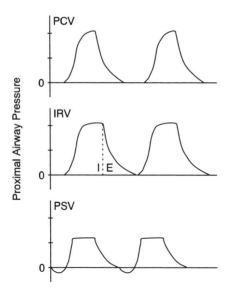

FIGURE 19.3 Ventilatory patterns during pressure-controlled ventilation (*PCV*), inverse ratio ventilation (*IRV*), and pressure-support ventilation (*PSV*).

C. Pressure-Support Ventilation

1. Pressure-support ventilation (PSV) is a method of augmenting the tidal volume during spontaneous breathing (5).

2. The ventilatory pattern during PSV is shown in the lower panel of Figure 19.3. Note that the inhaled gas is delivered at a constant pressure (usually 5 to 10 cm H_2O), which is accomplished by adjusting the inspiratory flow rate as needed. The inflation period is terminated when the inspiratory flow rate falls below 25% of the peak inspiratory flow.

3. PSV is used most often during weaning from mechanical ventilation. The goal of PSV in this setting is not to augment the tidal volume, but to provide enough pressure (5–10 cm H_2O) to overcome the resistance to flow in the tracheal tubes and ventilator tubing.

IV. POSITIVE END-EXPIRATORY PRESSURE

A. Basic Features

1. In conditions where the lungs are stiff or noncompliant (e.g., ARDS), there is a tendency for distal airspaces to collapse at the end of expiration, particularly during low-volume ventilation. To counteract this tendency, the pressure in the distal airspaces is not allowed to return to zero (atmospheric) pressure at the end of expiration. The resulting *positive end-expiratory pressure* (PEEP) acts like a stent to keep distal airspaces open at end-expiration.

2. PEEP is created by placing a pressure-relief valve in the expiratory limb of the ventilator circuit. Exhalation proceeds until the airways pressure reaches the pressure

level of the valve. Airflow ceases at this point, and the airways pressure remains constant (at the valve pressure) until the onset of the next lung inflation.

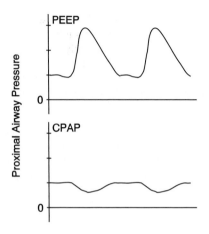

FIGURE 19.4 Upper panel shows positive-pressure lung inflations with positive end-expiratory pressure (*PEEP*), and lower panel shows spontaneous breathing with continuous positive airway pressure (*CPAP*).

3. The airway pressure pattern produced by PEEP is shown in the upper panel of Figure 19.4. Note that the entire pressure waveform is displaced upward. The implications of this displacement are as follows:

   a. The increase in peak airway pressure increases the risk of barotrauma (e.g., pneumothorax).

   b. The increase in mean airway (intrathoracic) pressure can retard venous return to the right side of the heart.

   c. When airway pressures are used to evaluate lung mechanics (see Figure 18.4), the amount of PEEP should be subtracted from the pressures.

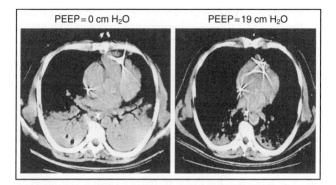

PEEP = 0 cm H$_2$O   PEEP = 19 cm H$_2$O

FIGURE 19.5 CT images from a patient with ARDS showing aeration of lung regions with atelectasis (recruitment) in response to PEEP. Images from Reference 6.

B. Lung Recruitment

1. The major benefit of PEEP is to keep the distal airspaces open. This is shown in Figure 19.5 (6). The increase in aerated lung is *lung recruitment*, and it improves pulmonary gas exchange.

2. The beneficial effect of PEEP on lung recruitment occurs only in areas of atelectasis that contain pockets of air (called "recruitable lung"). When the lungs contain areas of atelectasis that are airless ("nonrecruitable" lung), PEEP is distributed primarily to normal lung regions, resulting in overdistension and rupture of alveoli (7). CT images of the lungs can identify recruitable and nonrecruitable areas of lung (7).

3. The PaO$_2$/FIO$_2$ ratio (a measure of alveolar-capillary oxygen exchange) can be used to monitor the effects of PEEP on lung recruitment. ARDS is characterized by a PaO$_2$/FIO$_2$ ratio that is below 200 (see Table 16.2). An increase

in the PaO_2/FiO_2 ratio after the application of PEEP (like the response shown in Figure 19.6) indicates a favorable effect on lung recruitment.

B. Cardiac Performance

1. PEEP can decrease cardiac output by several mechanisms, including reduced venous return, reduced ventricular distensibility, and increased right ventricular outflow impedance (8,9).

2. The tendency for PEEP to reduce cardiac output is an important consideration because the beneficial effects of PEEP on gas exchange can be erased by a concurrent decrease in cardiac output. This is demonstrated by the equation for systemic oxygen delivery (DO_2):

$$DO_2 = Q \times 1.3 \times Hb \times SaO_2 \qquad (19.1)$$

Thus, PEEP can improve arterial oxygenation (SaO_2), but if there is a proportional decrease in cardiac output (Q), systemic oxygen delivery (DO_2) will remain unchanged.

3. An example of how PEEP can improve gas exchange but simultaneously reduce cardiac output is illustrated in Figure 19.6 (10). In this study of patients with ARDS, incremental PEEP was accompanied by a steady increase in the PaO_2/FiO_2 ratio and a steady decline in cardiac output. This demonstrates how the effects of PEEP on gas exchange can be misleading if the cardiac output is not monitored.

C. Clinical Uses

The use of PEEP should be reserved for the following situations:

1. In patients with ARDS who require toxic levels of inhaled oxygen (i.e., $FiO_2 \geq 60\%$) to maintain adequate arterial ox-

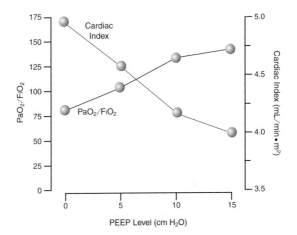

FIGURE 19.6 Opposing effects of positive end-expiratory pressure (PEEP) on pulmonary gas exchange (PaO_2/FiO_2) and cardiac output in patients with ARDS. From Reference 10.

ygenation (i.e., $SaO_2 \geq 88$–90%), PEEP-induced lung recruitment will increase the PaO_2/FiO_2 ratio and allow a decrease in the FiO_2 to less toxic or non-toxic levels.

2. During low-volume ventilation (see Tables 16.3 and 18.1), low-level PEEP (5–7 cm H_2O) is used routinely to prevent repeated closing and opening of distal airways, which is considered a source of lung injury (11).

V. CONTINUOUS POSITIVE AIRWAY PRESSURE

A. Basic Features

1. Spontaneous breathing from a pre-selected positive base-

line pressure is called *continuous positive airway pressure* (CPAP).

2. The airway pressure pattern during CPAP is shown in Figure 19.4. Note that the negative pressure deflection from the inspiratory effort does not fall below zero (atmospheric) pressure. This eliminates the extra work involved in generating a negative airway pressure to receive the inhaled gas.

B. Clinical Uses

The major uses of CPAP are in nonintubated patients, where CPAP is delivered through specialized face masks or nasal masks equipped with pressurized valves.

1. CPAP has been used as a method of noninvasive ventilation in patients with acute respiratory failure from a variety of disorders, including ARDS, cardiogenic pulmonary edema, and acute exacerbations of COPD (12–14).

2. In patients with cardiogenic pulmonary edema, CPAP may be particularly advantageous because of the actions of positive intrathoracic pressure to enhance ventricular emptying. (The cardiac effects of positive intrathoracic pressure are described in Chapter 18).

3. In patients with obstructive sleep apnea, CPAP is used to prevent collapse of the oropharynx during negative-pressure breathing efforts (15).

REFERENCES

1. Leung P, Jubran A, Tobin MJ. Comparison of assisted ventilator modes on triggering, patients' effort, and dyspnea. Am J Respir Crit Care Med 1997; 155:1940–1948.

2. Mathru M, Rao TL, El-Etr AA, Pifarre R. Hemodynamic responses to changes in ventilatory patterns in patients with nor-

tory patterns in patients with normal and poor left ventricular reserve. Crit Care Med 1982; 10:423–426.

3. Malarkkan N, Snook NJ, Lumb AB. New aspects of ventilation in acute lung injury. Anesthesia 2003; 58:647–667.

4. Wang SH, Wei TS. The outcome of early pressure-controlled inverse ratio ventilation on patients with severe acute respiratory distress syndrome in surgical intensive care unit. Am J Surg 2002; 183:151–155.

5. Hess DR. Ventilator waveforms and the physiology of pressure support ventilation. Respir Care 2005; 50:166–186.

6. Barbas CSV, Lung recruitment maneuvers in acute respiratory distress syndrome and facilitating resolution, Crit Care Med 2003; 31(Suppl):S265–S271.

7. Gattinoni L, Cairon M, Cressoni M, et al. Lung recruitment in patients with the acute respiratory distress syndrome. N Engl J Med 2006; 354:1775–1786.

8. Schmitt J-M, Viellard-Baron A, Augarde R, et al. Positive end-expiratory pressure titration in acute respiratory distress syndrome patients: Impact on right ventricular outflow impedance evaluated by pulmonary artery Doppler flow velocity measurements. Crit Care Med 2001; 29:1154–1158.

9. Takata M, Robotham JL. Ventricular external constraint by the lung and pericardium during positive end-expiratory pressure. Am Rev Respir Dis 1991; 43:872–875.

10. Gainnier M, Michelet P, Thirion X, et al. Prone position and positive end-expiratory pressure in acute respiratory distress syndrome. Crit Care Med 2003; 31:2719–2726.

11. Muscedere JG, Mullen JBM, Gan K, et al. Tidal ventilation at low airway pressures can augment lung injury. Am J Respir Crit Care Med 1994; 149:1327–1334.

12. Majid A, Hill NS. Noninvasive ventilation for acute respiratory failure. Curr Opin Crit Care 2005; 11(1):77–81.

13. Masip J, Roque M, Sanchez B, et al. Noninvasive ventilation in acute cardiogenic edema. JAMA 2005; 294:3124–3130.

14. de Lucas P, Tarancon C, Puente L, et al. Nasal continuous positive airway pressure in patients with COPD in acute respiratory failure. Chest 1993; 104:1694–1697.

15. Pack AI. Advances in sleep-disordered breathing. Am J Respir Crit Care Med 2006; 173(1):7–15.

Chapter 20

THE VENTILATOR-DEPENDENT PATIENT

This chapter describes the common practices and concerns in patients who require more than a few days of mechanical ventilation. The focus is on issues directly related to mechanical ventilation. Less specific issues in ventilator-dependent patients, such as nutritional support, are described elsewhere.

I. INDWELLING ENDOTRACHEAL TUBES

The following are some common concerns with indwelling endotracheal tubes.

A. Migration

1. Endotracheal tubes tend to migrate (in either direction) with time. Proximal migration can lead to vocal cord injury from the inflated balloon (cuff) at the distal end of the tube, and distal migration can lead to intubation of the right mainstem bronchus (which runs a straight course down from the main carina).

2. The position of endotracheal tubes should be monitored radiographically to prevent complications from migration. When the head is in a neutral position, the tip of the endotracheal tube should be 3 to 5 cm above the carina, or midway between the carina and vocal cords. (The carina is the point where the trachea bifurcates to form the right and left mainstem bronchi).

   a. If not visible, the carina is usually located over the in-

terspace between the fourth and fifth thoracic verte-
brae (T4–T5), and the vocal cords are situated over the
interspace between the fourh and fifth cervical verte-
brae (C4–C5) (1).

B. Paranasal Sinusitis

1. Nasotracheal (and nasogastric) tubes can obstruct the os-
tia that drain the paranasal sinuses, and this predisposes
to a purulent sinusitis (2). This complication has also been
reported with orotracheal intubation (3) for unclear reasons.

2. The maxillary sinus is almost always involved (2).

3. Opacification or air-fluid levels in the maxillary or ethmoid sinuses suggests the diagnosis of nosocomial sinusitis, but confirmation requires aspiration of infected material from the involved sinus (2).

4. Paranasal sinusitis is not a common cause of fever in the
ICU, but it should be considered in intubated patients who
have no other apparent cause of fever (see Chapter 32).

C. Laryngeal Damage

1. Injury of the larynx and vocal cords is a major concern
with indwelling endotracheal tubes, and is one of the
major reasons for the transition from endotracheal (translaryngeal) intubation to tracheostomy.

2. Some type of laryngeal damage (e.g., ulceration, edema)
is usually evident after 72 hours of translaryngeal intubation (4).

3. Fortunately, most cases of laryngeal injury resolve within weeks after extubation (5).

II. TRACHEOSTOMY

A. Transition to Tracheostomy

1. Tracheostomy offers several advantages over endotracheal intubation, including greater patient comfort, more effective clearing of secretions, reduced resistance for breathing, and the ability to vocalize and ingest food orally.

2. There is no consensus about the optimal time to switch from endotracheal intubation to tracheostomy. However, the following recommendation is reasonable (6):

   a. *After 5 to 7 days of endotracheal intubation, assess the likelihood of extubation in the following week: if the likelihood is low, proceed to tracheostomy.*

B. Techniques

1. Tracheostomy is traditionally performed as an open surgical procedure, but less invasive percutaneous techniques are gaining in popularity.

2. Percutaneous tracheostomy is very similar to the Seldinger technique for cannulating blood vessels (see Figure 5.2). A needle is used to puncture the trachea (in a space between the tracheal rings), and a guidewire is passed through the needle and into the trachea. The tracheostomy tube is then advanced over the guidewire (after a series of dilator tubes are used to increase the size of the tracheal stoma).

3. Emergency tracheostomy is usually performed through an opening in the cricothyroid membrane, just below the larynx. This technique, known as *cricothyroidotomy*, has a high incidence of laryngeal injury and subglottic stenosis, and patients who survive following a cricothyroido-

tomy should have a regular tracheostomy (surgical or percutaneous) as soon as they are stable (6).

C. Complications

1. Combining surgical and percutaneous tracheostomy, the mortality rate is less than 1%, and major adverse events occur in 5 to 10% of cases (6). The acute complications of most concern are bleeding and infection.

2. The pooled results of several studies comparing surgical and percutaneous tracheostomy show less bleeding and fewer infections with the percutaneous technique (7). However, the results of individual studies are conflicting.

3. Tracheal stenosis is a late complication that appears in the first 6 months after the tracheostomy tube is removed. Most cases of tracheal stenosis occur at the tracheotomy site and are caused by tracheal narrowing after the stoma closes. The incidence of tracheal stenosis ranges from zero to 15% (6), but most cases are asymptomatic.

III. CLEARING SECRETIONS

A. Respiratory Secretions

1. The mucosa of the respiratory tract is normally covered by a protective blanket of secretions. This blanket has a hydrophilic (water-soluble) layer, and a hydrophobic (water-insoluble) layer. The hydrophilic layer faces inward and keeps the mucosal surface moist. The hydrophobic layer, which faces toward the lumen of the airways, is composed of a meshwork of mucoprotein strands (called mucus threads) held together by disulfide

bridges. This meshwork traps particles and debris in the airways, and is responsible for the viscoelastic properties of sputum.

2. Under normal circumstances, the respiratory secretions are moved out of the lungs by the continuous action of cilia on the luminal surface of mucosal cells in the airways. This process is called *mucociliary clearance*, and it helps to clear dust and debris from the airways.

3. An abundance of particulate matter will increase the viscosity of respiratory secretions and hinder mucociliary clearance. When this occurs, coughing provides an additional means of clearing secretions.

4. These normal mechanisms of clearing respiratory secretions are defective in critically ill (e.g., ventilator-dependent) patients. Therefore, other measures such as tracheal suctioning are used to help clear secretions.

B. Tracheal Injections of Saline

Isotonic saline is routinely injected into the airways just prior to tracheal suctioning, presumably to facilitate the clearance of respiratory secretions. This practice is ill-advised for the following reasons.

1. The hydrophobic outer layer of respiratory secretions is responsible for their viscoelastic properties. This layer is not water soluble, which means that *saline cannot liquefy or reduce the viscosity of respiratory secretions*. Adding saline to thick, respiratory secretions is like pouring water over grease.

2. The injection of saline through tracheal tubes can predispose to pulmonary infections. Bacterial biofilms have been demonstrated on the inner surface of endotracheal tubes and tracheostomy tubes (8), and saline injections can dislodge these bacterial biofilms. Clinical studies

have shown that the injection of 5 mL of saline can dislodge up to 300,000 colonies of viable bacteria from the inner surface of endotracheal tubes (9). The dislodged bacteria can become a nidus of infection if they reach the lower airways.

TABLE 20.1 Mucolytic Therapy with *N*-Acetylcysteine (NAC)

Aerosol Therapy:	• Use 10% NAC solution.
	• Mix 2.5 mL NAC with 2.5 mL saline and place mixture (5 mL) in a small-volume nebulizer for aerosol delivery.
	• *Warning:* Can provoke bronchospasm, and is not recommended in asthmatics.
Tracheal Injection:	• Use 20% NAC solution.
	• Mix 2 mL NAC with 2 mL saline and inject 2 mL aliquots into the trachea.
	• *Warning:* Can promote bronchorrhea with repeated use.

C. Mucolytic Therapy

1. *N*-Acetylcysteine (Mucomyst) acts on the hydrophobic region of respiratory secretions to break the disulfide bridges between mucoprotein strands. By disrupting the elements responsible for the viscoelastic properties of respiratory secretions, *N*-acetylcysteine (NAC) acts as a *mucolytic agent* to liquefy secretions (10).

2. NAC can be used to relieve airways obstruction caused by tenacious secretions. The drug is available in a liquid preparation (10 or 20% solution) that can be given as an aerosol spray, or injected directly into the airways (Table 20.1). Direct injection into the airways is preferred because aerosolized NAC is irritating and can provoke coughing and bronchospasm (particularly in asthmatics).

3. If intratracheal injection of NAC does not relieve an obstruction, bronchoscopy is performed, and the NAC is applied directly to the mucous plug. Following relief of the obstruction, NAC can be instilled two or three times a day for the next few days. Repeated use of NAC is not advised because the drug solution is hypertonic (even with the saline additive) and can provoke bronchorrhea.

IV. ALVEOLAR DISRUPTION

Overdistension and rupture of alveoli is a common occurrence during mechanical ventilation and is clinically apparent in as many as 25% of ventilator-dependent patients (11).

A. Clinical Manifestations

Air that escapes from disrupted alveoli can produce a variety of clinical manifestations.

1. The air can dissect along tissue planes in the lungs and produce *pulmonary interstitial emphysema*, and air can move into the mediastinum to produce *pneumomediastinum*.

2. Air that reaches the mediastinum can move into the neck to produce *subcutaneous emphysema*, or can pass below the diaphragm to produce *pneumoperitoneum*.

3. If the alveolar disruption is close to the surface of the lung, air can enter the pleural space to produce a *pneumothorax*.

4. Each of these entities can occur alone or in combination with the others (11,12).

B. Pneumothorax

Radiographic evidence of pneumothorax is reported in 5 to

15% of ventilator-dependent patients (11,12). Predisposing factors include high inflation pressures and inflation volumes, intrinsic PEEP (described later in the chapter), and diffuse lung injury. Pneumothorax is particularly prevalent in patients with severe *Pneumocystis jirovecii* pneumonia.

1. *Clinical Presentation*

   Pneumothoraces are often clinically silent, at least initially.

   a. The most reliable clinical sign is *subcutaneous emphysema*, first apparent in the upper thorax and base of the neck.

   b. Pneumothorax may not be accompanied by diminished breath sounds in ventilator-dependent patients because sounds transmitted from the ventilator tubing can be mistaken as breath sounds.

   c. Continued accumulation of air in the pleural space will eventually produce a *tension pneumothorax*, which is characterized by a shift in the mediastinum toward the uninvolved hemithorax with hemodynamic instability.

2. *Radiographic Detection*

   The radiographic appearance of pneumothorax is atypical in ICU patients because the patients are usually supine and *pleural air does not collect at the lung apex in the supine position* (12,13).

   a. Pleural air can collect anterior to the lung in the supine position, and this may not be evident on portable chest films. This is demonstrated in Figure 20.1. In this case (a traumatic pneumothorax), the chest x-ray is unrevealing, but the CT image shows an anterior pneumothorax in the left hemithorax.

   b. Basilar and subpulmonic collections of air are also common features of pneumothorax in the supine position (13).

3. *Pleural Evacuation*

   The detection of a pneumothorax in a ventilator-depend-

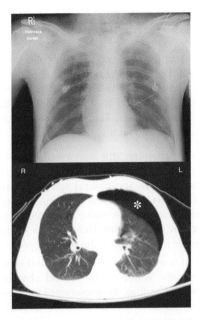

FIGURE 20.1 A portable chest x-ray and CT image of the thorax in a young male with blunt trauma to the chest. An anterior pneumothorax is evident on the CT image (indicated by the asterisk) but is not apparent on the chest x-ray.

ent patient should always prompt immediate insertion of a chest tube to evacuate the pleural air. Delays in pleural evacuation can lead to a tension pneumothorax.

a. Once the chest tube is inserted, the pleural drainage system described next is used for continued removal of air from the pleural space.

C. Pleural Drainage System

A triple-chamber system like the one shown in Figure 20.2 is used to drain both air and fluid from the pleural space (14). This is the same system used by the popular Pleur-Evac

Chest Drainage Systems (Teleflex Medical). The following is a brief description of how the system works.

1. The first chamber in the system (the collection bottle) collects fluid from the pleural space and allows air to pass through to the next bottle in the series. Because the inlet of this chamber is not in direct contact with the fluid, pleural fluid can accumulate in the bottle without imposing a back pressure on the pleural space.

2. The second chamber (the water-seal bottle) acts like a one-way valve that allows air to pass through to the next bottle (away from the pleural space) but prevents air from moving in the opposite direction (toward the pleural space). This one-way valve is created by submerging the inlet tube under water. This creates a "water-seal" that prevents air from entering the pleural space.

   a. Air that is evacuated from the pleural space will pass through the water in the second chamber, creating bubbles. Therefore, the presence of bubbles in the water-seal chamber is evidence of continued air leakage from the pleural space.

3. The third chamber in the system (the suction-control bottle) is attached to a negative-pressure source (suction), and the chamber is designed to set a maximum limit on the negative pressure imposed on the pleural space. This maximum pressure is determined by the height of the water column in the air-inlet tube. Negative pressure (from wall suction) draws the water down the air-inlet tube, and when the negative pressure exceeds the height of the water column, air is entrained from the atmosphere. Therefore, the pressure in the bottle can never become more negative than the height of the water column in the air-inlet tube.

   a. Water is added to the suction-control chamber to achieve a water level of 20 cm. The wall suction is then activated and slowly increased until bubbles appear in the water. This bubbling indicates that atmospheric air is being entrained, and thus the maximum allowable negative pressure has been achieved.

4. *Why Use Suction?*

The practice of using negative pressure to evacuate pleural air is unnecessary and potentially harmful.

a. Negative pressure is used to help re-inflate the lungs, but this is not necessary because the lungs will re-inflate when pleural air is evacuated and the intrapleural pressure drops to atmospheric (zero) pressure.

b. Creating a negative pressure in the pleural space is counterproductive in the presence of an air leak in the lungs because negative intrapleural pressure increases the transpulmonary pressure (the pressure difference between alveoli and the pleural space) that drives air out of the lungs and into the pleural space. Thus, *applying negative pressure to the pleural space promotes air leakage through a bronchopleural fistula.* Applying suction to the pleural space is not advised if there is a persistent air leak.

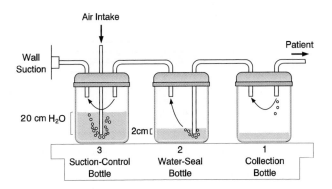

FIGURE 20.2 A triple-chamber drainage system for evacuating air and fluid from the pleural space.

V. INTRINSIC PEEP

As mentioned in Chapter 19, positive end-expiratory pressure (PEEP) is applied to the airways in certain conditions to prevent the distal airspaces from collapsing at the end of expiration. In addition to this applied or *extrinsic PEEP*, there is an internally generated or *intrinsic PEEP* that is produced by incomplete emptying of the lungs during expiration. The following is a description of the intrinsic form of PEEP and how it can be measured.

A. Pathogenesis

1. When the tidal volume is exhaled completely and there is no airflow at the end of expiration, the end-expiratory

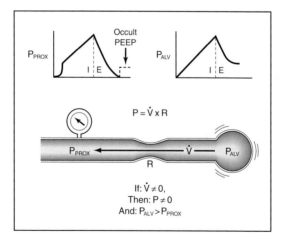

FIGURE 20.3 The features of intrinsic PEEP. The lower portion of the figure indicates that, when exhalation is incomplete and flow persists at end-expiration ($\dot{V} \neq 0$), alveolar pressure will be positive relative to proximal airway pressure ($P_{ALV} > P_{prox}$). This is depicted in the graphs in the upper portion of the figure. The positive alveolar pressure at end-expiration is intrinsic PEEP.

pressure returns to zero (atmospheric pressure) in both the alveoli and proximal airways.

2. When the tidal volume is not exhaled completely and there is persistent airflow at the end of expiration, the end-expiratory pressure in the alveoli will be positive while the end-expiratory pressure in the proximal airways returns to zero (see the graphs in the upper portion of Figure 20.3). This positive end-expiratory pressure (PEEP) in the alveoli is called intrinsic PEEP.

3. Because intrinsic PEEP is not apparent when monitoring proximal airways pressures, it is also called *occult PEEP* (15).

4. Intrinsic PEEP is the physiologic expression of hyperinflation from air trapping.

B. Predisposing Factors

Any condition that favors incomplete exhalation will predispose to the development of hyperinflation and intrinsic PEEP. These predisposing conditions can be separated into ventilator-related and disease-related conditions.

1. The ventilator-related conditions have been described in Chapter 19 and include volume-cycled ventilation with relatively large tidal volumes (10 to 12 mL/kg), and the use of assist-control ventilation for patients who are breathing rapidly.

2. The disease-related conditions include rapid breathing and obstructive airways disease; i.e., asthma and chronic obstructive pulmonary disease (COPD).

3. Most or all predisposing conditions can be present at the same time. In patients with asthma and COPD, intrinsic PEEP may be universal during conventional (large tidal volume) mechanical ventilation (16–18).

C. Consequences

The consequences of extrinsic PEEP described in Chapter 19 also apply to intrinsic PEEP. The following consequences deserve mention because of their possible impact on clinical outcomes.

1. *Reduced Cardiac Output*

   Intrinsic PEEP has been implicated as a cause of failed attempts at cardiopulmonary resuscitation (18). As described in Chapter 13, manual ventilation during CPR is often excessive (both in rate and inflation volume), which means that intrinsic PEEP may be commonplace during CPR, and the ability of PEEP to reduce venous return will impair the ability of chest compressions to promote cardiac output. The incidence and magnitude of intrinsic PEEP during CPR deserves further study.

2. *Increased Work of Breathing*

   Intrinsic PEEP can increase the work of breathing by increasing the pressure that must be generated to trigger a ventilator breath; e.g., if the ventilator breath is triggered at a negative pressure of 2 cm H_2O and there is 5 cm H_2O of intrinsic PEEP, the total pressure that must be generated by the patient to trigger the ventilator breath is 7 cm H_2O. This increased work of breathing can impede the ability to wean from mechanical ventilation.

D. Monitoring Intrinsic PEEP

The most accurate method of measuring intrinsic PEEP is to measure intraesophageal (pleural) pressure at end-expiration, but this measurement is difficult to perform and not readily available. The following methods can be used to detect intrinsic PEEP, but none of them provides an accurate quantitative measurement of the intrinsic PEEP level.

1. *End-Expiratory Air Flow*

   Expiratory flow tracings (available on many of the newer ventilator models) can be used to identify persistent flow at end-expiration. This confirms the presence of intrinsic PEEP, but provides no quantitative information.

2. *End-Expiratory Occlusion*

   During controlled ventilation (i.e., when the patient is completely passive), intrinsic PEEP can be detected by occluding the expiratory tubing at the end of expiration (16). This maneuver blocks airflow and allows the pressure in the proximal airways to equilibrate with alveolar pressure.

   a. A sudden rise in proximal airways pressure in response to end-expiratory occlusion is evidence of intrinsic PEEP (see the upper left panel in Fig. 20.3).

   b. This method does not provide accurate measurements of intrinsic PEEP because the occlusion cannot be timed to coincide with the very end of expiration.

3. *Response to Extrinsic PEEP*

   The application of extrinsic PEEP normally causes an equivalent increase in the peak inspiratory pressure. However, in the presence of intrinsic PEEP, the peak inspiratory pressure may be unaffected by extrinsic PEEP (this is explained below).

   a. Failure of extrinsic PEEP to produce an equivalent rise in peak airway pressure is evidence of intrinsic PEEP (19).

   b. The level of extrinsic PEEP that first produces a rise in peak airway pressures can be used as the measure of intrinsic PEEP (19).

E. Management

Maneuvers designed to promote exhalation (e.g., low-volume ventilation) can reduce the severity of intrinsic PEEP.

Adding extrinsic PEEP can also reduce intrinsic PEEP, as described below.

1. *Extrinsic PEEP*

When intrinsic PEEP is due to collapse of small airways at end-expiration (e.g., in asthma and COPD), extrinsic PEEP can help to keep the small airways open, and this will facilitate exhalation and reduce intrinsic PEEP. The amount of extrinsic PEEP should be enough to counterbalance the pressure causing small airways collapse (the *critical closing pressure*) but should not exceed the level of intrinsic PEEP (so expiratory flow is not impaired) (20). To accomplish this, *the amount of extrinsic PEEP should match the level of intrinsic PEEP.* Unfortunately, this is difficult to accomplish because of the difficulty in obtaining an accurate measure of intrinsic PEEP.

REFERENCES

1. Goodman LR. Pulmonary support and monitoring apparatus. In: Goodman LR, Putman CE, eds. Critical care imaging. 3rd ed. Philadelphia: WB Saunders, 1992;35–59.
2. Rouby J-J, Laurent P, Gosnach M, et al. Risk factors and clinical relevance of nosocomial maxillary sinusitis in the critically ill. Am J Respir Crit Care Med 1994; 150:776–783.
3. van Zanten AR, Dixon JM, Nipshagen MD, et al. Hospital-acquired sinusitis is a common cause of fever of unknown origin in orotracheally intubated critically ill patients. Crit Care 2005; 9:R583–R590.
4. Gallagher TJ. Endotracheal intubation. Crit Care Clin 1992; 8:665–676.
5. Colice GL. Resolution of laryngeal injury following translaryngeal intubation. Am Rev Respir Dis 1992; 145:361–364.
6. Tracheotomy: application and timing. Clin Chest Med 2003; 24:389–398.
7. Freeman BD, Isabella K, Lin N, Buchman TG. A meta-analysis of prospective trials comparing percutaneous and surgical tracheostomy in critically ill patients. Chest 2000; 118:1412–1418.

8. Adair CG, Gorman SP, Feron BM, et al. Implications of endotracheal tube biofilm for ventilator-associated pneumonia. Intensive Care Med 1999; 25:1072–1076.

9. Hagler DA, Traver GA. Endotracheal saline and suction catheters: sources of lower airways contamination. Am J Crit Care 1994; 3:444–447.

10. Holdiness MR. Clinical pharmacokinetics of *N*-acetylcysteine. Clin Pharmacokinet 1991; 20:123–134.

11. Gammon RB, Shin MS, Buchalter SE. Pulmonary barotrauma in mechanical ventilation. Chest 1992; 102:568–572.

12. Marcy TW. Barotrauma: detection, recognition, and management. Chest 1993; 104:578–584.

13. Tocino IM, Miller MH, Fairfax WR. Distribution of pneumothorax in the supine and semirecumbent critically ill adult. Am J Radiol 1985; 144:901–905.

14. Kam AC, O'Brien M, Kam PCA. Pleural drainage systems. Anesthesia 1993; 48:154–161.

15. Pepe P, Marini JJ. Occult positive end-expiratory pressure in mechanically ventilated patients with airflow obstruction. Am Rev Respir Dis 1982; 126:166–170.

16. Blanch L, Bernabe F, Lucangelo U. Measurement of air trapping, intrinsic positive end-expiratory pressure, and dynamic hyperinflation in mechanically ventilated patients. Respir Care 2005; 50:110–123.

17. Mughal MM, Culver DA, Minai OA, Arroliga AC. Auto-positive end-expiratory pressure: mechanisms and treatment. Cleve Clin J Med 2005; 72:801–809.

18 Rogers PL, Schlichtig R, Miro A, Pinsky M. Auto-PEEP during CPR. An "occult" cause of electromechanical dissociation. Chest 1991; 99:492–493.

19. Slutsky AS. Mechanical ventilation. Chest 1993; 104:1833–1859.

20. Tobin MJ, Lodato RF. PEEP, auto-PEEP, and waterfalls. Chest 1989; 96:449–451.

Chapter 21

DISCONTINUING MECHANICAL VENTILATION

This chapter describes the transition from ventilatory support to unaided breathing. This process is uneventful in most patients, but it can consume over half the time on a ventilator in problem patients.

I. IDENTIFYING CANDIDATES

A. Readiness Criteria

1. When ventilator-dependent patients show evidence of significant and continued clinical improvement, the checklist in Table 21.1 can be used to identify candidates for a trial of spontaneous (unaided) breathing off the ventilator.

2. Patients who satisfy the criteria in Table 21.1 should be removed from the ventilator briefly to obtain the measurements in Table 21.2 These measurements have been used to predict the likelihood that a patient will tolerate a trial of spontaneous breathing.

   a. No single measurement in Table 21.1 can predict with certainty which patients are ready to resume spontaneous breathing (1,2). However, when taken together, these measurements provide an impression of how difficult it will be for the patient to resume spontaneous breathing. Two of the more predictive measurements are described next.

TABLE 21.1 Checklist to Identify Candidates for a Trial of Spontaneous Breathing

Respiratory Criteria:
- ☑ $PaO_2 \geq 60$ mm Hg on $FiO_2 < 40-50\%$ and PEEP $\leq 5-8$ cm H_2O
- ☑ PaO_2 normal or baseline
- ☑ Patient is able to initiate an inspiratory effort

Cardiovascular Criteria:
- ☑ No evidence of myocardial ischemia
- ☑ Heart rate ≤ 140 beats/min
- ☑ Blood pressure normal without vasopressors or with minimum vasopressor support (e.g., dopamine < 5 μg/kg/min)

Adequate Mental Status:
- ☑ Patient is arousable, or Glasgow Coma Score ≥ 13

Absence of Correctable Comorbid Conditions:
- ☑ Patient is afebrile
- ☑ There are no significant electrolyte abnormalities.

From Reference 1.

A. Rapid-Shallow Breathing Index

1. Rapid, shallow breathing is common in patients who do not tolerate spontaneous breathing (6). The tendency for rapid shallow breathing is evaluated by the ratio of respiratory rate to tidal volume (RR/V_T), which is called the *rapid-shallow breathing index* (RSBI). For a healthy adult with a tidal volume of 500 mL (0.5 L) and a respiratory rate of 10 bpm, the RSBI is: $10/0.5 = 20/L$

2. The predictive value of the RSBI from a landmark study (2) showed the following:

   a. When the RSBI was above 105/L, 95% of the attempts to wean (discontinue) mechanical ventilation failed.

b. When the RSBI was below 105/L, 80% of the wean attempts were successful.

c. The results of this study have been used to establish a *threshold RSBI of 100/L for predicting success or failure to resume spontaneous breathing* (i.e., an RSBI below 100/L predicts success, and an RSBI above 100/L predicts failure).

TABLE 21.2 Identifying Patients Who Will Tolerate a Spontaneous Breathing Trial (SBT)

Measurement	Reference Range in Adults	Threshold for Successful SBT
Tidal Volume (V_T)	5–7 mL/kg	4–6 mL/kg
Respiratory Rate (RR)	10–18 bpm	30–38 bpm
Total Ventilation (V_E)	5–6 L/min	10–15 L/min
RR/V_T Ratio	20–40/L	100/L
Maximum Inspiratory Pressure (PImax)	-90 to -120 cm H_2O	-15 to -30 cm H_2O

All measurements should be obtained during spontaneous breathing.
From Reference 1.

B. Maximum Inspiratory Pressure

1. The strength of the respiratory muscles can be evaluated by having a patient exhale to residual lung volume and then inhale as forcefully as possible against a closed valve (8). The airway pressure generated by this maneuver is called the *maximum inspiratory pressure* (PImax).

2. Healthy adults can generate a negative PImax of 90 to 120 cm H_2O (see Table 21.2), with men generating higher pressures than women.

a. When the PImax is less than -20 cm H_2O, there is little or no chance of weaning from mechanical ventilation (2). However, a PImax greater than -20 cm H_2O does not ensure a successful attempt at weaning.

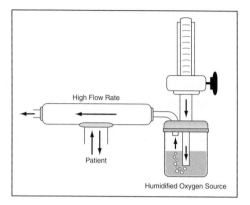

High Flow Rate

Patient

Humidified Oxygen Source

FIGURE 21.1 Diagram of the T-shaped circuit used for spontaneous breathing trials.

II. SPONTANEOUS BREATHING TRIALS

The spontaneous breathing trial (SBT) can be conducted while the patient is still connected to the ventilator circuit, or the patient can be removed completely from the ventilator and allowed to breathe from an independent source of oxygen. The advantages and disadvantages of each method are described next. There is no evidence that either method is superior to the other (1).

A. Breathing Through the Ventilator

1. Spontaneous breathing trials are usually conducted while the patient is attached to the ventilator. The advan-

tage of this method is the ability to monitor the tidal volume and respiratory rate during the trial. The drawback is the extra work of breathing imposed by the flow resistance of the ventilator tubing.

2. Pressure-support ventilation (described in Chapter 20) is used counteract the increased work of breathing through the ventilator circuit. A positive pressure of 5–7 cm H_2O will accomplish this goal without augmenting the patient's spontaneous tidal volume.

B. Breathing Through a T-Piece

1. Spontaneous breathing trials can be conducted with the patient disconnected from the ventilator using a T-shaped breathing circuit like the one in Figure 21.1. Oxygen-enriched gas is delivered at high flow rates through the horizontal arm of the T-shaped circuit. The rapid flow creates a suction that draws exhaled gas out of the lungs. This reduces the work of breathing and prevents rebreathing of exhaled gas.

2. Because of the T-shaped breathing circuit, spontaneous breathing trials with the patient disconnected from the ventilator are often called *T-piece trials*.

3. The advantage of T-piece trials is the reduced work of breathing. The disadvantage of T-piece trials is the inability to monitor the patient's tidal volume and respiratory rate.

C. Protocol

1. The initial trial of spontaneous breathing should last between 30 and 120 minutes (1). About 80% of patients who tolerate this amount of time without ventilatory support can be permanently removed from the ventilator (1).

2. For cases of short-term ventilatory support (e.g., cardiac surgery), a successful one-hour period of spontaneous breathing is enough to discontinue ventilatory support.

3. For prolonged mechanical ventilation (>72 hrs), longer periods of spontaneous breathing are needed before discontinuing mechanical ventilation. Patients should tolerate at least 8 hours (and sometimes up to 24 hours) of spontaneous breathing before removing the ventilator from the room.

D. Troubleshooting

Rapid breathing is common during spontaneous breathing trials, and can be a sign of failure to sustain unaided breathing. However, rapid breathing can also be a manifestation of anxiety, which is common when patients are removed from ventilatory support (3).

1. *The Tidal Volume*

The flow diagram in Figure 21.2 shows a simple approach to the patient with rapid breathing based on the patient's tidal volume. Anxiety causes hyperventilation, which is associated with an increase in tidal volume, whereas failure to sustain spontaneous breathing when rapid breathing develops is associated with a decrease in tidal volume (rapid, shallow breathing).

2. *The Arterial PCO$_2$*

In cases where anxiety is expected, the arterial PCO$_2$ (PaCO$_2$) can be a useful measurement.

a. A decrease in PaCO$_2$ is evidence of adequate ventilation, and suggests an underlying anxiety, whereas a normal or increasing PaCO$_2$ is evidence of respiratory failure. (Remember that a normal PaCO$_2$ in the face of a high minute ventilation is a sign of ventilatory failure).

III. FAILURE TO WEAN

A. Persistence

1. Failure to wean from mechanical ventilation is almost never an irreversible or permanent condition, and patients who fail initial wean attempts should continue to have daily trials of spontaneous breathing. The purpose of this is not to acclimate the patient to life off the ventilator, but simply to provide multiple opportunities to detect when the patient no longer needs ventilatory assistance (4).

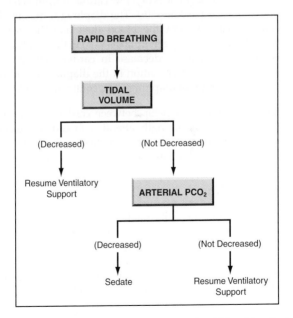

FIGURE 21.2 Flow diagram for the evaluation of rapid breathing during a spontaneous breathing trial.

2. Failure to wean should also prompt a search for conditions that might be responsible for the continued ventilator dependence. This search should include the conditions that follow.

B. Low Cardiac Output

1. The transition from positive-pressure ventilation to negative-pressure spontaneous breathing can prompt a decrease in cardiac stroke output (5). (The negative intrathoracic pressure holds the ventricles open and opposes ventricular emptying).

2. One of the consequences of a low cardiac output is respiratory muscle weakness (6). The diaphragm maximally extracts oxygen from the blood (just like the heart), which means that oxygen uptake (VO_2) in the diaphragm is flow-dependent. A decrease in cardiac output will jeopardize tissue oxygenation in the diaphragm and reduce the strength of diaphragmatic contractions (6).

3. Because of the relationship between cardiac output and respiratory muscle strength, attention should be directed to the cardiac output whenever a patient with known cardiac dysfunction is unable to wean from the ventilator.

C. Overfeeding

1. An increase in the daily intake of calories will increase metabolic CO_2 production, as demonstrated in Figure 21.3 (7). If the daily intake of calories exceeds the daily caloric requirements, the excess CO_2 that is produced will stimulate ventilation and increase the work of breathing, and this can jeopardize a spontaneous breathing trial (7,8).

2. In patients with lung disease and abnormal gas exchange, excess metabolic CO_2 production can lead to an increase in the arterial PCO_2 and acute respiratory acidosis.

3. To avoid this problem, the daily intake of calories should not exceed the daily requirement. (See Chapter 36 to learn how the daily caloric requirement is determined).

D. Neuromuscular Weakness

1. Ventilator-dependent patients can develop a specific type of neuromuscular weakness that is found only in ICU patients. There are 2 disorders that are responsible for most cases of ICU-acquired neuromuscular weakness, and they are known collectively as *critical illness polyneuropathy and myopathy* (9). These disorders are described in Chapter 41.

2. Respiratory muscle strength can be impaired by depletion of magnesium and phosphorus (8,10). The clinical significance of this is unclear, but correcting the problem will optimize the conditions for weaning.

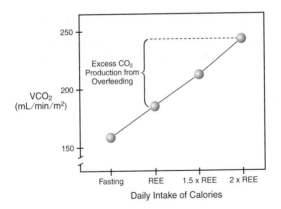

FIGURE 21.3 The influence of daily caloric intake on metabolic CO_2 production (VCO_2) in mechanically ventilated patients. REE is the resting energy expenditure (in kcal/24 hours), which is a measure of daily caloric requirements. Each data point represents a mean value. (From Reference 7).

IV. TRACHEAL DECANNULATION

When unaided breathing is no longer a concern, the next step is to consider removing the endotracheal tube or tracheostomy tube. At this point, there are 2 questions that must be answered:

1) Is the patient able to protect the airway and clear secretions?

2) Is there any evidence of laryngeal injury that would compromise breathing after the tube is removed?

A. Protecting the Airway

All of the conditions mentioned below are needed for optimal airway protection.

1. The patient should be awake or easily aroused and able to follow commands.

2. The volume of respiratory secretions should be minimal.

3. The gag and cough reflexes should be present, and cough strength should be adequate. The strength of coughing can be evaluated by placing a file card or piece of paper 1-2 cm from the end of the tracheal tube and asking the patient to cough. If wetness appears on the card, the cough strength is considered adequate (11).

4. The absence of a cough or gag reflex should delay tracheal decannulation if these reflexes are likely to return. If these protective mechanisms are permanently lost, the decision to decannulate the trachea is a complex one that is beyond the scope of this little book.

B. Laryngeal Edema

1. *Translaryngeal Intubation*

   Injury to the larynx is a common consequence of endotracheal (translaryngeal) intubation, and is often the result of a traumatic or prolonged intubation. The laryngeal edema that develops can obstruct the larynx after the endotracheal tube is removed.

a. Severe laryngeal edema is reported in as many as 40% of cases of prolonged translaryngeal intubation (12), and 5% of patients experience severe upper airway obstruction following extubation (13).

2. *The Cuff-Leak Test*

The cuff-leak test is used to identify patients with severe laryngeal edema prior to extubation. The test is performed while the patient is receiving volume-cycled ventilation.

a. The volume of exhaled gas is measured with the cuff inflated and again after the cuff is deflated. If there is no obstruction at the level of the larynx, cuff deflation will result in the escape of exhaled gas around the endotracheal tube, and the volume of gas exhaled through the endotracheal tube will decrease.

b. Unfortunately, there is a lack of agreement about the magnitude of the volume change that is significant. Volume changes of 110 mL, 140 mL, and 25% have been proposed as the threshold volume for identifying a patent larynx (12–14).

c. Despite this lack of agreement, the absence of a volume change after cuff deflation can be used as evidence of laryngeal obstruction.

3. *Tracheostomy*

Laryngeal edema also occurs with tracheostomy, and laryngeal obstruction can be a problem after removal of tracheostomy tubes (15). The laryngeal damage associated with tracheostomy tubes can be the result of an endotracheal intubation that preceded the tracheostomy, or can be the result of ischemic injury to the larynx during the tracheostomy procedure.

4. *Fenestrated Tube*

Breathing through a fenestrated (windowed) tracheostomy tube like the one in Figure 21.4 can be useful in detecting laryngeal obstruction. When the inner cannula is removed, the fenestration allows the patient's breathing efforts to move air through the larynx. If the opening of the tube is capped and the cuff is deflated, the patient must breathe entirely through the larynx. Difficulty breathing in this situation raises suspicion for a laryngeal obstruction, which can be confirmed using direct laryngoscopy.

5. *Steroids (for Anything That Swells)*

a. The antiinflammatory actions of steroids justifies their use to treat laryngeal edema associated with anaphylaxis, because this edema is produced by inflammation.

b. Steroids are also used to treat the laryngeal edema associated with tracheal intubation, but this does not seem justified because this edema is produced by trauma. There are 2 studies evaluating the use of steroids for

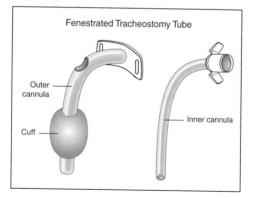

FIGURE 21.4 A fenestrated tracheostomy tube. When the inner cannula is removed, the fenestration (window) allows breathing efforts to move air through the larynx.

this type of (traumatic) laryngeal edema, and the results are conflicting (16,17).

c. The use of steroids for traumatic laryngeal edema is an
example of *steroids for anything that swells* (18).

V. THE POST-EXTUBATION PERIOD

A. A Paradox

1. The cross-sectional area of the glottis (the narrowest portion of the upper airway) is 66 mm^3 in the average-sized
adult, whereas the cross-sectional area of an average-
sized adult tracheal tube (8 mm internal diameter) is 50
mm^3 (19). The larger cross-sectional area of the glottis creates less resistance for airflow, so the work of breathing
should be reduced after extubation.

2. However, there is a paradoxical *increase* in the work of
breathing following extubation (20). This is a consistent
observation, and is unexplained.

B. Post-Extubation Stridor

1. Laryngeal obstruction following extubation can produce
a sonorous sound known as *stridor*. Because the obstruction is extrathoracic, the stridor occurs during inspiration
(i.e., the negative intrathoracic pressure is transmitted to
the larynx and causes inspiratory narrowing).

2. Post-extubation stridor is not always an indication for
immediate reintubation. If the patient is not exhibiting
signs of respiratory distress, inhalation of **aerosolized
epinephrine** (2.5 mL of 1% epinephrine) is a popular (but
unproven) treatment option. A racemic mixture of epinephrine (which has equal amounts of the *l*-isomer and

d-isomer) has been popular in this situation, but has no proven superiority over the standard (*l*-isomer) preparation (21).

REFERENCES

1. MacIntyre NR, Cook DJ, Ely EW Jr, et al. Evidence-based guidelines for weaning and discontinuing ventilatory support: A collective task force facilitated by the American College of Chest Physicians, the American Association for Respiratory Care, and the American College of Critical Care Medicine. Chest 2001; 120(Suppl):375S–395S.

2. Yang K, Tobin MJ. A prospective study of indexes predicting the outcome of trials of weaning from mechanical ventilation. N Engl J Med 1991; 324:1445–1450.

3. Bouley GH, Froman R, Shah H. The experience of dyspnea during weaning. Heart Lung 1992; 21:471–476.

4. Frutos-Vivar F, Esteban A. When to wean from a ventilator: an evidence-based strategy. Cleve Clin J Med 2003; 70:389-397.

5. Pinsky MR. Cardiovascular issues in respiratory care. Chest 2005; 128:592S–597S.

6. Nishimura Y, Maeda H, Tanaka K, et al. Respiratory muscle strength and hemodynamics in heart failure. Chest 1994; 105:355–359.

7. Talpers SS, Romberger DJ, Bunce SB, Pingleton SK. Nutritionally associated increased carbon dioxide production. Chest 1992; 102: 551–555.

8. Benotti PN, Bistrian B. Metabolic and nutritional aspects of weaning from mechanical ventilation. Crit Care Med 1989; 17:181–185.

9. Hudson LD, Lee CM. Neuromuscular sequelae of critical illness. N Engl J Med 2003; 348:745–747.

10. Malloy DW, Dhingra S, Solren F, et al. Hypomagnesemia and respiratory muscle power. Am Rev Respir Dis 1984; 129:427–431.

11. Khamiees M, Raju P, DeGirolamo A, et al. Predictors of extubation outcome in patients who have successfully completed a spontaneous breathing trial. Chest 2001; 120:1262–1270.

12. Chung Y-H, Chao T-Y, Chiu C-T, Lin M-C. The cuff-leak test is a simple tool to verify severe laryngeal edema in patients undergoing long-term mechanical ventilation. Crit Care Med 2006; 34:409–414.

13. Kriner EJ, Shafazand S, Colice GL. The endotracheal tube cuff leak test as a predictor for postextubation stridor. Respir Care 2005; 50:1632–1638.

14. Prinianakis G, Alexopoulou C, Mamidakis E, et al. Determinants of the cuff-leak test: a physiological study. Crit Care 2005; 9: R24–R31.

15. Colice C, Stukel T, Dain B. Laryngeal complications of prolonged intubation. Chest 1989; 96:877–884.

16. Cheng K-C, Hou C-C, Huang H-C, et al. Intravenous injection of methylprednisolone reduces the incidence of postextubation stridor in intensive care unit patients. Crit Care Med 2006; 34: 1345–1350.

17. Gaussorgues P, Boyer F, Piperno D, et al. Do corticosteroids prevent postintubation laryngeal edema? A prospective study of 276 adults. Crit Care Med 1988; 16:649–652.

18. Shemie, S. Steroids for anything that swells: Dexamethasone and postextubation airway obstruction. Crit Care Med: 1996; 24: 1613–1614.

19. Kaplan JD, Schuster DP. Physiologic consequences of tracheal intubation. Clin Chest Med 1991; 12:425–432.

20. Mehta S, Nelson DL, Klinger JR, et al. Prediction of post-extubation work of breathing. Crit Care Med 2000; 28:1341–1346.

21. Nutman J, Brooks LJ, Deakins K, et al. Racemic versus l-epinephrine aerosol in the treatment of postextubation laryngeal edema: results from a prospective, randomized, double-blind study. Crit Care Med 1994; 22:1591–1594.

Chapter 22

ACID-BASE INTERPRETATIONS

This chapter reviews some basic features of acid-base physiology, and then uses these features to present an organized approach to the identification of acid-base disorders.

I. BASIC CONCEPTS

A. Hydrogen Ion Concentration

1. The hydrogen ion concentration $[H^+]$ in extracellular fluid is determined by the balance between the PCO_2 and the bicarbonate concentration $[HCO_3]$ (1,2). The relationship between these variables is defined in Equation 22.1.

$$[H^+] = 24 \times PCO_2 / [HCO_3] \qquad (22.1)$$

The normal $[H^+]$ in arterial blood is shown below using a PCO_2 of 40 mm Hg and a $[HCO_3]$ of 24 mEq/L.

$$[H^+] = 24 \times (40/24) = 40 \text{ nEq/L} \qquad (22.2)$$

2. Note that $[H^+]$ is expressed in nanoequivalents per liter (nEq/L), while $[HCO_3]$ is expressed in milliequivalents per liter (mEq/L). This means that the H^+ concentration in extracellular fluid is *one-millionth* the HCO_3 concentration (i.e., one nanoequivalent is 10^{-6} milliequivalents).

3. Because the $[H^+]$ is so much lower (by 6 orders of magnitude) than the concentration of HCO_3 and other electrolytes, it is expressed in logarithmic terms as the pH:

$$pH = -\log[H^+] \qquad (22.3)$$

349

The pH varies inversely with the [H⁺], so an increase in the [H⁺] reduces the pH, and a decrease in [H⁺] raises the pH. The [H⁺] and corresponding pH values in arterial blood are shown in Table 22.1. The normal [H⁺] of 40 nEq/L corresponds to a pH of 7.40. Note that over the physiologic pH range, the [H⁺] varies by only 18 nEq/L. This is a testament to the acid-base control system.

TABLE 22.1 Relationship Between pH and [H⁺] in Arterial Blood

pH	[H⁺] (nEq/L)	
7.7	20	
7.6	26	
7.5	32	Physiologic
7.4 ← Normal →	40	Range
7.3	50	(Δ18 nEq/L)
7.2	63	
7.1	80	
7.0	100	

B. Types of Acid–Base Disorders

Acid-base disorders are characterized by a change in the PCO₂ or HCO₃ concentration in extracellular fluid (plasma).

1. A change in the PCO₂ represents a *respiratory* acid-base disorder: an increase in PCO₂ is a *respiratory acidosis*, and a decrease in PCO₂ is a *respiratory alkalosis*.

2. A change in HCO₃ is a *metabolic* acid-base disorder: a decrease in HCO₃ is a *metabolic acidosis*, and an increase in HCO₃ is a *metabolic alkalosis*.

3. Every acid-base disorder elicits a *compensatory response* that limits the impact of the disorder on the pH.

a. Compensatory responses operate by controlling the PCO_2/HCO_3 ratio. For example, if there is an increase in arterial PCO_2 (respiratory acidosis), the compensatory response will involve an increase in the plasma HCO_3 concentration, and this will keep the PCO_2/HCO_3 ratio (and the pH) relatively constant. Table 22.2 shows the compensatory adjustments for each of the primary acid-base disorders.

b. Compensatory responses do not correct the primary acid-base disorder; i.e., they limit, but do not prevent, the change in pH.

TABLE 22.2 Primary Acid-Base Disorders and Associated Compensatory Changes

$$[H^+] = 24 \times PCO_2/HCO_3$$

Primary Disorder	Primary Change	Compensatory Change*
Respiratory acidosis	Increased PCO_2	Increased HCO_3
Respiratory alkalosis	Decreased PCO_2	Decreased HCO_3
Metabolic acidosis	Decreased HCO_3	Decreased PCO_2
Metabolic alkalosis	Increased HCO_3	Increased PCO_2

*Compensatory changes are designed to keep the PCO_2/HCO_3 ratio constant.

II. PREDICTIVE EQUATIONS

The diagnosis of acid-base disorders requires that you not only identify the primary disorder, but also evaluate compensatory responses (to identify additional or secondary acid-base disorders). This latter task requires the equations included in this section, which define the expected compensation for primary acid-base disorders. These equations (which are also shown in Figure 22.1) will be incorporated into a diagnostic scheme that is presented in the next section.

A. Metabolic Acid-Base Disorders

The compensatory response to metabolic acid-base derangements is an immediate change in minute ventilation that changes the arterial PCO_2 ($PaCO_2$) in the same direction as the primary change in HCO_3 (see Table 22.2).

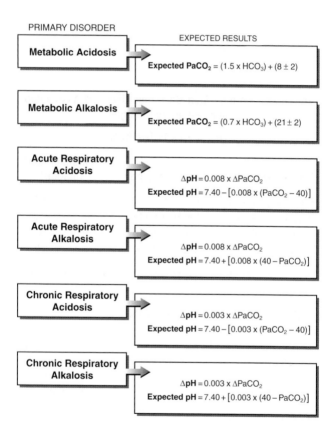

FIGURE 22.1 Useful formulas for acid-base interpretations.

1. *Metabolic Acidosis*

Metabolic acidosis is characterized by a primary decrease in the plasma HCO_3 concentration, and the compensatory response is an increase in minute ventilation, which decreases the arterial PCO_2 ($PaCO_2$) to a level that is predicted by Equation 22.4 (3). (The HCO_3 in Equations 22.4 and 22.5 is the measured concentration in plasma, in mEq/L).

a. COMPENSATION FOR METABOLIC ACIDOSIS:

$$\textbf{Expected PaCO}_2 = \textbf{(1.5} \times \textbf{HCO}_3\textbf{)} + \textbf{(8} \pm \textbf{2)} \qquad (22.4)$$

2. *Metabolic Alkalosis*

Metabolic alkalosis is characterized by a primary increase in the plasma HCO_3 concentration. The compensatory response is a decrease in minute ventilation, which increases the $PaCO_2$ to a level predicted by Equation 22.5 (4).

a. COMPENSATION FOR METABOLIC ALKALOSIS:

$$\textbf{Expected PaCO}_2 = \textbf{(0.7} \times \textbf{HCO}_3\textbf{)} + \textbf{(21} \pm \textbf{2)} \qquad (22.5)$$

B. Respiratory Acid-Base Disorders

The compensatory response to respiratory acid-base disorders takes place in the kidneys and involves an adjustment in HCO_3 reabsorption in the proximal tubules. This response is not immediate, but begins to appear in 6 to 12 hours, and is fully developed after a few days. Because of this delay, respiratory acid-base disorders are classified as acute (uncompensated) and chronic (fully compensated).

1. *Acute Respiratory Disorders*

Prior to the onset of renal compensation, a change in $PaCO_2$ of 1 mm Hg will produce a change in pH of 0.008 pH units (1,5).

$$\Delta \textbf{pH} = \textbf{0.008} \times \Delta \textbf{PaCO}_2 \qquad (22.6)$$

This relationship is incorporated into Equations 22.7 and 22.8 using 7.40 for the normal pH and 40 mm Hg for the normal $PaCO_2$.

a. ACUTE RESPIRATORY ACIDOSIS:

$$\text{Expected pH} = 7.40 - [0.008 \times (PaCO_2 - 40)] \quad (22.7)$$

b. ACUTE RESPIRATORY ALKALOSIS:

$$\text{Expected pH} = 7.40 + [0.008 \times (40 - PaCO_2)] \quad (22.8)$$

2. *Chronic Respiratory Disorders*

When renal compensation is fully developed, a change in $PaCO_2$ of 1 mm Hg will produce a change in pH of 0.003 pH units (5).

$$\Delta pH = 0.003 \times \Delta PaCO_2 \quad (22.9)$$

This relationship is incorporated into Equations 22.10 and 22.11 using 7.40 as a normal arterial pH and 40 mm Hg as a normal $PaCO_2$.

a. CHRONIC RESPIRATORY ACIDOSIS:

$$\text{Expected pH} = 7.40 - [0.003 \times (PaCO_2 - 40)] \quad (22.10)$$

b. CHRONIC RESPIRATORY ALKALOSIS:

$$\text{Expected pH} = 7.40 + [0.003 \times (40 - PaCO_2)] \quad (22.11)$$

II. SCHEME FOR ACID-BASE INTERPRETATIONS

The following is a structured approach to the diagnosis of acid-base disorders that proceeds in three stages. The first two stages are designed to identify primary and secondary acid-base disorders using only three variables: arterial pH, $PaCO_2$, and plasma HCO_3 concentration. The last stage involves the evaluation of metabolic acidosis. The detection of acid-base disorders requires the normal ranges for acid-base parameters, which are listed below.

$$\text{Arterial pH} = 7.36 - 7.44$$
$$\text{Arterial } PCO_2 = 36 - 44 \text{ mm Hg}$$
$$\text{Plasma } HCO_3 = 22 - 26 \text{ mEq/L}$$

A. Identify the Primary Acid-Base Disorder

This stage requires only the pH and $PaCO_2$. If either of these measurements is outside the normal range, there is an acid-base disorder, and you should proceed as follows:

1. If the pH and $PaCO_2$ are both abnormal, compare the directional change.

   a. If both change in the same direction, the primary acid-base disorder is metabolic.

   b. If both change in opposite directions, the primary acid-base disorder is respiratory.

   c. EXAMPLE: Consider a patient with a pH of 7.23 and a $PaCO_2$ of 23 mm Hg. The pH and $PaCO_2$ are both reduced (indicating a primary metabolic disorder), and the pH is low (indicating an acidosis), so this condition represents a *primary metabolic acidosis*.

2. If either the pH or $PaCO_2$ is normal, there is a *mixed* metabolic and respiratory acid-base disorder (one is an acidosis and the other is an alkalosis). There is no primary acid-base disorder in this instance because compensatory responses to primary acid-base disorders never fully correct the problem (i.e., never normalize the pH and $PaCO_2$).

   a. If the pH is normal, the direction of change in $PaCO_2$ identifies the respiratory disorder.

   b. If the $PaCO_2$ is normal, the direction of change in the pH identifies the metabolic disorder.

   c. EXAMPLE: Consider a patient with an arterial pH of

7.37 and a PaCO$_2$ of 55 mm Hg. The pH is normal, so there is a mixed metabolic and respiratory acid-base disorder. The PaCO$_2$ is elevated. so the respiratory disorder is an acidosis, and thus the metabolic disorder must be an alkalosis. Therefore, the acid-base disorder in this case is a *mixed respiratory acidosis and metabolic alkalosis*.

B. Evaluate Compensatory Responses

If there is a primary acid-base disorder, proceed as directed below. If there is a mixed acid-base disorder, skip this stage and go to the third stage (if applicable).

1. If there is a primary metabolic acidosis or alkalosis, use Equations 22.4 or 22.5 to calculate the expected PaCO$_2$.

   a. If the measured PaCO$_2$ is higher than predicted, there is an additional (secondary) respiratory acidosis.

   b. If the measured PaCO$_2$ is lower than predicted, there is an additional (secondary) respiratory alkalosis.

2. If there is a respiratory acidosis or alkalosis, use the PaCO$_2$ to calculate the expected pH using Equations 22.7–22.11. Compare the measured pH to the expected pH to determine if the condition is acute, partially compensated, or fully compensated.

   a. If the measured pH is between the expected pH for the acute (uncompensated) and chronic (compensated) condition, the disorder is called a *partially compensated* respiratory acidosis or alkalosis.

   b. For respiratory acidosis, if the pH is lower than expected for the acute condition, there is a secondary metabolic acidosis, and if the pH is higher than expected for the chronic (compensated) condition, there is a secondary metabolic alkalosis.

   c. For respiratory alkalosis, if the pH is higher than expected for the acute condition, there is a secondary

metabolic alkalosis, and if the pH is lower than expected for the chronic (compensated) condition, there is a
superimposed metabolic acidosis.

d. EXAMPLE: Consider a patient with a $PaCO_2$ of 23 mm
Hg and a pH of 7.57, which represents a primary respiratory alkalosis. The expected pH for an acute respiratory alkalosis is described in Equation 22.8, and is
$7.40 + [0.008 \times (40-23)] = 7.54$. The measured pH is higher than expected, so this condition represents an *acute
respiratory alkalosis with a secondary metabolic alkalosis.*

C. Evaluate Metabolic Acidosis

The final stage of this approach is for patients with a metabolic acidosis, and it involves two determinations known as
gaps.

1. The first is the *anion gap*, which is an estimate of unmeasured anions in the extracellular fluid that helps to identify the cause of a metabolic acidosis.

2. The second gap is a comparison of the change in the
   anion gap and the change in the serum HCO_3 concentration. The difference or "gap" between these two measurements (also known as the *gap-gap*) can uncover mixed
   metabolic disorders (e.g., a metabolic acidosis and alkalosis) that would otherwise go undetected.

3. These two measurements are described in the next section.

III. "THE GAPS"

A. Anion Gap

The anion gap is used to determine if a metabolic acidosis is
due to an accumulation of nonvolatile acids (e.g., lactic acid)
or a net loss of bicarbonate (e.g., diarrhea) (6–8).

1. *What is the Anion Gap?*

To achieve electrochemical balance, the concentration of negatively charged anions must equal the concentration of positively charged cations. All ions participate in this balance, including routinely measured ions like sodium (Na), chloride (CL), and bicarbonate (HCO_3), as well as unmeasured cations (UC) and unmeasured anions (UA). The electrochemical balance equation can thus be written as:

$$Na + UC = CL + HCO_3 + UA \qquad (22.12)$$

Rearranging the terms yields the following relationships:

$$Na - (CL + HCO_3) = UA - UC \qquad (22.13)$$

The difference (UA – UC) is a measure of the relative abundance of unmeasured anions and is called the *anion gap* (AG). The anion gap is measured as the difference between the plasma sodium concentration and the sum of the plasma chloride and bicarbonate concentrations.

2. *Reference Range*

The normal value of the AG was originally recorded at 12 ± 4 mEq/L (range = 8 to 16 mEq/L) (7). With the adoption of newer automated systems that more accurately measure serum electrolytes, *the normal value of the AG has decreased to 7 ± 4 mEq/L* (range = 3 to 11 mEq/L) (9). This newer reference range has not been universally adopted, and this is a source of error in the interpretation of the AG.

3. *Interpreting the Anion Gap*

Metabolic acidoses are characterized as having an elevated AG or a normal AG..

a. Elevated AG metabolic acidoses are caused by the addition of a fixed (nonvolatile) acid to the extracellular fluid (e.g., lactic acid, ketoacids).

b. Normal AG metabolic acidoses are characterized by a net loss of HCO_3 and a compensatory increase in chloride concentration. (In the high AG metabolic acidoses, the loss of HCO_3 is not accompanied by increased chloride because the anions from the dissociated acids balance the loss of HCO_3). This condition is also called *hyperchloremic metabolic acidosis.*

c. The clinical conditions responsible for elevated AG and normal AG metabolic acidoses are listed in Table 22.3.

TABLE 22.3 Interpretations of the Anion Gap

High AG Acidoses	Normal AG Acidoses
Lactic acidosis	Diarrhea
Ketoacidosis	Isotonic saline infusion
End-stage renal failure	Early renal insufficiency
Methanol ingestion	Renal tubular acidosis
Ethylene glycol ingestion	Acetazolamide
Salicylate toxicity	Ureterenterostomy

4. *Reliability*

The AG can be unreliable, as demonstrated by the numerous reports of lactic acidosis with a normal AG (10, 11). This discrepancy may be due to a disregard for the influence of plasma albumin on the AG (explained next).

5. *Influence of Albumin*

As indicated in Table 22.4, *albumin is the major unmeasured anion in plasma.* This means that a decrease in serum albumin will decrease the AG, and this can lead to errors in the interpretation of the AG (e.g., a high AG metabolic acidosis can present with a normal AG in the presence of hypoalbuminemia).

a. The spurious influence of hypoalbuminemia on the anion gap can be eliminated by calculating the AG as shown below using the albumin (g/dL) and phosphate (mg/dL) concentrations (12,13) (this is possible because albumin and phosphate are responsible for the majority of the normal anion gap).

$$AG = [2 \times albumin] + [0.5 \times PO_4] \qquad (22.14)$$

The albumin-derived AG is then compared to the traditional AG [Na – (CL = HCO₃)]. If the traditional AG is greater than the albumin-derived AG, the difference is a true measure of nonvolatile acids.

TABLE 22.4 Determinants of the Anion Gap	
Unmeasured Anions	**Unmeasured Cations**
Albumin (15 mEq/L)*	Calcium (5 mEq/L)
Organic Acids (5 mEq/L)	Potassium (4.5 mEq/L)
Phosphate (2 mEq/L)	Magnesium (1.5 mEq/L)
Sulfate (1 mEq/L)	
Total UA: (23 mEq/L)	Total UC: (11 mEq/L)
Anion Gap = UA – UC = 12 mEq/L	

*If albumin is reduced by 50%, anion gap = 4 mEq/L.

B. The "Gap-Gap"

1. *What is the Gap-Gap?*

   In the presence of a high AG metabolic acidosis, it is possible to detect another metabolic acid-base disorder (a normal AG metabolic acidosis or a metabolic alkalosis) by comparing the AG excess (the difference between the measured and normal AG) to the HCO₃ deficit (the difference between the measured and normal HCO₃ concentration in plasma). The AG excess/HCO₃ deficit ratio is shown below (12 mEq/L is the normal AG and 24 mEq/L is the normal plasma HCO₃ concentration).

AG Excess /HCO$_3$ Deficit = (AG − 12)/(24 − HCO$_3$)

(22.15)

This ratio is sometimes called the *gap-gap* because it is a measure of the difference (gap) between another gap (the anion gap) and the changes in HCO$_3$ concentration.

2. *Mixed Metabolic Acidoses*

When a fixed acid accumulates in extracellular fluid (i.e., high AG metabolic acidosis), the decrease in serum HCO$_3$ is equivalent to the increase in AG, and the AG excess/HCO$_3$ deficit ratio is unity (=1). However, when a hyperchloremic acidosis appears, the decrease in HCO$_3$ is greater than the increase in the AG, and the ratio (AG excess/HCO$_3$ deficit) falls below unity (<1).

a. Thus, in the presence of a high AG metabolic acidosis, a gap-gap (AG excess/HCO$_3$ deficit) <1 indicates the coexistence of a normal AG metabolic acidosis (5,14).

3. *Metabolic Acidosis and Alkalosis*

When alkali is added in the presence of a high AG acidosis, the decrease in serum bicarbonate is less than the increase in AG, and the gap-gap (AG excess/HCO$_3$ deficit) is greater than unity (>1).

a. Thus, in the presence of a high AG metabolic acidosis, a gap-gap (AG excess/HCO$_3$ deficit) >1 indicates the coexistence of a metabolic alkalosis (5,14).

REFERENCES

1. Narins RG, Emmett M. Simple and mixed acid-base disorders: a practical approach. Medicine 1980; 59:161–187.
2. Whittier WL, Rutecki GW. Primer on clinical acid-base problem solving. Dis Mon 2004; 50:117–162.
3. Albert M, Dell R, Winters R. Quantitative displacement of acid-base equilibrium in metabolic acidosis. Ann Intern Med 1967; 66:312–315.

4. Javaheri S, Kazemi H. Metabolic alkalosis and hypoventilation in humans. Am Rev Respir Dis 1987; 136:1011–1016.

5. Morganroth ML. An analytical approach to diagnosing acid-base disorders. J Crit Illness 1990; 5:138–150.

6. Casaletto JJ. Differential diagnosis of metabolic acidosis. Emerg Med Clin N Am 2005; 23:771–787.

7. Emmet M, Narins RG. Clinical use of the anion gap. Medicine 1977; 56:38–54.

8. Judge BS. Metabolic acidosis: differentiating the causes in the poisoned patient. Med Clin N Am 2005; 89:1107–1124.

9. Winter SD, Pearson JR, Gabow PA, et al. The fall of the serum anion gap. Arch Intern Med 1990; 150:311–313.

10. Iberti TS, Liebowitz AB, Papadakos PJ, et al. Low sensitivity of the anion gap as a screen to detect hyperlactatemia in critically ill patients. Crit Care Med 1990; 18:275–277.

11. Schwartz-Goldstein B, Malik AR, Sarwar A, Brandtsetter RD. Lactic acidosis associated with a normal anion gap. Heart Lung 1996; 25:79–80.

12. Kellum JA. Determinants of plasma acid-base balance. Crit Care Clin 2005; 21:329–346.

13. Kellum JA, Kramer DJ, Pinsky MJ. Closing the gap: a simple method of improving the accuracy of the anion gap. Chest 1996; 110:185.

14. Haber RJ. A practical approach to acid-base disorders. West J Med 1991; 155:146–151.

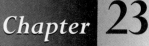

Chapter 23

ORGANIC ACIDOSES

This chapter describes the clinical disorders associated with the production of organic (carbon-based) acids, including lactic acid, ketoacids, oxalic acid (from ethylene glycol ingestion), and formic acid (from methanol ingestion) (1,2).

I. LACTIC ACIDOSIS

A. Clinical Presentation

1. Lactic acidosis typically presents as a high anion gap metabolic acidosis in association with one of the conditions presented in the next section. However, a normal anion gap has also been reported in cases of lactic acidosis (3), and thus *the anion gap should not be used as a screening test for lactic acidosis*. (See Chapter 22 for information on the anion gap.)

2. The diagnosis of lactic acidosis requires a blood lactate concentration. The blood sample should be placed on ice to retard lactate production by red blood cells. A lactate level above 2 mEq/L is considered abnormal.

B. Etiologies

1. *Circulatory Shock*

   In patients with a low cardiac output due to hypovolemia or heart failure, an increase in blood lactate levels is taken as evidence of impaired tissue oxygenation. This condition is generally known as *circulatory shock*. The degree of elevation in blood lactate levels is directly correlated with the mortality rate in circulatory shock, as shown in Figure 23.1 (4).

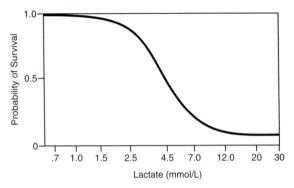

FIGURE 23.1 The relationship between blood lactate levels and survival in patients with circulatory shock. From Reference 4.

2. *Sepsis*

a. Some patients with sepsis have mild elevations of blood lactate (2 to 5 mEq/L) with a normal lactate:pyruvate ratio and a normal blood pH. These patients have *stress hyperlactatemia*, which is considered a result of hypermetabolism without impaired cellular oxygen utilization (5).

b. Patients with severe sepsis can have marked elevations in blood lactate with increased lactate:pyruvate ratios and a reduced blood pH. These patients have a defect in cellular oxygen utilization that has been called *cytopathic hypoxia* (6).

c. In severe sepsis, a blood lactate level above 4 mEq/L is associated with a poor prognosis (7).

3. *Thiamine Deficiency*

Lactic acidosis is one of the manifestations of thiamine deficiency (8). Thiamine is a cofactor for pyruvate dehydrogenase (the enzyme that catalyses the conversion of pyruvate to acetyl coenzyme A), and thiamine deficiency diverts glucose metabolism to the production of lactate. See Chapter 36 for more on thiamine deficiency.

4. *Drugs*

A variety of drugs can produce lactic acidosis, including (in alphabetical order) acetaminophen, epinephrine, linezolid, metformin, propofol, nitroprusside, and nucleoside reverse transcriptase inhibitors (9–12).

5. *Propylene Glycol*

Propylene glycol is a solvent that enhances the solubility of intravenous medications, including lorazepam, diazepam, esmolol, nitroglycerin, and phenytoin. The metabolism of propylene glycol takes place primarily in the liver, and the principal metabolites are lactate and pyruvate (13).

a. Propylene glycol toxicity has been reported in 19% to 66% of ICU patients receiving high-dose lorazepam or diazepam for more than 2 days (13,14). Signs of toxicity include agitation, coma, seizures, tachycardia, hypotension, and hyperlactatemia.

6. *Other Causes*

Other possible causes of hyperlactatemia in ICU patients include *seizures* (from increased lactate production), *hepatic insufficiency* (from reduced lactate clearance), and *acute asthma* (possibly from enhanced lactate production by the respiratory muscles) (15–17).

C. D-Lactic Acidosis

1. The lactate produced by mammalian tissues is a levo-isomer (bends light to the left). A dextro-isomer of lactate (bends light to the right) is produced by certain strains of bacteria that can populate the bowel.

2. D-lactate generated by bacterial fermentation in the bowel can enter the systemic circulation and produce a meta-

bolic acidosis, often combined with a metabolic encephalopathy (18). Most cases of d-lactic acidosis have been reported after extensive small bowel resection or after jejunoileal bypass for morbid obesity (18,19).

3. D-lactic acidosis can produce an elevated anion gap, but the standard laboratory assay for lactate measures only l-lactate. If d-lactic acidosis is suspected, you must request a specific d-lactate assay.

D. Alkali Therapy

1. The primary goal of therapy in lactic acidosis is to correct the underlying cause of the acidosis. *Alkali therapy to correct the acidosis has no proven value* (20) and is not recommended for the routine treatment of lactic acidosis.

2. For patients with severe acidosis (pH <7.1) who are hemodynamically unstable, a trial infusion of sodium bicarbonate (7.5% $NaHCO_3$, 0.9 mEq HCO_3 per liter) can be attempted by administering one-half of the estimated bicarbonate deficit (21).

$$\textbf{HCO}_3 \textbf{ deficit (mEq)} = \textbf{0.6} \times \textbf{wt (kg)} \times \textbf{(15} - \textbf{plasma HCO}_3\textbf{)} \quad (23.1)$$

(where 15 mEq/L is the target plasma HCO_3). If cardiovascular improvement occurs, bicarbonate therapy can be continued to maintain the plasma HCO_3 at 15 mEq/L. If there is no improvement, further bicarbonate administration is not warranted.

II. DIABETIC KETOACIDOSIS

A. Pathogenesis

1. In conditions of reduced nutrient intake (or reduced glucose entry into cells), adipose tissue releases free fatty

acids, which are taken up in the liver and metabolized to acetoacetate and β-hydroxybutyrate. These ketones are released from the liver and can be used as oxidative fuels by vital organs such as the heart and central nervous system.

2. Acetoacetate and β-hydroxybutyrate are strong acids, and their accumulation in blood can produce a metabolic acidosis (i.e., *ketoacidosis*). In diabetic ketoacidosis, the principal ketone in blood is β-hydroxybutyrate (see Figure 23.2).

B. Clinical Features

1. Diabetic ketoacidosis (DKA) is usually seen in insulin-dependent diabetics, but in 20% of cases, there is no previous history of diabetes mellitus.

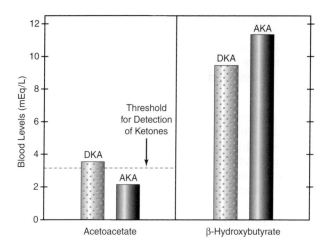

FIGURE 23.2 The concentrations of acetoacetate and β-hydroxybutyrate in the blood in diabetic ketoacidosis (DKA) and alcoholic ketoacidosis (AKA). The horizontal dashed line represents the minimum concentration of acetoacetate that will produce a positive nitroprusside reaction.

2. DKA is most often the result of inappropriate insulin dosing, but some patients have a concurrent illness, most commonly an infection.

3. The hallmark of DKA is the combination of hyperglycemia, a serum bicarbonate below 20 mEq/L, and an elevated anion gap. The blood glucose is usually above 250 mg/dL, but it may be lower or even normal in about 20% of cases (22).

4. The increase in ketoacids should produce an elevated anion gap; however, this is variable, and the anion gap can be normal in DKA (23). The renal excretion of ketones is accompanied by an increase in chloride reabsorption in the renal tubules, and the resulting hyperchloremia limits the increase in the anion gap.

C. Diagnosis

1. The diagnosis of DKA requires confirmation of elevated ketoacids in blood and urine. The assay used most often is the nitroprusside reaction, which is a colorimetric method for the detection of acetoacetate. A positive reaction requires a minimum acetoacetate concentration of 3 mEq/L.

2. The nitroprusside reaction *does not detect* β-*hydroxybutyrate* (22), which is the predominant ketoacid in DKA (30). As such, this reaction is insensitive for monitoring the severity of ketoacidosis. This is demonstrated in Figure 23.2. Note that the reaction is barely positive in DKA despite a total ketoacid concentration of 13–14 mEq/L in blood.

D. Management

The management of DKA is summarized in Table 23.1.

TABLE 23.1 Management of Diabetic Ketoacidosis

Insulin: 0.1U/kg IV push, then 0.1 U/kg/hr by continuous infusion. Decrease dose rate 50% when serum HCO_3 rises above 16 mEq.

Fluids: Start 0.9% saline, 1 L/hr for the first 2 hrs. Follow with 0.45% saline at 250–500 mL/hr. Total fluid deficit is usually 50–100 mL/kg.

Potassium: If serum K = ___ mEq/L, give ___ mEq over next hour.

<3	40
3–4	30
4–5	20
5–6	10
<6	0

Phosphate: If serum PO_4 is <1.0 mg/dL, give 7.7 mg/kg over 4 hrs.

1. *Insulin Therapy*

   a. Insulin is given intravenously, starting with a bolus dose of 0.1 units per kilogram body weight (some feel this is unnecessary) and followed with a continuous infusion of 0.1 units per kilogram per hour. Because *insulin adsorbs to intravenous tubing,* the initial 50 mL of infusate should be run through the IV setup before the insulin drip is started.

   b. The blood glucose levels should be measured every 1 to 2 hours during intravenous insulin therapy. The goal is to decrease the blood glucose by 50 to 75 mg/dL per hour (24). If this goal is not achieved, the insulin infusion rate should be doubled (24). Fingerstick glucose determinations can be performed if the blood glucose is below 500 mg/dL.

2. *Fluids*

   a. Volume deficits average 50 to 100 mL/kg (or 4 to 8 L for a 175 lb adult) in DKA.

   b. Fluid therapy usually begins with 0.9% (isotonic) saline infused at a rate of one liter per hour for the first 2 hours. This is followed by infusion of 0.45% saline at 250 to 500 mL/hour.

   c. When the blood glucose falls to 250 mg/dL, dextrose can be added to the intravenous fluids, and the infusion rate should then be slowed to 100 to 250 mL/hour.

   d. If there is evidence of hypovolemic shock (i.e., hypotension), colloid fluids may be preferred until the blood pressure normalizes. The preferred colloid in this situation is 5% albumin because 6% hetastarch produces an increase in serum amylase levels, and this can lead to confusion because low-grade pancreatitis may be common in DKA (22).

3. *Potassium*

   Potassium depletion is almost universal in DKA, and the average deficit is 3 to 5 mEq/kg. However, the serum potassium is usually normal (74% of patients) or even elevated (22% of patients) at presentation. The serum potassium falls during insulin therapy (transcellular shift), and this fall can be dramatic. Therefore, potassium replacement should be started as soon as possible (see Table 23.1), and the serum potassium should be monitored hourly for the first 4 to 6 hours of therapy.

4. *Phosphate*

   a. Phosphate depletion is common in DKA, and averages 1 to 1.5 mmol/kg. However, phosphate replacement has little impact on the outcome in DKA, and is not recommended as a routine measure (22).

   b. The serum phosphate level should be measured 4 hours after the start of therapy. If the level is severely depressed (less than 1 mg/dL), phosphate replacement is advised (see Table 23.1 for the recommended replacement dose).

5. *Alkali Therapy*

Alkali therapy with sodium bicarbonate does not improve the outcome in DKA and is not recommended, regardless of the severity of the acidemia (22).

E. Monitoring Acid-Base Status

1. The serum bicarbonate may not be a reliable parameter for following the acid-base changes in DKA. Aggressive fluid replacement often produces a hyperchloremic acidosis by promoting ketoacid excretion in the urine, which increases chloride reabsorption in the renal tubules. This prevents the bicarbonate from rising despite a resolving ketoacidosis. In this situation, the *pattern* of the acidosis is changing (i.e., changing from a high anion gap to a low anion gap acidosis).

2. The most appropriate parameter to monitor during the therapy of DKA is the gap-gap: i.e., the anion gap excess:bicarbonate deficit ratio (this parameter is described in Chapter 22). This ratio is 1.0 in pure ketoacidosis, and decreases toward zero as the ketoacidosis resolves and is replaced by the hyperchloremic acidosis. When the ketones have been cleared from the bloodstream, the ratio approaches zero.

III. ALCOHOLIC KETOACIDOSIS

A. Pathogenesis

Alcoholic ketoacidosis (AKA) is a complex disorder with several sources of ketosis, including reduced nutrient intake, hepatic oxidation of ethanol (which generates NADH and enhances β-hydroxybutyrate formation), and dehydration (which impairs ketone excretion in the urine).

B. Clinical Features

1. AKA is usually seen in chronic alcoholics, and typically appears 1 to 3 days after a period of heavy binge drinking (25).

2. The presentation usually includes nausea, vomiting, and abdominal pain. Electrolyte abnormalities are common, particularly the *hypos* (e.g., hyponatremia, hypokalemia, hypophosphatemia, hypomagnesemia, hypoglycemia).

3. Mixed acid-base disorders are common in AKA. More than half the patients can have lactic acidosis (caused by other conditions) (25), and metabolic alkalosis occurs in patients with protracted vomiting.

C. Diagnosis

1. The diagnosis of AKA is suggested by the appearance of a high anion gap metabolic acidosis in the appropriate clinical setting (i.e., after a period of binge drinking), and the diagnosis is confirmed by the presence of ketones in the blood and urine.

2. The ratio of β-hydroxybutyrate to acetoacetate in blood can be as high as 8:1 in AKA, and the plasma levels of acetoacetate may not be high enough to be detected by the nitroprusside reaction (see Figure 23.2). Therefore, *the nitroprusside reaction for detecting ketones can be negative in AKA.* When this occurs, the diagnosis of AKA requires elimination of the other conditions (e.g., lactic acidosis) that can produce a high anion gap metabolic acidosis.

D. Management

1. AKA is corrected simply by infusing dextrose-containing

saline solutions. The glucose helps retard hepatic ketone production, while the infused volume promotes the renal clearance of ketones. The ketoacidosis usually resolves within 24 hours.

2. Alkali therapy is not necessary in AKA (25).

IV. TOXIC ALCOHOLS

Two alcohols are noted for their ability to generate organic acids: ethylene glycol and methanol.

A. Ethylene Glycol Intoxication

1. *Pathophysiology*

Ethylene glycol is a solvent used primarily in antifreeze and deicing solutions. When ingested, ethylene glycol is rapidly absorbed from the GI tract, and 80% of the ingested dose is metabolized in the liver.

a. Metabolism by alcohol dehydrogenase in the liver produces glycolic acid, as shown in Figure 23.3. This is the major metabolite of ethylene glycol, and it produces a metabolic acidosis with an elevated anion gap (26).

b. The formation of glycolic acid involves the conversion of NAD to NADH, and this promotes the conversion of pyruvate to lactate. As a result, serum lactate levels are also elevated in ethylene glycol poisoning (26,27).

c. The final metabolite of ethylene glycol is oxalic acid, which can combine with calcium to form *calcium oxalate crystals* in the renal tubules. These crystals (which are recognizable on microscopic examination of the urine) can damage the renal tubules and produce acute renal failure.

2. *Clinical Presentation*

a. Early signs of ethylene glycol intoxication include nausea, vomiting, and apparent inebriation. Because ethylene glycol is odorless, there is no odor of alcohol on the breath.

b. Severe cases are accompanied by coma, generalized seizures, renal failure, pulmonary edema, and cardiovascular collapse (26).

c. Laboratory studies show a metabolic acidosis with an elevated anion gap.

d. Serum lactate levels can be elevated (usually 5–6 mEq /L). Hypocalcemia can be present, and calcium oxalate crystals are visualized in the urine in about 50% of cases (28).

e. A plasma assay for ethylene glycol is available, and a level >25 mg/dL is considered toxic (26,29). However, plasma levels can be negligible (due to metabolism of the parent compound) in patients who present late after ingestion.

3. *Treatment*

The results of the ethylene glycol assay are often not available immediately, and therapy is started based on a high clinical suspicion of ethylene glycol intoxication. Treatment involves inhibition of alcohol dehydrogenase, and hemodialysis if necessary.

a. The traditional use of ethanol to inhibit alcohol dehydrogenase has been replaced by the drug **fomepizole**, which inhibits alcohol dehydrogenase (see Figure 23.3) without the side effects that accompany ethanol. The best results are obtained when therapy begins within 4 hours after ingestion. The recommended dosage is 15 mg/kg IV as an initial dose, then 10 mg/kg every 12 hours for 48 hours, then 15 mg/kg every 12 hours until the plasma ethylene glycol level is 25 mEq/L or lower (26,30).

b. Hemodialysis increases the clearance of ethylene glycol and its metabolites. The indications for immediate hemodialysis include severe acidemia (pH <7.1), and evidence of end-organ damage (e.g., coma, seizures,

and renal failure) (26,30). Multiple courses of hemodialysis may be necessary. Fomepizole should be given
every 4 hours if hemodialysis is continued.

   c. ADJUNCTS. **Thiamine** (100 mg IV daily) and **pyridoxine** (100 mg IV daily) can divert glyoxylic acid to non-
toxic metabolites (see Figure 23.3).

B. Methanol Intoxication

Methanol is a common ingredient in shellac, varnish, wind-
shield washer fluid and solid cooking fuel (Sterno) (26,31).

   1. *Pathophysiology*

     a. Like ethylene glycol, methanol is rapidly absorbed from
the GI tract and is metabolized by alcohol dehydrogenase in the liver (see Figure 23.3).

     b. The metabolite, formic acid, is a mitochondrial toxin
that acts by inhibiting cytochrome oxidase. Tissues

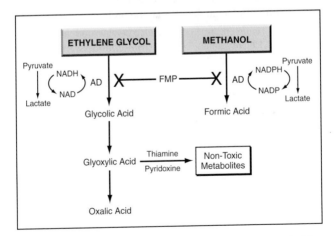

FIGURE 23.3 The metabolism of ethylene glycol and methanol. *AD* =
alcohol dehydrogenase. *FMP* = fomepizole.

that are particularly susceptible to damage are the retina, optic nerve, and basal ganglia (31).

   c. Serum lactate levels can be elevated for the same reason as explained for ethylene glycol, but the added mitochondrial toxicity of formic acid can result in higher serum lactate levels.

2. Clinical Presentation

a. Early signs (within 6 hours of ingestion) include apparent inebriation without the odor of ethanol (as in ethylene glycol intoxication).

b. Later signs (6 to 24 hours after ingestion) include visual disturbances (e.g., scotoma, blurred vision, complete blindness), depressed consciousness, coma, and generalized seizures. Pancreatitis has also been described (26).

c. Examination of the retina can reveal papilledema and generalized retinal edema.

d. Laboratory studies show the same acid-base abnormalities as described for ethylene glycol intoxication (although lactate levels may be higher).

e. Pancreatic enzymes can be also be elevated, and elevated CPK levels in blood (from rhabdomyolysis) has been reported (26).

f. A plasma assay for methanol is available, and a level above 25 mg/dL is considered toxic. As explained with ethylene glycol intoxication, plasma levels can be misleading late after ingestion because the parent compound may be completely degraded.

3. Treatment

Treatment is the same as described for ethylene glycol intoxication, except:

a. Visual impairment is an indication for dialysis.

b. Adjunctive therapy with thiamine and pyridoxine is not indicated.

REFERENCES

1. Gauthier PM, Szerlip HM. Metabolic acidosis in the intensive care unit. Crit Care Clin 2002; 18:289–308.

2. Judge BS. Metabolic acidosis: differentiating the causes in the poisoned patient. Med Clin N Am 2005; 89:1107–1124.

3. Iberti TS, Liebowitz AB, Papadakos PJ, et al. Low sensitivity of the anion gap as a screen to detect hyperlactatemia in critically ill patients. Crit Care Med 1990; 18:275–277.

4. Weil MH, Afifi AA. Experimental and clinical studies on lactate and pyruvate as indicators of the severity of acute circulatory failure (shock). Circulation 1970; 16:989–1001.

5. Mizock BA. Metabolic derangements in sepsis and septic shock. Crit Care Clin 2000; 16:319–336.

6. Fink MP. Cytopathic hypoxia. Crit Care Clin 2001; 17:219–238.

7. Aduen J, Bernstein WK, Khastgir T, et al. The use and clinical importance of a substrate-specific electrode for rapid determination of blood lactate concentrations. JAMA 1994; 272:1678–1685.

8. Campbell CH. The severe lactic acidosis of thiamine deficiency: acute, pernicious or fulminating beriberi. Lancet 1984; 1:446–449.

9. Judge BS. Metabolic acidosis: differentiating the causes in the poisoned patient. Med Clin North Am 2005; 89:1107–1124.

10. Ogedegbe AO, Thomas DL, Diehl AM. Hyperlactatemia syndromes associated with HIV therapy. Lancet Infect Dis 2003; 3:329–337.

11. Apodaca AA, Rakita RM. Linezolid induced lactic acidosis. N Engl J Med 2003; 348:86–87.

12. Yann-Erick C, Cariou A, Monchi M, et al. Detecting life-threatening lactic acidosis related to nucleoside-analog treatment of human immunodeficiency virus-infected patients and treatment with L-carnitine. Crit Care Med 2003; 31:1042–1047.

13. Wilson KC, Reardon C, Theodore AC, Farber HW. Propylene glycol toxicity: a severe iatrogenic illness in ICU patients receiving IV benzodiazepines. Chest 2005; 128:1674–1681.

14. Arroglia A, Shehab N, McCarthy K, Gonzales JP. Relationship of continuous infusion lorazepam to serum propylene glycol concentration in critically ill adults. Crit Care Med 2004; 32:1709–1714.

15. Kruse JA, Zaidi SAJ, Carlson RW. Significance of blood lactate levels in critically ill patients with liver disease. Am J Med 1987; 83:77–82.

16. Brivet F, Bernadin M, Cherin P, et al. Hyperchloremic acidosis during grand mal seizure acidosis. Intensive Care Med 1994; 20:27–31.

17. Mountain RD, Heffner JE, Brackett NC, Sahn SA. Acid-base disturbances in acute asthma. Chest 1990; 98:651–655.

18. Thurn JR, Pierpoint GL, Ludvigsen CW, Eckfeldt JH. D-lactate encephalopathy. Am J Med 1985; 79:717–720.

19. Bustos D, Ponse S, Pernas JC et al. Fecal lactate and the short bowel syndrome. Dig Dis Sci 1994; 39:2315–2319.

20. Forsythe SM, Schmidt GA. Sodium bicarbonate for the treatment of lactic acidosis. Chest 2000; 117:260–267.

21. Rose BD. Clinical physiology of acid-base and electrolyte disorders. 4th ed. New York: McGraw-Hill, 1994:590.

22. Charfen MA, Fernandez-Frackelton M. Diabetic ketoacidosis. Emerg Med Clin N Am 2005; 23:609–628.

23. Gamblin GT, Ashburn RW, Kemp DG, Beuttel SC. Diabetic ketoacidosis presenting with a normal anion gap. Am J Med 1986; 80:758–760.

24. Kitabachi AE, Umpierrez GE, Murphy MB, et al. American Diabetes Association. Hyperglycemic crisis in diabetes. Diabetes Care 2004; 27(Suppl):S94–S102.

25. Wrenn KD, Slovis CM, Minion GE, Rutkowsli R. The syndrome of alcoholic ketoacidosis. Am J Med 1991; 91:119–128.

26. Weiner SW. Toxic alcohols. In: Goldfrank LR, Flomenbaum NE, Hoffman RS, et al., eds. Goldfrank's toxicologic emergencies. 7th ed. New York, McGraw-Hill, 2002:1447–1459.

27. Gabow PA, Clay K, Sullivan JB, Lepoff R. Organic acids in ethylene glycol intoxication. Ann Intern Med 1986; 105:16–20.

28. Borkan SC. Extracorporeal therapies for acute intoxications. Crit Care Clin 2002; 18:393–420.

29. Caravati EM, Erdman AR, Christianson G, et al. Ethylene glycol exposure: an evidence-based consensus guideline for out-of-hospital management. Clin Toxicol 2005; 43:327–345.

30. Brent J, McMartin K, Phillips S, et al. Fomepizole for the treatment of ethylene glycol poisoning. N Engl J Med 1999; 340:832–838.

31. Barceloux DG, Bond GR, Krenzelok EP, et al. American Academy of Clinical Toxicology practice guidelines on the treatment of methanol poisoning. J Toxicol Clin Toxicol 2002; 40:415–446.

Chapter 24

METABOLIC ALKALOSIS

Although metabolic acidosis seems to get the most attention, one of every three acid-base disorders in hospitalized patients is a metabolic *alkalosis* (1). This chapter describes the causes, consequences, and correction of metabolic alkalosis (1–3).

I. ORIGINS OF METABOLIC ALKALOSIS

Metabolic alkalosis is characterized by an increase in extracellular bicarbonate (HCO_3) concentration, and is usually the result of one (or more) of the following conditions.

A. Loss of Gastric Secretions

1. Gastric secretions are rich in hydrogen and chloride ions (concentration of each is 50 to 100 mEq/L), and loss of these secretions from vomiting or nasogastric (NG) suction can produce a profound metabolic alkalosis.

2. Despite the loss of gastric acid, chloride depletion is the major factor responsible for the metabolic alkalosis from vomiting and NG suctioning. Chloride depletion stimulates HCO_3 reabsorption in the kidneys, and the resulting increase in extracellular HCO_3 creates a metabolic alkalosis. (The HCO_3 that is added to the extracellular fluid balances the chloride loss to maintain electrical neutrality).

3. Other factors that contribute to the alkalosis from loss of gastric secretions are hypovolemia and hypokalemia.

B. Diuretics

Thiazide diuretics and "loop" diuretics like furosemide promote metabolic alkalosis by increasing the urinary loss of sodium, chloride, potassium, and magnesium.

1. The principal action of these diuretics is to increase sodium and chloride loss in the urine. The chloride loss is accompanied by increased HCO_3 reabsorption in the kidneys (to maintain electrical neutrality), and the resulting increase in extracellular fluid HCO_3 concentration produces a metabolic alkalosis. Sodium loss promotes extracellular fluid loss, and this promotes metabolic alkalosis by mechanisms explained in the next section.

2. Diuretics increase urinary potassium excretion by the following mechanisms:

    a. Sodium delivery to the distal tubules is increased, and this promotes potassium secretion via the sodium–potassium exchange pump in the distal tubule.

    b. Magnesium reabsorption in the kidneys usually mirrors sodium reabsorption, so these diuretics also promote magnesium loss in the urine. Magnesium depletion plays an important role in diuretic-induced potassium depletion, as described in Chapter 28.

Potassium depletion promotes metabolic alkalosis by mechanisms explained later in this section.

C. Volume Depletion

1. Volume depletion promotes metabolic alkalosis in two ways.

    a. There is a direct link between the reabsorption of sodium and HCO_3 in the renal tubules, so the increased sodium reabsorption in response to volume depletion is accompanied by an increase in HCO_3 reabsorption.

b. Volume depletion also stimulates renin release, and the subsequent increase in aldosterone production serves to promote H^+ secretion in the distal tubules.

2. The importance of volume depletion as a cause of metabolic alkalosis is being questioned because volume replacement does not correct metabolic alkalosis without chloride repletion (2). Since volume replacement is usually accompanied by chloride replacement (i.e., in saline solutions), this distinction may not be clinically relevant.

D. Hypokalemia

1. Hypokalemia promotes metabolic alkalosis via two mechanisms:

   a. Transcellular shift of H^+ into cells.

   b. Increased H^+ secretion in the distal renal tubules.

2. The enhanced secretion of H^+ in the distal renal tubules involves a $Na^+ - H^+$ transporter that requires adequate delivery of sodium to the distal tubules. In the setting of hypovolemia, most of the filtered sodium is reabsorbed in the proximal tubules, and the effects of hypokalemia on H^+ secretion are minimal.

E. Chronic CO_2 Retention

The compensatory response to CO_2 retention is an increase in HCO_3 reabsorption in the proximal tubules of the kidneys. If chronic hypercapnia is corrected suddenly (e.g., by overventilation when mechanical ventilation is initiated), the compensatory metabolic alkalosis will become a primary acid-base disorder.

F. Administration of Organic Anions

The administration of organic anions such as lactate (in lactated Ringer's solution), acetate (in parenteral nutrition solutions), and citrate (in banked blood) could produce a metabolic alkalosis. However, only citrate administration in blood transfusions is capable of causing a metabolic alkalosis (4), and a minimum of 8 units of blood must be transfused before the plasma HCO₃ begins to rise (5).

II. CLINICAL CONSEQUENCES

Despite the potential for harm, metabolic alkalosis has no apparent deleterious effects in most patients. The following adverse effects are the ones most often mentioned.

A. Neurologic Manifestations

The neurologic manifestations attributed to alkalosis include depressed consciousness, generalized seizures, and carpopedal spasms. However, these manifestations are almost always associated with respiratory alkalosis, not metabolic alkalosis. This is explained by the greater tendency for respiratory alkalosis to influence the acid-base status of the central nervous system.

B. Hypoventilation

1. The respiratory compensation for metabolic alkalosis is described by the equation shown below (where $PaCO_2$ is the arterial PCO_2 and HCO_3 is the plasma HCO_3 in mEq/L) (6).

$$\textbf{Expected PaCO}_2 = \textbf{(0.7} \times \textbf{HCO}_3\textbf{)} + \textbf{(21} \pm \textbf{2)} \qquad (24.1)$$

This equation is used to plot the relationship between HCO_3 and arterial PCO_2 shown in Figure 24.1. Note that the threshold for hypercapnia ($PaCO_2$ of 46 mm Hg) is not reached until the HCO_3 rises above the range of 34 – 39 mEq/L.

2. Figure 24.1 demonstrates that *respiratory depression occurs only in severe cases of metabolic alkalosis.*

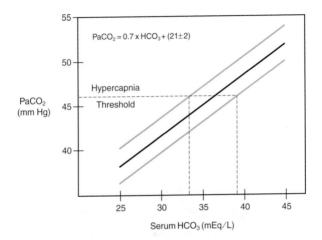

FIGURE 24.1 The relationship between plasma bicarbonate (HCO_3) and arterial PCO_2 ($PaCO_2$) based on the equation shown at the top of the graph. Note that the serum HCO_3 must rise above the range of 34–39 mEq/L to produce hypercapnia.

C. Systemic Oxygenation

Alkalosis has a number of effects that can threaten tissue oxygen availability (see Figure 24.2).

1. Alkalosis reduces myocardial contractility and promotes peripheral vasoconstriction (by decreasing ionized or free plasma calcium): both effects can lead to a decrease in cardiac output.

2. Alkalosis shifts the oxyhemoglobin dissociation curve to

the left (Bohr effect), which impairs the ability of hemoglobin to release oxygen to the tissues.

3. Intracellular alkalosis can increase cellular O_2 consumption by stimulating the activity of enzymes in the glycolytic pathway. However, this effect is predominantly seen with respiratory alkalosis (7).

The clinical significance of these effects is unclear, but they may be important in patients with circulatory failure or circulatory shock.

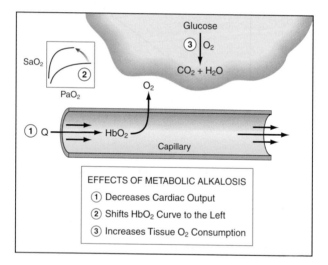

FIGURE 24.2 Effects of alkalosis on the determinants of systemic oxygenation.

III. THE EVALUATION

Metabolic alkaloses are traditionally classified as chloride-responsive or chloride-resistant, based on the urinary chloride concentration (see Table 24.1).

TABLE 24.1 Classification of Metabolic Alkalosis

Chloride-Responsive	Chloride-Resistant
Urinary chloride <15 mEq/L:	*Urinary chloride >25 mEq/L:*
1. Loss of gastric acid	1. Mineralocorticoid excess
2. Diuretics	2. Potassium depletion
3. Volume depletion	
4. Posthypercapnia	

A. Chloride-Responsive Alkalosis

1. A *chloride-responsive* metabolic alkalosis is characterized by a low urinary chloride concentration; i.e., less than 15 mEq/L.

2. This type of metabolic alkalosis is the result of gastric acid loss, diuretic therapy, volume depletion, or renal compensation for hypercapnia.

3. The majority of metabolic alkaloses in hospitalized patients are chloride-responsive.

B. Chloride-Resistant Alkalosis

1. A *chloride-resistant* metabolic alkalosis is characterized by an elevated urinary chloride concentration; i.e., above 25 mEq/L.

2. Most cases of chloride-resistant alkalosis are caused by primary mineralocorticoid excess (e.g., hyperadrenal conditions) or severe potassium depletion (these two conditions often co-exist).

3. This type of metabolic alkalosis is usually associated with volume expansion rather than volume depletion.

IV. MANAGEMENT

Most metabolic alkaloses in hospitalized patients are chloride-responsive, so chloride replacement is the mainstay of therapy for metabolic alkalosis. The chloride can be replaced as sodium chloride, potassium chloride, or hydrochloric acid (HCL).

A. Saline Infusion

1. Because volume depletion is common in chloride-responsive metabolic alkalosis, infusion of isotonic saline (0.9% sodium chloride) is the most common method of chloride replacement.

2. The volume of isotonic saline needed can be determined by estimating the chloride (CL) deficit in mEq/L, as shown below:

$$\text{CL deficit} = 0.2 \times \text{wt(kg)} \times (\text{normal} - \text{current } P_{CL}) \quad (24.2)$$

where P_{CL} is plasma chloride in mEq/L. The factor 0.2 represents the volume of distribution for chloride as a fraction of body weight.

3. The volume of isotonic saline needed to correct the chloride deficit is then determined as follows:

$$\text{Volume of 0.9\% NaCl (L)} = \text{CL deficit} / 154 \quad (24.3)$$

where 154 is the chloride concentration (in mEq/L) in isotonic saline.

EXAMPLE. A patient who weighs 70 kg has a metabolic alkalosis from repeated vomiting. The plasma chloride is 80 mEq/L. Using a normal serum chloride of 100 mEq/L, the chloride deficit is 0.2 x 70 x (100 – 80) = 280 mEq. The volume of isotonic saline needed to correct this deficit is 280/154 = 1.8 liters.

B. Potassium Chloride

1. Potassium chloride administration is indicated only when metabolic alkalosis is accompanied by hypokalemia.

2. It is important to emphasize that the administration of *potassium chloride will not replenish potassium stores if there is concurrent magnesium depletion* (8). (See Chapter 28 for more information on this topic.)

C. Hydrochloric Acid Infusion

Infusions of dilute solutions of hydrochloric acid (HCL) produce the most rapid correction of metabolic alkalosis (1). However, because of the risks involved (see later), HCL infusions are reserved only for the most severe and refractory cases of metabolic alkalosis.

1. The "dose" of HCL is determined by estimating the hydrogen ion (H^+) deficit in mEq/L using the equation below.

$$H^+ \text{ deficit} = 0.5 \times \text{wt(kg)} \times (\text{current} - \text{desired } P_{HCO_3})$$

(24.4)

where P_{HCO_3} is plasma HCO_3 in mEq/L. The factor 0.5 represents the volume of distribution for H^+ as a fraction of body weight. The desired HCO_3 should be above the normal range (the goal is not to correct the alkalosis, but to reduce the severity), and can be set halfway between the actual and normal HCO_3.

2. The H^+ deficit is corrected with 0.1N HCL, which contains 100 mEq H^+ per liter. The volume of 0.1N HCL needed to correct the H^+ deficit is determined as shown below.

$$\text{Volume of 0.1N HCL (L)} = H^+ \text{ deficit}/100 \qquad (24.5)$$

3. Because HCL solutions are sclerosing, they must be infused through a large, central vein (9), and the infusion rate should not exceed 0.2 mEq/kg/hr (3).

4. The corrosive effects of HCL solutions are a major concern. In addition to sclerosis, extravasation of HCL solutions can produce severe tissue necrosis (10). Because of their toxic potential, HCL infusions should be used very judiciously.

D. Chloride-Resistant Alkalosis

1. The management of chloride-resistant metabolic alkalosis is aimed at treating the underlying cause of the mineralocorticoid excess (e.g., hyperadrenalism, heart failure) and correcting potassium deficits.

2. The carbonic anhydrase inhibitor, **acetazolamide**, blocks HCO_3 reabsorption in the proximal tubule, and has been used successfully in treating cases of chloride-resistant metabolic alkalosis.

   a. The recommended dose is 5 to 10 mg/kg IV (or PO), and the maximum effect occurs after an average of 15 hours (11).

   b. Acetazolamide promotes both volume depletion and potassium depletion, and it should not be used in cases of chloride-resistant metabolic alkalosis that are accompanied by either of these conditions.

REFERENCES

1. Khanna A, Kurtzman NA. Metabolic alkalosis. Respir Care 2001; 46:354–365.
2. Galla JH. Metabolic alkalosis. J Am Soc Nephrol 2000; 11:360–375.
3. Androgue HJ, Madias N. Management of life-threatening acid-base disorders. Part 2. N Engl J Med 1998; 338:107–111.

4. Driscoll DF, Bistrian BR, Jenkins RL. Development of metabolic alkalosis after massive transfusion during orthotopic liver transplantation. Crit Care Med 1987; 15:905–908.

5. Rose BD, Post TW. Metabolic alkalosis. In: Clinical physiology of acid-base and electrolyte disorders. 5th ed. New York: McGraw-Hill, 2001:551–577.

6. Javaheri S, Kazemi H. Metabolic alkalosis and hypoventilation in humans. Am Rev Respir Dis 1987; 136:1011–1016.

7. Rastegar HR, Woods M, Harken AH. Respiratory alkalosis increases tissue oxygen demand. J Surg Res 1979; 26:687–692.

8. Whang R, Flink EB, Dyckner T, et al. Mg depletion as a cause of refractory potassium depletion. Arch Intern Med 1985; 145:1686–1689.

9. Brimioulle S, Vincent JL, Dufaye P, et al. Hydrochloric acid infusion for treatment of metabolic alkalosis: effects on acid-base balance and oxygenation. Crit Care Med 1985; 13:738–742.

10. Jankauskas SJ, Gursel E, Antonenko DR. Chest wall necrosis secondary to hydrochloric acid use in the treatment of metabolic alkalosis. Crit Care Med 1989; 17:963–964.

11. Marik PE, Kussman BD, Lipman J, Kraus P. Acetazolamide in the treatment of metabolic alkalosis in critically ill patients. Heart Lung 1991; 20:455–458.

Chapter 25

OLIGURIA AND ACUTE RENAL FAILURE

A decrease in urine output can be a normal adaptation to hypovolemia or a sign of acute renal failure. This chapter describes how to distinguish between these two conditions, and also describes the causes and management of acute renal failure.

I. OLIGURIA

A. Definition

1. Oliguria is traditionally defined as a urine output of less than 400 mL/day (1), but no one waits 24 hours to make the diagnosis, so this translates to an average urine output of less than 17 mL/hr.

B. Categories

The causes of oliguria are traditionally separated into three categories based on the anatomic location of the problem. The conditions in each category are listed in Table 25.1 (2).

1. *Prerenal Conditions*

The prerenal conditions are located proximal to the kidneys and are characterized by a decrease in renovascular flow. Prerenal disorders are responsible for about 30 to

40% of cases of oliguria in the ICU (1). This type of oliguria usually resolves when the underlying disorder (e.g., hypovolemia) is treated.

TABLE 25.1 Usual Causes of Acute Oliguria in the ICU

Prerenal Conditions	Renal Failure	Postrenal Obstruction
Hypovolemia	Circulatory shock	Papillary necrosis
Decompensated heart failure	Myoglobinuria	Retroperitoneal mass
Drugs that impair renal autoregulation*	Nephrotoxic drugs	Urethral stricture
	Radiocontrast dye	Prostatic hypertrophy
	Severe sepsis with multiorgan failure	
	Surgery†	

*Includes nonsteroidal antiinflammatory agents (ketorolac), angiotensin-converting enzyme inhibitors, and angiotensin receptor blockers.
†Cardiac surgery and abdominal aortic aneurysm repair.

2. *Renal Disorders*

   a. Acute renal failure is responsible for about 50% of cases of acute oliguria. The renal disorder most often involved is a condition known as *acute tubular necrosis* (ATN) (1).

   b. The hallmark of ATN is injury to the renal tubular epithelial cells. The injured cells are sloughed into the tubular lumen to create an obstruction that increases proximal pressure in the tubules. This decreases the net filtration pressure across the glomerular capillaries and reduces the glomerular filtration rate (GFR).

   c. The causes of ATN include severe sepsis, circulatory shock, and toxic injury from drugs (e.g., aminoglycosides), radiocontrast dye, and myoglobinuria.

3. *Postrenal Obstruction*

Obstruction distal to the renal parenchyma is responsible for only about 10% of cases of oliguria in the ICU (3). The obstruction can involve the most distal portion of the renal collecting ducts (papillary necrosis), the ureters (extraluminal obstruction from a retroperitoneal mass), or the ureters (strictures or extraluminal obstruction from prostatic enlargement). Ureteral obstruction from stones does not cause oliguria unless the patient has a solitary kidney.

TABLE 25.2 Prenatal Azotemia vs. Acute Renal Failure

Parameter	Acute Azotemia	Renal Failure
Urine Sodium	<10 mEq/L	>20 mEq/L
Fractional Excretion of Sodium	<1%	>2%
Urine Osmolality	>450 mosm/kg	290 ± 10 mosm/kg
BUN/Creatinine Ratio in Plasma	$\geq 20/1$	10/1

C. Evaluation

The following studies can help to distinguish prerenal conditions from intrinsic renal failure in cases of acute oliguria. (see Table 25.2).

1. *Urine Sodium*

   a. A decrease in renal perfusion is accompanied by sodium conservation and a decrease in urinary sodium excretion. *A urine sodium below 20 mEq/L usually indicates a prerenal cause of oliguria* (1).

   b. Intrinsic renal disease is usually accompanied by obligatory sodium loss in the urine and an increase in urinary sodium excretion. Therefore, *a urine sodium above 40 mEq/L suggests an intrinsic renal disorder as a cause of oliguria.*

CAVEAT. Prerenal conditions can be associated with a high urinary sodium (>40 mEq/L) when they are superimposed on chronic renal insufficiency (where there is obligatory sodium loss in the urine), or when there is ongoing diuretic therapy.

2. *Fractional Excretion of Sodium*

The *fractional excretion of sodium* (FE_{Na}) eliminates the influence of sodium intake on urinary sodium. The FE_{Na} is the fraction of filtered sodium that is excreted in the urine, and is equivalent to the sodium clearance divided by the creatinine clearance (see Table 25.3) (4).

a. The FE_{Na} is normally less than 1%; i.e., less than 1% of the filtered sodium is excreted in the urine.

b. *In the setting of oliguria, an FE_{Na} <1% suggests a prerenal condition, and an FE_{Na} >2% suggests intrinsic renal disease.*

c. One exception to the above criteria is ATN due to myoglobinuria, where the FE_{Na} can be less than 1% (1).

3. *Urine Osmolality*

a. The normal response to hypovolemia involves an increase in free water reabsorption in the kidneys (mediated, in part, by antidiuretic hormone.) This results in a relatively concentrated urine and an increase in urine osmolality.

b. Urinary concentrating ability is impaired in renal failure, and the urine osmolality tends to mirror the osmolality of plasma. This condition is known as *isosthenuria.*

c. In the setting of oliguria, *a urine osmolality >450 mosm /kg is evidence of a prerenal condition, and a urine osmolality of 280–300 mosm/kg is evidence of an intrinsic renal disorder* (5).

CAVEAT. Prerenal conditions may not cause the expected rise in urine osmolality if there is underlying renal disease, ongoing use of diuretics, or diabetes insipidus.

4. *Urine Microscopy*

Microscopic examination of the urine sediment can provide the following information:

a. The presence of abundant tubular epithelial cells with epithelial cell casts establishes the diagnosis of ATN.

b. The presence of white cell casts identifies an interstitial nephritis (see later).

c. The presence of pigmented casts identifies myoglobinuria.

TABLE 25.3 Quantitative Assessment of Renal Function

Creatinine Clearance (Men):

$$CL_{CR} \text{ (mL/min)} = \frac{(140 - age) \times weight \text{ (kg)}}{72 \times Serum\ creatinine \text{ (mg/dL)}}$$

Creatinine Clearance (Women):

$$CL_{CR} \text{ (mL/min)} = 0.85 \times Cl_{CR} \text{ for men}$$

Fractional Excretion of Sodium:

$$FE_{NA} = \frac{Urine\ [Na]/Plasma\ [Na]}{Urine\ [Cr]/Plasma\ [Cr]} \times 100$$

---

5. *BUN/Creatinine Ratio*

a. In normal subjects and patients with intrinsic renal failure, the ratio of blood urea nitrogen (BUN) to creatinine in plasma is about 10/1.

b. The reabsorption of urea in the proximal renal tubules is linked to the reabsorption of sodium, so in conditions where sodium reabsorption is increased (e.g., hypovolemia), increased urea reabsorption leads to an increase in plasma BUN and an increase in the BUN/creatinine ratio (5).

c. *A plasma BUN/creatinine ratio of 20 or higher suggests a prerenal cause for oliguria.* This condition is called *prerenal azotemia.*

CAVEAT. The BUN/creatinine ratio is also influenced by the rate of urea production. Therefore, conditions associated with an increase in urea production (e.g., GI bleeding) can also increase the BUN/creatinine ratio, and conditions associated with a decrease in urea production (e.g., hepatic insufficiency) can prevent the normal rise in the BUN/creatinine ratio in prerenal disorders.

6. *Creatinine Clearance*

Although not often used in the evaluation of oliguria, the creatinine clearance can be estimated using the equations in Table 25.3. The creatinine clearance is used as a *rough* estimate of the glomerular filtration rate (GFR), which is a measure of the functional renal mass. (The creatinine clearance overestimates GFR because creatinine is secreted by the renal tubules.

a. In acute oliguric renal failure, the creatinine clearance is less than 25% of normal. (The creatinine clearance varies with age, body size, and gender, but the normal range should be about 70–100 mL/min for most patients.)

b. In prerenal conditions, the creatinine clearance can decrease (if the condition is severe enough to cause a decrease in GFR), but the magnitude of change will be much less than in renal failure.

7. *Renal Ultrasound*

a. There are no laboratory tests that will identify postrenal obstruction as a cause of oliguria (acute obstruction has urinary indices similar to prerenal conditions, and chronic obstruction has urinary indices similar to intrinsic renal failure).

b. If postrenal obstruction is a possibility, ultrasound images of the kidneys can provide valuable information. Signs of obstruction include an increase in the size of the kidneys and enlargement of the renal calyces.

II. IMMEDIATE CONCERNS

The most immediate concerns in the oliguric patient are to identify and correct volume deficits and discontinue nephrotoxic drugs (if possible).

A. Correct Volume Deficits

1. Prompt correction of volume deficits is important because severe and prolonged hypovolemia can promote renal injury.

2. As mentioned in Chapter 10 (see Section I-B), oliguria due to hypovolemia usually involves a volume deficit of 20–30 mL/kg (ideal body weight).

3. Either colloid or crystalloid fluids can be used for volume replacement, but the volume of crystalloid fluids should be three to four times the estimated volume deficit (see Chapter 10, Section IV-B).

4. If the volume status of the patient is not clear, a fluid challenge is a reasonable measure (the risks of prolonged oliguria outweigh the risks of any retained volume). Fluid challenges should employ 500 ml to 1,000 mL for crystalloid fluids, or 300 mL to 500 mL for colloid fluids, infused over 30 minutes (6).

B. Dopamine & Furosemide

1. Low-dose dopamine (2 µg/kg/min), can promote renal vasodilation, but there is no associated improvement in

GFR in the setting of acute renal failure (7,8). As a result, low-dose dopamine is NOT recommended for the management of acute oliguric renal failure (8).

2. Furosemide has been used in oliguric renal failure in an attempt to promote urine output and limit volume retention. However, this effect is unlikely because less than 10% of the furosemide dose reaches the site of action in the renal tubules in patients with renal failure (9).

III. SPECIFIC RENAL DISORDERS

A. Inflammatory Renal Injury

1. Acute, oliguric renal failure occurs in 25% of patients with severe sepsis and 50% of patients with septic shock (10). The renal impairment in these disorders is just one part of a more widespread condition of multiorgan failure (11).

2. The culprit in this type of renal failure is the inflammatory response. The term *malignant intravascular inflammation* has been used to describe inflammation that results in multiorgan damage (12).

3. The management of inflammatory organ injury is supportive, and is described in Chapter 33.

B. Contrast-Induced Renal Failure

1. *General Features*
   a. Injection of iodinated radiocontrast dyes is the third leading cause of acute renal failure in hospitalized patients (13). The mechanism of injury is believed to involve hyperosmolar damage in the endothelium of small blood vessels and oxidative injury in renal tubular epithelial cells.

b. Predisposing conditions include diabetes, hypertension, pre-existing renal disease, congestive heart failure, and the osmolality and volume of the contrast agent.

c. The renal injury is usually apparent within 72 hours after dye administration. Oliguria is uncommon, but can occur in patients with pre-existing renal disease. Most cases resolve within 2 weeks, and few require hemodialysis (13).

2. *Preventive Measures*

The following regimen of intravenous hydration and N-acetylcysteine (an antioxidant) has proven successful in limiting the incidence and severity of contrast-induced nephropathy in high-risk patients (13,14):

Volume infusion: Isotonic saline at 100 to 150 mL/hr started at 3 to 12 hours before the procedure. For emergent procedures, at least 300 to 500 mL isotonic saline should be infused just prior to the procedure. Urine output should be maintained at 150 mL/hr for at least 6 hours after the procedure (13).

N-acetylcysteine: 600 mg by mouth twice daily from 24 hours before to 24 hours after the procedure (13). For emergent procedures (such as coronary angioplasty), give 600 mg IV just before the procedure, and follow with an oral dose of 600 mg twice daily for 48 hours after the procedure (15).

C. Acute Interstitial Nephritis (AIN)

1. AIN is an inflammatory condition that involves the renal interstitium and can progress to acute renal failure, usually without oliguria (16). Most cases are the result of a hypersensitivity drug reaction, but infections (usually viral or atypical pathogens) can also be involved.

2. The drugs most often implicated in AIN are listed in Ta-

ble 25.4. Antibiotics are the most frequent offenders (particularly the penicillins).

TABLE 25.4 Drugs That Can Cause Interstitial Nephritis

Antibiotics	CNS Drugs	Diuretics
Aminoglycosides	Carbamazepine	Acetazolamide
Amphotericin	Phenobarbital	Furosemide
Cephalosporins	Phenytoin	Thiazides
Fluoroquinolones	**NSAIDs**	**Others**
Penicillins	Aspirin	Acetaminophen
Sulfonamides	Ibuprofen	ACE Inhibitors
Vancomycin	Ketorolac	Iodinated dyes
	Naproxen	Ranitidine

NSAIDs = non-steroidal antiinflammatory drugs; *ACE* = angiotensin-converting enzyme. From Reference 16.

3. The diagnosis of AIN can be difficult. In cases of drug-induced AIN, the characteristic signs of a hypersensitivity reaction (e.g., fever, rash, eosinophilia) can be absent, and the onset of renal failure can be delayed for months after treatment with the offending drug is started (17). The presence of eosinophils and leukocyte casts on urine microscopy are the most characteristic findings. A renal biopsy can secure the diagnosis.

4. In cases of drug-induced AIN, immediate discontinuation of all possible offending drugs is mandatory. Oral prednisone at a dose of 0.5 to 1 mg/kg daily for one to four weeks may help to speed recovery (16,17). Complete resolution can take months.

D. Myoglobinuric Renal Failure

1. *General Features*

Acute renal failure develops in about one-third of patients

with diffuse muscle injury (rhabdomyolysis) (18,19). The culprit is myoglobin released by injured muscle cells, which is capable of damaging the renal tubular epithethial cells after it is filtered through the glomerulus. Predisposing factors for myoglobinuric renal failure include the extent of skeletal muscle injury and the added presence of hypovolemia, acidosis, or hypophosphatemia.

2. *Diagnosis*

Myoglobin can be detected in urine using the orthotoluidine dipstick reaction (Hemastix) that is used to detect blood in urine. If the test is positive, the urine should be centrifuged (to separate erythrocytes) and the supernatant should be passed through a micropore filter (to remove hemoglobin). A persistently positive test after these measures is evidence of myoglobin in urine.

3. *Management*

a. Avoiding and correcting hypovolemia is the most effective method for limiting the incidence and severity of myoglobinuric renal failure.

b. Alkalinizing the urine (with sodium bicarbonate infusions) has been effective in limiting the renal injury from myoglobin in animal studies, but this is difficult to accomplish and usually not necessary.

c. About 30% of patients who develop myoglobinuric renal failure will require dialysis (19), but the renal failure is rarely permanent.

IV. RENAL REPLACEMENT THERAPY

A. General Considerations

1. *Renal replacement therapy* (RRT) involves the use of semipermeable membranes to remove fluid and toxic substances from the bloodstream. The basic methods of RRT are *hemodialysis* and *hemofiltration*.

2. About 70% of patients with acute renal failure will require RRT. The indications for RRT in acute renal failure are uremic encephalopathy, volume overload, and life-threatening hyperkalemia or metabolic acidosis.

B. Hemodialysis

1. *Method*

   The basis of fluid and solute removal by hemodialysis is illustrated in Figure 25.1.

   a. Hemodialysis removes solutes by *diffusion* across a semipermeable dialysis membrane. Water (fluid) removal is passive, and follows solute removal.

   b. The removal of solutes by diffusion is driven by the concentration gradient of solutes across a semipermeable membrane. Normally, as solutes move from one compartment to another, the concentration gradient for the solute decreases, and this slows the rate of solute clearance. In hemodialysis, the concentration gradient for solute clearance is maintained by moving the blood and dialysis fluid in opposite directions (a technique known as *countercurrent exchange*) (20). The blood is moved (by a pump) at a rate of 200 to 300 mL/min (roughly 2–3 times faster than the normal GFR), and the dialysate moves even faster, at 500 to 800 mL/min (20).

2. *Vascular Access*

   a. Short-term hemodialysis is performed through specialized large-bore, double-lumen catheters like the one shown in Figure 4.2 (Chapter 4).

   b. These catheters are placed in the internal jugular or femoral veins. The subclavian vein cannulation is not advised because of a high incidence of vascular stenosis, which makes the ipsilateral arm veins unsuitable for chronic dialysis access (21).

c. During dialysis, blood is withdrawn from one lumen of the catheter, pumped through the dialysis chamber, and then returned to the patient through the other lumen. The large diameter of each lumen allows the rapid flow rates (200–300 ml/min) needed for effective dialysis.

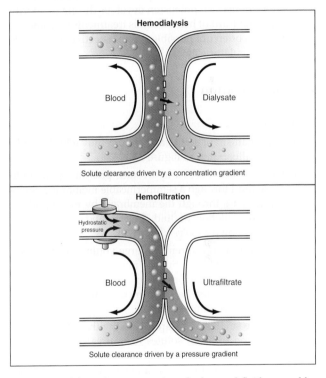

FIGURE 25.1. Schematic representation of solute and fluid removal by hemodialysis and hemofiltration. The smaller circles represent small solutes (e.g., urea) that are readily cleared from the bloodstream, and the larger circles represent larger molecules such as inflammatory cytokines that are partly cleared by hemofiltration but not by dialysis.

3. *Advantages & Disadvantages*

The rapid flow rates used during dialysis can be an advantage or a disadvantage.

a. The advantage is the ability to achieve a day's worth of solute clearance in just a few hours.

b. The disadvantage is the potential for hemodynamic compromise. Hypotension develops during or shortly after one-third of hemodialysis treatments (20), and dialysis is often not possible (or not effective) in patients with circulatory shock.

B. Hemofiltration

1. *Method*

The mechanism of solute and fluid removal by hemofiltration is illustrated in Figure 25.1.

a. Hemofiltration uses a hydrostatic pressure gradient to drive fluid through a semipermeable membrane. Small solutes pass through the membrane by moving along with the bulk flow of fluid. This method of solute clearance is known as *solvent drag* (20).

b. Hemofiltration can remove large volumes of fluid (up to 3 liters per hour), but the rate of solute clearance is much slower than during hemodialysis. As a result, hemofiltration must be performed continuously to provide effective solute clearance.

c. Because small solutes are cleared with water, the concentration of small solutes (e.g., urea) in blood does not decrease during hemofiltration unless a solute-free fluid is infused to replace some of the ultrafiltrate that is lost (this is often necessary because of the large volumes lost during hemofiltration).

2. *Vascular Access*

a. Hemofiltration was originally performed by cannulating an artery (radial, brachial, or femoral) and a large vein (internal jugular or femoral). This method of *arteriovenous hemofiltration* uses the mean arterial pressure as the filtration pressure (i.e., the pressure driving fluid across the hemofiltration membrane).

b. The more popular method at present is *venovenous hemofiltration*, where venous blood is withdrawn and replaced through a double-lumen catheter similar to the one used for hemodialysis. This method requires a pump to create an effective filtration pressure.

3. *Advantages & Disadvantages*

There are 2 major advantages with hemofiltration:

a. Hemofiltration allows more gradual fluid removal than hemodialysis, and thus is less likely to produce hemodynamic compromise.

b. Hemofiltration removes larger molecules than hemodialysis dialysis, and clinical trials have shown that hemofiltration can remove harmful cytokines from the bloodstream in patients with severe sepsis and multiorgan failure (22).

The major disadvantages of hemofiltration are as follows:

c. Hemofiltration must be used continuously to provide effective dialysis, and this is time-consuming and often not possible (because of mechanical problems). A method known as *hemodiafiltration* (which combines the features of dialysis and hemofiltration) is more suitable for patients with renal failure.

d. Hemofiltration requires anticoagulation to maintain patency in the circuit. Despite attempts to restrict anticoagulation to the hemofiltration circuit, systemic anticoagulation can occur, which increases the risk of hemorrhage.

e. Because hemofiltration requires a hydrostatic pressure gradient for solute clearance, it is not well-suited for hypotensive patients.

REFERENCES

1. Klahr S, Miller SB. Acute oliguria. N Engl J Med 1998; 338:671–675.
2. Bellomo R. Defining, quantifying, and classifying acute renal failure. Crit Care Clin 2005; 21:223–237.
3. Abernathy VE, Lieberthal W. Acute renal failure in the critically ill patient. Crit Care Clin 2002; 18:203–222.
4. Steiner RW. Interpreting the fractional excretion of sodium. Am J Med 1984; 77:699–702.
5. Rose BD, Post TW. Clinical physiology of acid-base and electrolyte disorders. 5th ed. New York: McGraw-Hill, 2001:426-428.
6. Vincent J-L, Gerlach H. Fluid resuscitation in severe sepsis and septic shock: an evidence-based review. Crit Care Med 2004; 32(Suppl):S451–S454.
7. Kellum JA, Decker JM. Use of dopamine in acute renal failure: a meta-analysis. Crit Care Med 2001; 29:1526–1531.
8. Holmes CL, Walley KR. Bad medicine: Low-dose dopamine in the ICU. Chest 2003; 123:1266–1275.
9. Brater DC, Anderson SA, Brown-Cartwright D. Response to furosemide in chronic renal insufficiency: rationale for limited doses. Clin Pharmacol Ther 1986; 40:134–139.
10. Schrier RW, Wang W. Acute renal failure and sepsis. N Engl J Med 2004; 351:159–169.
11. Balk RA. Pathogenesis and management of multiple organ dysfunction or failure in severe sepsis and septic shock. Crit Care Clin 2000; 16:337–352, 2000.
12. Pinsky MR, Vincent J-L, Deviere J, et al. Serum cytokine levels in human septic shock: Relation to multiple-system organ failure and mortality. Chest 1993; 103:565–575.
13. McCullough PA, Soman S. Contrast-induced nephropathy. Crit Care Clin 2005; 21:261–280.
14. Liu R, Nair D, Ix J, et al. N-acetylcysteine for the prevention of contrast-induced nephropathy. A systematic review and meta-analysis. J Gen Intern Med 2005; 20:193–200.
15. Marenzi G, Assanelli E, Marana I, et al. N-acetylcysteine and contrast-induced nephropathy in primary angioplasty. N Engl J Med 2006; 354:2772–2782.
16. Taber SS, Mueller BA. Drug-associated renal dysfunction. Crit Care Clin 2006; 22:357–374.

17. Ten RM, Torres VE, Millner DS, et al. Acute interstitial nephritis. Mayo Clin Proc 1988; 3:921–930.

18. Beetham R. Biochemical investigation of suspected rhabdomyolysis. Ann Clin Biochem 2000; 37:581–587.

19. Sharp LS, Rozycki GS, Feliciano DV. Rhabdomyolysis and secondary renal failure in critically ill surgical patients. Am J Surg 2004; 188:801–806.

20. O'Reilly P, Tolwani A. Renal replacement therapy III. IHD, CRRT, SLED. Crit Care Clin 2005; 21:367-378.

21. Hernandez D, Diaz F, Rufino M, et al. Subclavian vascular access stenosis in dialysis patients: natural history and risk factors. J Am Soc Nephrol 1998; 9:1507–1511.

22. Morgera S, Haase M, Kuss T, et al. Pilot study on the effects of high cutoff hemofiltration on the need for norepinephrine in septic patients with acute renal failure. Crit Care Med 2006; 34:2099–2104.

Chapter 26

HYPERTONIC AND HYPOTONIC CONDITIONS

This chapter describes conditions that alter the osmotic properties of extracellular fluid. In most of these conditions, the primary problem is an imbalance between sodium and water in the extracellular fluid, and the presenting feature is an abnormal sodium concentration in plasma (i.e., hypernatremia or hyponatremia). The chapter begins with a quick review of the factors that determine the osmotic activity of extracellular fluid.

I. OSMOTIC ACTIVITY

The distribution of water in the intracellular and extracellular fluids is governed by the osmotic activity of the extracellular fluid, which is determined primarily by the sodium concentration in extracellular fluid (plasma).

A. Definitions

1. The concentration of solutes in a solution can be expressed in terms of osmotic activity, which is a reflection of the number of solute particles in a solution. The unit of measurement is the osmole (osm), which is 6×10^{23} particles (Avogadro's number) for a nondissociable substance (1).

2. Osmotic activity can be expressed in relation to the volume of water in a solution, or the total volume of the solution.

    a. Osmotic activity per volume of solution is called *osmolarity*, and is expressed as milliosmoles per liter (mosm/L).

    b. Osmotic activity per volume of water is called *osmolality*, and is expressed as milliosmoles per kilogram of H_2O (mosm/kg H_2O).

3. The importance of osmotic activity in biological systems is the ability to influence water movement between fluid compartments. Therefore, osmolality (i.e., osmotic activity per volume of water) is the appropriate measure of osmotic activity in the biological world.

4. Extracellular fluid is mostly water (e.g., plasma is 93% water), so there is little difference between osmolality and osmolarity in extracellular fluid (plasma) ,and the two terms are often used interchangeably (2).

B. Osmotic Activity of Plasma

1. The osmotic activity of plasma is determined by the factors in the equation shown below

$$P_{osm} = 2 \times \text{Plasma } [Na^+] + \frac{[Glucose]}{18} + \frac{[BUN]}{2.8}$$

(26.1)

where P_{osm} is the osmolarity of plasma in mosm/L, $[Na^+]$ is the plasma sodium concentration in mEq/L, [glucose] and [BUN] are the plasma concentrations of glucose and urea in mg/dL, and the factors 18 and 2.8 are conversion factors that express glucose and urea concentrations in milliosmoles per liter (mosm/L). Note the following:

    a. The plasma sodium concentration is doubled to include the osmotic activity of chloride.

    b. The plasma concentrations in this equation are measured in relation to the total plasma volume, so the calculated P_{osm} is expressed as osmolarity instead of osmolality. (The osmotic activity measured in the clinical laboratory is the osmolality.)

2. If the normal plasma concentrations of sodium (140 mEq/L), glucose (90 mg/dL), and BUN (14 mg/dL) are used in Equation 26.1, the plasma osmolarity is $(2 \times 140) + 90/18 + 14/2.8 = 290$ mosm/L.

C. Effective Osmotic Activity

1. The driving force for water movement between two fluid compartments is the *difference* in osmotic activity in the two compartments. This difference is called *effective osmotic activity.*

2. The osmotic relationship between two fluids is described by the term *tonicity* — the fluid with the higher osmotic activity is described as *hypertonic*, the fluid with the lower osmotic activity is described as *hypotonic*, and fluids with the same osmotic activity are described as *isotonic.*

3. The effective osmotic activity of plasma does not include the osmotic activity of urea because urea passes readily across cell membranes. This is reflected in Equation 26.2.

$$\textbf{Effective P}_{\textbf{osm}} = \textbf{2} \times \textbf{Plasma [Na}^+\textbf{]} + \frac{\textbf{[Glucose]}}{\textbf{18}}$$

(26.2)

The osmolar concentration of urea is only $14/1.8 = 7.7$ mosm/L, which is less than 3% of the total plasma osmolarity (290 mosm/L), so there is little difference between total and effective plasma osmolarity.

4. Equation 26.2 demonstrates that sodium is the principal factor that determines the effective osmolarity of plasma (extracellular fluid). The effective osmolality of extracellular fluid governs the movement of water between intracellular and extracellular fluids, which means that *the sodium concentration in plasma is the principal factor that governs the distribution of water in the intracellular and extracellular fluids.*

II. HYPERNATREMIA

Hypernatremia (i.e., plasma sodium concentration >145 mEq/L) is a condition of sodium excess relative to water in the extracellular fluid (3).

TABLE 26.1 Changes in Total Body Sodium and Water in Hypernatremia and Hyponatremia

Condition	Extracellular Volume	Total Body	
		Sodium	Free Water
Hypernatremia	Decreased	↓	↓↓
	Normal	—	↓
	Increased	↑↑	↑
Hyponatremia	Decreased	↓↓	↓
	Normal	—	↑
	Increased	↑	↑↑

A. Causes of Hypernatremia

Hypernatremia can be the result of any of the following conditions:

1. Loss of hypotonic fluids; i.e., fluids that have a lower sodium concentration than extracellular fluid.

2. Net loss of free water; i.e., when sodium lost in hypotonic fluids is replaced, leaving a free water deficit.

3. Gain of hypertonic fluids; i.e., fluids with a higher sodium concentration than extracellular fluid.

Each of these conditions is associated with a specific extracellular volume (i.e., low, normal, or high), as shown in Table 26.1. Therefore, evaluating the extracellular volume can be used to identify the source of hypernatremia in individual patients.

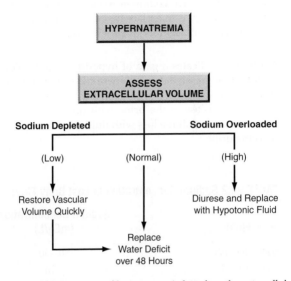

FIGURE 26.1 Management of hypernatremia based on the extracellular volume.

B. Extracellular Volume

The condition of the extracellular volume (ECV) provides the following diagnostic and therapeutic information. (see Figure 26.1).

1. **Low ECV** indicates loss of hypotonic fluids. Common causes are excessive diuresis, vomiting, and diarrhea. The management strategy is to replace the sodium deficit quickly (to maintain plasma volume) and to replace the free water deficit slowly (to prevent intracellular overhydration).

2. **Normal ECV** indicates a net loss of free water. This can be seen in diabetes insipidus, or when loss of hypotonic fluids (e.g., diuresis) is treated by replacement with isotonic saline in a 1:1 volume-to-volume ratio. The management strategy is to replace the free water deficit slowly (to prevent intracellular overhydration).

3. **High ECV** indicates a gain of hypertonic fluids. This is seen with aggressive use of hypertonic saline or sodium bicarbonate solutions. The management strategy is to induce sodium loss in the urine with diuresis and to replace the urine volume loss with fluids that are hypotonic to the urine.

TABLE 26.2 Sodium Concentration in Lost Body Fluids

Body Fluid	Sodium Concentration (mEq/L)
Sweat (normal)	20–80
Urine (normal)†	<10
Urine (furosemide diuresis)	70–80
Gastrointestinal Fluids:	
Gastric secretions	70–80
Pancreatic secretions	140–145
Small bowel secretions	60–70
Stool (diarrhea)	30–40

†Urinary sodium secretion varies with sodium intake.

III. HYPOVOLEMIC HYPERNATREMIA

The most common cause of hypernatremia is exaggerated loss of one or more of the fluids listed in Table 26.2.

A. Consequences of Hypotonic Fluid Loss

1. *Hypovolemia*

   All body fluids that are lost contain sodium, as shown in Table 26.1, so hypotonic fluid loss will eventually lead to sodium depletion if the lost sodium is not replaced. The major consequence of sodium depletion is hypovolemia.

2. *Hypertonicity*

   Hypernatremia from hypotonic fluid loss increases the effective osmolality of the extracellular fluid, and this draws water out of cells and promotes cellular dehydration.

   a. The principal manifestation of cellular dehydration is *hypernatremic encephalopathy*, which can be accompanied by coma, seizures, and focal neurologic deficits (4).

   b. Dehydrated cells regain volume after several hours by somehow generating an additional osmotic force, and this osmotic adaptation can create problems during free water replacement (see later).

B. Volume Replacement

1. Volume (sodium) replacement is an immediate priority because hypovolemia can impair organ perfusion.

2. Crystalloid fluids are preferred for sodium replacement in hemodynamically stable patients because these fluids will replenish sodium uniformly throughout the extracellular fluid. Isotonic saline is preferred because more dilute solutions can promote cell swelling and cerebral edema (see later).

C. Free Water Replacement

When plasma volume is restored, the next step is to determine the free water deficit and correct the deficit over a period of 3 to 4 days.

1. *The Free Water Deficit*

   The calculation of free water deficit is based on the reciprocal relationship between the total body water (TBW) and the plasma sodium concentration ($P[Na^+]$); i.e., when one parameter changes, the other changes in the opposite direction. The product of these two variables (TBW x $P[Na^+]$) remains constant, regardless of conditions in the extracellular fluid. This allows the following relationships.

   $$\text{Current (TBW} \times P[Na^+]) = \text{Normal (TBW} \times P[Na^+])$$

   (26.3)

   Using 140 mEq/L for a normal $P[Na^+]$ and rearranging terms yields the following relationship:

   $$\text{Current TBW} = \text{Normal TBW} \times (140/\text{Current } P[Na^+])$$

   (26.4)

   The normal TBW (in liters) is 60% of lean body weight (in kg) in men and 50% of lean body weight in women. Once the current TBW is determined, the free water deficit is simply the difference between the normal and current TBW .

   $$\text{Water deficit (L)} = \text{Normal TBW} - \text{Current TBW}$$
   (26.5)

   EXAMPLE. For an adult male with a lean body weight of 70 kg and a plasma $[Na^+]$ of 160 mEq/L, the normal TBW is 0.6 x 70 = 42 liters, the current TBW is 42 x 140/160 = 36.8 liters, and the free water deficit is 42 − 36.8 = 5.2 liters.

2. *Replacing the Free Water Deficit*

   Hypotonic saline solutions (usually half-normal saline) are used to replace water deficits, and the volume needed to accomplish this is identified using the equation shown below. (5).

   $$\text{Replacement volume (L)} = \text{Water deficit} \times (1/1 - X)$$ (26.6)

where X is the ratio of the sodium concentration in the resuscitation fluid to the sodium concentration in isotonic saline (154 mEq/L).

EXAMPLE. If the replacement fluid is half-normal saline (Na=75 mEq/L), and the water deficit is 5.2 liters, as calculated previously, the replacement volume will be $5.2 \times (1/0.5) = 10.4$ liters.

3. *Risk of Cerebral Edema*

a. Acute hypernatremia draws fluid out of brain cells and promotes cellular dehydration. This effect is only transient, and after several hours, there is an increase in brain cell osmolality that draws fluid back into the cells (3).

b. The osmotic adaptation in brain cells can be problematic during free water replacement because hypotonic fluids can accumulate in brain cells and produce cellular overhydration and cerebral edema. To limit this risk, free water deficits should be replaced slowly; i.e., *the decrease in plasma sodium should not exceed 0.5 mEq/L per hour* (3,4).

IV. OTHER HYPERTONIC CONDITIONS

A. Diabetes Insipidus

1. *General Features*

Diabetes insipidus (DI) is a condition of impaired water conservation that results in hypernatremia without apparent volume deficits. (6,7) The underlying abnormality in DI is loss of the actions of antidiuretic hormone (ADH) in the kidneys, which results in a marked increase in free water excretion in the urine. There are two types of DI based on the cause of the lost ADH activity.

a. CENTRAL DI is characterized by the absence of ADH release from the posterior pituitary. This condition is most often the result of traumatic brain injury, anoxic encephalopathy, and brain death. The onset is heralded by polyuria that usually is evident within 24 hours of the inciting event.

b. NEPHROGENIC DI is characterized by defective end-organ responsiveness to ADH. This condition can be caused by drugs (i.e., amphotericin, aminoglycosides, dopamine, and lithium), radiocontrast dyes, hypokalemia, and the polyuric phase of ATN (7,8).

2. *Diagnosis*

The hallmark of DI is a dilute urine in the face of hypertonic plasma.

a. In central DI, the urine osmolarity is often below 200 mosm/L, whereas in nephrogenic DI, the urine osmolarity is usually between 200 and 500 mosm/L (9).

b. The diagnosis of DI is confirmed by noting the urinary response to fluid restriction. Failure of the urine osmolarity to increase more than 30 mosm/L in the first few hours of complete fluid restriction is diagnostic of DI.

c. Once the diagnosis of DI is confirmed, the response to vasopressin (5 units intravenously) will differentiate central from nephrogenic DI. In central DI, the urine osmolality promptly increases by at least 50% after vasopressin administration, whereas in nephrogenic DI, the urine osmolality remains unchanged.

3. *Management*

a. The fluid loss in DI is almost pure water, so the the goal of management is to replace free water deficits only. The free water deficit is calculated as described earlier.

b. In central DI, **vasopressin** administration is required to prevent ongoing free water losses. The usual dose is 2 to 5 units of aqueous vasopressin by subcutaneous injection every 4 to 6 hours (7).

B. Nonketotic Hyperglycemia

1. *General Features*

Nonketotic hyperglycemia (NKH) is a condition of progressive hyperglycemia without ketoacidosis. Because glucose contributes to the effective osmolality of extracellular fluid (see Equation 26.2), the progressive hyperglycemia in NKH promotes hypertonic cell dehydration in the brain and produces a hypertonic encephalopathy similar to the one described for hypernatremia (4). This condition is usually seen in patients who have enough endogenous insulin to prevent ketosis. There may be no prior history of diabetes (10).

2. *Clinical Presentation*

   a. Depressed consciousness is very common at presentation, and a rise in plasma osmolality above 330 mosm/kg H_2O can precipitate coma and generalized seizures (10).

   b. Hypovolemia may be evident, and can be profound (from the glycosuria-induced osmotic diuresis).

   c. The hyperglycemia in NKH is typically very severe, with plasma glucose levels of 1000 mg/dL or higher.

3. *Fluid Management*

The fluid management of NKH is similar to that described for hypovolemic hypernatremia. Volume deficits are more profound in NKH (because of the osmotic diuresis).

4. *The Free Water Deficit*

The plasma sodium concentration is not an accurate reflection of free water deficits in NKH because the hyperglycemia draws water from the intracellular space, and this creates a dilutional effect on the plasma sodium concentration. The magnitude of this effect depends on the severity of the hyperglycemia.

   a. *For every 100 mg/dL increment in the plasma glucose, the plasma sodium will decrease 1.6 to 2.4 mEq/L* (the lower number is more accurate when the blood glucose is below 400 mg/dL, and the higher number is more accurate when the blood glucose is above 400 mg/dL) (10,11).

b. To calculate the free water deficit in NKH (or any patient with hyperglycemia), the plasma sodium concentration must be adjusted using the dilutional factors just mentioned. For example, if the blood glucose is 800 mg/dL, the sodium concentration should be adjusted upward by 7 x 2.4 = 16.8 mEq/L.

5. *Insulin Therapy*

a. The insulin requirements in NKH and diabetic keto-acidosis (DKA) are roughly the same (10), so the insulin regimen for DKA described in Chapter 23 (see Section II-D) is also appropriate for NKH.

b. Insulin therapy drives water into cells along with glucose, and this effect can aggravate hypovolemia. Therefore in patients with severe volume deficits (which is common in NKH), volume replacement should be started before insulin is given.

V. HYPONATREMIA

Hyponatremia (serum sodium concentration <135 mEq/L) is the result of excess water relative to sodium in the extracellular fluid (12).

A. Pseudohyponatremia

1. Plasma is 93% water, and the remaining 7% is made up of circulating lipids and proteins. Sodium is confined to the aqueous portion of plasma, but the standard method of measuring sodium concentration uses total plasma volume (aqueous and nonaqueous portions). The meas-

ured sodium concentration will therefore underestimate the actual (aqueous phase) sodium concentration, but the difference is normally small because water makes up over 90% of plasma..

2. In conditions where there is an abundance of circulating lipids and plasma proteins (e.g., severe hyperlipidemias or hyperproteinemias), the nonaqueous portion of plasma will increase in volume, and can grow to 30% of the plasma volume. In this situation, the measured plasma sodium can be considerably lower than the actual sodium concentration. This condition is called *pseudohyponatremia* (13), but it is really a laboratory artifact.

3. The hallmark of pseudohyponatremia is the combination of hyponatremia and a normal plasma osmolality. The diagnosis is confirmed if the plasma sodium concentration is measured with an ion-specific electrode (which measures the aqueous phase sodium), and the hyponatremia disappears.

B. Diagnostic Approach

As is the case with hypernatremia, the extracellular volume (ECV) can be high, normal, or low in hyponatremia (see Table 26.1), and the status of the ECV can be used to organize the diagnostic approach to hyponatremia, as shown in Figure 26.2.

1. *Hypovolemic Hyponatremia*

Volume depletion predisposes to hyponatremia by stimulating the release of antidiuretic hormone (ADH), which promotes water retention. The conditions associated with hypovolemic hyponatremia can be grouped according to the urinary sodium concentration, as shown below (see also Figure 26.2).

Urine [Na+]	Site of Na+ Loss	Conditions
>20 mEq/L	Renal	Diuresis
		Adrenal Insufficiency
		Cerebral Salt Wasting
<20 mEq/L	Extrarenal	Vomiting
		Diarrhea

2. *Isovolemic Hyponatremia*

   When hyponatremia is associated with an apparently normal ECV, the principal disorders to consider include inappropriate secretion of antidiuretic hormone (ADH), water intoxication (also known as psychogenic polydipsia), and hypothyroidism (rare). The urine sodium and urine osmolality can help to distinguish water intoxication from inappropriate ADH release, as shown below.

Clinical Disorder	Urine Sodium	Urine Osmolality
Inappropriate ADH	>20 mEq/L	>100 mOsm/kg H_2O
Water Intoxication	<10 mEq/L	<100 mOsm/kg H_2O

   INAPPROPRIATE ADH RELEASE. The inappropriate (nonosmotic) release of ADH is characterized by an inappropriately concentrated urine (urine osmolality above 100 mOsm/kg H_2O) in the face of a hypotonic plasma (<290 mosm/kg H_2O). This condition is a common cause of hyponatremia in hospitalized patients, and is considered the result of "stress-induced" release of ADH. This condition differs from the *syndrome of inappropriate ADH* (SIADH), which is associated with a variety of neoplasms, infections, and drugs (see Reference 14 for a recent review of SIADH).

3. *Hypervolemic Hyponatremia*

   Hypervolemic hyponatremia is usually the result of salt and water retention in patients with heart failure, renal failure, or hepatic failure.

C. Symptoms

1. Hyponatremia promotes cerebral edema, and the result-

ing encephalopathy produces the symptoms of hyponatremia. Symptoms range from lethargy and somnolence to seizures, coma, and brain death.

2. Acute hyponatremia (<48 hrs) is more likely to produce symptoms, probably because the severity of the cerebral edema and cell swelling diminish with time (osmotic adaptation).

3. Hyponatremic encephalopathy carries a poor prognosis, particularly for women. One-third of patients who develop hyponatremic encephalopathy do not survive, and 80% of deaths involve women (15).

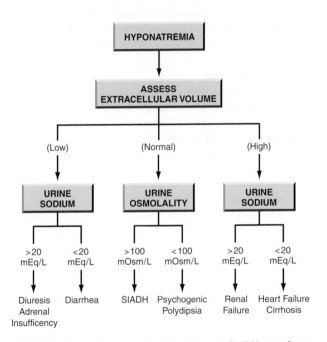

FIGURE 26.2 Diagnostic approach to hyponatremia. *SIADH* = syndrome of inappropriate antidiuretic hormone.

D. Management

1. *Extracellular Volume*

The management of hyponatremia is guided by the status of the ECV (i.e., low, normal, or high), and the presence or absence of symptoms related to hyponatremia.

LOW ECV: Infuse hypertonic saline (3% NaCl) in symptomatic patients, and isotonic saline in asymptomatic patients.

NORMAL ECV: Combine furosemide diuresis with infusion of hypertonic saline in symptomatic patients, or isotonic saline in asymptomatic patients.

HIGH ECV: Use furosemide-induced diuresis in asymptomatic patients. In symptomatic patients, combine furosemide diuresis with judicious use of hypertonic saline.

2. *Rate of Correction*

Rapid correction of hyponatremia has been reported to cause a demyelinating disorder known as *central pontine myelinolysis* (16). The following recommendations are designed to prevent osmotic demyelination by limiting the rate of rise of the plasma

a. For asymptomatic hyponatremia, the increase in plasma sodium should not exceed 0.5 mEq/L per hour (12 mEq/L in 24 hours) (17).

b. For symptomatic hyponatremia, particularly when the symptoms suggest severe cerebral impairment (e.g., obtundation, coma, seizures), hypertonic saline should be used to raise the plasma sodium concentration by 1.5 to 2 mEq/L per hour for 3 to 4 hours (17). Subsequent replacement should be adjusted so that the total rise in sodium does not exceed 12 mEq/L in the first 24 hours. (Rapid correction of plasma sodium can be guided by the calculated sodium deficit, which is described next).

3. *Sodium Deficit*

When hypertonic saline is used for rapid correction of symptomatic hyponatremia, the volume of fluid that is required can be determined by estimating the sodium deficit in mEq (17).

Na^+ deficit = Normal TBW $\times$ (Desired $P[Na^+]$ − Current $P[Na^+]$)

(26.7)

The desired $P[Na^+]$ is obtained by adding the expected increment in plasma sodium (e.g., 2 mEq/L per hour x 4 hours = 8 mEq/L) to the current $P[Na^+]$.

a. The sodium deficit is divided by 513 (the concentration of sodium in 3% NaCl) to determine the volume of hypertonic saline (in liters) needed to produce the desired increment in plasma sodium.

REFERENCES

1. Rose BD, Post TW. The total body water and the plasma sodium concentration. In: Clinical physiology of acid-base and electrolyte disorders. 5th ed. New York: McGraw-Hill, 2001:241–257.

2. Erstad BL. Osmolality and osmolarity: narrowing the terminology gap. Pharmacotherapy 2003; 23:1085–1086.

3. Adrogue HJ, Madias NE. Hypernatremia. N Engl J Med 2000; 342:1493–1499.

4. Arieff AI, Ayus JC. Strategies for diagnosing and managing hypernatremic encephalopathy. J Crit Illness 1996; 11:720–727.

5. Marino PL, Krasner J, O'Moore P. Fluid and electrolyte expert, Philadelphia: WB Saunders, 1987.

6. Makaryus AN, McFarlane SI. Diabetes insipidus: diagnosis and treatment of a complex disease. Cleve Clin J Med 2006; 73:65–71.

7. Blevins LS Jr, Wand GS. Diabetes insipidus. Crit Care Med 1992; 20:69–79.

8. Garofeanu CG, Weir M, Rosas-Arellano MP, et al. Causes of reversible nephrogenic diabetes insipidus: a systematic review. Am J Kidney Dis 2005; 45:626–637.

9. Geheb MA. Clinical approach to the hyperosmolar patient. Crit Care Clin 1987; 3:797–815.

10. Rose BD, Post TW. Hyperosmolal states: hyperglycemia. In: Clinical physiology of acid-base and electrolyte disorders. 5th ed. New York: McGraw-Hill, 2001:794–821.

11. Hillier TA, Abbott RD, Barrett EJ. Hyponatremia: evaluating the correction factor for hyperglycemia. Am J Med 1999; 106:399–403.

12. Adrogue HJ, Madias NE. Hyponatremia. N Engl J Med 2000; 342:1581–1589.

13. Weisberg LS. Pseudohyponatremia: A reappraisal. Am J Med 1989; 86:315–318.

14. Ellison DH, Berl T. The syndrome of inappropriate antidiuresis. N Engl J Med 2007; 356:2064-2072.

15. Arieff A. Influence of hypoxia and sex on hyponatremic encephalopathy. Am J Med 2006; 119:559–564.

16. Brunner JE, Redmond JM, Haggar AM, et al. Central pontine myelinolysis and pontine lesions after rapid correction of hyponatremia: a prospective magnetic resonance imaging study. Ann Neurol 1990; 27:61–66.

17. Rose BD, Post TW. Hypoosmolal states—hyponatremia. In: Clinical physiology of acid-base and electrolyte disorders. 5th ed. New York: McGraw-Hill, 2001:696–745.

Chapter 27

POTASSIUM

Monitoring the potassium (K^+) level in plasma as an index of total body potassium is similar to evaluating an iceberg by its tip, because less than 1% of the total amount of K^+ in the body is located in plasma. With this shortcoming in mind, this chapter describes the causes and consequences of hypokalemia and hyperkalemia.

I. POTASSIUM DISTRIBUTION

A. Total Body vs. Serum K^+

1. The total body K^+ in healthy adults is about 50 mEq/kg (1,2), so a 70 kg adult will have 3,500 mEq of total body K^+. However, only 70 mEq (2% of the total amount) is located in extracellular fluid.

2. The plasma accounts for approximately 20% of the extracellular fluid, so the K^+ content of plasma (serum) will be $0.2 \times 70 = 14$ mEq, which is about 0.4% of the total amount of K^+ in the body.

B. Changes in Serum K^+

1. The relationship between changes in total body and serum K^+ is curvilinear, as shown in Figure 27.1 (3,4). The slope of the curve decreases on the "deficit" side of the graph, indicating that the change in serum K^+ is much smaller when K^+ is depleted than when it accumulates.

2. In an average-sized adult with a normal serum K^+ (i.e.,

3.5 to 5.5 mEq/L), a total body K^+ deficit of 200 to 400 mEq is required to produce a 1 mEq/L decrease in serum K^+, whereas a total body excess of 100 to 200 mEq is required to produce a 1 mEq/L rise in serum K^+ (4).

3. Thus, K^+ depletion must be twice as great as K^+ accumulation to produce a significant (1 mEq/L) change in serum K^+. This difference is due to the large pool of intracellular K^+, which can replenish extracellular stores when K^+ is lost.

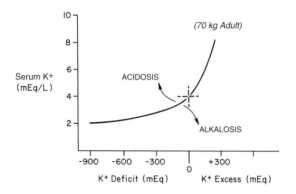

FIGURE 27.1 The relationship between changes in serum and total body potassium. (Redrawn from Reference 3.)

II. HYPOKALEMIA

Hypokalemia (defined as a serum K^+ below 3.5 mEq/L) can be the result of an intracellular shift of K^+ (transcellular shift) or total body K^+ depletion.

A. Transcellular Shift

The following conditions can result in hypokalemia from K^+ movement into cells:

1. Inhaled β-agonist bronchodilators can cause a mild decrease in serum K^+ (0.5 mEq/L or less) in the usual therapeutic doses (5). The mechanism of action is stimulation of β-receptors on the cell membranes of skeletal muscle cells. The hypokalemic effect of inhaled β-agonists is magnified when they are given with glucose and insulin (5) or diuretics (6).

2. Alkalosis (respiratory or metabolic) can promote the exchange of K^+ for intracellular H^+ via a membrane H^+–K^+ exchange pump. However, alkalosis has a variable and unpredictable effect on serum K^+ (7).

3. Hypothermia (accidental or induced) causes a transient drop in serum K^+ that usually resolves during rewarming (8). Lethal cases of hypothermia can be accompanied by *hyper*kalemia because of widespread cell death (9).

4. Insulin drives K^+ into cells via the glucose transporter, and the effect lasts 1–2 hours.

B. K^+ Depletion

Potassium depletion can be the result of either renal or extrarenal K^+ losses. The site of K^+ loss can often be identified by using a combination of urinary K^+ and chloride concentrations, as shown in Figure 27.2.

1. *Renal Loss*
   a. The leading cause of renal K^+ loss is diuretic therapy. Other causes include nasogastric drainage, alkalosis, and magnesium depletion.
   b. The urinary chloride is low (less than 15 mEq/L) when nasogastric drainage or alkalosis is involved, and it is high (greater than 25 mEq/L) when magnesium depletion or diuretics are responsible.
   c. Magnesium depletion impairs potassium reabsorption across the renal tubules and may play a very important

role in promoting and sustaining potassium depletion, particularly in patients receiving diuretics (10).

2. *Extrarenal Loss*

The major cause of extrarenal K^+ loss is diarrhea. The K^+ concentration in stool is 75 mEq/L, and in diarrheal states, the daily volume of stool can rise from <200 mL/day to >10 L/day, so severe or prolonged diarrhea can result in profound K^+ losses.

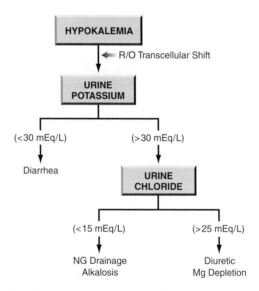

FIGURE 27.2 Diagnostic approach to hypokalemia.

C. Clinical Manifestations

Severe hypokalemia (serum K^+ below 2.5 mEq/L) can be accompanied by diffuse muscle weakness (2). Milder degrees of hypokalemia (serum K^+ 2.5 to 3.5 mEq/L) are often asymptomatic.

1. *ECG Abnormalities*

   a. Abnormalities in the ECG, including prominent U waves (more than 1 mm in height), flattening and inversion of T waves, and prolongation of the QT interval, can be present in more than 50% of cases of hypokalemia (11).

   b. None of the ECG changes is specific for hypokalemia. The T wave changes and U waves can be seen with digitalis or left ventricular hypertrophy, and QT prolongation can be seen with hypocalcemia and hypomagnesemia.

2. *Arrhythmias*

   There is a misconception about the ability of hypokalemia to promote cardiac arrhythmias. *Hypokalemia alone does not produce serious ventricular arrhythmias* (2,11). Hypokalemia is often combined with other conditions that can promote arrhythmias (e.g., magnesium depletion, digitalis, myocardial ischemia), and the hypokalemia may enhance the proarrhythmic effects of these other conditions; e.g., hypokalemia is well known for the ability to promote digitalis-induced arrhythmias.

D. Management

The first concern in hypokalemia is to eliminate or treat any condition that promotes transcellular shift of K^+ (2). If the hypokalemia is due to K^+ depletion, proceed as described next.

1. *Estimating Deficits*

   A deficit of 10% of the total body K^+ is expected for every 1 mEq/L decrease in the serum K^+ (12). The correlation between K^+ deficits and the severity of hypokalemia is shown in Table 27.1.

2. *Replacement Fluids*

   a. The usual replacement fluid is potassium chloride (KCL), which is available with K^+ concentrations of

1 and 2 mEq/mL, and comes in ampules containing 10, 20, 30, and 40 mEq of KCL. These solutions are extremely hyperosmotic (the 2 mEq/L solution has an osmolality of 4000 mosm/L) and must be diluted (13).

b. A potassium phosphate solution is also available (contains 4.5 mEq K^+ and 3 mmol phosphate per mL) and is preferred by some for K^+ replacement in diabetic ketoacidosis (because of the phosphate depletion that accompanies ketoacidosis).

TABLE 27.1 Potassium Deficits in Hypokalemia*

Serum K+ (mEq/L)	Potassium Deficit	
	mEq	% Total Body K+
3.0	175	5
2.5	350	10
2.0	470	15
1.5	700	20
1.0	875	25

*Estimated deficits for a 70 kg adult with a total body K+ of 50 mEq/kg.

3. *Infusion Rate*
   a. The standard method of intravenous K^+ replacement is to add 20 mEq of K^+ to 100 mL of isotonic saline and infuse this mixture over 1 hour (14).
   b. The maximum rate of intravenous K^+ replacement is usually set at 20 mEq/hour (14), but dose rates up to 40 mEq/hour occasionally may be necessary (e.g., with serum K^+ below 1.5 mEq/L or serious arrhythmias), and dose rates as high as 100 mEq/hour have been used safely (15).
   c. A large central vein should be used for infusion because of the irritating properties of the hyperosmotic

K⁺ solutions. However, if the desired replacement rate is greater than 20 mEq/hour, the infusion should not be given through a central vein because of the risk of local hyperkalemia in the right heart chambers, which can predispose to cardiac standstill. In this situation, the potassium dose can be split and administered via two peripheral veins.

4. *Response*

a. The serum potassium may be slow to rise at first, because of the position on the flat part of the curve in Figure 27.1. Full replacement usually takes a few days, particularly if potassium losses are ongoing.

b. If the hypokalemia is refractory to K⁺ replacement, check for magnesium depletion because *magnesium depletion* promotes urinary K⁺ losses and *can cause refractory hypokalemia* (16). The evaluation for magnesium depletion is described in Chapter 28.

III. HYPERKALEMIA

While hypokalemia is often well tolerated, hyperkalemia (serum K⁺ > 5.5 mEq/L) can be a life-threatening condition (17).

A. Pseudohyperkalemia

Local release of K⁺ can lead to spurious elevations of the serum K⁺ in the following situations:

1. Traumatic hemolysis during the venipuncture has been reported as a cause of the elevated serum K⁺ in 20% of blood samples showing hyperkalemia (18).

2. In cases of severe leukocytosis (>50,000/mm³) or thrombocytosis (platelet count >106/mm³), K⁺ release from cells during clot formation in the specimen tube can pro-

duce spurious hyperkalemia. When this condition is suspected, the serum K^+ should be measured in an unclotted blood sample.

3. Muscle contraction distal to a tourniquet (during fist clenching) can lead to K^+ release from muscle cells (19).

TABLE 27.2 Drugs That Can Cause Hyperkalemia

ACE Inhibitors[†]	NSAIDs
Angiotensin Receptor Blockers[†]	Pentamidine
ß-Blockers	Penicillin
Cyclosporine	Tacrolimus
Digitalis	TMP–SMX
Diuretics (K^+-sparing)	Succinylcholine
Heparin	

ACE = Angiotensin-converting enzyme; NSAIDs = nonsteroidal anti-inflammatory drugs; TMP–SMX = trimethoprim–sulfamethoxazole.
[†]Especially when combined with K^+-sparing diuretics.

B. Enhanced Cellular Release

The following conditions can result in hyperkalemia from enhanced K^+ release from cells.

1. Acidosis is often listed as a cause of hyperkalemia because of the tendency for acidosis to enhance K^+ release from cells and reduce renal K^+ excretion. However, hyperkalemia does not always accompany respiratory acidosis (7), and there is no clear evidence that organic acidoses (i.e., lactic acidosis and ketoacidosis) produce hyperkalemia (7).

2. Rhabdomyolysis can release large amounts of K^+ into the extracellular fluid, but if renal function is normal, the extra K^+ is promptly cleared by the kidneys.

3. Certain drugs can promote hyperkalemia via transcellular K^+ shifts, such as β-receptor antagonists and digitalis (Table 27.2). Digitalis toxicity can cause severe hyperkalemia (i.e., serum $K^+ >7$ mEq/L).

4. Massive blood transfusions (i.e., when the transfusion volume exceeds the normal blood volume) can promote hyperkalemia, but only in patients with circulatory shock (20). Potassium leaks from erythrocytes in stored blood, but the amounts are small (see Table 30.2) (21).

C. Impaired Renal Excretion

Impaired renal excretion of K^+ is the most common cause of hyperkalemia, and is characterized by a urinary $K^+ <30$ mEq/L in the face of hyperkalemia.

1. Renal insufficiency can produce hyperkalemia when the glomerular filtration rate (GFR) falls below 10 mL/minute (22). Hyperkalemia is seen relatively early when renal insufficiency is due to interstitial nephritis, or is associated with hyporeninemic hypoaldosteronism (22). The latter condition is seen in elderly diabetic patients who have defective renin release in response to reduced renal blood flow.

2. Adrenal insufficiency is a well-known cause of hyperkalemia from impaired renal K^+ excretion, but is not a common cause of hyperkalemia in the ICU.

3. Drugs that impair renal K^+ excretion are among the leading causes of hyperkalemia (2,23). A list of possible offenders is shown in Table 27.2.

   a. The drugs most often implicated are angiotensin-converting enzyme inhibitors, angiotensin receptor blockers, K^+-sparing diuretics, and nonsteroidal antiinflammatory drugs (23,24). The potential for hyperkalemia is magnified when these drugs are given along with potassium supplements.

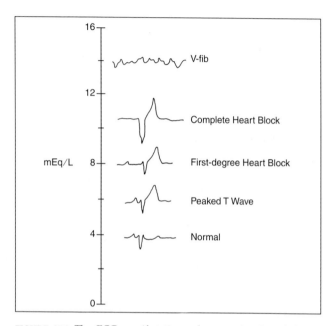

FIGURE 27.3 The ECG manifestations of progressive hyperkalemia. (Adapted from Burch GE, Winsor T. A primer of electrocardiography. Philadelphia: Lea & Febiger, 1966:143.)

D. ECG Abnormalities

1. The most serious consequence of hyperkalemia is the slowing of electrical conduction in the heart.

2. The ECG can begin to change when the serum K$^+$ reaches 6.0 mEq/L, and it is always abnormal when the serum

K^+ reaches 8.0 mEq/L (22). Figure 27.3 shows the ECG changes associated with progressive hyperkalemia.

3. The earliest change in the ECG is a tall, tapering (tented) T wave that is most evident in precordial leads V_2 and V_3. As the hyperkalemia progresses, the P wave amplitude decreases and the PR interval lengthens. The P waves eventually disappear and the QRS duration becomes prolonged. The final event is ventricular asystole or ventricular fibrillation.

E. Acute Management

The acute management of hyperkalemia is guided by the serum K^+ level and the ECG (2,17). The therapeutic maneuvers are outlined in Table 27.3.

1. *Membrane Antagonism*

   Calcium directly antagonizes the membrane actions of potassium.

   a. When hyperkalemia is severe (i.e., above 7 mEq/L) or accompanied by advanced ECG changes (i.e., loss of P waves and prolonged QRS duration), calcium gluconate is given in the dose shown in Table 27.3. A second dose can be given if there is no response within a few minutes.

   b. When hyperkalemia is accompanied by circulatory compromise, *calcium chloride* is preferred to calcium gluconate because 10% calcium chloride contains three times more elemental calcium (per mL) than 10% calcium gluconate, and the extra calcium could help to promote cardiac contraction and maintain peripheral vascular tone.

   c. Calcium must be given cautiously to patients on digitalis because hypercalcemia can potentiate digitalis cardiotoxicity. For patients receiving digitalis, the calcium gluconate should be added to 100 mL of isotonic

saline and infused over 20 to 30 minutes. If the hyperkalemia is a manifestation of digitalis toxicity, calcium
is contraindicated.

d. The response to calcium lasts only 20 or 30 minutes, so
other therapies should be initiated to enhance potassium clearance.

TABLE 27.3 Acute Management of Hyperkalemia

Condition	Treatment	Comments
ECG changes or serum K^+ >7 mEq/L	Calcium gluconate (10%): 10 mL IV over 3 min; can repeat in 5 min.	Response lasts only 20–30 min. *Do not* give bicarbonate after calcium.
ECG changes and circulatory compromise	Calcium chloride (10%): 10 mL IV over 3 min.	Calcium chloride contains 3 times more calcium than calcium gluconate.
AV block refractory to calcium treatment	1. 10 U regular insulin in 500 mL of 20% dextrose: infuse over 1 hr. 2. Transvenous pacemaker	Insulin-dextrose treatment should drop the serum K by 1 mEq/L for 1–2 hrs.
Digitalis cardiotoxicity	1. Magnesium sulfate: 2 g as IV bolus. 2. Digitalis-specific antibodies if necessary.	*Do not* use calcium for the hyperkalemia of digitalis toxicity.
After acute phase or when no ECG changes	Kayexalate: oral dose of 30 g in 50 mL of 20% sorbitol, or 50 g in 200 mL 20% sorbitol as a retention enema.	Oral dosing is preferred. Enemas poorly tolerated by patients and nurses.

2. *Transcellular Shift*

Combined therapy with insulin and dextrose will drive potassium into muscle cells and decrease the serum potassium by an average of 1 mEq/L, but this effect is temporary (lasts 1–2 hours), and should be combined with measures designed to enhance potassium excretion.

3. *Enhanced Clearance*

Measures aimed at enhancing the removal of K^+ from the body can be used alone (in mild cases of hyperkalemia without advanced ECG changes) or as a follow-up to calcium and insulin-dextrose therapy.

a. Sodium polystyrene sulfonate (Kayexalate) is a cation-exchange resin that promotes K^+ clearance across the gastrointestinal mucosa. It can be given orally or by retention enema, and it is mixed with 20% sorbitol to prevent concretion. For each mEq of K^+ removed, 2 to 3 mEq of sodium is added. If there is concern about the added sodium, one or two doses of furosemide can be used to enhance natriuresis (except in the presence of renal failure).

b. The loop diuretics (e.g., furosemide) enhance urinary potassium excretion, but are ineffective if renal failure is the cause of hyperkalemia.

c. Hemodialysis is the most effective method of removing K^+ in patients with renal failure.

REFERENCES

1. Rose BD, Post TW. Potassium homeostasis. In: Clinical physiology of acid-base and electrolyte disorders. 5th ed. New York: McGraw-Hill, 2001:372–402.

2. Schaefer TJ, Wolford RW. Disorders of potassium. Emerg Med Clin North Am 2005; 23:723–747.

3. Brown RS. Extrarenal potassium homeostasis. Kidney Int 1986; 30:116–127.

4. Sterns RH, Cox M, Feig PU, et al. Internal potassium balance and the control of the plasma potassium concentration. Medicine 1981; 60:339–354.

5. Allon M, Copkney C. Albuterol and insulin for treatment of hyperkalemia in hemodialysis patients. Kidney Int 1990; 38:869–872.

6. Lipworth BJ, McDevitt DG, Struthers AD. Prior treatment with diuretic augments the hypokalemic and electrocardiographic effects of inhaled albuterol. Am J Med 1989; 86:653–657.

7. Adrogue HJ, Madias NE. Changes in plasma potassium concentration during acute acid-base disturbances. Am J Med 1981; 71:456–467.

8. Bernard SA, Buist M. Induced hypothermia in critical care medicine: a review. Crit Care Med 2003 ;31:2041–2051.

9. Schaller MD, Fischer AP, Perret CH. Hyperkalemia: A prognostic factor during acute severe hypothermia. JAMA 1990; 264:1842–1845.

10. Salem M, Munoz R, Chernow B. Hypomagnesemia in critical illness. A common and clinically important problem. Crit Care Clin 1991; 7:225–252.

11. Flakeb G, Villarread D, Chapman D. Is hypokalemia a cause of ventricular arrhythmias? J Crit Illness 1986; 1:66–74.

12. Stanaszek WF, Romankiewicz JA. Current approaches to management of potassium deficiency. Drug Intell Clin Pharm 1985; 19:176–184.

13. Trissel LA. Handbook on Injectable Drugs. 13th ed. Bethesda, MD: American Society of Health System Pharmacists, 2005:1230.

14. Kruse JA, Carlson RW. Rapid correction of hypokalemia using concentrated intravenous potassium chloride infusions. Arch Intern Med 1990; 150:613–617.

15. Kim GH, Han JS. Therapeutic approach to hypokalemia. Nephron 2002; 92(Suppl 1):28–32.

16. Whang R, Flink EB, Dyckner T, et al. Magnesium depletion as a cause of refractory potassium repletion. Arch Intern Med 1985; 145:1686–1689.

17. Evans KJ, Greenberg A. Hyperkalemia: a review. J Intensive Care Med 2005; 20:272–290.

18. Rimmer JM, Horn JF, Gennari FJ. Hyperkalemia as a complication of drug therapy. Arch Intern Med 1987; 147:867–869.

19. Don BR, Sebastian A, Cheitlin M, et al. Pseudohyperkalemia caused by fist clenching during phlebotomy. N Engl J Med 1990; 322:1290–1292.

20. Leveen HH, Pasternack HS, Lustrin I, et al. Hemorrhage and transfusion as the major cause of cardiac arrest. JAMA 1960; 173:770–777.

21. Michael JM, Dorner I, Bruns D, et al. Potassium load in CPD-preserved whole blood and two types of packed red blood cells. Transfusion 1975; 15:144–149.

22. Williams ME, Rosa RM. Hyperkalemia: disorders of internal and external potassium balance. J Intensive Care Med 1988; 3:52-64.

23. Perazella MA. Drug-induced hyperkalemia: old culprits and new offenders. Am J Med 2000; 109:307–314.

24. Palmer BF. Managing hyperkalemia caused by inhibitors of the renin-angiotensin-aldosterone system. N Engl J Med 2004; 351:585–592.

Chapter 28

MAGNESIUM

Magnesium is the second most abundant intracellular cation, and it serves as a cofactor for all reactions involving ATPase enzymes (including the membrane pump that generates the electrical gradient across cell membranes). Unfortunately, the "tip of the iceberg" analogy used for potassium also applies to magnesium; i.e., only a minor fraction (0.3%) of total body magnesium is located in plasma (1–3), so monitoring the plasma magnesium provides little information about total body magnesium.

I. MAGNESIUM BALANCE

A. Serum Magnesium

1. The normal range for serum magnesium depends on the daily magnesium intake, which varies according to geographic region. The normal range for healthy adults residing in the United States is shown in Table 28.1 (4).

2. Only 67% of the magnesium in plasma is in the ionized (active) form, and the remaining 33% is either bound to plasma proteins (19% of the total) or chelated with divalent anions such as phosphate and sulfate (14% of the total) (5).

3. The standard assay for magnesium measures the total concentration in plasma. Therefore, when the total magnesium is abnormally low, it is not possible to determine if the problem is a decrease in the ionized (active) fraction or a decrease in the bound fractions (e.g., hypoproteinemia).

4. The level of ionized magnesium can be measured with an ion-specific electrode. However, since the total amount of magnesium in plasma is small, the difference between the ionized and bound magnesium *content* may not be large enough to be clinically relevant.

	TABLE 28.1 Reference Ranges for Magnesium*	
Parameter	**Traditional Units**	**SI Units**
Serum magnesium:		
Total	1.4–2.0 mEq/L	0.7–1.0 mmol/L
Ionized	0.8–1.1 mEq/L	0.4–0.6 mmol/L
Urinary magnesium	5–15 mEq/24 hr	2.5–7.5 mmol/24 hr

*Pertains to healthy adults residing in the United States. From Reference 4.

Conversions: mmol x 2 = mEq or mEq x 0.5 = mmol

B. Urinary Magnesium

1. The normal range for urinary magnesium excretion is shown in Table 28.1. Under normal circumstances, only small quantities of magnesium are excreted in the urine.

2. When magnesium intake is deficient, the kidneys conserve magnesium, and urinary magnesium excretion falls to negligible levels. This is shown in Figure 28.1. Note that, after the start of a magnesium-deficient diet, the urinary magnesium excretion promptly falls to negligible levels, while the serum magnesium remains in the normal range. This illustrates the relative value of urinary magnesium over serum magnesium levels in the detection of magnesium deficiency.

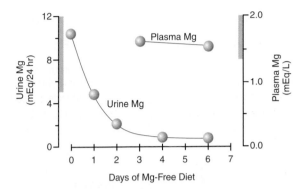

FIGURE 28.1 Urinary and plasma magnesium levels in a healthy volunteer placed on a magnesium-free diet. Solid bars on the vertical axes indicate the normal range for urine and plasma magnesium. (Adapted from Shils ME. Experimental human magnesium deficiency. Medicine 1969; 48:61–82).

II. MAGNESIUM DEFICIENCY

A. Incidence

Hypomagnesemia is reported in as many as 60 to 70% of ICU patients (1,6), but this underestimates the true incidence of magnesium deficiency because the serum magnesium concentration can be normal in patients with magnesium deficiency (2,3).

B. Predisposing Conditions

Because serum magnesium levels have a limited ability to detect magnesium depletion, recognizing the conditions that predispose to magnesium depletion may be the only clue to an underlying magnesium imbalance. The conditions that most often promote magnesium depletion are listed in Table 28.2.

TABLE 28.2 Markers of Possible Magnesium Depletion

Predisposing Conditions	Clinical Findings
Drug therapy:*	Electrolyte abnormalities:*
Furosemide (50%)	Hypokalemia (40%)
Aminoglycosides (30%)	Hypophosphatemia (30%)
Amphotericin, pentamidine	Hyponatremia (27%)
Digitalis (20%)	Hypocalcemia (22%)
Cisplatin, cyclosporine	
	Cardiac manifestations:
Diarrhea (secretory)	Torsades de pointes
	Digitalis toxicity
Alcohol abuse (chronic)	
Diabetes mellitus	Hyperactive CNS Syndrome

*Numbers in parentheses indicate incidence of associated hypo-magnesemia.

1. *Diuretic Therapy*

   a. Diuretics are the leading cause of magnesium deficiency. Diuretic-induced inhibition of sodium reabsorption also interferes with magnesium reabsorption, and the urinary magnesium losses can parallel urinary sodium losses.

   b. The diuretic effect is most pronounced with loop diuretics like furosemide, and *magnesium deficiency has been reported in 50% of patients receiving chronic therapy with furosemide* (7).

   c. The thiazide diuretics also promote magnesium depletion, but primarily in elderly patients (8).

   d. Magnesium depletion is not a complication of therapy with "potassium-sparing" diuretics (9).

2. *Antibiotic Therapy*

   The antibiotics that promote magnesium depletion are the aminoglycosides, amphotericin and pentamidine (10, 11). The aminoglycosides block magnesium reabsorption in the ascending loop of Henle, and hypomagnesemia has been reported in 30% of patients receiving aminoglycoside therapy (11).

3. *Other Drugs*

A variety of other drugs have been associated with magnesium depletion, including digitalis, and the chemotherapeutic agents cisplatin and cyclosporine (10,12). Digitalis shifts magnesium into cells, and the chemotherapeutic agents promote renal magnesium excretion.

4. *Alcohol-Related Illness*

Hypomagnesemia is reported in 30% of hospital admissions for alcohol abuse, and in 85% of admissions for delirium tremens (13,14). Malnutrition and chronic diarrhea may play a role in the magnesium depletion in these conditions.

5. *Secretory Diarrhea*

Secretions from the lower GI tract have a high magnesium concentration (10 to 14 mEq/L) (15), so a secretory diarrhea can be accompanied by profound magnesium depletion.

6. *Diabetes Mellitus*

Magnesium depletion is common in insulin-dependent diabetics, probably as a result of glycosuria-induced urinary magnesium loss (16). Hypomagnesemia is reported in only 7% of admissions for diabetic ketoacidosis, but the incidence increases to 50% over the first 12 hours after admission (17), probably as a result of insulin-induced movement of magnesium into cells.

C. Clinical Manifestations

There are no specific clinical manifestations of magnesium deficiency, but the following clinical findings should raise suspicion of an underlying magnesium deficiency.

1. *Electrolyte Abnormalities*

   Magnesium depletion is often accompanied by abnormal levels of other electrolytes in blood (See Table 28.2) (18).

   a. Magnesium depletion enhances renal potassium excretion, and hypokalemia is reported in almost half of patients with magnesium depletion (18). The hypokalemia that accompanies magnesium depletion can be refractory to potassium replacement therapy, and magnesium repletion is often necessary before potassium repletion is possible (19).

   b. Hypocalcemia is common in magnesium depletion and is due to a combination of impaired parathormone release (20) and impaired end-organ response to parathormone (21). As is the case with hypokalemia, the hypocalcemia that accompanies magnesium deficiency is difficult to correct unless magnesium deficits are corrected.

   c. Hypophosphatemia can be associated with magnesium depletion, but is a cause (rather than an effect) of magnesium depletion. The mechanism is enhanced renal excretion of magnesium (22).

2. *Arrhythmias*

   a. Magnesium depletion prolongs the QT interval on the ECG and can provoke a polymorphous ventricular tachycardia known as *torsades de pointes* (see Chapter 15, Section VI).

   b. Because both digitalis and magnesium deficiency act to inhibit the sodium-potassium pump on cell membranes, magnesium deficiency promotes digitalis cardiotoxicity. Intravenous magnesium can abolish digitalis-toxic arrhythmias, even when serum magnesium levels are normal (23,24).

3. *Neurologic Findings*

   a. The neurologic manifestations of magnesium deficiency can include altered mentation, generalized seizures, tremors, and hyperreflexia.

b. A neurologic syndrome described recently that can abate with magnesium therapy deserves mention. The clinical presentation is characterized by ataxia, slurred speech, metabolic acidosis, excessive salivation, diffuse muscle spasms, generalized seizures, and progressive obtundation (25). The clinical features are often triggered by loud noises or bodily contact, hence the term *reactive central nervous system magnesium deficiency* has been used to describe this disorder.

TABLE 28.3 Magnesium Retention Test

Indications
1. For suspected Mg^{++} deficiency when the serum Mg^{++} concentration is normal.
2. For identifying the end-point of Mg^{++} replacement therapy.

Contraindications
1. Renal failure or ongoing renal magnesium wasting.

Method
1. Add 24 mmol (48 mEq) of Mg^{++} (6 g of $MgSO_4$) to 250 mL of isotonic saline and infuse over 1 hour.
2. Collect urine for 24 hrs. after the Mg^{++} infusion is started.

Results
1. Urinary Mg^{++} excretion <12 mmol (24 mEq) in 24 hrs (<50% of the infused Mg^{++}) is evidence of Mg^{++} depletion.
2. Urinary Mg^{++} excretion >19 mmol (38 mEq) in 24 hrs (>80% of the infused Mg^{++}) is evidence *against* Mg^{++} depletion.

From Reference 26.

D. Diagnosis

As mentioned several times, the serum magnesium level is an insensitive marker of magnesium depletion. The most sensitive index of total body magnesium stores is a specialized test described next.

1. *Magnesium Retention Test*

   Magnesium reabsorption in the renal tubules is close to the maximum tubular reabsorption rate (T_{max}), so most of an infused magnesium load will be excreted in the urine when total body magnesium stores are normal. However when magnesium stores are deficient, magnesium is reabsorbed in the renal tubules, and a smaller fraction of an infused magnesium load is excreted in the urine.

   a. The magnesium retention test, which is outlined in Table 28.3, measures the fraction of an intravenous magnesium load that is excreted in the urine (26,27).

   b. When less than 50% of the infused magnesium is recovered in the urine, magnesium deficiency is likely, and when more than 80% of the infused magnesium is excreted in the urine, magnesium deficiency is unlikely.

   c. This test is reliable only when renal function is not impaired and when there is no ongoing renal magnesium wasting.

E. Magnesium Preparations

1. The magnesium preparations available for oral and parenteral use are listed in Table 28.4. The oral preparations can be used for daily maintenance therapy (5 mg/kg in normal subjects). Intravenous magnesium is preferred for replacing deficits because intestinal absorption of magnesium can be erratic.

2. The standard intravenous preparation is magnesium sulfate ($MgSO_4$). Each gram of $MgSO_4$ has 8 mEq (4 mmol) of elemental magnesium.

3. The 50% $MgSO_4$ solution (500 mg/mL) has an osmolarity of 4000 mosm/L, so it must be diluted to a 10% (100 mg/mL) or 20% (200 mg/mL) solution for intravenous use (28). Saline solutions should be used as the diluent. Ringer's solutions are not advised because the calcium in

Ringer's solutions will counteract the actions of the infused magnesium.

TABLE 28.4 Oral and Parenteral Magnesium Preparations

Preparations	Elemental Mg^{++}	
Oral preparations:		
Magnesium chloride enteric-coated tablets	64 mg	(5.3 mEq)
Magnesium oxide tablets (400 mg)	241 mg	(19.8 mEq)
Magnesium oxide tablets (140 mg)	85 mg	(6.9 mEq)
Magnesium gluconate tablets (500 mg)	27 mg	(2.9 mEq)
Parenteral solutions:		
Magnesium sulfate (50%)*	500 mg/mL	(4 mEq/mL)
Magnesium sulfate (12.5%)	120 mg/mL	(1 mEq/mL)

*Should be diluted to a 20% solution for intravenous injection.

F. Replacement Protocols

The following magnesium replacement protocols are recommended for patients with normal renal function (29).

1. *Mild, Asymptomatic Hypomagnesemia*
   a. Assume a total magnesium deficit of 1 to 2 mEq/kg.
   b. Because 50% of the infused magnesium can be lost in the urine, assume that the total magnesium requirement is twice the magnesium deficit.
   c. Replace 1 mEq/kg for the first 24 hours, and 0.5 mEq/kg daily for the next 3 to 5 days.

2. *Moderate Hypomagnesemia*

   The following therapy is intended for patients with a serum magnesium level less than 1 mEq/L or when hypomagnesemia is accompanied by other electrolyte abnormalities:

    a. Add 6 g MgSO$_4$ (48 mEq Mg) to 250 or 500 mL isotonic saline and infuse over 3 hours.

    b. Follow with 5 g MgSO$_4$ (40 mEq Mg) in 250 or 500 mL isotonic saline infused over the next 6 hours.

    c. Continue with 5 g MgSO$_4$ every 12 hours (by continuous infusion) for the next 5 days.

3. *Life-Threatening Hypomagnesemia*

The following protocol is recommended when hypomagnesemia is accompanied by serious cardiac arrhythmias (e.g., torsades de pointes) or generalized seizures.

    a. Infuse 2 g MgSO$_4$ (16 mEq Mg) intravenously over 2–5 minutes.

    b. Follow with 5 g MgSO$_4$ (40 mEq Mg) in 250 or 500 mL isotonic saline infused over the next 6 hours.

    c. Continue with 5 g MgSO$_4$ every 12 hours (by continuous infusion) for the next 5 days.

Serum magnesium levels will rise after the initial magnesium bolus but will begin to fall after 15 minutes. Therefore, it is important to follow the bolus dose with a continuous magnesium infusion. Serum magnesium levels may normalize after 1 to 2 days, but it will take several days to replenish the total body magnesium stores.

4. *Renal Insufficiency*

When magnesium is replaced in the setting of renal insufficiency, no more than 50% of the magnesium in the standard replacement protocols should be administered (29), and the serum magnesium should be monitored carefully.

III. HYPERMAGNESEMIA

Hypermagnesemia (i.e., serum Mg^{++} >2 mEq/L) is reported in 5% of hospitalized patients (30) and is found almost exclusively in patients with renal insufficiency.

A. Etiologies

1. *Hemolysis*

The magnesium concentration in erythrocytes is approximately three times greater than that in serum (31). Traumatic disruption of erythrocytes can produce a spurious hypermagnesemia. In hemolytic anemia, the serum magnesium is expected to rise by 0.1 mEq/L for every 250 mL of erythrocytes that lyse completely (31), so hypermagnesemia is expected only with massive hemolysis.

2. *Renal Insufficiency*

The renal excretion of magnesium becomes impaired when the creatinine clearance falls below 30 mL/minute (32). However, hypermagnesemia is not a prominent feature of renal insufficiency unless magnesium intake is increased.

3. *Other Conditions*

Other conditions that can be associated with hypermagnesemia include diabetic ketoacidosis (transient), adrenal insufficiency, hyperparathyroidism, and lithium intoxication (32). The hypermagnesemia in these conditions is usually mild.

B. Clinical Manifestations

1. The clinical consequences of progressive hypermagnesemia are listed below (32).

Manifestation	Serum Mg^{++}
Hyporeflexia	>4 mEq/L
1st° AV Block	>5 mEq/L
Complete Heart Block	>10 mEq/L
Cardiac Arrest	>13 mEq/L

2. The serious consequences of hypermagnesemia are due to calcium antagonism in the cardiovascular system. The

predominant effect is delayed cardiac conduction (contractility and vascular tone are relatively unaffected).

C. Management

1. Hemodialysis is the treatment of choice for severe hypermagnesemia.

2. Intravenous calcium gluconate (1 g IV over 2 to 3 minutes) can be used to antagonize the cardiovascular effects of hypermagnesemia, but the effects are transient and should not delay hemodialysis (33).

REFERENCES

1. Noronha JL, Matuschak GM. Magnesium in critical illness: metabolism, assessment, and treatment. Intensive Care Med 2002; 28:667–679.
2. Elin RJ. Assessment of magnesium status. Clin Chem 1987; 33:1965–1970.
3. Reinhart RA. Magnesium metabolism. A review with special reference to the relationship between intracellular content and serum levels. Arch Intern Med 1988; 148:2415–2420.
4. Lowenstein FW, Stanton MF. Serum magnesium levels in the United States, 1971–1974. J Am Coll Nutr 1986; 5:399–414.
5. Altura BT, Altura BM. A method for distinguishing ionized, complexed and protein-bound Mg in normal and diseased subjects. Scand J Clin Lab Invest 1994; 217:83–87.
6. Tong GM, Rude RK. Magnesium deficiency in critical illness. J Intensive Care Med 2005; 20:3–17.
7. Dyckner T, Wester PO. Potassium/magnesium depletion in patients with cardiovascular disease. Am J Med 1987; 82:11–17.
8. Hollifield JW. Thiazide treatment of systemic hypertension: effects on serum magnesium and ventricular ectopic activity. Am J Cardiol 1989; 63:22G–25G.
9. Ryan MP. Diuretics and potassium/magnesium depletion. Directions for treatment. Am J Med 1987; 82:38–47.
10. Atsmon J, Dolev E. Drug-induced hypomagnesaemia: scope and management. Drug Safety 2005; 28:763–788.

11. Zaloga GP, Chernow B, Pock A, et al. Hypomagnesemia is a common complication of aminoglycoside therapy. Surg Gynecol Obstet 1984; 158:561–565.

12. Whang R, Oei TO, Watanabe A. Frequency of hypomagnesemia in hospitalized patients receiving digitalis. Arch Intern Med 1985; 145:655–656.

13. Balesteri FJ. Magnesium metabolism in the critically ill. Crit Care Clin 1985; 5:217–226.

14. Martin HE. Clinical magnesium deficiency. Ann NY Acad Sci 1969; 162:891–900.

15. Kassirer J, Hricik D, Cohen J. Repairing body fluids: Principles and practice. 1st ed. Philadelphia: WB Saunders, 1989:118–129.

16. Sjogren A, Floren CH, Nilsson A. Magnesium deficiency in IDDM related to level of glycosylated hemoglobin. Diabetes 1986; 35:459–463.

17. Lau K. Magnesium metabolism: normal and abnormal. In: Arieff AI, DeFronzo RA, eds. Fluids, electrolytes, and acid base disorders. New York: Churchill Livingstone, 1985:575–623.

18. Whang R, Oei TO, Aikawa JK, et al. Predictors of clinical hypomagnesemia. Hypokalemia, hypophosphatemia, hyponatremia, and hypocalcemia. Arch Intern Med 1984; 144:1794–1796.

19. Whang R, Flink EB, Dyckner T, et al. Magnesium depletion as a cause of refractory potassium repletion. Arch Intern Med 1985; 145:1686–1689.

20. Anast CS, Winnacker JL, Forte LR, et al. Impaired release of parathyroid hormone in magnesium deficiency. J Clin Endocrinol Metab 1976; 42:707–717.

21. Rude RK, Oldham SB, Singer FR. Functional hypoparathyroidism and parathyroid hormone end-organ resistance in human magnesium deficiency. Clin Endocrinol 1976; 5:209–224.

22. Dominguez JH, Gray RW, Lemann J Jr. Dietary phosphate deprivation in women and men: effects on mineral and acid balances, parathyroid hormone and the metabolism of 25-OH-vitamin D. J Clin Endocrinol Metab 1976; 43:1056–1068.

23. Cohen L, Kitzes R. Magnesium sulfate and digitalis-toxic arrhythmias. JAMA 1983; 249:2808–2810.

24. French JH, Thomas RG, Siskind AP, et al. Magnesium therapy in massive digoxin intoxication. Ann Emerg Med 1984; 13:562–566.

25. Langley WF, Mann D. Central nervous system magnesium deficiency. Arch Intern Med 1991; 151:593–596.

26. Clague JE, Edwards RH, Jackson MJ. Intravenous magnesium loading in chronic fatigue syndrome. Lancet 1992; 340:124–125.

27. Hebert P, Mehta N, Wang J, et al. Functional magnesium deficiency in critically ill patients identified using a magnesium-loading test. Crit Care Med 1997; 25:749–755.

28. Trissel LA. Handbook on injectable drugs. 13th ed. Bethesda, MD: American Society of Health System Pharmacists, 2005.

29. Oster JR, Epstein M. Management of magnesium depletion. Am J Nephrol 1988; 8:349–354.

30. Whang R, Ryder KW. Frequency of hypomagnesemia and hypermagnesemia: Requested vs. routine. JAMA 1990; 263:3063–3064.

31. Elin RJ. Magnesium metabolism in health and disease. Dis Mon 1988; 34:161–218.

32. Van Hook JW. Hypermagnesemia. Crit Care Clin 1991; 7:215–223.

33. Mordes JP, Wacker WE. Excess magnesium. Pharmacol Rev 1977; 29:273–300.

Chapter 29

CALCIUM AND PHOSPHORUS

Calcium and phosphorus are responsible for much of the structural integrity of the bony skeleton. Although neither is found in abundance in the soft tissues, both play an important role in vital cell functions. Phosphorus participates in aerobic energy production, while calcium has a vital role in several diverse processes, including blood coagulation, neuromuscular transmission, and cardiovascular performance.

I. CALCIUM IN PLASMA

A. Plasma Fractions

1. The calcium in plasma is present in three forms, as depicted in Figure 29.1.

2. About half of the calcium is ionized and biologically active, while the other half is bound to other molecules and is biologically inactive [1,2]. Most (80%) of the bound calcium is bound to albumin, and the remainder is complexed to small anions like sulfates and phosphates.

B. Total vs. Ionized Calcium

1. The concentration of total and ionized calcium in plasma is shown in Table 29.1.

2. Although only the ionized calcium is biologically important, most clinical laboratories measure the total plasma calcium, and this can be misleading.

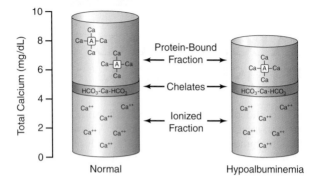

FIGURE 29.1 The three fractions of calcium in plasma and their contribution to the total plasma calcium concentration. The column on the right shows how a decrease in plasma albumin can reduce the total plasma calcium without affecting the ionized calcium.

3. The problem with measuring total serum calcium is illustrated in Figure 29.1. The column on the right demonstrates the effect of a decrease in the concentration of plasma albumin. The total calcium in plasma decreases, but the ionized calcium remains unchanged. Thus, the decrease in total serum calcium is not physiologically significant because the physiologically active (ionized) calcium is not affected.

TABLE 29.1 Normal Ranges for Calcium & Phosphorus in Blood

Serum Fraction	Traditional Units (mg/dL)	SI Units[†] (mmol/L)
Total calcium	9 – 10	2.2–2.5
Ionized calcium	4.5 – 5	1.1–1.3
Phosphorus	2.5 – 5	0.8–1.6

[†]mmol/L = (mg/dL x 10)/molecular weight.
Molecular weight is 40 for calcium and 31 for phosphorus.

4. A variety of correction factors have been proposed for adjusting the plasma calcium concentration in the setting of hypoalbuminemia, but none is reliable (3,4).

5. Ionized calcium can be measured with ion-specific electrodes that are now available in most clinical laboratories, and this is the only reliable measure of serum calcium in patients with hypoalbuminemia.

II. IONIZED HYPOCALCEMIA

Ionized hypocalcemia has been reported in 15 to 50% of admissions to the ICU (5). The common causes of this disorder are listed in Table 29.2. Hypoparathyroidism is a leading cause of hypocalcemia in outpatients, but is not a consideration in the ICU unless neck surgery has been performed recently.

A. Etiologies

1. *Magnesium Depletion*

    a. Magnesium depletion promotes hypocalcemia by inhibiting parathormone secretion and reducing end-organ responsiveness to parathormone.

    b. Hypocalcemia from magnesium depletion is refractory to calcium replacement therapy, and magnesium repletion often corrects the hypocalcemia without calcium replacement.

2. *Sepsis*

    Sepsis is a common cause of hypocalcemia in the ICU (5,6). The mechanism is unclear. The significance of the hypocalcemia is also unclear since it has a causal role in the vasodilation that accompanies sepsis (6).

3. *Alkalosis*

    Alkalosis can reduce the ionized fraction of calcium in

blood by promoting the binding of calcium to albumin. Symptomatic hypocalcemia is more common with respiratory alkalosis than with metabolic alkalosis.

4. *Blood Transfusions*

   a. Ionized hypocalcemia has been reported in 20% of patients receiving blood transfusions (5). The culprit is calcium binding by the citrate anticoagulant in banked blood. The hypocalcemia is short-lived, and resolves when the infused citrate is metabolized by the liver and kidneys (5).

   b. Hypocalcemia from blood transfusions has no apparent consequences (particularly on blood coagulation), and calcium infusions are no longer recommended to correct this abnormality.

5. *Drugs*

   A number of drugs can bind calcium and promote ionized hypocalcemia (5). The ones most often used in the ICU are aminoglycosides, cimetidine, heparin, and theophylline.

6. *Renal Failure*

   a. Ionized hypocalcemia can accompany renal failure as a result of phosphate retention and impaired conversion of vitamin D to its active form in the kidneys. Treatment is aimed at lowering phosphate levels in blood with antacids that block phosphorus absorption in the small bowel.

   b. The acidosis in renal failure can decrease the binding of calcium to albumin, so a decrease in total serum calcium in renal failure does not always indicate the presence of ionized hypocalcemia.

7. *Pancreatitis*

   Severe pancreatitis can produce ionized hypocalcemia through several mechanisms. The appearance of hypocalcemia carries a poor prognosis (7), although it may not contribute to the poor prognosis.

TABLE 29.2 Causes of Ionized Hypocalcemia in the ICU

Alkalosis	Drugs:
Blood transfusions (15%)	Aminoglycosides (40%)
Cardiopulmonary bypass	Cimetidine (30%)
Fat embolism	Heparin (10%)
Magnesium depletion (70%)	Theophylline (30%)
Pancreatitis	
Renal insufficiency (50%)	
Sepsis (30%)	

*Numbers in parentheses show the frequency of ionized hypocalcemia reported in each condition.

B. Clinical Manifestations

1. *Neuromuscular Excitability*

   a. Hypocalcemia can be accompanied by hyperreflexia, paresthesias, tetany (of peripheral or laryngeal muscles), and seizures (8).

   b. Chvostek's and Trousseau's signs are often listed as manifestations of hypocalcemia. However, *Chvostek's sign is nonspecific* (it is present in 25% of normal adults), and *Trousseau's sign is insensitive* (it can be absent in 30% of patients with hypocalcemia) (9).

2. *Cardiovascular Effects*

   Advanced stages of ionized hypocalcemia (i.e., ionized calcium <0.65 mmol/L) can be associated with heart block, ventricular tachycardia, and refractory hypotension (5).

C. Calcium Replacement Therapy

The treatment of ionized hypocalcemia should be directed at the underlying cause of the problem.   ·

TABLE 29.3 Intravenous Calcium Replacement Therapy

Solution	Elemental Calcium	Unit Volume	Osmolarity
10% Calcium chloride	27 mg/mL	10-mL ampules	2,000 mosm/L
10% Calcium gluconate	9 mg/mL	10-mL ampules	680 mosm/L

For symptomatic hypocalcemia:

1. Infuse calcium into a large central vein if possible. If a peripheral vein is used, calcium gluconate should be used.

2. Give a bolus dose of 200 mg elemental calcium (8 mL of 10% calcium chloride or 22 mL of 10% calcium gluconate) in 100 mL isotonic saline over 10 minutes.

3. Follow with a continuous infusion of elemental calcium at 1–2 mg/kg/hr for 6–12 hours.

1. Intravenous calcium replacement is recommended for symptomatic hypocalcemia or when the ionized calcium is below 0.65 mmol/L (5). The calcium solutions and dosage recommendations are shown in Table 29.3.

2. There are 2 calcium solutions for intravenous use: 10% calcium chloride and 10% calcium gluconate. Both solutions have the same concentration of calcium salt (i.e., 100 mg/mL), but *calcium chloride contains three times more elemental calcium than calcium gluconate.*

3. The intravenous calcium solutions are hyperosmolar and should be given through a large central vein if possible. If a peripheral vein is used, calcium gluconate is the preferred solution because of its lower osmolarity.

4. A bolus dose of 200 mg elemental calcium (diluted in 100 mL isotonic saline and given over 5–10 minutes) should

raise the total serum calcium by 0.5 mg/dL, but levels will begin to fall after 30 minutes (5). Therefore, the bolus dose of calcium should be followed by a continuous infusion at a dose rate of 0.5 to 2 mg/kg/hr (elemental calcium) for at least 6 hours.

5. Individual responses to calcium infusion will vary, so calcium dosing should be guided by the level of ionized calcium in blood (5).

III. HYPERCALCEMIA

Hypercalcemia is uncommon in hospitalized patients, with a reported incidence of less than 1% (10).

A. Etiologies

1. Ninety percent of cases of hypercalcemia are caused by hyperparathyroidism or malignancy, and malignancy is the most common cause of severe hypercalcemia (i.e., total serum calcium above 14 mg/dL or ionized calcium above 3.5 mmol/L) (11,12).

2. Less common causes of hypercalcemia include thyrotoxicosis, prolonged immobilization, and drugs (lithium, thiazide diuretics).

B. Clinical Manifestations

The manifestations of hypercalcemia usually are nonspecific and can be categorized as follows (11):

1. **Gastrointestinal (GI):** nausea, vomiting, constipation, ileus, and pancreatitis

2. **Cardiovascular:** hypovolemia, hypotension, and shortened QT interval

3. **Renal:** polyuria and nephrocalcinosis

4. **Neurologic:** confusion and depressed consciousness, including coma

5. The above manifestations can appear when the total serum calcium rises above 12 mg/dL (or the ionized calcium rises above 3 mmol/L), and they are almost always present when the serum calcium is greater than 14 mg/dL (or the ionized calcium is above 3.5 mmol/L) (17).

C. Management

Treatment is indicated when the hypercalcemia is associated with adverse effects, or when the serum calcium is greater than 14 mg/dL (ionized calcium above 3.5 mmol/L). The management of hypercalcemia is summarized in Table 29.4.

1. *Saline Infusion*

   Hypercalcemia usually is accompanied by an osmotic diuresis (from hypercalciuria). This eventually leads to hypovolemia, which reduces calcium excretion in the urine and precipitates a rapid rise in the serum calcium.

   a. Volume infusion (with isotonic saline) to correct hypovolemia and promote renal calcium excretion is an immediate priority in the management of hypercalcemia.

   b. However, saline infusion alone will not return the calcium to normal levels.

2. *Furosemide*

   a. Natriuresis increases urinary calcium excretion, and adding furosemide to the saline infusion will promote natriuresis and thus facilitate urinary calcium excretion.

   b. The usual furosemide dose is 40 to 80 mg IV every 2 hours to achieve an hourly urine output of 100 to 200 mL/minute.

   c. During furosemide diuresis, the hourly urine output

must be replaced with isotonic saline. Failure to replace urinary volume losses is counterproductive because it promotes hypovolemia.

TABLE 29.4 Management of Severe Hypercalcemia

Agent	Dose	Comments
Isotonic saline	Variable	Initial treatment of choice. Goal is rapid correction of hypovolemia.
Furosemide	40–80 mg IV every 2 hrs.	Add to isotonic saline to maintain a urine output of 100–200 mL/hr.
Calcitonin	4 Units/kg IM or SC every 12 hrs.	Response is evident within a few hours. Maximum drop in serum calcium is only 0.5 mmol/L.
Hydrocortisone	200 mg IV daily in 2–3 divided doses.	Used as an adjunct to calcitonin.
Biphosphonates:		
Pamidronate	90 mg IV over 2 hrs.	Reduce dose to 60 mg in renal impairment.
Zoledronate	4 mg IV over 15 min.	Equivalent to pamidronate in efficacy.
Plicamycin	25 µg/kg IV over 4 hrs; can repeat every 2 hrs.	More rapid effect than pamidronate, but can have toxic side effects.

3. *Calcitonin*

    Saline and furosemide can correct the hypercalcemia acutely, but will not correct the underlying cause of the hypercalcemia, which (in malignancy) is enhanced bone resorption. Calcitonin is a naturally occurring hormone that inhibits bone resorption.

a. Salmon calcitonin can be given for hypercalcemia due to enhanced bone resorption. The dose is 4 Units/kg given subcutaneously or intramuscularly every 12 hours.

b. The response to calcitonin is rapid (onset within a few hours), but the effect is mild (the maximum drop in serum calcium is 0.5 mmol/L).

4. *Hydrocortisone*

Corticosteroids can reduce the serum calcium by impeding the growth of lymphoid neoplastic tissue and enhancing the actions of vitamin D. Steroids are usually combined with calcitonin and can be particularly useful in the hypercalcemia associated with multiple myeloma or renal failure (11,12). The standard regimen uses hydrocortisone, 200 mg IV daily in 2 or 3 divided doses.

5. *Biphosphonates*

Calcitonin can be used for rapid reduction of serum calcium, but the mild response will not keep the calcium in the normal range.

a. A group of compounds known as *biphosphonates* are more potent inhibitors of bone resorption and are capable of maintaining a normal serum calcium. However, their onset of action is delayed, and they are not useful when rapid control of serum calcium is desirable.

b. **Zoledronate** (4 mg IV over 5 minutes) and **pamidronate** (90 mg IV over 2 hours) are currently the preferred biphosphonates for the management of severe hypercalcemia (12). Their peak effect is seen in 2 to 4 days, and normalization of the serum calcium occurs within 4 to 7 days in up to 90% of cases. The dose may be repeated in 4 to 10 days if necessary.

6. *Plicamycin*

Plicamycin (formerly mithramycin) is an antineoplastic

agent that inhibits bone resorption. It is more potent than calcitonin, but the potential for serious side effects (e.g., bone marrow suppression) has limited its popularity. Biphosphonates are currently preferred to plicamycin because of their safety profile.

7. *Dialysis*

Dialysis (hemodialysis or peritoneal dialysis) is effective in removing calcium in patients with renal failure (12).

IV. HYPOPHOSPHATEMIA

Hypophosphatemia (serum PO_4 less than 2.5 mg/dL or 0.8 mmol/L) can be found in up to one-third of ICU patients (13,14). Most cases are due to movement of PO_4 into cells, and the remainder are the result of increased renal excretion or decreased GI absorption of phosphorus.

A. Etiologies

1. *Glucose Loading*

a. Glucose loading is the most common cause of hypophosphatemia in hospitalized patients (13,15), and is the result of a link between glucose and PO_4 entry into cells. The drop in serum PO_4 is usually seen during refeeding in alcoholic, malnourished, or debilitated patients, and it can occur with any type of feeding regimen (i.e., oral, enteral tube feedings, or parenteral nutrition).

b. The influence of total parenteral nutrition (TPN) on serum PO_4 levels is shown in Figure 29.2. Note the severe drop in serum PO_4 (to <1 mg/dL) after one week of TPN. The risk of hypophosphatemia is one reason that TPN regimens are advanced gradually for the first few days.

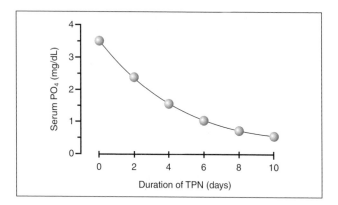

FIGURE 29.2 The influence of total parenteral nutrition (*TPN*) on the serum PO_4. (Data from Knochel JP. Arch Intern Med 1977; 137:203–220).

2. *Respiratory Alkalosis*

   Respiratory alkalosis increases the rate of glycolysis, and this prompts an increase in glucose (and PO_4) movement into cells (16). This mechanism is a potential offender in ventilator-dependent patients because overventilation and respiratory alkalosis is common in these patients.

3. *β-Receptor Agonists*

   Stimulation of β-adrenergic receptors can shift PO_4 into cells and promote hypophosphatemia. In one study of patients with acute asthma who were treated aggressively with nebulized β-agonists, the serum PO_4 decreased by 1.25 mg/dL (0.4 mmol/L) (17).

4. *Phosphate-Binding Agents*

   Aluminum can form insoluble complexes with inorganic phosphates. As a result, aluminum-containing compounds such as sucralfate (Carafate) can impede the absorption of phosphate in the upper GI tract and promote phosphate depletion (18).

5. *Diabetic Ketoacidosis*

As mentioned in Chapter 23, phosphate depletion is almost universal in diabetic ketoacidosis, but it does not become evident until insulin therapy drives PO_4 into cells. Because phosphate supplementation does not alter the outcome in diabetic ketoacidosis (see Chapter 23), the significance of the phosphate depletion in this disorder is unclear.

B. Clinical Manifestations

1. *Oxidative Energy Production*

Hypophosphatemia has a number of effects that could impair oxidative energy production in cells, and these are indicated in Figure 29.3. Each of the following determinants of systemic oxygen transport can be adversely affected by hypophosphatemia.

a. CARDIAC OUTPUT. Phosphate depletion can impair myocardial contractility and reduce cardiac output. Hypophosphatemic patients with heart failure have shown improved cardiac performance after phosphate supplementation (19).

b. HEMOGLOBIN. Hemolysis is a recognized effect of severe hypophosphatemia (18), presumably as a result of impaired RBC deformability.

c. OXYHEMOGLOBIN DISSOCIATION. Phosphate depletion is accompanied by depletion of 2,3-diphosphoglycerate, and this shifts the oxyhemoglobin dissociation curve to the left. When this occurs, hemoglobin is less likely to release oxygen to the tissues.

In addition to the adverse effects on tissue oxygen availability, phosphate depletion can directly impede cellular energy production by reducing the availability of inorganic phosphorus for high-energy phosphate production.

2. *Muscle Weakness*

Muscle weakness is usually mentioned as an adverse effect

of hypophosphatemia. However, the following observations suggest that muscle weakness is NOT a major complication of hypophosphatemia.

a. Biochemical evidence of skeletal muscle disruption (e.g., elevated creatine kinase levels in blood) is common in patients with hypophosphatemia, but overt muscle weakness is usually absent (20).

b. Respiratory muscle weakness has been reported in association with hypophosphatemia (21), but it is not clinically significant.

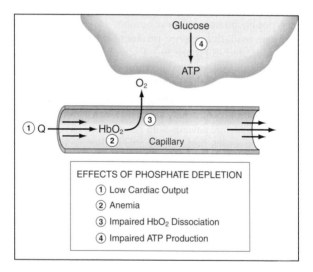

FIGURE 29.3 The effects of hypophosphatemia on factors that influence oxidative energy production.

3. *Apparent Lack of Harm*

Most of the adverse effects of hypophosphatemia have no proven clinical significance. In fact, hypophosphatemia is usually clinically silent, even when the serum PO_4 falls to extremely low levels. *In one study of patients with severe hypophosphatemia* (i.e., serum PO_4 <1.0 mg/dL), *none of the patients showed evidence of harm* (22).

C. Phosphorus Replacement

Despite the apparent lack of harm in most cases of hypophosphatemia, intravenous phosphorus replacement is recommended for all patients with severe hypophosphatemia (i.e., serum PO_4 below 1.0 mg/dL or 0.3 mmol/L) and for patients with hypophosphatemia and cardiac dysfunction, respiratory failure, muscle weakness, or impaired tissue oxygenation. The phosphate solutions and dosage recommendations are shown in Table 29.5 (23,24).

TABLE 29.5 Intravenous Phosphate Replacement Therapy

Solution	Phosphorus[†] Content	Other Content
Sodium phosphate	93 mg/mL	Na^+: 4.0 mEq/L
Potassium phosphate	93 mg/mL	K^+: 4.3 mEq/L

Dosage Recommendations:[*]

For severe hypophosphatemia (PO_4 <1 mg/dL) without adverse effects:
   IV dose is 0.6 mg/kg/hr.

For hypophosphatemia (PO_4 <2 mg/dL) with adverse effects:
   IV dose is 0.9 mg/kg/hr.

Monitor serum PO_4 level every 6 hrs.

[†]For phosphorus 1 mmol = 31 mg.
[*]In patients with renal dysfunction, slower dose rates are advised.
From Reference 9.

1. *Oral Replacement*

Once the serum PO_4 rises above 2 mg/dL, phosphate replacement can be continued using oral phosphate preparations like Neutra-Phos or K-Phos. The oral replacement dosage is 1,200–1,500 mg phosphorus daily.

2. *Daily Maintenance*

The normal daily maintenance dose of phosphate is 1,200 mg if given orally, and 800 mg if the PO_4 is given intravenously (24). Higher oral doses are required because only 70% of orally administered phosphate is absorbed from the GI tract.

V. HYPERPHOSPHATEMIA

A. Etiologies

Hyperphosphatemia (serum PO_4 >5 mg/dL or >1.6 mmol/L) is usually the result of one of the conditions listed below.

1. Impaired urinary excretion of PO_4 in patients with renal insufficiency.

2. Exaggerated PO_4 release from cells in conditions of prominent cell necrosis (e.g., rhabdomyolysis or tumor lysis).

B. Clinical Manifestations

The clinical manifestations of hyperphosphatemia include formation of insoluble calcium–phosphate complexes (with deposition into soft tissues) and acute hypocalcemia (with tetany) (8). The incidence and clinical significance of these effects is unclear.

C. Management

There are two approaches to lowering the serum PO_4.

1. Aluminum-containing antacids (or sucralfate) can be used

to bind phosphorus in the upper GI tract (25). This can lower phosphorus even in the absence of oral phosphorus intake (i.e., GI dialysis).

2. Hemodialysis can clear phosphorus from the bloodstream, but this is rarely necessary.

REFERENCES

1. Baker SB, Worthley LI. The essentials of calcium, magnesium and phosphate metabolism: part I. Physiology. Crit Care Resusc 2002; 4:301–306.

2. Forman DT, Lorenzo L. Ionized calcium: its significance and clinical usefulness. Ann Clin Lab Sci 1991; 21:297–304.

3. Slomp J, van der Voort PH, Gerritsen RT, et al. Albumin-adjusted calcium is not suitable for diagnosis of hyper- and hypocalcemia in the critically ill. Crit Care Med 2003; 31:1389–1393.

4. Byrnes MC, Huynh K, Helmer SD, et al. A comparison of corrected serum calcium levels to ionized calcium levels among critically ill surgical patients. Am J Surg 2005; 189:310-314.

5. Zaloga GP. Hypocalcemia in critically ill patients. Crit Care Med 1992; 20:251–262.

6. Burchard KW, Simms HH, Robinson A, et al. Hypocalcemia during sepsis. Relationship to resuscitation and hemodynamics. Arch Surg 1992; 127:265–272.

7. Steinberg W, Tenner S. Acute pancreatitis. N Engl J Med 1994; 330:1198–1210.

8. Baker SB, Worthley LI. The essentials of calcium, magnesium and phosphate metabolism: part II. Disorders. Crit Care Resusc 2002; 4:307–315.

9. Marino PL. Calcium and magnesium in serious illness: A practical approach. In: Sivak ED, Higgins TL, Seiver A, eds. The high risk patient: management of the critically ill. Philadelphia: Williams & Wilkins, 1995:1183–1195.

10. Shek CC, Natkunam A, Tsang V, et al. Incidence, causes and

mechanism of hypercalcaemia in a hospital population in Hong Kong. Q J Med 1990; 77:1277–1285.

11. Ziegler R. Hypercalcemic crisis. J Am Soc Nephrol 2001; 12 (Suppl 17):S3–9.

12. Stewart AF. Clinical practice. Hypercalcemia associated with cancer. N Engl J Med 2005; 352:373–379.

13. French C, Bellomo R. A rapid intravenous phosphate replacement protocol for critically ill patients. Crit Care Resusc 2004; 6:175–179.

14. Fiaccadori E, Coffrini E, Fracchia C, et al. Hypophosphatemia and phosphorus depletion in respiratory and peripheral muscles of patients with respiratory failure due to COPD. Chest 1994; 105:1392–1398.

15. Marinella MA. Refeeding syndrome and hypophosphatemia. J Intensive Care Med 2005; 20:155-159.

16. Paleologos M, Stone E, Braude S. Persistent, progressive hypophosphataemia after voluntary hyperventilation. Clin Sci 2000; 98:619–625.

17. Bodenhamer J, Bergstrom R, Brown D, et al. Frequently nebulized beta-agonists for asthma: effects on serum electrolytes. Ann Emerg Med 1992; 21:1337–1342.

18. Brown GR, Greenwood JK. Drug- and nutrition-induced hypophosphatemia: mechanisms and relevance in the critically ill. Ann Pharmacother 1994; 28:626–632.

19. Davis SV, Olichwier KK, Chakko SC. Reversible depression of myocardial performance in hypophosphatemia. Am J Med Sci 1988; 295:183–187.

20. Singhal PC, Kumar A, Desroches L, et al. Prevalence and predictors of rhabdomyolysis in patients with hypophosphatemia. Am J Med 1992; 92:458–464.

21. Gravelyn TR, Brophy N, Siegert C, et al. Hypophosphatemia-associated respiratory muscle weakness in a general inpatient population. Am J Med 1988; 84:870–876.

22. King AL, Sica DA, Miller G, et al. Severe hypophosphatemia in a general hospital population. South Med J 1987; 80:831–835.

23. Clark CL, Sacks GS, Dickerson RN, et al. Treatment of hypophosphatemia in patients receiving specialized nutrition support using a graduated dosing scheme: results from a prospective clinical trial. Crit Care Med 1995; 23:1504–1511.

24. Knochel JP. Phosphorus. In: Shils ME, et al., eds. Modern nutri-

tion in health and disease. 10th ed. Philadelphia: Lippincott Williams & Wilkins, 2006:211–222.

25. Lorenzo Sellares V, Torres Ramirez A. Management of hyper-phosphataemia in dialysis patients: role of phosphate binders in the elderly. Drugs Aging 2004; 21:153–165.

Chapter 30

ANEMIA AND ERYTHROCYTE TRANSFUSIONS

Close to one-half of all patients admitted to ICUs are given an erythrocyte transfusion at some time during their ICU stay (1). The current practice of transfusing erythrocytes to correct anemia is being scrutinized because there is no scientific basis for the practice; i.e., erythrocyte transfusions are usually given without evidence that tissue oxygenation is impaired or threatened.

I. ANEMIA IN THE ICU

A. Anemia of Critical Illness

1. Anemia is almost a universal finding in patients who require ICU care for more than a few days (1,2). (See Table 30.1 for the normal range of values for hemoglobin, hematocrit, and other erythrocyte parameters). In fact, anemia is so common in ICU patients that it has been given a name: i.e., *anemia of critical illness*.

2. The anemia of critical illness is very similar to the *anemia of chronic disease*. In both conditions, there is a defect in iron incorporation into hemoglobin, and both conditions are associated with a decrease in iron and transferrin levels in plasma, an increase in ferritin levels in plasma, and iron sequestration in reticuloendothelial cells (3,4).

TABLE 30.1 Normal Range of Values for Red Cell Parameters

Red Blood Cell Count Males: $4.6 - 6.2 \times 10^{12}$/L Females: $4.2 - 5.4 \times 10^{12}$/L	**Mean Cell Volume** Males: $80 - 100 \times 10^{-15}$L Females: same
Reticulocyte Count Males: $25 - 75 \times 10^{9}$/L Females: same	**Hematocrit** Males: 40–54% Females: 38–47%
Red Blood Cell Volume† Males: 26 mL/kg Females: $4.2 - 5.4 \times 10^{12}$/L	**Hemoglobin‡** Males: 14–18 g/dL Females: 12–16 g/dL

†Normal values are 10% lower in the elderly (≥65 yrs. of age).

‡Normal values are 0.5 g/dL lower in blacks.

From References (17,26).

B. Contributing Factors

Two factors are implicated in the anemia of critical illness: systemic inflammation, and aggressive blood-letting for laboratory tests.

1. *Inflammation*

    Inflammatory cytokines have several effects that can promote anemia, including inhibition of erythropoietin release from the kidneys, diminished marrow responsiveness to erythropoietin, iron sequestration in macrophages, and increased destruction of RBCs (3,4).

2. *Phlebotomy*

    The volume of blood withdrawn for laboratory tests averages 40 to 70 mL each day for ICU patients (5,6). At a daily blood loss of 70 mL, one unit of whole blood (500 mL) will be lost each week of the ICU stay. The following measures have been used to reduce phlebotomy-associated blood loss.

a. When blood is withdrawn from central venous catheters, the initial 5 mL of blood is discarded to eliminate contamination of the sample with intravenous fluids. Returning this initial aliquot to the patient has been shown to reduce blood loss from phlebotomy by 50% (7).

b. Laboratory instruments used for pediatric blood analysis require a much smaller blood sample than instruments used for adults. Utilizing pediatric instrumentation for laboratory tests in adult ICU patients has resulted in a 47% decrease in blood loss from phlebotomy (8).

C. Anemia & Systemic Oxygenation

The driving force behind all erythrocyte transfusions is the fear than anemia will impair tissue oxygenation. However, the risk of impaired tissue oxygenation from anemia is greatly exaggerated, as demonstrated next.

1. *Oxygen Transport*

    The effects of progressive anemia on the oxygen transport parameters are shown in Figure 30.1 (The oxygen transport parameters are described in Chapter 9). The observed effects are explained by the following relationship between oxygen delivery (DO_2), oxygen uptake (VO_2), and O_2 extraction from systemic capillaries.

    $$VO_2 = DO_2 \times O_2 \text{ Extraction} \qquad (30.1)$$

    a. Progressive anemia is accompanied by a steady decrease in systemic O_2 delivery (DO_2). However, there is also a steady rise in peripheral O_2 extraction, and the reciprocal changes in DO_2 and O_2 extraction keep the VO_2 constant.

    b. When the hematocrit drops below 10% (corresponding to a serum hemoglobin below 3 g/dL), the O_2 extraction begins to level off, and the decrease in DO_2 is accompanied by a decrease in VO_2. The point where the VO_2 begins to drop marks the onset of impaired tissue oxygenation, as confirmed by the increase in blood lactate level.

c. Thus, Figure 30.1 demonstrates that anemia does not threaten tissue oxygenation until the hemoglobin and hematocrit fall to extremely low levels.

2. *Tolerance to Anemia*

Figure 30.1 reveals a tolerance to even severe degrees of anemia. The data in this study are from anesthetized animals breathing pure oxygen, but similar results have been reported in awake animals breathing room air (9).

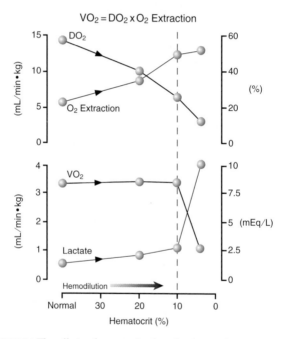

FIGURE 30.1 The effects of progressive isovolemic anemia on systemic oxygen transport and blood lactate levels. *DO₂* is the rate of oxygen delivery in arterial blood, and *VO₂* is the rate of oxygen uptake into tissues. (From Reference 15.)

a. The lowest hemoglobin or hematocrit capable of supporting tissue oxygenation in humans in not known, but one study in healthy adults shows that hemoglobin levels as low as 5 g/dL have no adverse effects on tissue oxygenation (10).

b. The tolerance to anemia is made possible by the ability of O_2 extraction to increase in response to anemia. When O_2 extraction is already elevated (e.g., from heart failure), tolerance to anemia will diminish.

II. TRANSFUSION TRIGGER

The practice of transfusing erythrocytes to alleviate anemia has one serious flaw; i.e., the inability to identify the point where anemia threatens tissue oxygenation (the *transfusion trigger*). Transfusion decisions are usually based on the serum hemoglobin concentration, which provides no information about the state of tissue oxygenation, and undoubtedly leads to excessive transfusions.

A. Hemoglobin

1. The first transfusion trigger, which dates back to 1942, was a hemoglobin concentration of 10 g/dL and a corresponding hematocrit of 30% (11). This "10/30 rule" became the standard for over half a century.

2. There is now evidence that a lower hemoglobin of 7 g/dL (which corresponds to a hematocrit of 21%) is safe in most patients (12,13), and this *lower hemoglobin (7 g/dL) has been adopted as a transfusion trigger for most ICU patients*. The higher hemoglobin of 10 g/dL is still advised for the following situations:

   a. For hospitalized patients with symptomatic coronary insufficiency.

   b. For the early management of patients with severe sepsis or septic shock who have a central venous O_2 saturation below 70% (see Chapter 33, Section II-A) (14).

B. Oxygen Extraction

1. As described in Chapter 9 and illustrated in Figures 9.1 and 30.1, a progressive decrease in systemic O_2 delivery (e.g., from anemia) impairs tissue oxygenation only after the O_2 extraction from systemic capillaries increases to a maximum level of about 50%. Thus, *an O_2 extraction of 50% can be used as evidence of threatened tissue oxygenation* (15).

2. Systemic O_2 extraction is roughly equivalent to the difference between arterial O_2 saturation (SaO_2) and "central venous" O_2 saturation ($ScvO_2$).

$$\textbf{O}_2 \textbf{ Extraction (\%) = (SaO}_2 - \textbf{ScvO}_2\textbf{)} \qquad (30.2)$$

The SaO_2 is routinely monitored with pulse oximetry, and the $ScvO_2$ can be monitored continuously using fiberoptic central venous catheters (available from Edwards Lifesciences, Irvine, CA) (16).

3. Thus, systemic O_2 extraction can be monitored continuously, and seems far superior to the serum hemoglobin for identifying when anemia becomes a threat to tissue oxygenation.

III. ERYTHROCYTE TRANSFUSIONS

A. Erythrocyte Products

Whole blood is stored only on request and is otherwise fractionated into erythrocyte, platelet, and plasma fractions within a few hours of collection.

1. *Packed Cells*

   Erythrocyte concentrates, also called *packed cells,* are prepared by centrifuging whole blood and removing the plasma supernatant.

a. Each unit of packed cells has about 200 mL of cells (mostly erythrocytes) and 50 to 100 mL of plasma and preservative. The hematocrit is usually 60–80%, and the hemoglobin concentration is 23–27 g/dL (17).

b. Packed cells are refrigerated at 1–6°C and have a shelf life of up to 35 days. The effects of storage time are described later.

2. *Leukocyte-Poor Red Cells*

A majority of the leukocytes in packed cells can be removed by passing the blood through specialized filters. Removal of 50% or more of the leukocytes can prevent transfusion-related nonhemolytic fevers (17), which are caused by antibodies to leukocytes in donor blood (see later).

3. *Washed Red Cells*

a. For patients with a history of transfusion-related urticaria or anaphylaxis (caused by antibodies to plasma proteins in donor blood), washing the packed cells with isotonic saline (to remove leukocytes and residual plasma) will reduce the incidence of future reactions.

b. For patients with IgA deficiency, who have a high risk of transfusion-related anaphylactic reactions (caused by anti-IgA antibodies in the recipient), multiple washings (x 5) of packed cells can be protective (17).

B. Storage Effects

The effects of storage time on red cell preparations is shown in Table 30.2.

1. *2,3-Diphosphoglycerate*

The tendency for hemoglobin to release O_2 to the tissues is regulated, in part, by the concentration of 2,3-diphosphoglycerate (2,3-DPG) in RBCs. A decrease in 2,3-DPG will decrease O_2 release by hemoglobin.

TABLE 30.2 Effects of Storage on Packed Cells

	Days of Storage	
Parameter	**0**	**35**
% viable RBCs 24 hrs post-transfusion[†]	100	71
pH	7.55	6.71
2,3-DPG (% initial value)	100	<10
Plasma K+ (mEq/L)	5.1	78.5 (!)

[†]An acceptable storage time requires that at least 70% of the transfused RBCs remain viable after 24 hours.

From Reference 17.

a. The concentration of 2,3-DPG in stored RBCs is normal for the first 10 days of storage. Thereafter, there is a 90% decrease in 2,3-DPG levels over the next 3 weeks (see Table 30.2).

b. The decrease in 2,3-DPG with prolonged storage will adversely affect the O_2 transport function of transfused RBCs, but this may have little consequence because transfused RBCs regenerate 2,3-DPG, and levels return to normal 24 hours after the transfusion (17).

2. *Other Changes*

Prolonged storage is associated with marked acidosis and astronomic elevations in plasma K+ (see Table 30.2). However, because the volume of plasma in packed cells is small (<100 mL), these abnormalities will have little impact on the corresponding variables in the recipient's plasma.

C. Response to RBC Transfusions

1. *Hemoglobin & Hematocrit*

Each unit of packed cells should increase the hemoglobin concentration and hematocrit by 1 g/dL and 3%, respectively. However, appropriate changes in hemoglobin and hematocrit should not be the end-point of RBC transfusions. The ultimate goal of RBC transfusions is to improve tissue oxygenation, so the oxygen transport parameters are more appropriate for evaluating the response to RBC transfusions (see next).

2. *Oxygen Transport*

The effects of erythrocyte transfusions on systemic oxygen transport are shown in Figure 30.2. These effects are summarized below.

a. The rate of systemic oxygen delivery (DO₂) increases in response to RBC transfusions, but the rate of oxygen uptake into tissues (VO₂) is not similarly affected because the increase in DO₂ is accompanied by a propor-

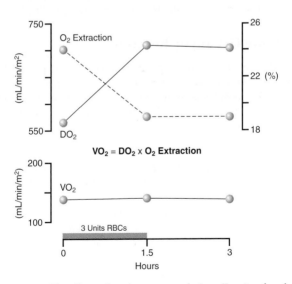

FIGURE 30.2 The effects of erythrocyte transfusions (3 units of packed cells) on oxygen delivery (*DO₂*), oxygen extraction, and oxygen uptake (*VO₂*) in anemic ICU patients with sepsis. From Reference 18.

tional decrease in O_2 extraction. This pattern of response is a reversal of the response to anemia.

b. Thus, a decrease in systemic O_2 extraction can be used as a measure of responsiveness to RBC transfusions.

c. The most important observation in Figure 30.2 is the lack of a post-transfusion increase in oxygen uptake (VO_2) because it implies that RBC transfusions do not improve tissue oxygenation.

IV. TRANSFUSION RISKS

Adverse reactions are reported in 2 to 4% of RBC transfusions (1,19). The most notable reactions are listed in Table 30.3, along with the frequency of each reaction expressed in relation to the number of units transfused. The following is a brief description of acute transfusion reactions (19–21).

A. Acute Hemolytic Reactions

Transfusion of ABO-incompatible blood is accompanied by prompt lysis of donor RBCs, which incites a systemic inflammatory response that can progress to multiorgan failure. These reactions occur once every 35,000 transfusions, and are the result of human error.

1. *Clinical Manifestations*

   a. Symptoms typically appear soon after the onset of transfusion, and they can appear after infusion of only 5 mL of donor blood (19).

   b. The clinical presentation is marked by fever, dyspnea, chest pain, and low back pain. Severe reactions are marked by hypotension, consumptive coagulopathy, and progressive multiorgan failure.

2. *Management*

   a. For any suspected hemolytic reaction, you must STOP the transfusion immediately because the severity of hemolytic reactions is directly related to the volume of incompatible blood transfused (19). The entire infusion system should be disconnected from the patient and replaced.

b. You must notify the blood bank immediately and compare the ABO type of the patient's blood with the donor blood for a mismatch.

c. The remainder of the approach involves an evaluation for hemolysis and bacterial contamination, and hemodynamic support if necessary. A decreasing blood pressure should prompt immediate volume infusion followed by vasopressors (e.g., dopamine starting at 5 µg/kg/min) if necessary.

TABLE 30.3 Adverse Consequences of RBC Transfusions[†]

Immune Reactions	Other Consequences
Acute hemolytic reaction (1 per 35,000)	*Infections:* Bacterial (1 per 500,000)
Fatal hemolytic reaction (1 per million)	Hepatitis B virus (1 per 220,000)
Acute lung injury (1 per 5,000)	Hepatitis C virus (1 per 1.6 million)
Allergic reactions: Urticaria (1 per 100)	HIV (1 per 1.9 million)
Anaphylaxis (1 per 1,000)	
Anaphylactic shock (1 per 50,000)	*Transfusion Errors:* Wrong person transfused (1 per 15,000)
Nonhemolytic fever (1 per 200)	Incompatible transfusion (1 per 35,000)

[†]Incidence per number of units transfused is shown in parentheses. From References 19–21.

B. Non–Hemolytic Fever

Patients who have received prior blood transfusions can develop transfusion-related fever that is not the result of an acute hemolytic reaction. This reaction is caused by antibodies to leukocytes in donor blood.

1. *Clinical Manifestations*

   a. The fever usually appears 1 to 6 hours after starting the transfusion (later than the onset of fever from hemolytic transfusion reactions).

   b. There are no specific features of the clinical presentation. The temperature elevation can be mild to severe, and patients can be asymptomatic or toxic.

2. *Management*

   a. The same approach described previously for suspected hemolytic transfusion reactions should be used for all cases of transfusion-related fever.

   b. If the diagnosis is nonhemolytic fever, nothing further is required. Fever suppression should not be necessary (see Chapter 32, Section IV-C for more information on antipyretic therapy).

   c. Leukocyte-poor RBCs are recommended for transfusing patients with recurrent nonhemolytic febrile reactions, but recurrent febrile reactions are not common; i.e., 20% of patients with one episode of fever will have a second episode, and only 8% will have a third episode (20).

C. Allergic Reactions

Immediate hypersensitivity reactions are the result of prior sensitization to plasma proteins. Patients with IgA deficiency are prone to transfusion-related hypersensitivity reactions without prior exposure to plasma products.

1. *Clinical Manifestations*

   a. Reactions usually appear within one hour after the transfusion is started.

    b. The most common reaction is urticaria (one episode per 100 units transfused) (21). Anaphylaxis (e.g., wheezing) is one-tenth as common, and anaphylactic shock is rare (one episode per 50,000 units) (21).

    c. Transfusion-related anaphylactic shock can have a similar presentation to severe hemolytic reactions. However, anaphylactic reactions tend to occur later than hemolytic reactions, and they are not typically accompanied by fever.

2. *Management*

    a. Mild urticaria without fever does not require interruption of the transfusion.

    b. Anaphylaxis should be managed as described in Chapter 33. Patients with anaphylaxis should be tested for IgA deficiency.

    c. Future transfusions should be avoided if possible for all cases of anaphylaxis. For less severe allergic reactions, washed RBC preparations (plasma removed) are advised for subsequent transfusions.

D. Acute Lung Injury

1. *General Features*

    a. Transfusion-related acute lung injury (TRALI) is an inflammatory lung injury that is indistinguishable from the acute respiratory distress syndrome (ARDS).

    b. The reported incidence is 1 per 5,000 transfusions (20).

    c. The presumed mechanism involves anti-leukocyte antibodies in donor blood that bind to circulating granulocytes in the recipient. The activated granulocytes become trapped in the pulmonary microcirculation and migrate into the lung parenchyma to incite inflammatory injury (22).

    d. This disorder is considered the leading cause of death from blood transfusions (19,20).

2. *Clinical Manifestations*

    a. TRALI has the same clinical manifestations as ARDS (see Chapter 16).

    b. Signs of respiratory compromise (dyspnea, hypoxemia) usually appear in the first 6 hours after the transfusion begins.

    c. The acute syndrome can be severe, but the condition usually resolves within a week (23).

3. *Management*

    a. The transfusion, if still ongoing, should be stopped at the first sign of respiratory compromise.

    b. There is no specific therapy for TRALI, and care is supportive (as in ARDS).

    c. There are no firm recommendations about future transfusions in patients with TRALI. If transfusion is absolutely necessary, washed RBC preparations (plasma and leukocytes removed) are theoretically the best choice.

E. Immune Suppression

Blood transfusions can depress the immune response (24), and this may explain why *patients who receive blood transfusions have an increased incidence of nosocomial infections* (24,25). Immunosuppression may be the most significant risk of RBC transfusions, and should be a consideration in the decision to transfuse RBCs in septic patients.

REFERENCES

1. Corwin HL, Gettinger A, Pearl R, et al. The CRIT study: Anemia and blood transfusion in the critically ill – Current clinical practice in the United States. Crit Care Med 2004; 32:39–52.

2. Vincent JL, Baron J-F, Reinhart K, et al. Anemia and blood transfusion in critically ill patients. JAMA 2002; 288:1499–1507.

3. Shander A. Anemia in the critically ill. Crit Care Clin 2004; 20:159–178.

4. Scharte M, Fink MP. Red blood cell physiology in critical illness. Crit Care Med 2003; 31(Suppl):S651–S657.

5. Smoller BR, Kruskall MS. Phlebotomy for diagnostic laboratory tests in adults: Pattern of use and effect on transfusion requirements. N Engl J Med 1986; 314: 1233–1235.

6. Corwin HL, Parsonnet KC, Gettinger A, et al. RBC transfusion in the ICU: Is there a reason? Chest 1995; 108: 767–771.

7. Silver MJ, Li Y-H, Gragg LA, et al. Reduction of blood loss from diagnostic sampling in critically ill patients using a blood-conserving arterial line system. Chest 1993; 104:1711–1715.

8. Smoller BR, Kruskall MS, Horowitz GL. Reducing adult phlebotomy blood loss with the use of pediatric-sized blood collection tubes. Am J Clin Pathol 1989; 91:701–703.

9. Levine E, Rosen A, Sehgal L, et al. Physiologic effects of acute anemia: implications for a reduced transfusion trigger. Transfusion 1990; 30:11–14.

10. Weiskopf RB, Viele M, Feiner J, et al. Human cardiovascular and metabolic response to acute, severe, isovolemic anemia. JAMA 1998; 279:217–221.

11. Adam RC, Lundy JS. Anesthesia in cases of poor risk: Some suggestions for decreasing the risk. Surg Gynecol Obstet 1942; 74: 1011–1101.

12. Hebert PC, Wells G, Blajchman MA, et al. A multicenter, randomized, controlled clinical trial of transfusion requirements in critical care. N Engl J Med 1999; 340:409–417.

13. Hebert PC, Yetisir E, Martin C, et al. Is a low transfusion threshold safe in critically ill patients with cardiovascular disease. Crit Care Med 2001; 29:227–234.

14. Dellinger RP, Carlet JM, Masur H, et al. Surviving Sepsis Campaign guidelines for the management of severe sepsis and septic shock. Crit Care Med 2004; 32:858–873.

15. Wilkerson DK, Rosen AL, Gould SA, et al. Oxygen extraction ratio: a valid indicator of myocardial metabolism in anemia. J Surg Res 1987; 42:629–634.

16. Rivers EP, Ander DS, Powell D. Central venous oxygen saturation monitoring in the critically ill patient. Curr Opin Crit Care 2001; 7:204–211.

17. Walker RH. ed. American Association of Blood Banks Technical Manual. 10th ed. Arlington, VA: American Association of Blood

Banks, 1990; 37–58, 635–637, 649–651.

18. Marik PE, Sibbald W. Effect of stored-blood transfusion on oxygen delivery in patients with sepsis. JAMA 1993; 269:3024–3029.

19. Kuriyan M, Carson JL. Blood transfusion risks in the intensive care unit. Crit Care Clin 2004; 237–253.

20. Goodnough LT. Risks of blood transfusion. Crit Care Med 2003; 31:S678–686.

21. Greenberger PA. Plasma anaphylaxis and immediate-type reactions. In: Rossi EC, Simon TL, Moss GS, eds. Principles of transfusion medicine. Philadelphia: Williams & Wilkins, 1991:635–639.

22. Curtis BR, McFarland JG. Mechanisms of transfusion-related acute lung injury (TRALI): Anti-leukocyte antibodies. Crit Care Med 2006; 34(Suppl):S118–S123.

23. Moore SB. Transfusion-related acute lung injury (TRALI): Clinical presentation, treatment, and prognosis. Crit Care Med 2006; 34(Suppl):S114–S117.

24. Landers DF, Hill GE, Wong KC, et al. Blood transfusion-induced immunomodulation. Anesth Analg 1996; 82:187–204.

25. Vamvakas EC. Pneumonia as a complication of blood product transfusion in the critically ill: Transfusion-related immunomodulation (TRM). Crit Care Med 2006; 34(Suppl):S151–S159.

26. Hillman RS, Finch CA. Red cell manual. 6th ed. Philadelphia: FA Davis, 1994:46.

Chapter 31

THROMBOCYTOPENIA AND PLATELET TRANSFUSIONS

Thrombocytopenia is defined as a platelet count below 150,000/μL, but the ability to form a hemostatic plug is retained until the platelet count falls below 100,000/μL, so "hemostatically significant" thrombocytopenia is defined as a platelet count below 100,000/μL. In the ICU setting, significant thrombocytopenia (<100,000/μL) has been reported in 23 to 35% of patients, and severe thrombocytopenia (<50,000/μL) has been reported in 10 to 17% of patients (1,2).

This chapter presents the usual causes of significant thrombocytopenia in the ICU setting, and then describes the indications, methods, and complications of platelet transfusion therapy.

I. ETIOLOGIES

The usual causes of thrombocytopenia in the ICU setting are listed in Table 31.1. Systemic sepsis is the most common cause of thrombocytopenia in ICU patients (1) and is the result of increased platelet destruction. This section describes 3 thrombocytopenia "syndromes" that deserve attention. These conditions share one important feature; i.e., thrombosis plays an important role in the thrombocytopenia, and in the clinical presentation of the syndrome.

493

TABLE 31.1 Causes of Significant Thrombocytopenia in the ICU

Condition	Drugs*
Systemic sepsis	Heparin
Disseminated intravascular coagulation	Antibiotics (linezolid, rifampin, sulfonamides, vancomycin)
Thrombotic thrombocytopenia purpura	Platelet glycoprotein (IIb-IIIa) inhibitors
Hypersplenism	Acetaminophen
Chronic ethanol abuse	Phenytoin
Post-transfusion purpura	Quinidine

*Includes drugs implicated in at least 5 reports.

From Aster R, Bougie D. Drug-induced immune thrombocytopenia. N Engl J Med 2007; 357:580–587.

A. Heparin-Induced Thrombocytopenia

1. *Pathogenesis*

   Heparin can bind to a protein (platelet factor 4) on platelets to form an antigenic complex that induces the formation of IgG antibodies. These antibodies bind to the antigen complex on the platelet surface and form cross-bridges between contiguous platelets. This promotes platelet aggregation, which can lead to symptomatic thrombosis and a consumptive thrombocytopenia (3,4).

2. *Clinical Features*

   Heparin-induced thrombocytopenia (HIT) typically appears as a ≥50% decrease in platelet count that develops 5 to 14 days after the first exposure to heparin (the onset is earlier in patients with a prior exposure to heparin).

   a. HIT is not a dose-dependent phenomenon, and has been reported as a result of heparin flushes and heparin-coated pulmonary artery catheters (5).

b. The thrombocytopenia is mild (>100,000/μL) in 20% of cases, moderate (30–100,000/μL) in 60% of cases, and severe (<30,000/μL) in 20% of cases (3).

c. The major complication of HIT is thrombosis, not bleeding. Over 50% of patients with HIT can develop symptomatic thrombosis, including deep vein thrombosis in the legs (50% of cases), acute pulmonary embolism (25% of cases), arterial thrombosis involving a limb (5–10% of cases), and thrombotic stroke (3–5% of cases) (4).

3. *Risk Factors*

The risk of HIT varies with the patient population and the type of heparin preparation. Unfractionated heparin (UFH) has a higher risk of HIT than low-molecular-weight heparin (LMWH).

a. The risk of HIT from UFH is greatest following orthopedic surgery (3 to 5%) and cardiac surgery (1 to 3%), and is least (1%) in medical patients (4).

b. The risk of HIT from LMWH is about 1% in orthopedic surgery, and <1% in other clinical settings (4).

4. *Diagnosis*

The diagnosis of HIT requires a positive assay for IgG antibodies to the heparin-platelet factor 4 complex (6). However, this assay can be falsely positive, so a positive assay must be combined with a high-risk clinical setting to secure the diagnosis of HIT.

5. *Acute Management*

Heparin must be discontinued immediately (don't forget to discontinue heparin flushes and remove heparin-coated intravascular catheters). If anticoagulation is necessary, two direct thrombin inhibitors are available: lepirudin and argatroban. The dose recommendations for each are shown in Table 31.2.

a. **Lepirudin** (Refludan) is a recombinant protein that has been used for both prophylaxis and treatment of thromboembolism in patients with HIT (7,8). Dose adjustments are required in renal failure. Anaphylaxis has been reported after IV bolus doses of lepirudin, especially in patients who have received the drug previously (3).

b. **Argatroban** is a synthetic analogue of *L*-arginine that has been successful in treating thromboembolism in patients with HIT (8,9). Dose adjustments are necessary in hepatic insufficiency. Anaphylaxis has not been reported with argatroban.

TABLE 31.2 Anticoagulation with Direct Thrombin Inhibitors

	Lepirudin	Argatroban
Prophylactic Dose	0.10 mg/kg/hr IV or 25 mg SC every 12 h.	———
Therapeutic Dose	0.4 mg/kg IV bolus, then 0.15 mg/kg/hr (max. wt = 110 kg). Adjust dose to PTT of 1.5–3 x control	Start at 2 µg/kg/min and adjust dose to PTT of 1.5–3 x control Max. rate = 10 µg/kg/min.
Dose Adjustments:		
Renal Failure	0.1 mg/kg IV bolus on alternate days. Hold dose if PTT > 1.5 x control	No dose adjustment
Liver Failure	No dose adjustment	↓ initial dose rate to 0.5 µg/kg/min.

From References 7–9

6. *Long-Term Management*

Heparin antibodies can persist for longer than 100 days after the initial exposure, long after the thrombocytopenia has resolved (8). **Coumadin** can be used for long-term anticoagulation if necessary. Coumadin should NEVER be used during the active phase of HIT because there is an increased risk of limb gangrene (8).

B. Disseminated Intravascular Coagulation

Disseminated intravascular coagulation (DIC) is a thrombotic microangiopathy characterized by widespread microvascular thrombosis that is severe enough to deplete circulating platelets and procoagulant proteins (10). The culprit is a protein known as *tissue factor* that is released by the endothelium and activates the coagulation cascade.

1. *Clinical Features*

    a. DIC is not a primary disorder, and is most often a complication of severe sepsis, trauma, and obstetric emergencies (e.g., abruptio placentae).

    b. The microvascular thrombosis in DIC can produce multiorgan failure (e.g., oliguric renal failure, ARDS), while depletion of platelets and coagulation factors can promote bleeding, particularly from the GI tract.

    c. DIC can be accompanied by symmetrical necrosis and ecchymosis involving the limbs; a condition known as *purpura fulminans*. This condition can develop in any case of overwhelming sepsis but is most characteristic of meningococcemia (11).

3. *Diagnosis*

    The diagnosis of DIC is based on the presence of a predisposing condition combined with laboratory evidence of widespread coagulation deficits. Table 31.3 shows a scoring system for the diagnosis of DIC proposed by the International Society on Thrombosis and Haemostasis (12).

4. *Management*

    a. There is no effective treatment for DIC other than that directed against the predisposing condition.

    b. Bleeding from DIC often prompts the replacement of

platelets and coagulation factors (10 units of cryoprecipitate provides about 2.5 grams of fibrinogen), but this rarely helps, and consumption of the administered platelets and coagulation proteins can aggravate the microvascular thrombosis.

c. Advanced cases of DIC have a mortality rate in excess of 80% (10,11).

TABLE 31.3 Scoring System for the Diagnosis of DIC

Variable	Points*			
	0	1	2	3
Platelet Count/nL	>100	≥50	<50	—
D-dimer (µg/mL)	≤1	—	1–5	>5
Fibrinogen (g/L)	>1	≤1	—	—
Prothrombin Index (%)	>70	40–70	<40	—

*A score of ≥5 is consistent with the diagnosis of DIC.
From Reference 12.

C. Thrombotic Thrombocytopenia Purpura

Thrombotic thrombocytopenia purpura (TTP) is thrombotic microangiopathy (like DIC) that often follows a nonspecific illness like a viral syndrome. The culprit in this case is immune-mediated platelet aggregation.

1. Clinical Features

TTP presents with *five clinical features* (pentad): fever, change in mental status, acute renal failure, thrombocytopenia, and microangiopathic hemolytic anemia. All 5 are required for diagnosis.

a. Depressed consciousness can progress rapidly to coma and seizures.

    b. The microangiopathic hemolytic anemia is detected by the presence of schistocytes in the blood smear.

    c. Laboratory tests of coagulation (e.g., prothrombin time) are usually normal in TTP, which helps to distinguish it from DIC.

2. *Management*

The treatment of choice for TTP is *plasma exchange* (13,14). This is achieved with a technique called *plasmapheresis,* where aliquots of blood are removed from the patient and centrifuged to separate the plasma from the RBCs. The plasma is discarded, and the RBCs are reinfused with fresh frozen plasma. This is continued until 1.5 times the plasma volume is exchanged, and this process is repeated daily for 3–7 days.

    a. Acute fulminant TTP is almost always fatal if untreated, but if plasma exchange is started early (within 48 hours of symptom onset), as many as 90% of patients can survive the illness (13,14).

II. TRANSFUSION TRIGGER

The platelet count that should initiate platelet transfusions (i.e., the *transfusion trigger*) is dependent on a number of factors (e.g., the presence of bleeding, additional coagulation abnormalities, etc). The following are some general guidelines taken from published reviews (15,16).

A. Contraindications

1. Platelet transfusions are contraindicated in patients with HIT and TTP because the primary problem in these conditions is thrombosis from enhanced platelet aggregation, and transfused platelets will promote further thrombosis.

2. Even though transfused platelets can aggravate the microvascular thrombosis in DIC, platelet transfusions are not contraindicated in DIC if there is significant bleeding (15).

B. Active Bleeding

In the presence of active bleeding other than ecchymoses or petechiae, platelet transfusions are indicated when:

1. The platelet count is below 100,000/µL and:
   a. There is intracranial bleeding or a risk of intracranial bleeding (e.g., head trauma), or
   b. Hemostasis is otherwise impaired (e.g., platelet adhesion is impaired).

2. The platelet count is below 50,000/µL and:
   a. There is no intracranial bleeding or risk of intracranial bleeding, and
   b. Hemostasis is otherwise normal (e.g., platelet function is normal).

C. No Active Bleeding

Despite evidence that spontaneous bleeding through an intact vascular system is uncommon with platelet counts down to 5,000/µL (16), most experts are reluctant to adopt a platelet transfusion trigger as low as 5,000/µL. In the absence of bleeding (other than ecchymoses or petechiae), prophylactic platelet transfusions are usually recommended when (15,16):

1. The platelet count is below 10,000/µL and there is no risk of hemorrhage.

2. The platelet count is below 20,000/µL and there is a risk of hemorrhage from a pre-existing lesion (e.g., peptic ulcer disease).

D. Procedures

In the absence of associated coagulation abnormalities:

1. Platelet counts >40,000/μL are sufficient to perform laparotomy, craniotomy, tracheotomy, percutaneous liver biopsy, and bronchoscopic or endoscopic biopsy (16).

2. Platelet counts >20,000/μL are sufficient to perform lumbar punctures (16).

3. Platelet counts >10,000/μL are sufficient to perform central venous cannulation safely (17,18).

III. PLATELET TRANSFUSIONS

A. Random Donor Platelets

1. Platelet concentrates are prepared from fresh whole blood by differential centrifugation. Each platelet concentrate contains an average of 80×10^9 platelets in 50 mL of plasma (16), and can be stored for up to 5 days.

2. Platelet concentrates are rich in leukocytes, and this feature is responsible for the high frequency of febrile reactions to platelet transfusions (see later).

3. Platelet transfusions are given as multiples of 4 to 6 platelet concentrates (units), each one from a different donor. The total volume is 200 to 300 mL.

B. Response to Transfused Platelets

1. In an average-sized adult with no ongoing blood loss, *each platelet concentrate should raise the circulating platelet count by*

7,000 to 10,000/μL at one hour post-transfusion (16). This number is reduced by about 40% at 24 hours post-transfusion. The increment can be lower in thrombocytopenia patients; however, an increment of <6000/μL at one hour post-transfusion is considered an inadequate response (16).

3. Patients who receive multiple platelet transfusions often (up to 70% of the time) become refractory to platelet transfusions because of a buildup of antibodies to ABO antigens on random donor platelets (15,16). This problem can be alleviated by transfusing ABO-compatible platelets from a single donor.

C. Complications

1. *Bacterial Transmission*

   a. Bacteria are much more likely to flourish in platelet concentrates than in RBC concentrates (packed cells) because platelets are stored at room temperature (22°C) while RBCs are refrigerated at about 1–6°C.

   b. It is estimated that one in every 2,000 to 3,000 platelet concentrates harbors bacteria and that one in 5,000 of these concentrates will produce sepsis in the recipient (16).

   c. Cultures of all platelet concentrates are now required, (16) but, since platelets can be stored for only 5 days, the platelets can be transfused before the culture results are available.

2. *Fever*

   a. Febrile nonhemolytic reactions have been reported in as many as 30% of platelet transfusions (15), which is much greater than the 1% rate of similar reactions reported with RBC transfusions (see Chapter 30).

   b. Reducing or eliminating the leukocytes in platelet concentrates will help to alleviate this problem, but the leukoreduction process also reduces the number of platelets (by about 25%) available for transfusion.

3. *Allergic Reactions*

Hypersensitivity reactions (urticaria, anaphylaxis, anaphylactic shock) are also more more common with platelet transfusions than with erythrocyte transfusions (16). These reactions are caused by sensitization to proteins in donor plasma, and removing the plasma from platelet concentrates will reduce the incidence of these reactions.

REFERENCES

1. Stephan F, Hollande J, Richard O, et al. Thrombocytopenia in a surgical ICU. Chest 1999; 115:1363-1379.
2. Strauss R, Wehler M, Mehler K, et al. Thrombocytopenia in patients in the medical intensive care unit: Bleeding prevalence, transfusion requirements, and outcome. Crit Care Med 2002; 30:1765–1771.
3. Napolitano LM, Warkentin TE, AlMahameed A, Nasraway SA. Heparin-induced thrombocytopenia in the critical care setting: diagnosis and management. Crit Care Med 2006; 34:2898–2911.
4. Warkentin TE, Cook DJ. Heparin, low molecular weight heparin, and heparin-induced thrombocytopenia in the ICU. Crit Care Clin 2005; 21:513–529.
5. Laster J, Silver D. Heparin-coated catheters and heparin-induced thrombocytopenia. J Vasc Surg 1988; 7:667–672.
6. Warkentin TE. New approaches to the diagnosis of heparin-induced thrombocytopenia. Chest 2005; 127(Suppl):35S–45S.
7. Greinacher A, Janssens U, Berg G, et al. Lepirudin (recombinant hirudin) for parenteral anticoagulation in patients with heparin-induced thrombocytopenia. Circulation 1999; 100:587–593.
8. Hassell K. The management of patients with heparin-induced thrombocytopenia who require anticoagulant therapy. Chest 2005; 127(Suppl):1S–8S.
9. Levine RL, Hursting MJ, McCollum D. Argatroban therapy in heparin-induced thrombocytopenia with hepatic dysfunction. Chest 2006; 129:1167–1175.
10. Senno SL, Pechet L, Bick RL. Disseminated intravascular coagulation (DIC). Pathophysiology, laboratory diagnosis, and management. J Intensive Care Med 2000; 15:144–158.

11. DeLoughery TG. Critical care clotting catastrophies. Crit Care Clin 2005; 21:531–562.

12. Angstwurm MWA, Dempfle C-E, Spannagl M. New disseminated intravascular coagulation score: A useful tool to predict mortality in comparison with Acute Physiology and Chronic Health Evaluation II and Logistic Organ Dysfunction Scores. Crit Care Med 2006; 34:314–320.

13. Rock GA, Shumack KH, Buskard NA, et al. Comparison of plasma exchange with plasma infusion in the treatment of thrombotic thrombocytopenia purpura. N Engl J Med 1991; 325:393–397.

14. Hayward CP, Sutton DMC, Carter WH Jr, et al. Treatment outcomes in patients with adult thrombotic thrombocytopenic purpura-hemolytic uremic syndrome. Arch Intern Med 1994; 154:982–987.

15. Gelinas J-P, Stoddart LV, Snyder EL. Thrombocytopenia and critical care medicine. J Intensive Care Med 2001; 16:1–21.

16. Slichter SJ. Platelet transfusion therapy. Hematol Oncol Clin N Am 2007; 21:697–29.

17. Doerfler ME, Kaufman B, Goldenberg AS. Central venous catheter placement in patients with disorders of hemostasis. Chest 1996; 110:185–188.

18. DeLoughery TG, Liebler JM, Simonds V, et al. Invasive line placement in critically ill patients: Do hemostatic defects matter? Transfusion 1996; 36:827–831.

Chapter 32

FEVER IN THE ICU

The evaluation of new-onset fever is (unfortunately) part of everyday life in the ICU. This chapter describes the usual sources of ICU-acquired fever (1,2). The final section focuses on the early management of patients with fever and includes an evaluation of antipyretic therapy.

I. BODY TEMPERATURE

A. Normal Body Temperature

The normal body temperature is usually defined as a single point; i.e., 37°C or 98.6°F (see Appendix 1 for the correlation between the Celsius and Fahrenheit scales). The problem with this definition is demonstrated by the following observations.

1. There is a diurnal variation in body temperature, with the nadir in the early morning (between 4 and 8 a.m.) and the peak in the late afternoon (between 4 and 6 p.m.). The extent of the diurnal variation varies in individual subjects. The highest reported diurnal variation is 1.3° C (2.4° F) (3).

2. Elderly subjects have a body temperature that averages 0.5° C (0.9° F) below that of younger adults (4).

3. Core body temperature can be 0.5° C (0.9° F) higher than oral temperatures (5), and 0.2° C to 0.3° C lower than rectal temperatures (1).

4. These observations indicate that the normal body temperature is influenced by age, time of day, and measurement site.

B. Fever

1. Fever is defined as a body temperature that exceeds the normal daily temperature range for an individual subject. This is not a practical definition because the body temperature is not monitored continuously in hospitalized patients, so it is not possible to determine the diurnal temperature variation for each patient.

2. The Society of Critical Care Medicine, in their practice guideline (1), proposes that a *body temperature above 38.3°C (101°F) represents a fever*. The time of day or measurement site is not specified in this definition.

II. NONINFECTIOUS SOURCES

Fever is the result of inflammatory cytokines (called endogenous pyrogens) that act on the hypothalamus to elevate the body temperature. Therefore, any condition that incites a systemic inflammatory response can produce a fever. The noninfectious sources of fever in the ICU setting are listed in Table 32.1. The following conditions deserve mention.

A. Postoperative Fever

1. Fever in the first day following major surgery is reported in 15% to 40% of patients, (6,7), and in most of these cases, there is no associated infection. These fevers are short-lived and usually resolve within 24 to 48 hours.

2. There is a general belief that atelectasis is a common cause of fever in the early postoperative period. However, the following observations indicate that *atelectasis is not a cause of postoperative fever*.

   a. An animal study has shown that lobar atelectasis (produced by ligation of a bronchus) is not accompanied by fever (8).

b. A clinical study has shown that 75% of patients with post-op atelectasis do not develop a fever (9).

3. The tissue injury caused by major surgery can trigger a systemic inflammatory response, and this inflammatory reponse is the most likely cause of fever in the early post-operative period.

TABLE 32.1 Noninfectious Causes of ICU-Acquired Fever

1. Major surgery	a. Postoperative fever
	b. Malignant hyperthermia
2. Other procedures	a. Hemodialysis
	b. Bronchoscopy
3. Drugs	a. Drug fever
	b. Neuroleptic malignant syndrome
4. Infarctions	a. Bowel
	b. Cerebral
	c. Myocardial
5. Transfusions	a. Erythrocytes
	b. Platelets
6. Venous thromboembolism	
7. Systemic inflammatory response syndrome	
8. Iatrogenic fever	

B. Malignant Hyperthermia

Malignant hyperthermia (MH) is an inherited disorder characterized by high fever, muscle rigidity, and autonomic instability in response to halogenated inhalational anesthetics (e.g., halothane, isoflurane, servoflurane, and desflurane) and depolarizing neuromuscular blockers (e.g., succinylcholine) (10,11). The culprit in this disorder is excessive release of calcium from the sarcoplasmic reticulum of skeletal muscles.

1. The first sign of MH may be an unexplained elevation in

exhaled PCO_2 in the operating room (reflecting hypermetabolism in skeletal muscle).

2. Muscle rigidity is usually evident within minutes to a few hours, and the heat generated by the muscle activity can raise the body temperature above 40°C (104°F). Autonomic instability can produce cardiac arrhythmias, fluctuating blood pressure, or persistent hypotension.

3. The treatment of MH is **dantrolene sodium**, a muscle relaxant that inhibits calcium release from the sarcoplasmic reticulum of skeletal muscle cells.

   a. The dose of dantrolene is 1 to 2 mg/kg given as an IV bolus and repeated every 15 minutes if needed to a total dose of 10 mg/kg. The initial dosing regimen is followed by a dose of 1 mg/kg IV four times daily for 3 days to prevent recurrences.

   b. Dantrolene can cause hepatocellular injury, but this is uncommon when the initial dose is less than 10 mg/kg (10).

   c. When given early in the course of MH, dantrolene can reduce the mortality rate from 70% or higher (in untreated cases) to 10% or less (10,11).

C. Other Procedures

1. *Hemodialysis*

   Febrile reactions during hemodialysis are attributed to endotoxin contamination of the dialysis equipment, but bacteremia occurs on occasion (12).

2. *Bronchoscopy*

   Fiberoptic bronchoscopy is followed by fever in 5% of cases (13). The fever usually appears 8 to 10 hours after the procedure, and it subsides spontaneously in 24 hours. The fever is often associated with leukocytosis (13), but pneumonia and bacteremia are rare (14).

D. Drug Fever

1. Drug-induced fever can be the result of a hypersensitivity reaction, an idiosyncratic reaction, or infusion-related phlebitis.

2. Almost any drug can cause fever, but the ones most often implicated are listed in Table 32.2. Antibiotics are the most common offenders.

3. The onset of the fever varies from a few hours to a few weeks after initial drug exposure. The fever can appear as an isolated finding or can be accompanied by the other findings listed in Table 32.2 (15). Note the about 50% of patients have rigors, and close to 20% develop hypotension, indicating that *patients with a drug fever can appear seriously ill.*

4. Drug fever is usually suspected only when other causes of fever have been excluded. The fever should disappear in 2 to 3 days after stopping the offending drug, but on occasion the fever can take as long as 7 days to disappear (16).

TABLE 32.2 Drug-Associated Fever

Common Offenders	Clinical Findings*
Amphotericin	Rigors (53%)
Cephalosporins	Myalgias (25%)
Penicillins	Leukocytosis (22%)
Phenytoin	Eosinophilia (22%)
Procainamide	Rash (18%)
Vancomycin	Hypotension (18%)

1From Reference 15.

TABLE 32.3 Causes of Neuroleptic Malignant Syndrome

Antipsychotic agents:	Butyrophenones (e.g., haloperidol), phenothiazines, clozapine, olanzapine, respiradone
Antiemetic agents:	Metaclopramide, droperidol, prochlorperazine
CNS stimulants:	Amphetamines, cocaine
Other:	Lithium, overdose with tricyclic antidepressants

E. Neuroleptic Malignant Syndrome

1. The *neuroleptic malignant syndrome* (NMS) is similar to malignant hyperthermia in that it is a drug-induced disorder characterized by increased body temperature, muscle rigidity, altered mentation, and autonomic instability (17).

2. The drugs most often implicated in NMS are listed in Table 32.3. The drug of most concern is haloperidol, which is used as a sedative for ICU patients (see Chapter 43).

3. There is no relationship between the intensity or duration of drug therapy and the risk of NMS (17).

4. In 80% of cases of NMS, the initial manifestation is muscle rigidity or altered mental status (17). Clinical manifestations begin to appear 24 to 72 hours after the onset of drug therapy, and are almost always apparent in the first 2 weeks of drug therapy.

5. Fever (which can exceed 41°C) is required for the diagnosis of NMS (17), and can help to distinguish NMS from dystonic reactions to neuroleptic agents.

6. The management of NMS mandates immediate removal

of the offending drug. **Dantrolene sodium** (the same muscle relaxant used in the treatment of MH) can be used for severe cases of muscle rigidity. The optimal dose is not clearly defined, but one suggestion is to start with a single IV dose of 2–3 mg/kg and repeat this dose every few hours if needed to a total dose of 10 mg/kg/day (17).

F. Other Sources

1. Acute pulmonary embolism can produce a fever that lasts up to 1 week (18).

2. Acute infarction of the heart, brain, or GI tract can be accompanied by fever. Unexplained fever and metabolic (lactic) acidosis may be the only signs of bowel infarction in elderly patients or patients with depressed consciousness.

3. Iatrogenic fever can be caused by faulty thermal regulators in water mattresses and aerosol humidifiers (19).

III. NOSOCOMIAL INFECTIONS

A. Prevalence & Pathogens

1. The prevalence of different nosocomial infections in medical and surgical ICU patients in the United States is shown in Table 32.4 (20). Note that four infections account for over three-quarters of the cases: pneumonia, urinary tract infection, bloodstream infection, and surgical site infection. Three of these infections are related to indwelling devices: i.e., 83% of pneumonias occur in intubated patients, 97% of urinary tract infections occur in catheterized patients, and 87% of bloodstream infections originate from intravascular catheters (20).

TABLE 32.4 Nosocomial Infections in the ICU Setting[†]

Nosocomial Infection	% Total Infections	
	Medical Patients	Surgical Patients
Pneumonia	30% ⎫	33% ⎫
Urinary Tract Infection	30% ⎬ 76%	18% ⎪
Bloodstream Infection	16% ⎭	13% ⎬ 78%
Surgical Site Infection	—	14% ⎭
Cardiovascular Infection	5%	4%
GI Tract Infection	5%	4%
Ear, Nose & Throat Infection	4%	4%
Skin & Soft Tissue Infection	3%	3%
Others	7%	7%

[†]Pertains to ICUs in the United States. From Reference 20.

2. The pathogens isolated in three of the common ICU-acquired infections are shown in Table 32.5 (21). The microbial spectrum of these infections provides a valuable guide for selecting empiric antibiotic regimens.

B. Selected Infections

The diagnosis and management of ICU-related pneumonias, urinary tract infections, catheter-related bloodstream infections, and GI tract infections are described elsewhere in the book, and will not be presented here. The following descriptions include the remaining ICU-related infections that deserve attention.

1. *Surgical Wound Infections*

Surgical wounds are classified as clean (abdomen and chest unopened), contaminated (abdomen or chest opened), or dirty (direct contact with pus or bowel contents) (22).

TABLE 32.5 Pathogens in ICU-Related Infections

| Pathogen | Pneumonia | % of Infections | |
		Urinary Tract Infection	Bloodstream Infection
Staph. aureus	20	2	13
Staph. epidermidis	1	2	36
Enterococci	2	14	16
P. aeruginosa	21	10	3
Klebsiella pneumoniae	8	6	4
Enterobacter	9	5	3
Escherichia coli	4	14	3
Candida albicans	5	23	6

From Reference 21.

a. Wound infections typically appear at 5 to 7 days after surgery.

b. Most infections do not extend beyond the skin and subcutaneous tissues and can be managed with debridement only. Antimicrobial therapy (to cover streptococcus, staphylococcus, and anaerobes) can be reserved for cases with persistent erythema or evidence of deep tissue involvement (6).

c. Sternal wound infection with spread to the mediastinum is a prominent concern following median sternotomy (23). Sternal instability can be an early sign of sternal wound infections.

2. *Necrotizing Wound Infections*

Necrotizing wound infections are produced by *Clostridia* or β-hemolytic streptococci.

a. These infections are usually evident in the first few postoperative days (earlier than other types of wound infection).

b. There is often marked edema around the incision, and the skin may have crepitance and fluid-filled bullae.

c. Spread to deeper structures is often rapid and produces progressive rhabdomyolysis and myoglobinuric renal failure.

d. Treatment involves extensive debridement and intravenous penicillin. The mortality is high (above 60%) when treatment is delayed.

3. *Paranasal Sinusitis*

Paranasal sinusitis from indwelling nasogastric and nasotracheal tubes is described briefly in Chapter 20 (see Section I-B). The significance of sinusitis as a cause of ICU-related fever is unclear, but it should always be considered in patients with indwelling nasal (and oral) tubes who have unexplained fever.

a. This type of sinusitis produces opacification of the maxillary (and sometimes ethmoid) sinus (usually on CT scan). However, 30 to 40% of patients with radiographic evidence of sinusitis do not have a documented infection (35,36). Therefore, the diagnosis requires sinus puncture and isolation of pathogens by quantitative culture ($\geq 10^3$ colony forming units per milliliter) (24,25).

b. The presence of organisms on Gram stain can be used to guide empiric antibiotic therapy. Common isolates include aerobic gram-negative bacilli (especially *Pseudomonas aeruginosa*) in 60% of cases, and aerobic gram-positive cocci (particularly *Staphylococcus aureus*) in 30% of cases (1).

c. Nasal tubes should be removed in confirmed cases of sinusitis.

4. *Other Infections*

The following ICU-related infections should be considered in select patient populations.

a. Endocarditis — in patients with prosthetic valves.

b. Meningitis — in neurosurgical patients.

c. Spontaneous bacterial peritonitis — in patients with cirrhosis and ascites.

IV. INITIAL APPROACH

A. Blood Cultures

1. *Venipuncture Sites*

   No more than one set of blood cultures should be obtained from each venipuncture site (26). The appropriate number of venipunctures is determined by the likelihood of septicemia.

   a. Two venipunctures are adequate for blood cultures if the likelihood of septicemia is low (e.g., when pneumonia or urinary tract infection is suspected).

   b. Three venipunctures are recommended if the probability of septicemia is high (e.g., when endocarditis is suspected).

   c. For suspected catheter-related septicemia, one blood sample can be drawn through the indwelling central venous catheter if quantitative blood cultures are obtained (see Chapter 6, Section III-E, and Figure 6.2).

2. *Volume of Blood*

   Increasing the volume of blood that is cultured will increase the likelihood of a positive blood culture. To achieve optimal results, a volume of 20 to 30 mL of blood has been recommended for each venipuncture site (26). The volume of blood added to each culture bottle should be kept at the usual 1:5 ratio (blood volume:broth volume).

B. Empiric Antimicrobial Therapy

1. *Indications*

   Empiric antibiotic therapy is indicated in the following situations:

   a. When the likelihood of infection is high.

   b. When there is evidence of progressive dysfunction in two or more vital organs.

   c. When the patient is immunocompromised.

2. *Suggested Antibiotics*

   Empiric antibiotic therapy should be selected on the basis of common isolates (see Table 32.5) and antibiotic susceptibility patterns in each ICU.

   a. For ICUs where resistant pathogens are common, empiric coverage for gram-positive infections should include either **vancomycin** (for methicillin-resistant *Staph. aureus*—MRSA) or **linezolid** (for vancomycin-resistant strains of enterococci or MRSA).

   b. Empiric coverage of gram-negative infections can include either a carbepenem (e.g., **meropenem**), an antipseudomonal cephalosporin (e.g., **ceftazidime**), or an antipseudomonal penicillin (e.g., **pipericillin tazobactam**). In immunocompromised patients, an aminoglycoside can be added for gram-negative (particularly pseudomonal) coverage (27).

   c. See Table 34.4 (Chapter 34) for suggested starting doses of empiric antibiotics. For more detailed dosing information, see Chapter 44.

C. Antipyretic Therapy

1. *Fever as a Defense Mechanism*

   The popular perception that fever is harmful and should be suppressed is at odds with the emerging concept of fever as an adaptive response that enhances host defenses against infection. The following observations support this concept.

a. An increase in body temperature inhibits bacterial growth, as demonstrated in Figure 32.1 (28,29).

b. Increased body temperature enhances immune function by increasing the production of antibodies and cytokines, activating T-lymphocytes, and enhancing chemotaxis and phagocytosis by neutrophils and macrophages (2,30,31).

c. Patients with severe sepsis who develop hypothermia have more than twice the mortality rate of septic patients who develop a fever (32).

d. These observations indicate that fever helps to eradicate infection, which means that *suppressing fever* (antipyretic therapy) *can be counterproductive in patients with infectious fever.*

2. ***When Is Fever Harmful?***

The only clinical situation where fever has proven to be harmful is in the early period following ischemic brain injury (i.e., ischemic stroke or cardiac arrest). This topic is

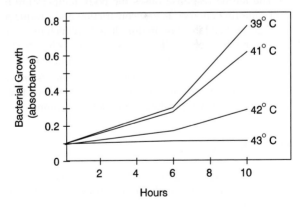

FIGURE 32.1 The influence of temperature on the growth of *Pasteurella multocida* from the blood of infected laboratory animals. The temperature range in the figure corresponds to the usual range of febrile temperatures for the study animal (rabbits). From Reference 28.

described in more detail in Chapters 13 and 42.

3. *Antipyretic Drugs*

The actions of endogenous pyrogens that raise body temperature are mediated by prostaglandin E, and drugs that interfere with prostaglandin E synthesis are effective in suppressing fever (33). These drugs include aspirin, acetaminophen, and the nonsteroidal anti-inflammatory agents (NSAIDs).

  a. Acetaminophen is given orally or by rectal suppository. The antipyretic dose is 325 to 650 mg every 4 to 6 hours, and the total daily dose should not exceed 10 grams to prevent acetaminophen hepatotoxicity (see Chapter 46).

  b. The NSAID ibuprofen can be given intravenously. A dose of 10 mg/kg up to 800 mg every 6 hours has proven safe in ICU patients with sepsis (34).

4. *Don't Use Cooling Blankets*

The use of cooling blankets to suppress fever is inappropriate for the following reasons.

  a. The febrile response raises the body temperature by promoting cutaneous vasoconstriction and producing a generalized increase in muscle tone (which increases internal heat production). This response is identical to the physiologic response to a cold environment.

  b. Thus, *the febrile response makes the body behave like it is wrapped in a cooling blanket.* Adding a cooling blanket can actually raise the body temperature by promoting shivering.

REFERENCES

1. O'Grady NP, Barie PS, Bartlett J, et al. Practice parameters for evaluating new fever in critically ill adult patients. Crit Care Med 1998; 26:392–408.
2. Marik PE. Fever in the ICU. Chest 2000; 117:855–869.
3. Mackowiak PA, Wasserman SS, Levine MM. A critical appraisal of 98.6° F, the upper limit of the normal body temperature, and other lega-

cies of Carl Reinhold August Wunderlich. JAMA 1992; 268:1578–1580.

4. Marion GS, McGann KP, Camp DL. Core body temperature in the elderly and factors which influence its measurement. Gerontology 1991; 37:225–232.

5. Tandberg D, Sklar D. Effect of tachypnea on the estimation of body temperature by an oral thermometer. N Engl J Med 1983; 308:945–946.

6. Fry DE. Postoperative fever. In: Mackowiak PA, ed. Fever: basic mechanisms and management. New York: Raven Press, 1991:243–254.

7. Freischlag J, Busuttil RW. The value of postoperative fever evaluation. Surgery 1983; 94:358–363.

8. Shields RT. Pathogenesis of postoperative pulmonary atelectasis: an experimental study. Arch Surg 1949; 48:489–503.

9. Engoren M. Lack of association between atelectasis and fever. Chest 1995; 107:81–84.

10. Rusyniakn DE, Sprague JE. Toxin-induced hyperthermic syndromes. Med Clin N Am 2005; 89:1277–1296.

11. Litman RS, Rosenberg H. Malignant hyperthermia. JAMA 2005; 293:2918–2924.

12 Pollack VE. Adverse effects and pyrogenic reactions during hemodialysis. JAMA 1988; 260:2106–2107.

13. Um SW. Prospective analysis of clinical characteristics and risk factors for postbronchoscopy fever. Chest 2004; 125:945–952.

14. Spach DH, Silverstein FE, Stamm WE. Transmission of infection by gastrointestinal endoscopy and bronchoscopy. Ann Intern Med 1993; 118:117–128.

15. Mackowiak PA, LeMaistre CF. Drug fever: a critical appraisal of conventional concepts. Ann Intern Med 1987; 106:728–733.

16. Cunha B. Drug fever: The importance of recognition. Postgrad Med 1986; 80:123–129.

17. Bhanushali NJ, Tuite PJ. The evaluation and management of patients with neuroleptic malignant syndrome. Neurol Clin N Am 2004; 22:389–411.

18. Murray HW, Ellis GC, Blumenthal DS, et al. Fever and pulmonary thromboembolism. Am J Med 1979; 67:232–235.

19. Gonzalez EB, Suarez L, Magee S. Nosocomial (water bed) fever. Arch Intern Med 1990; 150:687 (letter).

20. Richards MJ, Edwards JR, Culver DH, Gaynes RP. The National Nosocomial Infections Surveillance System. Nosocomial infections in combined medical-surgical intensive care units in the United States. Infect Control Hosp Epidemiol 2000; 21:510–515.

21. Richards MJ, Edwards JR, Culver DH, Gaynes RO. The National Nosocomial Infection Surveillance System. Nosocomial infections in medical intensive care units in the United States. Crit Care Med 1999; 27:887–892.

22. Ehrenkranz NJ, Meakins JL. Surgical infections. In: Bennet JV, Brachman PS, eds. Hospital infections. 3rd ed. Boston: Little, Brown, 1992:685–710.

23. Loop FD, Lytle BW, Cosgrove DM, et al. Sternal wound complications after isolated coronary artery bypass grafting: early and late mortality, morbidity, and cost of care. Ann Thorac Surg 1990; 49:179–187.

24. Holzapfel L, Chevret S, Madinier G, et al. Influence of long-term oro- or nasotracheal intubation on nosocomial maxillary sinusitis and pneumonia: results of a prospective, randomized, clinical trial. Crit Care Med 1993; 21:1132–1138.

25. Rouby J-J, Laurent P, Gosnach M, et al. Risk factors and clinical relevance of nosocomial maxillary sinusitis in the critically ill. Am Rev Respir Dis 1994; 150:776–783.

26. Aronson MD, Bor DH. Blood cultures. Ann Intern Med 1987; 106:246–253.

27. Hughes WH, Armstrong D, Bodey GP, et al. 2002 guidelines for the use of antimicrobial agents in neutropenic patients with cancer. Clin Infect Dis 2002; 34:730–751.

28. Kluger M, Rothenburg BA. Fever and reduced iron: their interaction as a host defense response to bacterial infection. Science 1979; 203:374–376.

29. Small PM, Tauber MG, Hackbarth CJ, Sande MA. Influence of body temperature on bacterial growth rates in experimental pneumococcal meningitis in rabbits. Infect Immun 1986; 52:484–487.

30. van Oss CJ, Absolom DR, Moore LL, et al. Effect of temperature on the chemotaxis, phagocytic engulfment, digestion, and O_2 consumption of human polymorphonuclear leukocytes. J Reticuloendothel Soc 1980; 27:561–565.

31. Azocar J, Yunis EJ, Essex M. Sensitivity of human natural killer cells to hyperthermia. Lancet 1982; 1:16–17.

32. Clemmer TP, Fisher CJ, Bone RC, et al. Hypothermia in the sepsis syndrome and clinical outcome. Crit Care Med 1990; 18:801–806.

33. Plaisance KI, Mackowiak PA. Antipyretic therapy. Physiologic rationale, diagnostic implications, and clinical consequences. Arch Intern Med 2000; 160:449–456.

34. Bernard GR, Wheeler AP, Russell JA, et al. The effects of ibuprofen on the physiology and survival of patients with sepsis. N Engl J Med 1997; 336:912–918.

INFECTION, INFLAMMATION, AND MULTIORGAN INJURY

The most significant discovery in critical care medicine in the past 20 years is the prominent role played by the inflammatory response in the morbidity and mortality associated with severe sepsis and septic shock. This chapter describes the relationship between infection, inflammation, and multiorgan failure, and the clinical syndromes that reflect this relationship (1–3).

I. INFLAMMATORY INJURY

A. The Two Sides of Inflammation

1. The inflammatory response can be triggered by a variety of physical, chemical, or infectious insults to the host, and it serves to protect the host in some way from the insult (e.g., eradicating invading organisms or remodeling areas of traumatic injury).

2. Although the inflammatory response generates a variety of noxious substances (e.g., proteolytic enzymes, oxygen metabolites), these substances do not damage the tissues of the host under normal circumstances.

3. When the inflammatory response is sustained, the normal protective mechanisms of the host are somehow lost, and the inflammatory response begins to damage the tissues of the host organism (1).

4. Once started, inflammatory tissue injury becomes a self-sustaining process; i.e., the tissue damage triggers more inflammation, which produces more tissue damage, and so on. This process becomes clinically apparent as progressive dysfunction in multiple organs, culminating in multiorgan failure (2).

5. The condition where an unregulated and persistent systemic inflammatory response produces progressive damage in multiple organs has been called *malignant intravascular inflammation* (3).

B. Clinical Conditions

The clinical conditions defined here were introduced in the early 1990s to emphasize the distinctions between infection, inflammation, and inflammatory organ injury (4).

1. The presence of two or more clinical manifestations of systemic inflammation is a clinical entity known as the *systemic inflammatory response syndrome* (SIRS). The dominant feature of this condition is systemic (disseminated) inflammation. An underlying infection may or may not be present.

2. When SIRS is the result of an infection, the condition is called *sepsis*.

3. When sepsis is associated with dysfunction in one or more vital organs, the condition is called *severe sepsis*.

4. When severe sepsis is accompanied by hypotension that is refractory to volume infusion, the condition is called *septic shock*.

C. Systemic Inflammatory Response Syndrome

1. *Diagnostic Criteria*

   The clinical criteria for the diagnosis of SIRS are shown in

Table 33.1. Some of these findings are nonspecific for inflammation, and this can produce false-positive diagnoses. (For example, an anxiety attack can produce a heart rate above 90 and a respiratory rate above 20, and would qualify as a case of SIRS using the criteria in Table 33.1).

a. The overdiagnosis of SIRS is demonstrated by one report showing that 93% of patients in a surgical ICU satisfied the diagnostic criteria for SIRS (5).

TABLE 33.1 Diagnostic Criteria for (SIRS)

The diagnosis of SIRS requires at least 2 of the following:

1. Temperature $> 38°$ or $< 36°C$

2. Heart rate > 90 beats/min

3. Respiratory rate > 20 breaths/min or arterial $PCO_2 < 32$ mm Hg

4. WBC count $> 12,000/mm^3$ or $< 4,000/mm^3$, or $> 10\%$ of neutrophils are immature (band) forms

From Reference 4.

---

2. *Significance*

SIRS is important as a clinical entity not because it identifies infection, but because it emphasizes that fever, leukocytosis, etc., are signs of *inflammation*, not infection.

a. Infection is identified in 25 to 50% of patients with SIRS (5,6), which means that the majority of ICU patients with fever, leukocytosis, etc., will not have an identifiable infection. This observation is important when considering the use of empiric antibiotics for patients with new-onset fever.

D. Multiorgan Injury

1. *Organs Affected*

Several organs can be adversely affected by inflammato-

ry injury, and Table 33.2 lists each organ and the corresponding clinical entity. The organs most often involved
are the lungs, kidneys, and nervous system (central and
peripheral).

a. The most common site of inflammatory organ injury is
the lungs, and the clinical manifestation of inflammatory lung injury is the *acute respiratory distress syndrome*
(ARDS). This condition is the most common cause of
acute respiratory failure in ICU patients and has been
reported in 40% of patients with severe sepsis (7). (See
Chapter 16 for more information on ARDS).

**TABLE 33.2 Clinical Consequences of Inflammatory
Organ Injury**

Injured Organ or System	Clinical Entity
Brain	Septic encephalopathy
Lungs	ARDS
Kidneys	Acute tubular necrosis
Peripheral nerves	Critical illness neuropathy
Skeletal muscle	Critical illness myopathy
Bone marrow	Anemia of critical illness
Coagulation system	Disseminated intravascular coagulation

---

2. *Mortality Rate*

When inflammatory injury results in failure of one or more
vital organs, the likelihood of survival is determined by
the number of organs involved and not by the severity of
functional impairment in individual organs. This is shown
in Figure 33.1 (7,8). Note that the mortality rate is 30–40%
with 2 organs failed, and it increases steadily to 70–80%
with 4 or more organ failures.

II. SEVERE SEPSIS & SEPTIC SHOCK

Severe sepsis and septic shock are among the leading causes of death in ICU patients (9), and the mortality rate in these conditions has changed little over the years (10). The approach to management presented here is based on evidence-based recommendations from an exhaustive international effort known as the "Surviving Sepsis Campaign" (11).

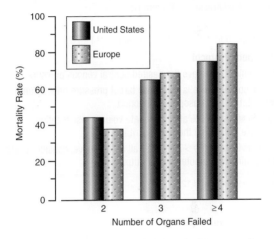

FIGURE 33.1 Direct relationship between mortality rate and number of organ failures in critically ill patients. Data from References 7 and 8.

A. Early Goal-Directed Therapy

The hemodynamic management outlined in Table 33.3 has proven effective in reducing the mortality in patients with septic shock (12). This protocol is designed to achieve four hemodynamic goals, as specified in the table. Therapy should should be started as soon as possible after the problem is clinically apparent, and all hemodynamic goals should be reached within 6 hours after the therapy is started. The major features of this approach are described next.

TABLE 33.3 Early Goal-Directed Therapy of Septic Shock

Hemodynamic Goals

1. Central venous pressure (CVP):
   a. 8–12 mm Hg in spontaneously breathing patients
   b. 12–15 mm Hg in ventilator-dependent patients
2. Mean arterial pressure ≥ 65 mm Hg
3. Urine output ≥ 0.5 mL/kg/hr
4. O_2 saturation in central venous blood ($ScvO_2$) ≥ 70%

Management Protocol

1. Infuse fluids to achieve the desired central venous pressure.
2. If the blood pressure is below the target pressure after volume resuscitation, use vasopressor support.
3. If the $ScvO_2$ is < 70% after adequate volume resuscitation, transfuse RBCs until the hematocrit is ≥ 30%.
4. If the $ScvO_2$ remains > 70% after all of the above, consider using dobutamine to promote cardiac output.

From References 11 and 12.

---

1. *Central Venous Catheters*

   Early goal-directed therapy requires frequent measurements of the central venous pressure (CVP) and the oxyhemoglobin saturation in central venous blood ($ScvO_2$). The latter measurement is best obtained with specially designed *central venous oximetry* catheters (available from Edwards Lifesciences, Irvine, CA) that monitor $ScvO_2$ continuously. See Chapter 9 for information on venous O_2 saturation as an indirect measure of tissue oxygenation.

2. *Volume Resuscitation*

   Circulatory support in septic shock always begins with volume resuscitation because sepsis is often accompanied by hypovolemia from fluid movement into the interstitial space (through leaky capillaries), and from systemic vasodilation, which creates a relative hypovolemia by increasing the fluid capacity of the intravascular space.

a. Volume resuscitation usually involves 500 mL bolus infusions of a crystalloid fluid (e.g., isotonic saline) every 30 minutes to achieve the desired CVP.

b. Because sepsis is often accompanied by hypoalbuminemia, 5% albumin solutions (250 mL every 30 minutes to attain the desired CVP) have a theoretical advantage over crystalloid fluids for volume resuscitation in sepsis. (See Chapter 11 for a description of colloid vs. crystalloid resuscitation).

3. *Vasopressors*

a. If volume resuscitation does not raise the mean arterial pressure to the desired end-point (≥65 mm Hg), then vasopressor support with either **dopamine** (starting at 5 µg/kg/min) or **norepinephrine** (starting at 2 µg/min) is warranted. (See Chapter 45 for more information on these vasopressors).

b. In cases of hypotension that are refractory to standard vasopressors, **vasopressin** can occasionally be effective. The recommended infusion rate is 0.01 to 0.04 units per minute (11).

4. *Other Interventions*

If the central venous O_2 saturation ($ScvO_2$) does not reach the desired level (≥70%) after volume resuscitation and vasopressors, the following interventions are recommended.

a. Transfuse erythrocytes (packed cells) to a target hematocrit of 30% or higher.

b. Start **dobutamine** infusions (at 2.5 µg/kg/min) until the $ScvO_2$ ≥70% or the dobutamine infusion rate reaches 20 µg/kg/min. (See Chapters 12 and 45 for more information on dobutamine).

B. Empiric Antimicrobial Therapy

1. Intravenous antibiotics should be started within one hour after the diagnosis is first suspected, and at least 2 sets of blood cultures should be obtained before starting antibiotics (11).

2. Empiric antibiotic therapy should be selected on the basis of common isolates (see Table 32.5) and antibiotic susceptibility patterns in each ICU.

   a. For ICUs where resistant pathogens are common, empiric coverage for gram-positive infections should include either **vancomycin** (for methicillin-resistant *Staph. aureus*—MRSA) or **linezolid** (for vancomycin-resistant strains of enterococci or MRSA).

   b. Empiric coverage of gram-negative infections can include either a carbepenem (e.g., **meropenem**), an antipseudomonal cephalosporin (e.g., **ceftazidime**), or an antipseudomonal penicillin (e.g., **pipericillin tazobactam**). In immunocompromised patients, an aminoglycoside can be added for gram-negative (particularly pseudomonal) coverage (13).

   c. See Table 34.4 (Chapter 34) for suggested starting doses of empiric antibiotics. For more detailed dosing information, see Chapter 44.

C. Corticosteroids

1. Intravenous steroids are recommended for all patients with septic shock who require vasopressor support (11).

2. A popular steroid regimen is **hydrocortisone**, 200–300 mg IV daily in 2 or 3 divided doses for 7 days (11).

D. Oxygen Transport

Management aimed at optimizing the oxygen transport variables (i.e., oxygen delivery, oxygen uptake) is not advised in severe sepsis and septic shock for the following reasons.

1. There is no evidence that tissue oxygenation is impaired in sepsis. In fact, there is evidence that tissue oxygenation is *increased* in sepsis, as demonstrated in Figure 33.2 (14).

2. The metabolic derangement in sepsis appears to be a defect in oxygen utilization in mitochondria; a condition known as *cytopathic hypoxia* (15).

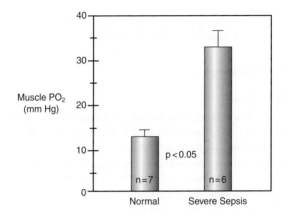

FIGURE 33.2 Tissue PO$_2$ (mean) recorded in the forearm muscles of 6 healthy volunteers and 7 patients with severe sepsis. Crossbars represent the standard error of the mean. Data from Reference 14.

III. ANAPHYLAXIS

The inflammatory response is also involved in hypersensitivity reactions, and anaphylaxis is the most life-threatening expression of these reactions. Common offenders are antimicrobial agents, anesthetics, radiocontrast dyes, nutrients, and insect venoms (16).

A. Clinical Presentation

Anaphylactic reactions vary in presentation and severity. Clinical manifestations appear within minutes to a few hours after exposure to the offending agent.

1. Less serious reactions include flushing, erythematous rashes, urticaria, abdominal cramping, and diarrhea.

2. More severe reactions include angioedema, laryngeal edema, bronchospasm, and hypotension.

3. The most life-threatening reaction is rapid-onset cardiovascular collapse known as *anaphylactic shock*.

B. Management

1. *Epinephrine*

   Epinephrine blocks the release of inflammatory mediators from sensitized cells and is the drug of choice for severe anaphylactic reactions.

   a. Epinephrine is available in strengths of 1:100 (10 mg/mL), 1:1,000 (1 mg/mL), and 1:10,000 (0.1 mg/mL).

   b. For anaphylactic reactions other than anaphylactic shock, the usual dose of epinephrine is 0.3–0.5 mg (or 0.3–0.5 mL of 1:1000 solution) by deep IM injection in the thigh.

   c. For laryngeal edema, epinephrine can be nebulized using an inhalant made up of 0.25 mL of the 1:100 strength epinephrine solution added to 2 mL isotonic saline.

   d. For anaphylactic shock, epinephrine is given intravenously (see later).

2. *Histamine Blockers*

   Histamine blockers have little effect in preventing or speeding the resolution of anaphylactic reactions, but they can help to relieve pruritis in skin reactions. The histamine H_1 blocker **diphenhydramine** (25–50 mg PO, IM, or IV) is a popular choice for alleviating pruritis.

3. *Steroids*

a. Twenty percent of anaphylactic reactions recur within 1 to 8 hours after the initial symptoms have resolved (16).

b. Steroids are used primarily to reduce the risk of these recurrent or "second-phase" reactions, but the response is inconsistent (16).

c. **Prednisone** (50 mg PO) or **methylprednisolone** (125 mg IV) are equivalent in efficacy and can be repeated every 6 hours when second-phase reactions appear.

4. *Bronchodilators*

Inhaled β_2-agonists (e.g., **albuterol**, 2.5 mL of 0.5% solution via nebulizer) can be used as an adjunct to epinephrine for persistent bronchospasm.

C. Anaphylactic Shock

Anaphylactic shock is a life-threatening condition that requires prompt intervention using the following measures (16):

1. **Epinephrine** is given intravenously in a dose of 0.3–0.5 mg (3–5 mL of a 1:10,000 dilution). This can be followed by an epinephrine infusion of 2–8 µg/min.

a. For patients treated with β-receptor antagonists, the response to epinephrine may be attenuated. In this situation, **glucagon** (5–15 µg/min by intravenous infusion) can prove beneficial by producing sympathomimetic effects that are independent of β-receptor stimulation (16). (See Chapter 46 for a description of glucagon use in β-blocker overdose).

2. Aggressive volume resuscitation is important in anaphylactic shock because there is profound systemic vasodilation (creating a relative hypovolemia) often accompanied by extravasation of plasma. Either colloid or crystalloid fluids can be used.

3. Persistent hypotension can be managed with **dopamine**

(starting at 5 µg/kg/min) or **norepinephrine** (starting at 2 µg/min). (See Chapter 45 for more information on these vasopressor agents).

REFERENCES

1. Fujishima S, Aikawa N. Neutrophil-mediated tissue injury and its modulation. Intensive Care Med 1995; 21:277–285.

2. Pinsky MR, Matuschak GM. Multiple systems organ failure: failure of host defense mechanisms. Crit Care Clin 1989; 5:199–220.

3. Pinsky MR. Multiple systems organ failure: malignant intravascular inflammation. Crit Care Clin 1989; 5:195–198.

4. American College of Chest Physicians/Society of Critical Care Medicine Consensus Conference Committee. Definitions of sepsis and organ failure and guidelines for the use of innovative therapies in sepsis. Chest 1992; 101:1644–1655.

5. Pittet D, Rangel-Frausto S, Li N, et al. Systemic inflammatory response syndrome, sepsis, severe sepsis, and septic shock: incidence, morbidities and outcomes in surgical ICU patients. Intensive Care Med 1995; 21:302–309.

6. Rangel-Frausto MS, Pittet D, Costigan M, et al. Natural history of the systemic inflammatory response syndrome (SIRS). JAMA 1995; 273:117–123.

7. Angus DC, Linde-Zwirble WT, Lidicker J, et al. Epidemiology of severe sepsis in the United States: Analysis of incidence, outcome, and associated costs of care. Crit Care Med 2001; 29:1303–1310.

8. Vincent J-L, de Mendonca A, Cantraine F, et al. Use of the SOFA score to assess the incidence of organ dysfunction/failure in intensive care units: Results of a multicenter, prospective study. Crit Care Med 1998; 26:1793–1800.

9. Balk RA. Severe sepsis and septic shock. Definitions, epidemiology, and clinical manifestations. Crit Care Clin 2000; 16:179–192.

10. Friedman C, Silva E, Vincent J-L. Has the mortality of septic shock changed with time? Crit Care Med 1998; 26:2078–2086.

11. Dellinger RP, Carlet JM, Masur H, et al. Surviving Sepsis Campaign guidelines for management of severe sepsis and septic shock. Crit Care Med 2004; 32:858–873.

12. Rivers E, Nguyen B, Havstad S, et al. Early goal-directed therapy in the treatment of severe sepsis and septic shock. N Engl J Med 2001; 345:1368–1377.

13. Hughes WH, Armstrong D, Bodey GP, et al. 2002 guidelines for the use of antimicrobial agents in neutropenic patients with cancer. Clin Infect Dis 2002; 34:730–751.

14. Sair M, Etherington PJ, Winlove CP, Evans TW. Tissue oxygenation and perfusion in patients with systemic sepsis. Crit Care Med 2001; 29:1343–1349.

15. Fink MP. Cytopathic hypoxia. Mitochondrial dysfunction as mechanism contributing to organ dysfunction in sepsis. Crit Care Clin 2001; 17:219–237.

16. Ellis AK, Day JH. Diagnosis and management of anaphylaxis. Can Med Assoc J 2003; 169:307–311.

Chapter 34

PNEUMONIA IN THE ICU

Pneumonia is the most common infection acquired in the ICU (see Table 32.4), but the prevalence is overstated because postmortem studies show that over 50% of cases of ICU-acquired pneumonia are false-positive diagnoses (see later). This points to one of the major problems in the approach to pneumonia; i.e., there is no "gold standard" method for the clinical diagnosis of pneumonia. This chapter will describe the variety of diagnostic approaches to ICU-acquired pneumonia, and some empiric antimicrobial regimens for suspected cases of pneumonia. The final section describes a preventive approach to pneumonia that deserves more attention.

I. CLINICAL FEATURES

A. Ventilator-Associated Pneumonia

1. Over 90% of ICU-acquired pneumonias occur during mechanical ventilation (1), and thus most of the information in this chapter pertains to *ventilator-associated pneumonia* (VAP). About 50% of cases of VAP occur in the first 4 days after intubation (1).

2. The predominant pathogens in VAP are *Staphylococcus aureus, Pseudomonas aeruginosa*, and other gram-negative aerobic bacilli (see Table 34.1) (2). These pathogens are believed to originate from colonization of the oropharynx (see later).

3. The mortality rate in VAP varies from as high as 50% (1) to as low as zero (3) in different reports. This variability probably reflects the lack of uniform diagnostic criteria for VAP.

TABLE 34.1 Pathogens Implicated in Ventilator-Associated Pneumonia

Organism	Frequency
Bacilli	**56.5%**
Pseudomonas aeruginosa	18.9%
Escherichia coli	9.2%
Hemophilus spp.	7.1%
Enterobacter spp.	3.8%
Proteus spp.	3.8%
Klebsiella pneumoniae	3.2%
Others	10.5%
Cocci	**42.1%**
Staphylococcus aureus	18.9%
Streptococcus pneumoniae	13.2%
Enterococcus faecalis	1.4%
Others	8.6%
Fungi	**1.3%**

From Reference 2.

B. Clinical Manifestations

1. Bacterial pneumonias typically present with fever, leukocytosis, purulent sputum production, and a new infiltrate on the chest x-ray. However, these clinical manifestations are nonspecific in ventilator-dependent patients.

2. In ventilator-dependent patients who are suspected of having pneumonia based on clinical findings (the pres-

ence of a pulmonary infiltrate plus any combination of fever, leukocytosis, or purulent sputum production), the actual incidence of pneumonia on postmortem exam is only 30% to 40% (4).

3. Pneumonia accounts for only 1/3 of all pulmonary infiltrates in ICU patients (5,6). The noninfectious causes of pulmonary infiltrates include pulmonary edema, acute respiratory distress syndrome (ARDS), and atelectasis.

4. Because of the nonspecific nature of the clinical presentation, the diagnosis of VAP is not possible based on the clinical presentation.

II. DIAGNOSTIC EVALUATION

The diagnosis of pneumonia requires isolation of pathogenic organisms. The variety of methods used for this purpose are described next.

A. Blood Cultures

1. Blood cultures have a limited value in the diagnosis of VAP because they are positive in only 25% of cases with suspected VAP (1), and the isolated pathogens can originate from extrapulmonary sites (7).

B. Tracheal Aspirates

1. *Qualitative Cultures*
   a. Qualitative cultures of respiratory secretions aspirated through an endotracheal or tracheostomy tube have a high sensitivity (usually >90%) but a very low specificity (15 to 40%) for the diagnosis of VAP (8).
   b. When using qualitative cultures, *a negative tracheal aspirate (TA) culture can be used to exclude the diagnosis of*

VAP, but a positive culture can not be used to confirm the diagnosis of VAP.

TABLE 34.2 Quantitative Cultures for the Diagnosis of Pneumonia*

	Method of Specimen Collection		
	TA	**PSB**	**BAL**
Diagnostic Threshold (cfu/mL)	10^5 to 10^6	10^3	10^4 to 10^5
Sensitivity (mean)	76%	66%	73%
Specificity (mean)	75%	90%	82%
Relative Performance	Most Sensitive	Most Specific	Most Reliable

*Data pertain to the diagnosis of ventilator-assisted pneumonia.
Abbreviations: TA = tracheal aspirates, PSB = protected specimen brushings, BAL = bronchoalveolar lavage.
From References 1,8,10.

2. *Quantitative Cultures*

For quantitative cultures, growth is reported as the number of colony-forming units per mL (cfu/mL). To obtain quantitative TA cultures, at least 1 mL of a TA sample should be collected in a sterile trap without adding saline.

a. The threshold for a positive TA culture is 10^5 to 10^6 cfu/mL. The lower threshold is used for samples obtained during antibiotic therapy (1).

b. As shown in Table 34.2, quantitative TA cultures have a sensitivity and specificity of 76% and 75%, respectively, for the diagnosis of VAP (1,8).

c. Thus, quantitative TA cultures are less sensitive, but more specific, than qualitative TA cultures for the diagnosis of VAP.

C. Protected Specimen Brush

The protected specimen brush (PSB) is passed through a bronchoscope to collect secretions from the distal airways (the brush is enclosed in a catheter to protect it from contamination as it is passes through the bronchoscope). PSB specimens are cultured quantitatively.

1. The threshold for a positive PSB culture is 10^3 cfu/mL (1).

2. As shown in Table 34.2, positive PSB cultures have the highest specificity (90%) of any culture method used for the diagnosis of VAP (1,8). *A positive PSB culture confirms the presence of pneumonia with 90% certainty.* However, a negative PSB culture does not exclude the presence of pneumonia (sensitivity only 66%).

C. Bronchoalveolar Lavage

Bronchoalveolar lavage (BAL) is performed by wedging the bronchoscope in a distal airway and lavaging the distal lung segment with sterile (isotonic) saline. The minimum lavage volume is 120 mL (9), and less than 25% of the instilled volume is returned. BAL cultures are performed quantitatively.

1. *Quantitative Cultures*
   a. The threshold for a positive BAL culture is 10^4 to 10^5 cfu/mL (the lower threshold is for patients who are on antibiotic therapy) (1).
   b. As shown in Table 34.2, BAL cultures are neither more sensitive nor more specific than the other culture methods (1,10). However, when sensitivity and specificity are considered together, *BAL cultures have the highest overall reliability for the diagnosis of VAP.*

2. *Intracellular Organisms*

Inspection of BAL specimens for intracellular organisms

can help in guiding initial antibiotic therapy until culture results are available.

a. *When intracellular organisms are present in more than 3% of the cells in the lavage fluid, the likelihood of pneumonia is over 90%* (11).

3. **BAL Without Bronchoscopy**

BAL can be performed without bronchoscopy by inserting BAL catheters through tracheal tubes and advancing the catheters blindly until they are wedged in the lower airways. A variety of catheters and techniques have been tested (see References 12 and 13).

a. In general, the sensitivity and specificity of nonbronchoscopic BAL cultures are equivalent to those of cultures from bronchoscopic BAL specimens (1,14).

D. Which Culture Method is Preferred?

There is little agreement about which culture method is preferred for the diagnosis of VAP. The following points are pertinent.

1. The diagnostic yield from all culture methods is adversely affected by ongoing antibiotic therapy (1). When possible, cultures should be obtained before antibiotics are started.

2. If tracheal aspirates are cultured, quantitative cultures are preferred to qualitative cultures because of the higher specificity. The low specificity of qualitative cultures means that *treatment based on qualitative cultures of tracheal aspirates will result in excessive use of antibiotics* (1,15).

3. PSB cultures are the most reliable for confirming the diagnosis of pneumonia, while BAL cultures are the most reliable for confirming *and* excluding the diagnosis of pneumonia.

4. For those interested in evidence-based practice, *there is no evidence that any culture method has an impact on survival in VAP* (1,15).

III. ANTIMICROBIAL THERAPY

Antibiotic treatment for pneumonia accounts for half of all antibiotic use in the ICU (16). However, 60% of antibiotic use for pneumonias involve suspected pneumonias that are not confirmed by bacteriologic studies (16). This latter observation highlights the importance of discontinuing antibiotics when culture results do not confirm the presence of pneumonia.

A. Empiric Antimicrobial Therapy

The choice of empiric antibiotics should be dictated by the likelihood that the patient's oropharynx is colonized with *Staphylococcus aureus* and gram-negative aerobic bacilli (the same pathogens listed in Table 34.1). The types of patients who are likely and unlikely to be colonized with these pathogens is shown in Table 34.3, along with recommended empiric antibiotic regimens for each type of patient. The recommended starting doses for each antibiotic are shown in Table 34.4.

1. *Colonization Unlikely*

    a. The typical patient who is not colonized by the pathogens in Table 34.1 has been admitted recently (within 5 days) from home, has no debilitating chronic illness (e.g., renal failure that requires dialysis), and has no other hospital admissions in the past 3 months (1).

    b. Patients like this can be treated with a single antibiotic like ceftriaxone or a quinolone (levofloxacin or moxifloxacin). This treatment is similar to the treatment of community-acquired pneumonia (17).

TABLE 34.3 Empiric Therapy of Ventilator-Associated Pneumonia Based on Likelihood of Colonization with Pathogenic Organisms

Colonization Unlikely	Colonization Likely
Type of Patient	**Type of Patient**
Admitted <5 days ago and	Admitted <5 days ago, or
Admitted from home, and	Admitted from a nursing home, or
No other admissions in past 3 mos., &	Other admissions in past 3 mos., or
Not a dialysis patient.	A dialysis patient.
Empiric Antibiotics	**Empiric Antibiotics**
Ceftriaxone or a quinolone	Pipericillin tazobactam, or
	Carbepenem, or
	Ceftazidime or cefepime
	plus
	Vancomycin or linezolid[†]
	and consider
	Quinolone or aminoglycoside*

[†]When colonization with methicillin-resistant *S. aureus* is likely.
*Double coverage for *Pseudomonas aeruginosa*.
From Reference 1.

2. *Colonization Likely*

   a. Colonization of the oropharynx with the pathogens in Table 34.1 is likely in nursing home residents, in patients who have been in the hospital for 5 days or longer, in patients with a chronic debilitating illness, and in patients with multiple hospital admissions.

   b. The empiric antibiotic regimen for these patients, which is shown in Table 34.4, is designed to cover staphylococci (particularly methicillin-resistant *S. aureus*—MRSA) and gram-negative aerobic bacilli (particularly *Pseudomonas aeruginosa*).

   The empiric regimen I favor is **meropenem** (covers most gram-positive and gram-negative pathogens except MRSA) and **vancomycin** (for gram-positive coverage, including MRSA) or **linezolid** (if vancomycin resistance is a problem).

TABLE 34.4 Initiating Therapy with Empiric Antibiotics

Antibiotic	Intravenous Dose*
Aminoglycosides	
Gentamicin	7 mg/kg once daily
Tobramycin	7 mg/kg once daily
Amikacin	20 mg/kg once daily
Antistaphylococcal agents	
Vancomycin	15 mg/kg every 12 hrs
Linezolid	600 mg/kg every 12 hrs
ß-Lactam/ß-lactamase inhibitor	
Pipericillin/tazobactam	4.5 g every 6 hrs
Carbapenem	
Imipenem	1 g every 8 hrs
Meropenem	1 g every 8 hrs
Cephalosporins	
Ceftriaxone	2 g every 12 hrs
Cefepime	1–2 g every 8–12 hrs
Ceftazidime	2 g every 8 hrs
Quinolones	
Levofloxacin	750 mg once daily
Ciprofloxacin	400 mg every 8 hrs

*Dose recommendations from Reference 1, and pertain only to patients with normal renal and hepatic function. For dose recommendations in renal and hepatic insufficiency, see Chapter 44.

  c. Double coverage for *Pseudomonas aeruginosa* (by adding a quinolone or aminoglycoside) is sometimes recommended for empiric antibiotic coverage (1). However, the benefit of this practice in immunocompetent patients is not supported by clinical studies (18).

B. Duration of Antimicrobial Therapy

1. Empiric antibiotics should be discontinued if all cultures are sterile.

2. For cases of VAP documented by culture, the traditional duration of antibiotic therapy has been 14 to 21 days (1). However, 8 days of antibiotic therapy for VAP has the same clinical outcome as 15 days of therapy (2).

3. The popular opinion at present is that one week of antibiotic therapy is adequate for most ICU-acquired pneumonias.

IV. ORAL DECONTAMINATION

A. Colonization of the Oropharynx

1. The oropharynx is normally colonized with saprophytic organisms that do little harm (other than producing bad breath).

2. In critically ill patients, the oropharynx becomes colonized with pathogenic organisms like those listed in Table 34.1, and aspiration of these organisms into the upper airway is believed to be the inciting event in the development of VAP (19).

3. The importance of colonization of the oropharynx in the pathogenesis of VAP has led to clinical studies evaluating the role of oropharyngeal decontamination as a preventive measure for VAP (see next).

B. Decontamination Regimens

Clinical studies have shown that decontamination of the oral mucosa with the topical application of nonabsorbable antibiotics (20) or the antiseptic agent chlorhexidine (21) is an effective measure for reducing the incidence of VAP.

1. *Antibiotic Regimen*

   One successful antibiotic regimen consists of a methylcellulose paste (Orabase, Squibb Pharmaceuticals) containing **2% polymyxin, 2% tobramycin, and 2% amphotericin B,** which is applied to the inside of the mouth with a gloved finger every 6 hours (20). There is minimal absorption of these antimicrobial agents, so systemic toxicity is not a concern.

2. *Chlorhexidine Regimen*

   The fear of antimicrobial resistance has prompted an evaluation of the antiseptic agent chlorhexidine for oral decontamination.

   a. The use of **2% chlorhexidine** in petroleum jelly (Vaseline), applied to the oral mucosa every 6 hours, has proven successful in reducing the incidence of VAP (21).

   b. Because chlorhexidine is active primarily against gram-positive cocci, **2% colistin can be added** for enhanced gram-negative coverage (21). (Colistin has little therapeutic use, so acquired resistance to colistin will be less of a problem than acquired resistance to more commonly used antibiotics.)

3. *Recommendations*

   a. Oral decontamination is advised for any patient who is likely to be ventilator dependent for more than a few days, and it should be continued as long as the patient stays in the ICU.

   b. The regimen of choice for oral decontamination has yet to be determined. The chlorhexidine regimen (with or without colistin) has a theoretical advantage over the antibiotic regimen, but this advantage is unproven, and the clinical experience with chlorhexidine is limited.

REFERENCES

1. American Thoracic Society and Infectious Disease Society of America. Guidelines for the management of adults with hospital-acquired, ventilator-associated, and healthcare-associated pneumonia. Am J Respir Crit Care Med 2005; 171:388–416.

2. Chastre J, Wolff M, Fagon J-Y, et al. Comparison of 8 vs. 15 days of antibiotic therapy for ventilator-associated pneumonia in adults. JAMA 2003; 290:2588–2598.

3. Bregeon F, Cias V, Carret V, et al. Is ventilator-associated pneumonia an independent risk factor for death? Anesthesiology 2001; 94:554–560.

4. Wunderink RG. Clinical criteria in the diagnosis of ventilator-associated pneumonia. Chest 2000; 117: 191S–194S.

5. Louthan FB, Meduri GU. Differential diagnosis of fever and pulmonary densities in mechanically ventilated patients. Semin Resp Infect 1996; 11:77–95.

6. Singh N, Falestiny MN, Rogers P, et al. Pulmonary infiltrates in the surgical ICU. Chest 1998; 114:1129–1136.

7. Luna CM, Videla A, Mattera J, et al. Blood cultures have limited value in predicting severity of illness and as a diagnostic tool in ventilator-associated pneumonia. Chest 1999; 116:1075–1084.

8. Cook D, Mandell L. Endotracheal aspiration in the diagnosis of ventilator-associated pneumonia. Chest 2000; 117:195S–197S.

9. Meduri GU, Chastre J. The standardization of bronchoscopic techniques for ventilator-associated pneumonia. Chest 1992; 102:557S–564S.

10. Torres A, El-Ebiary M. Bronchoscopic BAL in the diagnosis of ventilator-associated pneumonia. Chest 2000; 117:198S–202S.

11. Veber B, Souweine B, Gachot B, et al. Comparison of direct examination of three types of bronchoscopy specimens used to diagnose nosocomial pneumonia. Crit Care Med 2000; 28:962–968.

12. Kollef MH, Bock KR, Richards RD, Hearns ML. The safety and diagnostic accuracy of minibronchoalveolar lavage in patients with suspected ventilator-associated pneumonia. Ann Intern Med 1995; 122:743–748.

13. Perkins GD, Chatterjee S, Giles S, et al. Safety and tolerability of nonbronchoscopic lavage in ARDS. Chest 2005; 127:1358–1363.

14. Campbell CD, Jr. Blinded invasive diagnostic procedures in ventilator-associated pneumonia. Chest 2000; 117:207S–211S.

15. Shorr AF, Sherner JH, Jackson WL, Kollef MH. Invasive ap-

proaches to the diagnosis of ventilator-associated pneumonia: a meta-analysis. Crit Care Med 2005; 33:46–53.

16. Bergmanns DCJJ, Bonten MJM, Gaillard CA, et al. Indications for antibiotic use in ICU patients: a one-year prospective surveillance. J Antimicrob Chemother 1997; 111:676–685.

17. American Thoracic Society. Guidelines for the management of adults with community-acquired pneumonia. Am J Respir Crit Care Med 2001; 163:1730–1754.

18. Cometta A, Baumgartner JD, Lew D, et al. Prospective, randomized comparison of imipenem monotherapy with imipenem plus netilmicin for treatment of severe infections in nonneutropenic patients. Antimicrob Agents Chemother 1994; 38:1309–1313.

19. Bonten MJM, Gaillard CA, de Leeuw PW, Stobberingh EE. Role of colonization of the upper intestinal tract in the pathogenesis of ventilator-associated pneumonia. Clin Infect Dis 1997; 24:309–319.

20. Bergmans C, Bonten M, Gaillard C, et al. Prevention of ventilator-associated pneumonia by oral decontamination. Am J Respir Crit Care Med 2001; 164:382–388.

21. Koeman M, van der Ven A, Hak E, et al. Oral decontamination with chlorhexidine reduces the incidence of ventilator-associated pneumonia. Am J Respir Crit Care Med 2006; 173:1348–1355.

Chapter 35

SEPSIS FROM THE ABDOMEN & PELVIS

The GI, biliary, and urinary tracts are important sources of sepsis in critically ill patients, and this chapter describes the conditions that generate this infectious risk.

I. BOWEL SEPSIS

The gastrointestinal (GI) tract is considered the single most important source of severe sepsis in ICU patients. In fact, the GI tract has been called the "motor" of multiorgan dysfunction associated inflammation and infection (1). Two conditions predispose to bowel sepsis in critically ill patients: bacterial colonization of the upper GI tract, and disruption of the bowel mucosa.

A. Gastric Colonization

1. Because bacteria do not thrive in an acidic environment (see Chapter 2, Figure 2.1), gastric acid helps to maintain a sterile environment in the stomach.

2. Loss of gastric acidity promotes colonization of the upper GI tract with pathogenic organisms, and this colonization may be responsible for the increased incidence of nosocomial pneumonia and postoperative sepsis associated with loss of gastric acidity (2,3).

B. Mucosal Disruption

1. Disruption of the mucosal barrier in the GI tract may be

common in critically ill patients, and the disrupted mucosa allows pathogens in the bowel lumen to gain access to the systemic circulation. This breach of the mucosal barrier is called *translocation*.

2. Translocation of intestinal bacteria has been documented in 15% of postoperative patients, and 40% of these patients develop postoperative sepsis (4).

3. Conditions that promote mucosal disruption and translocation include splanchnic hypoperfusion, bowel rest, and malnutrition.

C. Preventive Measures

1. *Avoid Acid-Suppressing Drugs*

   Limiting or avoiding the use of acid-suppressing drugs for stress ulcer prophylaxis will reduce the risk of gastric colonization with pathogenic organisms. The following strategies can help to achieve this goal.

   a. Restrict the prophylaxis of stress ulcer bleeding to the conditions listed in Table 2.1.

   b. Consider the cytoprotective agent sucralfate (which does not reduce gastric pH) as an alternative method of stress ulcer prophylaxis. (See Chapter 2, Sections II-C and II-D).

2. *Alimentary Decontamination*

   Decontamination of the alimentary canal (from mouth to anus) using the antibiotic regimen in Table 35.1 has been shown to reduce the incidence of nosocomial infections and reduce the mortality rate in critically ill patients (4). Unfortunately, the fear of antibiotic resistance has limited the popularity of this regimen.

TABLE 35.1 Selective Digestive Decontamination†

A. Oral Decontamination

Have the pharmacy make a paste containing 2% polymyxin E, 2% tobramycin, and 2% amphotericin B, and apply the paste (with a gloved finger) to the buccal mucosa four times daily.

B. GI Tract Decontamination

Give the following non-absorbable antibiotics orally or via a feeding tube four times daily:
1. Polymyxin E, 100 mg
2. Tobramycin, 80 mg
3. Amphotericin B, 500 mg

C. Systemic Prophylaxis

Give intravenous cefotaxime, 1 g every 6 hrs, for the first 4 days of the decontamination regimen.

---

†The term "selective" is used because this regimen does not eradicate the indigenous anaerobic flora of the alimentary tract.

From Reference 4.

II. *CLOSTRIDIUM DIFFICILE* COLITIS

A. Pathogenesis

1. Eradication of indigenous bowel flora from antibiotic use leads to colonization of the lower GI tract with pathogenic organisms, and the most troublesome intruder is *Clostridium difficile*, a spore-forming gram-positive anaerobic bacillus (5,6).

2. *C. difficile* is not usually invasive, but it elaborates cytotoxins that damage the bowel mucosa. The inflammatory response can result in plaque-like lesions called pseudomembranes, and these lesions are responsible for the term *pseudomembranous enterocolitis* that is sometimes applied to cases of *C. difficile* enterocolitis.

3. This pathogen is readily transmitted from patient to patient, usually via the hands of hospital personnel. As a result, as many as 40% of hospitalized patients can harbor *C. difficile* in their stool (7); most are asymptomatic.

B. Clinical Presentation

1. Symptomatic *C. difficile* colitis usually presents with fever, abdominal pain, and watery diarrhea. Bloody diarrhea is seen in 5 to 10% of cases.

2. A rare presentation is toxic megacolon, which is characterized by abdominal distension, ileus, and clinical shock. This can be fatal and requires emergent subtotal colectomy (8).

C. Diagnosis

1. The diagnosis of *C. difficile* enterocolitis requires laboratory tests for the presence of the cytotoxins in stool. (Stool cultures are unreliable because they do not distinguish toxigenic from nontoxigenic strains of the organism.)

2. Most laboratories use an ELISA (enzyme-linked immunosorbent assay) method to detect the cytotoxins. The sensitivity of this test is about 85% for one stool specimen and up to 95% for 2 stool specimens (5,6,9). The specificity of this test is up to 98% (6), so false-positive results are uncommon.

3. Direct visualization of the lower GI mucosa is indicated for the few cases of suspected *C. difficile* enterocolitis where the toxin assay is negative. The presence of pseudomembranes confirms the diagnosis. Colonoscopy is preferred to proctosigmoidoscopy for optimal results.

D. Treatment

The first step in treatment is to discontinue the offending antibiotic(s) if possible. Antibiotic therapy to eradicate *C. difficile* is recommended if the diarrhea is severe and associated with signs of systemic inflammation (fever, leukocytosis, etc.) The following recommendations are standard practice (5,6,10,11).

1. Oral or intravenous **metronidazole** (500 mg three times daily) is the treatment of choice, and should be continued for 10 days. The oral route is preferred, but both routes are equally effective.

2. Oral **vancomycin** (125 mg four times daily) is as effective as metronidazole, but is used as a second-line agent because of the efforts to curtail vancomycin use and limit the emergence of vancomycin-resistant enterococci and staphylococci. Vancomycin is not effective when given intravenously.

3. *Antiperistaltic agents are contraindicated* (5,11) because reduced peristalsis can prolong exposure to the cytotoxins.

4. The expected response is loss of fever by 24 hours and resolution of diarrhea in 4 to 5 days (5). Most patients show a favorable response. For the few who do not respond by 3 to 5 days, a switch from metronidazole to vancomycin is indicated.

5. Relapses following antibiotic treatment occur in about 25% of cases (5,6,9). Most relapses are evident within 3 weeks after antibiotic therapy is completed. Repeat therapy using the same antibiotic is successful in about 75% of relapses, and another relapse is expected in about 25% of cases (11). A few (5%) patients experience more than 6 relapses (5).

III. ACALCULOUS CHOLECYSTITIS

Acalculous cholecystitis is a condition that could be described as an ileus of the gallbladder.

A. Clinical Features

1. Conditions that predispose to acalculous cholecystitis include circulatory shock, trauma, parenteral nutrition, abdominal surgery, and opioid analgesia (12,13).

2. Clinical manifestations can include fever, nausea and vomiting, abdominal pain, and right upper quadrant tenderness. Abdominal findings can be minimal or absent, and fever may be the only manifestation.

3. Laboratory studies can show elevated blood levels of bilirubin, alkaline phosphatase, and amylase, but these findings are variable and nonspecific (12,13).

B. Diagnosis & Management

1. Ultrasound examination of the right upper quadrant shows gallbladder sludge and distension of the gallbladder. More specific findings include a gallbladder wall thickness of at least 3.5 mm and submucosal edema (12,13). If ultrasound visualization is hampered, computed tomography (CT) is a suitable alternative.

2. Prompt intervention is necessary. Rupture of the gallbladder occurs in 40% of cases when treatment is delayed for 48 hours or longer after the onset of symptoms (12).

3. The treatment of choice is cholecystectomy, but percutaneous cholecystostomy is a suitable alternative for patients who are too unstable for surgery.

IV. ABDOMINAL ABSCESS

A. Clinical Features

1. Abdominal abscess is a consideration in any case of unexplained sepsis following blunt abdominal trauma or abdominal surgery (14,15).

2. The clinical examination is often unrevealing. Localized abdominal tenderness is present in only one-third of cases, and a palpable abdominal mass is present in fewer than 10% of cases (15).

B. Diagnosis and Treatment

1. Routine films of the abdomen show extraluminal air or air-fluid levels in fewer than 15% of cases (15).

2. Computed tomography (CT) of the abdomen is the diagnostic procedure of choice, with a sensitivity and specificity ≥90% (14,15). CT imaging in the first few postoperative days can be misleading because collections of blood or irrigant solutions in the peritoneal cavity can be misread as an abscess.

3. Immediate drainage is mandatory for all abdominal abscesses (16). Many abscesses can be drained percutaneously following CT-guided insertion of drainage catheters.

4. Empiric antibiotic therapy is recommended pending the results of abscess fluid cultures. Single-drug therapy with **ampicillin–sulbactam** (Unasyn) or **imipenem** is as effective as multiple-drug regimens (17).

V. URINARY TRACT INFECTIONS

Urinary tract infection (UTI) accounts for 30% of ICU-acquired infections, and 95% of UTIs occur in patients with indwelling urethral catheters (18). The following material applies to UTI in the catheterized patient.

A. Diagnostic Criteria

The criteria for the diagnosis of UTI in catheterized patients are shown in Table 35.2 (19,20).

1. *Clinical Findings*

The diagnosis of UTI based on urine cultures alone is misleading in catheterized patients because half of these patients have positive urine cultures after 5 days, and virtually all patients have positive urine cultures after 30 days (19).

a. The usual manifestations of UTI in catheterized patients are fever and/or suprapubic tenderness (see Table 35.2).

b. About 50% of elderly patients develop a change in mental status in association with UTIs (21).

2. *Urine Cultures*

The threshold for significant bacteriuria in catheterized patients is 10^5 colony-forming units per mL (cfu/mL). However, colony counts as low as 10^2 cfu/mL can represent infection if growth is sustained in more than one urine sample (collected on different days) (22).

3. *Urine Microscopy*

Urine microscopy is diagnostic only if an unspun urine specimen shows organisms on Gram stain or at least 3 leukocytes per high-powered field.

TABLE 35.2 Diagnostic Criteria for UTI in Catheterized Patients

I. One of the following must be present:
- Body temperature >38° C
- Suprapubic tenderness

AND

II. Urine culture grows ≥10^5 cfu/mL, with no more than 2 pathogens isolated.

OR

III. One of the following is present:
- Positive urine dipstick for leukocyte esterase or nitrates
- ≥3 WBCs per high-power field in unspun urine sample
- Organisms present on Gram stain in unspun urine sample
- 2 urine cultures with ≥10^2 cfu/mL of the same organism

From References 19,20.

B. Empiric Antibiotics

Empiric antibiotic therapy is recommended for patients with suspected UTI who are immunocompromised, have evidence of multiorgan dysfunction, or have a prosthetic or damaged heart valve.

1. *Microbiology*

The predominant pathogens in UTI are gram-negative aerobic bacilli. Enterococci and staphylococci are isolated in 15% and 5% of cases, respectively (18). *Candida albicans* is isolated in 20% of urine cultures, but almost 50% of cases of candiduria are asymptomatic (18) and might not represent infection.

2. *Recommendations*

The urine Gram stain should be used to guide antibiotic selection. The following are some suggestions.

a. **Imipenem** or **meropenem** should suffice for empiric coverage of gram-negative bacilli.

b. Gram-positive cocci on Gram stain of urine are most likely enterococci. If the patient is not seriously ill, enterococcal UTI can be treated effectively with **ciprofloxacin**. In seriously ill patients or those with a risk of endocarditis, ampicillin or **vancomycin** is preferred (add gentamicin if endocarditis is a risk). Ampicillin resistance is reported in 10 to 15% of nosocomial enterococcal infections (23), so vancomycin may be the better choice. If vancomycin-resistant enterococci are a concern, **linezolid** is an appropriate choice. (See Chapter 44 for more information on linezolid).

C. Candiduria

The presence of *Candida* in the urine often represents colonization, but candiduria can also be a sign of disseminated candidiasis (the candiduria in this case is the result, not the cause, of the disseminated candidiasis). Disseminated candidiasis can be an elusive diagnosis because blood cultures are sterile in more than 50% of cases (24), and candiduria may be the only sign of disseminated disease. The following recommendations are from recent guidelines published by the Infectious Disease Society of America (25).

1. Asymptomatic candiduria in immunocompetent patients does not require antifungal therapy. However, the urinary catheter should be removed if possible because this can eradicate candiduria in 40% of cases (26).

2. Candiduria should be treated in symptomatic patients (i.e., fever or suprapubic tenderness), and patients with neutropenia or a renal allograft.

3. Persistent candiduria in immunocompromised patients should prompt further investigation with ultrasonography of CT images of the kidney.

4. *Antifungal Therapy*

   a. For non-neutropenic patients with symptomatic candiduria, **fluconazole** (200 to 400 mg daily) for 7 to 14 days is often effective.

   b. For patients with renal insufficiency or for infection with species other than *Candida albicans*, the new antifungal agent **capsofungin** (50 mg daily) is a reasonable choice (see Chapter 44 for a description of capsofungin).

   c. For all other patients, **amphotericin B** (0.3 to 1 mg/kg daily) for 1 to 7 days can be effective in eradicating organisms (more prolonged therapy is needed for disseminated candidiasis). Bladder irrigation with amphotericin B is not recommended because recurrence of candiduria is common (25).

REFERENCES

1. Leaphart CL, Tepas JJ. The gut is a motor of organ system dysfunction. Surgery 2007; 141:563–569.

2. Messori A, Trippoli S, Vaiani M, et al. Bleeding and pneumonia in intensive care patients given ranitidine and sucralfate for prevention of stress ulcer: meta-analysis of randomized controlled trials. Br Med J 2000; 321:1–7.

3. MacFie J, Reddy BS, Gatt M, et al. Bacterial translocation studied in 927 patients over 13 years. Br J Surg 2006; 93:87–93.

4. de Jonge, Schultz MJ, Spanjaard PMM, et al. Effects of selective decontamination of the digestive tract on mortality and acquisition of resistant bacteria in intensive care: a randomised controlled trial. Lancet 2003; 362:1011–1016.

5. Bartlett JG. Antibiotic-associated diarrhea. N Engl J Med 2002; 346:334-339.

6. Mylonakis E, Ryan ET, Calderwood SB. *Clostridium difficile*-associated diarrhea. Arch Intern Med 2001; 161:525–533.

7. Fekety R, Kim F-H, Brown D, et al. Epidemiology of antibiotic associated colitis. Am J Med 1981; 70:906–908.

8. Lipsett PA, Samantaray DK, Tam ML, et al. Pseudomembranous colitis: A surgical disease? Surgery 1994; 116:491–496.

9. Yassin SF, Young-Fadok TM, Zein NN, Pardi DS. *Clostridium difficile*-associated diarrhea and colitis. Mayo Clin Proc 2001; 76:725–730.

10. Guerrant RL, Van Gilder T, Steiner TS, et al. Practice guidelines for the management of infectious diarrhea. Infectious Disease Society of America. Clin Infect Dis 2001; 32:331–350.

11. Aslam S, Hamill RJ, Musher DM. Treatment of *Clostridium difficile*-associated disease: old therapies and new strategies. Lancet Infect Dis 2005; 5:549–557.

12. Walden D, Urrutia F, Soloway RD. Acute acalculous cholecystitis. J Intensive Care Med 1994; 9:235–243.

13. Imhof M, Raunest J, Ohmann Ch, Rohrer H-D. Acute acalculous cholecystitis complicating trauma: a prospective sonographic study. World J Surg 1992; 1160–1166.

14. Mirvis SE, Shanmuganthan K. Trauma radiology: part I. Computerized tomographic imaging of abdominal trauma. J Intensive Care Med 1994; 9:151–163.

15. Fry DE. Noninvasive imaging tests in the diagnosis and treatment of intra-abdominal abscesses in the postoperative patient. Surg Clin North Am 1994; 74:693–709.

16. Oglevie SB, Casola G, van Sonnenberg E, et al. Percutaneous abscess drainage: current applications for critically ill patients. J Intensive Care Med 1994; 9:191–206.

17. Mosdell DM, Morris DM, Voltura A, et al. Antibiotic treatment for surgical peritonitis. Ann Surg 1991; 214:543–549.

18. Richards MJ, Edwards JR, Culver D, Gaynes RP. Nosocomial infections in medical intensive care units in the United States. Crit Care Med 1999; 27:887–892.

19. Calandra T, Cohen J, for the International Sepsis Forum Definition of Infection in the ICU Consensus Conference. Crit Care Med 2005; 33:1538–1548.

20. Garner JS, Jarvis WR, Emori TG, et al. CDC definitions for nosocomial infections, 1988. Am J Infect Control 1988; 16:128–140.

21. McCue JD. How to manage urinary tract infections in the elderly. J Crit Illness 1996; 11(Suppl):S30–S40.

22. Stamm WE, Hooten TM. Management of urinary tract infection in adults. N Engl J Med 1993; 329:1328–1334.

23. Jenkins SG. Changing spectrum of uropathogens: implications for treating complicated UTIs. J Crit Illness 1996; 11(Suppl):S7–S13.

24. British Society for Antimicrobial Chemotherapy Working Party. Management of deep *Candida* infection in surgical and intensive

care unit patients. Intensive Care Med 1994; 20:522–528.

25. Pappas PG, Rex JH, Sobel JD, et al. Guidelines for treatment of candidiasis. Infectious Disease Society of America. Clin Infect Dis 2004; 38:161–189.

26. Sobel JD, Kauffman CA, McKinsey D, et al. Candiduria: a randomized double-blind study of treatment with fluconazole or placebo. Clin Infect Dis 2000; 30:19–24.

Chapter 36

NUTRITIONAL REQUIREMENTS

Although neglected in most medical school programs, nutritional support is an integral part of patient care in the ICU. The next 3 chapters will introduce you to the fundamentals of nutritional support for ICU patients. This chapter describes the daily nutritional needs of the critically ill patient.

I. DAILY ENERGY EXPENDITURE

A. Oxidation of Nutrient Fuels

1. The business of oxidative metabolism is to use the energy stored in nutrient fuels (carbohydrates, lipids, and proteins) to perform the work needed to sustain the organism. This process consumes oxygen, and generates carbon dioxide, water, and heat. Table 36.1 shows the quantities involved in the oxidation of one gram of each nutrient fuel (carbohydrate, lipid, protein). The following points deserve mention.

   a. The energy yield (in kcal per gram) of each nutrient fuel is equivalent to the heat production associated with the complete oxidation of one gram of substrate.

   b. Lipids have the highest energy yield (9.1 kcal/gram), while glucose has the lowest energy yield (3.7 kcal/gram).

2. The summed metabolism of all three nutrient fuels determines the whole-body O_2 consumption (VO_2), CO_2 production (VCO_2), and heat production for any given time period. The 24-hour heat production is then equivalent to

the daily energy requirement (in kcal) for each patient. This daily energy requirement can be calculated or measured, as described next.

TABLE 36.1 Oxidative Metabolism of Nutrient Fuels

Substrate	Liters O_2 Consumed	Liters CO_2 Produced	kcal Heat Produced[†]
Glucose (1 gram)	0.74	0.74	3.7
Lipid (1 gram)	2	1.4	9.1
Protein (1 gram)	0.96	0.78	4

[†]Used as the energy yield (kcal per gram) for each nutrient fuel.

B. Predictive Equations

1. *Healthy Adults*

   a. The standard equations used to predict daily energy requirements are taken from experiments in healthy adults (1), and are based on height (in inches), weight (in kg), and age (see Table 36.2).

   b. Daily energy expenditure is expressed as *basal energy expenditure* (BEE), which is the heat production of basal metabolism in the resting and fasted state.

   c. Both actual and ideal body weight have been used when these equations are applied to ICU patients (2). In edematous patients, ideal body weight (or pre-edematous body weight) seems most appropriate.

2. *ICU Patients*

   a. The BEE in ICU patients is usually estimated by calculating the BEE for healthy adults and adding at least 20% to account for the stress of critical illness. Adjustments of BEE that exceed 20% often lead to overestimates of daily energy expenditure (2).

b. An alternative (and much easier) method for estimating the BEE in ICU patients is shown below :

$$\textbf{BEE (kcal/day)} = \textbf{25} \times \textbf{weight (in kg)} \qquad (36.1)$$

This simplified method has proven to be remarkably accurate for most ICU patients (3).

c. The daily energy expenditure in ICU patients can vary widely (4), so measurements of daily energy expenditure are superior to predictive equations.

TABLE 36.2 Equations for Estimating Basal Energy Expenditure

Healthy Men
BEE (kcal/24 h) = 66 + [13.7 x wt (kg)] + [5.0 x ht (in)] − (6.7 x age)

Healthy Women
BEE (kcal/24 h) = 655 + [9.6 x wt (kg)] + [1.8 x ht (in)] − (4.7 x age)

ICU Patients
BEE (kcal/24 h) = 25 x wt (kg)

Abbreviations: BEE = basal energy expenditure, wt = weight, ht = height.
From References 1 and 3.

C. Indirect Calorimetry

1. *The Principle*

It is not possible to measure metabolic heat production in clinical practice, so daily energy expenditure is measured indirectly by measuring the whole-body VO_2 and VCO_2 (5,6). The *resting energy expenditure* (REE) is then determined using the following equation (6):

$$\textbf{REE} = \textbf{(3.6} \times \textbf{VO}_2\textbf{)} + \textbf{(1.1} \times \textbf{VCO}_2\textbf{)} - \textbf{61} \qquad (36.2)$$

The REE (in kcal/min) is multiplied by 1440 (the number of minutes in 24 hours) to derive the 24-hour (daily) energy expenditure. This method of measuring daily energy expenditure is called *indirect calorimetry*.

2. *Methodology*

Indirect calorimetry is performed with specially designed "metabolic carts" that measure the whole-body VO_2 and VCO_2 directly (i.e., by measuring the concentrations of O_2 and CO_2 in inhaled and exhaled gas), and then calculate and display the REE using Equation 36.2. The steady-state REE is usually measured for 15 to 30 minutes, and the 24-hour energy expenditure is extrapolated as just described.

a. Indirect calorimetry is usually performed on intubated patients (although it can be used in spontaneously breathing patients).

b. The O_2 sensor in metabolic carts is not reliable at inspired O_2 levels above 50%, so indirect calorimetry is not advised for patients who require more than 50% O_2 in inhaled gas (5).

II. SUBSTRATE REQUIREMENTS

A. Nonprotein Intake

The daily energy requirements should be provided entirely by *nonprotein calories*.

1. *Carbohydrates*

Standard nutritional regimens use simple carbohydrates (dextrose) to provide 70% of the daily energy requirements. The relative abundance of carbohydrate intake compensates for the the limited stores of endogenous carbohydrates. As demonstrated in Table 36.3, endogenous carbohydrates (stored as glycogen) provide only 900 kcal in the fasting state.

TABLE 36.3 Endogenous Fuel Stores in Healthy Adults

Fuel Source	Amount (kg)	Energy Yield (kcal)
Adipose tissue fat	15.0	141,000
Muscle protein	6.0	24,000
Total glycogen	0.09	900
		165,900

Data from Cahill GF Jr. N Engl J Med 1970; 282:668–675.

2. *Lipids*

Lipids are used to provide 30% of the daily energy requirement. Lipids are provided as triglycerides (which are composed of a glycerol molecule linked to three fatty acids) or free fatty acids.

a. LINOLEIC ACID. The only dietary lipid that is essential (i.e., must be provided in the diet) is linoleic acid, a polyunsaturated fatty acid. Linoleic acid deficiency produces a clinical disorder characterized by a scaly dermopathy, cardiac dysfunction, and increased susceptibility to infections (7). Providing 0.5% of the dietary fatty acids as linoleic acid is enough to prevent linoleic acid deficiency. (Safflower oil is rich in linoleic acid).

B. Protein Intake

The daily intake of protein is determined by the rate of protein catabolism in individual patients.

1. *Estimating Daily Protein Needs*

Protein intake can be estimated by using the following generalized predictions for normal and hypercatabolic patients (8):

    a. Normal metabolism: Daily protein intake = 0.8 to 1.0 grams per kg body weight.

    b. Hypercatabolism: Daily protein intake = 1.2 to 1.6 grams per kg body weight.

2. *Nitrogen Balance*

The nitrogen balance (the difference between intake and excretion of protein-derived nitrogen) is the preferred method of evaluating the adequacy of protein intake.

    a. Two-thirds of the nitrogen derived from protein breakdown is excreted in the urine (8), and about 85% of this nitrogen is contained in urea (the remainder is in ammonia and creatinine). Thus the urinary urea nitrogen (UUN), measured in grams excreted in 24 hours, represents the bulk of nitrogen derived from protein breakdown. The remainder of the protein-derived nitrogen (usually about 4–6 grams/day) is excreted in the stool. Protein-derived nitrogen (N_2) excretion (in grams/24 h) can thus be expressed as follows:

$$\textbf{N}_2 \textbf{ Excretion (g/24 h) = UUN + (4–6)} \qquad (36.3)$$

If the UUN is greater than 30 g/24 h, 6 grams is more appropriate for the estimated nonurinary nitrogen losses (9).

    b. Because protein is 16% nitrogen, each gram of protein contains 1/6.25 grams of nitrogen. Therefore, protein-derived nitrogen intake (in grams/24 h) is derived as follows:

$$\textbf{N}_2 \textbf{ Intake (g/24 h) = Protein Intake / 6.25} \qquad (36.4)$$

    c. The equations for nitrogen intake and nitrogen excretion are combined to determine the daily nitrogen balance (10).

$$\textbf{N}_2 \textbf{ Balance = N}_2 \textbf{ Intake } - \textbf{ N}_2 \textbf{ Excretion} \qquad (36.5)$$

d. The goal of nutritional support is a positive nitrogen balance of 4 to 6 grams.

3. *Nitrogen Balance & Nonprotein Calories*

The first step in achieving a positive nitrogen balance is to provide enough nonprotein calories to spare proteins from being degraded to provide energy. This is demonstrated in Figure 36.1. When the daily protein intake is constant, the nitrogen balance becomes positive only when the intake of nonprotein calories is sufficient to meet the daily energy needs (i.e., the REE). Therefore, increasing protein intake will not achieve a positive nitrogen balance unless the intake of nonprotein calories is adequate.

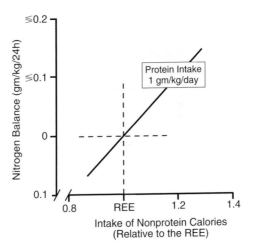

FIGURE 36.1 Graph showing the relationship between nitrogen balance and the daily intake of nonprotein calories relative to daily energy expenditure. Protein intake is constant. *REE* = resting energy expenditure.

IV. VITAMIN REQUIREMENTS

A. Daily Requirements

1. Thirteen vitamins are considered an essential part of the daily diet, and Table 36.4 shows the recommended daily dose of these vitamins for enteral tube feedings and total parenteral nutrition.

2. It is important to emphasize that the daily vitamin requirements in critically ill patients may be much higher than indicated in Table 36.4. In fact, deficiencies in several vitamins have been reported in hospitalized patients despite the daily provision of vitamins in nutritional support regimens (11,12).

B. Thiamine Deficiency

1. *Carbohydrate Metabolism*

   Thiamine (vitamin B_1) plays an essential role in carbohydrate metabolism, where it serves as a coenzyme (thiamine pyrophosphate) for pyruvate dehydrogenase, the enzyme that allows pyruvate to enter mitochondria and undergo oxidative metabolism. Thiamine deficiency can thus have an adverse effect on cellular energy production, particularly in tissues like the brain that rely heavily on glucose metabolism.

2. *Predisposing Factors*

   Thiamine deficiency may be much more common than suspected in ICU patients because of the following predisposing factors.

   a. Thiamine utilization is increased in hypercatabolic states like sepsis and trauma (14), and urinary thiamine excretion is increased by furosemide (15), a commonly used drug in the ICU. These factors will increase daily thiamine requirements above the normal daily requirement (1 mg).

TABLE 36.4 Recommended Daily Intake of Vitamins

Vitamin	Enteral RDA[†]	Parenteral Dose[‡]
Vitamin A	800 μg	1,000 μg
Vitamin B_{12}	2 μg	5 μg
Vitamin C	83 mg	200 mg
Vitamin D	10 μg	5 μg
Vitamin E	15 mg	10 mg
Vitamin K	105 μg	150 μg
Thiamine (B_1)	1 mg	6 mg
Riboflavin (B_2)	1 mg	4 mg
Niacin (B_3)	15 mg	40 mg
Pyridoxine (B_6)	2 mg	6 mg
Pantothenic acid	5 mg	15 mg
Biotin	30 μg	60 μg
Folate	400 μg	600 μg

[†]Food & Nutrition Board. Dietary Reference Intakes for Vitamins, 2002. Available at www.nal.usda.gov/fnic/etext/000105.html (accessed on June 13, 2006).

[‡]FDA. Parenteral Multivitamin Products. Federal Register 2000; 65:21200–21201.

Doses are rounded off to the nearest whole number.

    b. Magnesium is necessary for the conversion of thiamine into thiamine pyrophosphate, and magnesium depletion (which is common in ICU patients) causes a functional thiamine deficiency that is independent of thiamine intake (16).

    c. Thiamine is degraded by sulfites (used as preservatives) in parenteral nutrition solutions (17), so the multivitamin preparations used in total parenteral nutrition (TPN) are not suitable if infused with the TPN solutions.

3. *Clinical Manifestations*

Thiamine deficiency can produce any of the following

clinical disorders (13,18–20):

a. Cardiomyopathy (beriberi heart disease).

b. Metabolic (Wernicke's) encephalopathy, which is often accompanied by ophthalmoplegia (e.g., lateral gaze paralysis).

c. Unexplained lactic acidosis.

d. Peripheral neuropathy.

Conditions like cardiomyopathy and metabolic encephalopathy are common in ICU patients, and the possible contribution of thiamine deficiency to these conditions should not be overlooked.

TABLE 36.5 Laboratory Evaluation of Thiamine Status

Plasma Thiamine:

Thiamine Fraction	Normal Range
Total	3.4 – 4.8 µg/dL
Free	0.8 – 1.1 µg/dL
Phosphorylated	2.6 – 3.7 µg/dL

Erythrocyte Transketolase Activity[†]
Enzyme activity measured in response to TPP.
1. <20% increase in activity indicates normal thiamine stores.
2. >25% increase in activity indicates thiamine deficiency.

[†]From Reference 21. TPP = thiamine pyrophosphate.

---

4. *Diagnosis*

The laboratory evaluation of thiamine status is shown in Table 36.5. Plasma levels of thiamine can be useful in detecting thiamine depletion, but the most reliable measure of functional thiamine stores is the *erythrocyte transketolase assay* (21). This assay measures the activity of a thiamine pyrophosphate–dependent (transketolase) enzyme in the patient's red blood cells in response to the addition of thiamine pyrophosphate (TPP). An increase in enzyme activity of greater than 25% after the addition of TPP indicates functional thiamine deficiency.

C. Antioxidant Vitamins

a. Two vitamins serve as important endogenous antioxidants: *vitamin C and vitamin E*. Vitamin E is the major lipid-soluble antioxidant in the body, and vitamin C is one of the major antioxidants in the extracellular fluid.

b. Biological oxidation may play an important role in the pathogenesis of inflammatory-mediated organ injury (see Chapter 33) (22), and thus attention to the status of the antioxidant vitamins may be important in these conditions. (See Appendix 2 for the normal plasma levels of vitamins C and E).

TABLE 36.6 Daily Intake of Essential Trace Elements

Trace Element	Enteral Dose	Parenteral Dose
Chromium	200 µg	15 µg
Copper	3 mg	1.5 mg
Iodine	150 µg	150 µg
Iron	10 mg	2.5 mg
Manganese	5 mg	100 µg
Selenium	200 µg	70 µg
Zinc	15 mg	4 mg

Doses represent the maximum daily maintenance doses for each element. From Reference 24.

V. ESSENTIAL TRACE ELEMENTS

A. Daily Requirements

A trace element is a substance that is present in the body in amounts less than 50 µg per gram of body tissue (23).

   a. Seven trace elements are considered essential in humans (i.e., are associated with deficiency syndromes), and these are listed in Table 36.6 along with the recommended daily requirement for each element (24).

   b. As mentioned for daily vitamin requirements, the published trace element requirements are meant for healthy adults. The requirements in critically ill patients are not known.

B. Selenium

1. Selenium is an endogenous antioxidant by virtue of its role as a cofactor for glutathione peroxidase, an enzyme in the glutathione redox system, the major source of intracellular antioxidant activity in the human body.

2. The daily requirement for selenium in critically ill patients is not known. The minimum daily requirement is 55 µg in healthy adults (25), but selenium utilization is increased in acute illness (26), so daily requirements are likely higher in critically ill patients. The maximum daily dose of selenium that is considered safe is 200 µg.

3. Because of the uncertain selenium requirement in ICU patients, and the potential for selenium deficiency to promote oxidant stress, monitoring plasma selenium levels seems justified in patients with likely oxidant stress. The normal range of plasma selenium is 89–113 µg/L (27).

REFERENCES

1. Harris JA, Benedict FG. A biometric study of human basal metabolism. Proc Natl Acad Sci U S A 1918; 4:370–373.
2. Mann S, Westenskow DR, Houtchens BA. Measured and predicted caloric expenditure in the acutely ill. Crit Care Med 1985; 13:173–177.
3. Paauw JD, McCamish MA, Dean RE, et al. Assessment of caloric

needs in stressed patients. J Am Coll Nutr 1984; 3:51–59.

4. Weissman C, Kemper M, Askanazi J, et al. Resting metabolic rate of the critically ill patient: measured versus predicted. Anesthesiology 1986; 64:673–679.

5. McClave S, Snider H. Use of indirect calorimety in clinical nutrition. Nutr Clin Pract 1992; 7:207–221.

6. Bursztein S, Saphar P, Singer P, et al. A mathematical analysis of indirect calorimetry measurements in acutely ill patients. Am J Clin Nutr 1989; 50:227–230.

7. Jones PJH, Kubow S. Lipids, sterols, and their metabolites. In: Shils ME, et al., eds. Modern nutrition in health and disease. 10th ed. Philadelphia: Lippincott, Williams & Wilkins, 2006:92–121.

8. Matthews DE. Proteins and amino acids. In: Shils ME, et al., eds. Modern nutrition in health and disease. 10th ed. Philadelphia: Lippincott, Williams & Wilkins, 2006:23–61.

9 Velasco N, Long CL, Otto DA, et al. Comparison of three methods for the estimation of total nitrogen losses in hospitalized patients. J Parenter Enteral Nutr 1990; 14:517–522.

10. Blackburn GL, Bistrian BR, Maini BS, et al. Nutritional and metabolic assessment of the hospitalized patient. J Parenter Enteral Nutr 1977; 1:11–22.

11. Dempsey DT, Mullen JL, Rombeau JL, et al. Treatment effects of parenteral vitamins in total parenteral nutrition patients. J Parenter Enteral Nutr 1987; 11:229–237.

12. Beard ME, Hatipov CS, Hamer JW. Acute onset of folate deficiency in patients under intensive care. Crit Care Med 1980; 8:500–503.

13. Butterworth RF. Thiamin. In: Shils ME, et al., eds. Modern nutrition in health and disease. 10th ed. Philadelphia: Lippincott, Williams & Wilkins, 2006:426–433.

14. McConachie I, Haskew A. Thiamine status after major trauma. Intensive Care Med 1988; 14:628–631.

15. Seligmann H, Halkin H, Rauchfleisch S, et al. Thiamine deficiency in patients with congestive heart failure receiving long-term furosemide therapy: a pilot study. Am J Med 1991; 91:151–155.

16. Dyckner T, Ek B, Nyhlin H, et al. Aggravation of thiamine deficiency by magnesium depletion: A case report. Acta Med Scand 1985; 218:129–131.

17. Scheiner JM, Araujo MM, DeRitter E. Thiamine destruction by sodium bisulfite in infusion solutions. Am J Hosp Pharm 1981; 38:1911–1916.

18. Tan GH, Farnell GF, Hensrud DD, et al. Acute Wernicke's enceph-alopathy attributable to pure dietary thiamine deficiency. Mayo Clin Proc 1994; 69:849–850.

19. Oriot D, Wood C, Gottesman R, et al. Severe lactic acidosis relat-ed to acute thiamine deficiency. J Parenter Enteral Nutr 1991; 15:105–109.

20. Koike H, Misu K, Hattori N, et al. Postgastrectomy polyneuro-pathy with thiamine deficiency. J Neurol Neurosurg Psychiatry 2001; 71:357–362.

21. Boni L, Kieckens L, Hendrikx A. An evaluation of a modified erythrocyte transketolase assay for assessing thiamine nutrition-al adequacy. J Nutr Sci Vitaminol (Tokyo) 1980; 26:507–514.

22. Anderson BO, Brown JM, Harken AH. Mechanisms of neutro-phil-mediated tissue injury. J Surg Res 1991; 51:170–179.

23. Fleming CR. Trace element metabolism in adult patients requir-ing total parenteral nutrition. Am J Clin Nutr 1989; 49:573–579.

24. Dark DS, Pingleton SK. Nutritional support in critically ill patients. Intensive Care Med 1993; 8:16–33.

25. National Institutes of Health, Office of Dietary Supplements. Dietary Supplement Fact Sheet: Selenium. Available at http://dietarysup-plements.info.nih.gov/factsheets/Selenium_pf.asp (accessed on Nov. 30, 2007).

26. Hawker FH, Stewart PM, Snitch PJ. Effects of acute illness on selenium homeostasis. Crit Care Medicine 1990; 18:442–446.

27. Geoghegan M, McAuley D, Eaton S, et al. Selenium in critical ill-ness. Curr Opin Crit Care 2006; 12:136–141.

Chapter 37

ENTERAL TUBE FEEDING

For patients who are unable to eat, the preferred method of nutrition support involves liquid feeding formulas that are delivered directly into the stomach.

I. GENERAL FEATURES

A. Trophic Effects

1. The presence of nutrients in the bowel lumen has a trophic effect on the bowel mucosa (1). This effect is partly due to the presence of luminal bulk and partly due to individual nutrients like glutamine, which is a preferred fuel for epithelial cells in the bowel (2).

2. The trophic effects of enteral feeding are lost during periods of bowel rest, and this results in progressive atrophy and disruption of the intestinal mucosa (1). Total parenteral nutrition (TPN) does not prevent the epithelial degeneration that accompanies bowel rest.

3. Because the bowel mucosa serves as a barrier to microbial invasion (as described in Chapter 35), enteral feedings may play an important role in bolstering host defenses against infection. This notion is supported by clinical studies showing translocation of enteric pathogens across the bowel mucosa during periods of bowel rest (1,3).

4. The apparent role of enteral feedings as an *infection con-*

trol measure has secured the preference for enteral feedings over TPN.

B. Patient Selection

1. *Indications*

   The typical candidate for enteral tube feedings is the patient who is at risk for malnutrition (or is already malnourished) from impaired oral intake, and the situation is unlikely to improve over the next few days.

2. *Contraindications*

   a. Absolute contraindications to enteral feeding include circulatory shock, intestinal ischemia, complete bowel obstruction, and ileus (4).

   b. Full nutritional support via tube feedings is not advised in patients with partial bowel obstruction, severe or unrelenting diarrhea, pancreatitis, or high-volume (more than 500 mL daily) enterocutaneous fistulas. However, limited infusion of tube feedings is often permissible in these conditions, if tolerated. For cases of pancreatitis, tube feedings can be delivered into the jejunum.

II. FEEDING FORMULAS

A. Caloric Density

1. Most feeding formulas provide 1 to 1.3 kilocalories (kcal) per mL (see Table 37.1), and a few provide as much as 2 kcal/mL (see Table 37.2). The formulas with high caloric densities are intended for patients with severe hypermetabolism (e.g., multisystem trauma and burns), and for patients who are volume restricted.

2. The caloric density of feeding formulas includes the contribution of proteins, but daily caloric needs should be

provided by nonprotein calories (as described in Chapter 36). The adjustment of caloric density to reflect nonprotein calories is described later in the chapter.

TABLE 37.1 Standard Caloric Density Feeding Formulas

Feeding Formula	Caloric Density (kcal/mL)	Nonprotein Calories (%)	Protein (g/L)	Osmolality (mosm/kg H_2O)
Enrich	1.1	85	40	480
Glucerna	1	83	42	375
Isocal	1.1	87	34	300
Isocal HN	1.1	83	44	300
Jevity	1.1	83	44	300
Osmolite	1.1	86	37	300
Osmolite HN	1.1	83	44	300
Peptamen	1	84	40	270
Resource	1.1	86	37	430
Ultracal	1.1	83	43	310

TABLE 37.2 High Caloric Density Feeding Formulas

Feeding Formula	Caloric Density (kcal/mL)	Nonprotein Calories (%)	Protein (g/L)	Osmolality (mosm/kg H_2O)
Isocal HCN	2	85	75	690
Magnacal	2	86	70	590
Nepro	2	86	70	635
Suplena	2	94	15	615
Twocal HN	2	83	84	690

B. Osmolality

1. The osmotic activity of feeding solutions, which is expressed as osmolality (mosm/kg H_2O), varies directly with caloric density, and with the addition of "specialty" molecules like glutamine.

2. The osmolality of standard feeding formulas (i.e., caloric density of 1 kcal/mL and no additional specialty molecules) is a close approximation of plasma osmolality (280–300 mosm/kg H_2O). High caloric density solutions, like the ones in Table 37.2, show a two-fold increase in osmolality that matches the increase in caloric density.

3. Hypertonic feeding formulas have two undesirable effects: delayed gastric emptying and osmotic diarrhea. Gastric instillation is always advised for hypertonic feedings to take advantage of the diluting effects of gastric secretions.

C. Protein Content

1. Standard feeding formulas provide 35 to 45 grams of protein per liter.

2. High-protein formulas, often designated by the suffix HN (for "high nitrogen") provide only 20% more protein than the standard formulas.

3. Most enteral formulas provide intact proteins that are broken down into amino acids in the upper GI tract. Some feeding formulas contain small peptides (e.g., Peptamen, Vital HN), which are absorbed more rapidly than intact protein. Peptide-based formulas promote water reabsorption from the bowel and can be used in patients with troublesome diarrhea.

D. Lipid Content

The lipids in most feeding formulas are derived from vegetable oils. The lipid content is adjusted to provide about 30% of the caloric density of the formula.

1. *Omega-3 Fatty Acids*

   Polyunsaturated fatty acids from vegetable oils (which make up the lipid content of most feeding formulas) can serve as precursors for pro-inflammatory mediators (eicosanoids) that are capable of promoting inflammatory cell injury (9). This concern has prompted the introduction of feeding solutions that contain polyunsaturated fatty acids from fish oils (omega-3 fatty acids), which do not promote the production of pro-inflammatory mediators. Three of these feeding solutions are shown in Table 37.3. The use of feeding solutions like these to manipulate the inflammatory response is known as *immunonutrition* (5,6).

TABLE 37.3 Immune-Modulating Enteral Feeding Formulas

| Product | kcal/mL | grams per 1000 kcal | | |
		n-3 Fatty Acids	Arginine	Glutamine
Altraq	1	<1	5	14
Immun-Aid	1	11	14	9
Impact	1	17	13	0
Oxepa	1.5	63	0	0

From Reference 5. n-3 Fatty Acids = omega-3 fatty acids.

E. Conditionally Essential Nutrients

Nonessential nutrients (do not require exogenous support) can become essential (require exogenous support) in conditions where nutrient depletion is evident. Three of these *conditionally essential* nutrients deserve mention because the conditions where they become essential are common in ICU patients.

1. *Glutamine*

   Glutamine is the principal fuel for the bowel mucosa (2), and it is a precursor for glutathione, the principal intracellular antioxidant in the human body.

   a. More than 10 enteral feeding formulas are enriched with glutamine, and two of them are shown in Table 37.3. The optimal glutamine intake is not defined because there is no daily requirement for glutamine.

2. *Arginine*

   a. Arginine seems best suited for postoperative patients and trauma victims because it is a preferred metabolic substrate for injured muscle and also promotes wound healing.

   b. There are at least five enteral feeding formulas that provide arginine, and three of these are shown in Table 37.3. Clinical studies suggest a benefit with feeding formulas containing at least 12 g/L of arginine (5).

3. *Carnitine*

   Carnitine is necessary for the transport of fatty acids into mitochondria for fatty acid oxidation.

   a. Hypercatabolic conditions can promote carnitine deficiency (7), which is characterized by a myopathy involving the heart and skeletal muscle. A deficiency state is suggested by plasma carnitine levels that fall below 20 mmol/L.

   b. The recommended daily dose of carnitine is 20–30 mg/kg in adults (8). Feeding formulas that provide supplemental carnitine include Glucerna, Isocal HN, Jevity, and Peptamen.

IV. CREATING A FEEDING REGIMEN

This section describes the process of creating a feeding regimen. The major features are presented in sequence, and the variables involved are highlighted in Table 37.4.

TABLE 37.4 Creating a Feeding Regimen

1. *Estimate daily calorie and protein requirements:*

   kcal/day = 25 x wt (kg)

   Protein (g/day) = (1.2–1.6) x wt (kg)

2. *Determine daily feeding volume and infusion rate:*

   $$\text{Daily volume (mL)} = \frac{\text{kcal/day required}}{\text{kcal/mL in feedings}}$$

   $$\text{Infusion rate (mL/hr)} = \frac{\text{daily volume (mL)}}{\text{feeding time (hr)}}$$

3. *Evaluate protein intake:*

   Protein intake (g/day) = daily volume (L) x protein in feedings (g/L)

   $$\frac{\text{Desired protein intake (g/day)}}{\text{Actual protein intake (g/day)}} = <1 \text{ or } 1 \text{ or } >1$$

A. Daily Protein and Calorie Requirements

The first concern in nutrition support is to determine the daily requirements for protein and calories. These requirements can be estimated or measured, as described in Chapter 36. The predictive equations in Table 37.4 should suffice in most patients.

B. Nonprotein Calories

The caloric density of feeding formulas represents total calories from carbohydrates, lipids, and proteins, but only nonprotein calories should be used to provide needed calories (as described in Chapter 36). Therefore, the caloric density of feeding formulas should be adjusted to reflect only nonprotein calories.

1. As shown in Table 37.1, nonprotein calories represent 80 to 85% of the calories in standard feeding formulas, so

adjusting for nonprotein calories will reduce the caloric yield from feeding solutions by 15 to 20%.

C. Daily Volume and Infusion Rate

1. The daily caloric requirement that is defined in Step 1 can be divided by the (nonprotein) caloric density of a feeding formula to determine the volume of enteral feedings that will provide the desired calories (see Table 37.4). For feeding formulas that have a caloric density close to 1 kcal/min, the daily volume of enteral feedings (in mL) will be 15–20% greater than the desired number of daily calories.

2. Enteral feedings are infused continuously into the upper GI tract for 16 hours each day, and each feeding period is followed by 8 hours of bowel rest before the feedings resume. The desired infusion rate for feedings (mL/hr) is determined using the daily volume of feedings (in mL) and the duration of the feeding period (in hours) (see Table 37.4).

D. Protein Intake

The final step is to determine if the daily volume of feedings is providing enough protein.

1. The daily protein intake is determined by the protein concentration in the feeding formula and the volume of feeding formula infused each day.

2. The daily protein intake is then compared to the desired protein intake from Step 1. If the daily intake is less than desired, powdered protein (from the hospital pharmacy) is added to the tube feedings to correct the discrepancy.

3. The best method of evaluating protein intake is the 24-hour *nitrogen balance*, which is described in Chapter 36,

Section II-B. However, this method is reserved for patients receiving long-term nutrition support who are clinically stable.

IV. INITIATING TUBE FEEDINGS

A. Feeding Tube Insertion

1. Feeding tubes used for short-term (up to a few weeks) nutrition support are inserted through the nares and advanced blindly into the stomach or duodenum. The distance required to reach the stomach can be estimated by measuring the distance from the tip of the nose to the earlobe and then to the xiphoid process (typically 50–60 cm) (9).

2. Feeding tubes end up in the trachea during 1% of insertions (10). Because patients are often asymptomatic, feeding tubes can be advanced deep into the lungs and can puncture the visceral pleura and create a pneumothorax (11,12).

3. A portable chest x-ray should be performed after each insertion (see Figure 37.1) The common practice of pushing air through the feeding tube and listening for bowel sounds in the upper abdomen is not a reliable method for determining tube position because sounds emanating from a feeding tube in the lower airways can be transmitted into the upper abdomen (11,12).

4. Advancing the tip of the feeding tube into the duodenum to reduce the risk of aspiration of tube feedings is not necessary because clinical studies have shown that *the incidence of aspiration is the same with duodenal and gastric feedings* (4,13).

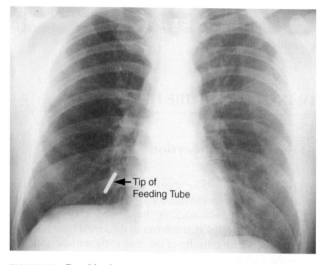

FIGURE 37.1 Portable chest x-ray taken after uneventful insertion of a feeding tube.

B. Gastric Residuals

1. Before feedings commence, the contents of the stomach should be aspirated to measure the gastric residual volume. (This may be difficult because small-bore, flexible feeding tubes tend to collapse when suction is applied).

2. If the volume aspirated is less than 150 mL, the feeding can commence. If the aspirated volume is greater than 150 mL, wait another two hours and repeat the gastric aspiration. If the second aspiration yields less than 150 mL, commence feedings. If more than 150 mL is aspirated a second time, the following options are available:

   a. Advance the feeding tube into the duodenum to begin feedings (recommended).

   b. Administer the prokinetic drug **metoclopramide** (10

mg IV), and check gastric residuals in 2 hours (but usually doesn't work).

C. Starter Regimens

1. The traditional approach to initiating tube feedings is to begin with dilute formulas and a slow infusion rate and gradually advance to the desired nutrient intake over one or two days. This practice accomplishes little other than extending the period of inadequate nutrition.

2. Studies involving intragastric feedings show that full feedings can be delivered immediately without troublesome vomiting or diarrhea (14,15).

3. Tube feedings are usually infused for 16 hours followed by 8 hours of bowel rest. Continuous feedings without a period of bowel rest is an unrelenting stress to the bowel mucosa and promotes malabsorption and diarrhea.

V. COMPLICATIONS

The complications associated with enteral feedings include occlusion of the feeding tube, reflux of gastric contents into the airways, and diarrhea.

A. Tube Occlusion

Narrow-bore feeding tubes can become occluded by protein precipitates that form when acidic gastric secretions reflux into the feeding tubes (16). Standard preventive measures include flushing the feeding tubes with 30 mL of water every 4 hours, and using a 10 mL water flush after medications are instilled.

1. *Restoring Patency*

If there is still some flow through the tube, warm water

should be injected into the tube and agitated with a syringe. This can relieve the obstruction in 30% of cases (22). If this is ineffective, **pancreatic enzyme** (Viokase) can be used as follows (17):

a. Dissolve 1 tablet of Viokase and 1 tablet of sodium carbonate (324 mg) in 5 mL of water. Inject this mixture into the feeding tube and clamp for 5 minutes. Follow with a warm-water flush.

b. This should relieve the obstruction in approximately 75% of cases (17). If the tube is completely occluded, an attempt should be made to insert a flexible wire or drum-cartridge catheter to clear the obstruction.

B. Aspiration

1. Retrograde regurgitation of feeding formula is reported in as many as 80% of patients receiving gastric or duodenal feedings (18). Elevating the head of the bed to 45° can reduce (but not eliminate) the problem.

2. Aspiration of feeding formulas into the airways can be detected by testing tracheal aspirates with glucose oxidase reagent strips. The results are measured with an automated glucose meter. A glucose concentration greater than 20 mg/dL in tracheal aspirates is evidence of aspiration (19).

3. Adding food coloring to the feeding formulas and inspecting the color of tracheal secretions is an insensitive method for detecting aspiration (19).

C. Diarrhea

1. Diarrhea occurs in approximately 30% of patients receiving enteral tube feedings (20). The hyperosmolality of feeding formulas is responsible for some but not all cases.

2. One important and often overlooked cause of diarrhea is sorbitol, which is added to liquid drug preparations to

improve palatability (20,21). Sorbitol causes an osmotic diarrhea.

3. Antibiotic-associated diarrhea, including *Clostridium difficile* enterocolitis, can also appear during tube feedings and should not be mistaken for the feeding-related osmotic diarrhea. Signs of systemic inflammation should not accompany the diarrhea from tube feedings.

REFERENCES

1. Alpers DH. Enteral feeding and gut atrophy. Curr Opin Clin Nutr Metab Care 2002; 5:679–683.
2. Herskowitz K, Souba WW. Intestinal glutamine metabolism during critical illness: a surgical perspective. Nutrition 1990; 6:199–206.
3. Wiest R, Rath HC. Gastrointestinal disorders of the critically ill: Bacterial translocation in the gut. Best Pract Res Clin Gastroenterol 2003; 17:397–425.
4. Kreymann KG, Berger MM, Deutz NE, et al. ESPEN Guidelines on Enteral Nutrition: Intensive care. Clin Nutr 2006; 25:210–223.
5. Bistrian BR, McCowen KC. Nutritional and metabolic support in the adult intensive care unit: key controversies. Crit Care Med 2006; 34:1525–1531.
6. Heyland DK, Novak F, Drover JW, et al. Should immunonutrition become routine in critically ill patients? JAMA 2007; 286:944–953.
7. Rebouche CJ. Carnitine. In: Shils ME, et al., eds. Modern nutrition in health and disease. 10th ed. Philadelphia: Lippincott, Williams & Wilkins, 2006:537–544.
8. Karlic H, Lohninger A. Supplementation of L-carnitine in athletes: does it make sense? Nutrition (Burbank, CA) 2004; 20:709–715.
9. Stroud M, Duncan H, Nightingale J. Guidelines for enteral feeding in adult hospital patients. Gut 2003; 52(Suppl 7):vii1–vii12.
10. Baskin WN. Acute complications associated with bedside placement of feeding tubes. Nutr Clin Pract 2006; 21:40–55.
11. Kolbitsch C, Pomaroli A, Lorenz I, et al. Pneumothorax following nasogastric feeding tube insertion in a tracheostomized patient after bilateral lung transplantation. Intensive Care Med 1997; 23:440–442.

12 Fisman DN, Ward ME. Intrapleural placement of a nasogastric tube: an unusual complication of nasotracheal intubation. Can J Anaesth 1996; 43:1252–1256.

13. Strong RM, Condon SC, Solinger MR, et al. Equal aspiration rates from postpylorus and intragastric-placed small-bore nasoenteric feeding tubes: a randomized, prospective study. J Parenter Enteral Nutr 1992; 16:59–63.

14. Rees RG, Keohane PP, Grimble GK, et al. Elemental diet administered nasogastrically without starter regimens to patients with inflammatory bowel disease. J Parenter Enteral Nutr 1986; 10:258–262.

15. Mizock BA. Avoiding common errors in nutritional management. J Crit Illness 1993; 10:1116–1127.

16. Marcuard SP, Perkins AM. Clogging of feeding tubes. J Parenter Enteral Nutr 1988; 12:403–405.

17. Marcuard SP, Stegall KS. Unclogging feeding tubes with pancreatic enzyme. J Parenter Enteral Nutr 1990; 14:198–200.

18. Metheny N. Minimizing respiratory complications of nasoenteric tube feedings: state of the science. Heart Lung 1993; 22:213–223.

19. Potts RG, Zaroukian MH, Guerrero PA, et al. Comparison of blue dye visualization and glucose oxidase test strip methods for detecting pulmonary aspiration of enteral feedings in intubated adults. Chest 1993; 103:117–121.

20. Edes TE, Walk BE, Austin JL. Diarrhea in tube-fed patients: feeding formula not necessarily the cause. Am J Med 1990; 88:91–93.

21. Cheng EY, Hennen CR, Nimphius N. Unsuspected source of diarrhea in an ICU patient. Clin Intensive Care 1992; 3:33–36.

Chapter 38

TOTAL PARENTERAL NUTRITION

When full nutritional support is not possible with enteral tube feedings, the intravenous route can be used to supplement enteral nutrition or provide *total parenteral nutrition* (TPN). This chapter describes the basic features of TPN and demonstrates how to create a TPN regimen for individual patients.

I. SUBSTRATE SOLUTIONS

A. Dextrose Solutions

1. Intravenous nutrition regimens use dextrose solutions like those in Table 38.1 to provide carbohydrate calories.

2. Because dextrose has a low energy yield (3.4 kcal/g), the dextrose solutions used for TPN must be concentrated to provide enough calories to satisfy daily requirements (50% dextrose solutions are standard in TPN). These solutions are hyperosmolar and should be infused through large, central veins.

B. Amino Acid Solutions

Protein is provided as amino acid solutions that contain varying mixtures of essential (N=9), semiessential (N=4) and nonessential (N=10) amino acids. These solutions are mixed with dextrose solutions in a 1:1 volume ratio. Examples of standard and "specialty"amino acid solutions are shown in Table 38.2.

TABLE 38.1 Intravenous Dextrose Solutions

Strength	Concentration (g/L)	Energy Yield* (kcal/L)	Osmolality (mosm/L)
5%	50	170	253
10%	100	340	505
20%	200	680	1010
50%	500	1700	2525
70%	700	2380	3530

*Based on an oxidative energy yield of 3.4 kcal/g for dextrose.

TABLE 38.2 Standard and Specialty Amino Acid Solutions

	Aminosyn	Aminosyn-HBC	Aminosyn RF
Available Concentrations	3.5%, 5%, 7%, 8.5%, 10%	7%	5.2%
Indications	Standard TPN	Hypercatabolism	Renal Failure
% EAA	50%	63%	89%
% BCAA	25%	46%	33%

EAA = essential amino acids, BCAA = branched chain amino acids.

1. *Standard Solutions*

   Standard amino acid solutions (e.g., Aminosyn in Table 38.2) are balanced mixtures of 50% essential amino acids and 50% nonessential and semiessential amino acids. These solutions are available in strengths that provide 35 to 100 grams of protein per liter.

2. *Hypercatabolism*

   Amino acid solutions designed for hypercatabolic conditions (e.g., Aminosyn-HBC in Table 38.2) are enriched with branched-chain amino acids (isoleucine, leucine, and va-line), which are preferred fuels in skeletal muscle when metabolic demands are heightened.

3. *Renal Failure*

Amino acid solutions designed for use in renal failure (e.g., Aminosyn RF in Table 38.2) are rich in essential amino acids because the nitrogen in essential amino acids is partially recycled to produce nonessential amino acids, which results in smaller increments in blood urea nitrogen (BUN) than produced by breakdown of nonessential amino acids.

4. *Hepatic Failure*

Amino acid solutions designed for use in hepatic failure (e.g., HepaticAid) are enriched with branched-chain amino acids (like solutions designed for renal failure) because these amino acids block the transport of aromatic amino acids (implicated in hepatic encephalopathy) across the blood-brain barrier.

5. *Glutamine*

The potential benefits of the amino acid glutamine are mentioned in Chapter 37 (Section II-E). Amino acid solutions enriched with glutamate (e.g., Aminosyn II) are used as an exogenous source of glutamine because glutamate can combine with ammonia to form glutamine.

6. *Efficacy*

a. None of the specialty amino acid solutions (i.e., those designed for hypercatabolism, renal or hepatic failure) has been shown to improve clinical outcomes (1).

b. There is some evidence that glutamine-enhanced TPN can reduce infectious complications in ICU patients (2), and glutamine supplementation has been recommended as a routine practice for ventilator-dependent patients (3).

C. Lipid Emulsions

Lipids are provided as emulsions consisting of submicron droplets (≤0.45 μm) of cholesterol, phospholipids, and triglycerides. The triglycerides are derived from vegetable oils (safflower and soybean oils) and are rich in linoleic acid, an essential fatty acid.

1. Lipids are used to provide 15 to 30% of daily calorie requirements, and 4% of the daily calories should be provided as linoleic acid to prevent essential fatty acid deficiency (4).

2. As shown in Table 38.3 (5), lipid emulsions are available in 10% and 20% strengths (the percentage refers to grams of triglyceride per 100 mL of solution). The 10% emulsions provide about 1 kcal/mL, and the 20% emulsions provide 2 kcal/mL. They can be infused separately (maximum rate = 50 ml/hr) or in combination with the dextrose–amino acid mixtures.

TABLE 38.3 Intravenous Lipid Emulsions for Clinical Use

Feature	Intralipid		Liposyn II	
	10%	**20%**	**10%**	**20%**
Calories (kcal/mL)	1.1	2	1.1	2
% calories as EFA (Linoleic acid)	50%	50%	66%	66%
Cholesterol (mg/dL)	250–300	250–300	13–22	13–22
Osmolarity (mosm/L)	260	260	276	258
Unit volumes (mL)	50	50	100	200
	100	100	200	500
	250	250	500	
	500	500		

Adapted from Reference 5. EFA = Essential fatty acid.

3. Unlike the hypertonic dextrose solutions, lipid emulsions are roughly isotonic to plasma and can be infused through peripheral veins.

TABLE 38.4 Trace Element Preparations & Daily Requirements

Trace Element	Daily Parenteral[†] Requirement	MTE-5[‡] concentrated	MTE-6[‡] concentrated
Chromium	10–15 µg	10 µg	10 µg
Copper	0.5–1.5 mg	1 mg	1 mg
Iodine	150 µg	—	75 µg
Iron	0.5 mg	—	—
Manganese	150–800 µg	500 µg	500 µg
Selenium	50–200 µg	60 µg	60 µg
Zinc	2.5–4 mg	5 mg	5 mg

†Adapted from Reference 7.
‡From Reference 5.

D. Additives

Commercially available mixtures of electrolytes, vitamins, and trace elements are added directly to the dextrose–amino acid mixtures.

1. *Electrolytes*

There are more than 15 electrolyte mixtures available. Most have a volume of 20 mL and contain sodium, chloride, potassium, and magnesium. Check the mixture used at your hospital to determine if additional electrolytes must be added. Additional requirements for potassium or other electrolytes can be specified in the TPN orders.

2. *Vitamins*

Aqueous multivitamin preparations are designed to provide normal daily requirements (see Chapter 36, Table 36.4). Enhanced vitamin requirements in hypermetabolic patients may not be satisfied. Some vitamins (e.g., thiamine) are degraded before they are delivered (6).

3. *Trace Elements*

A variety of trace-element additives are available, and Table 38.4 shows two of them, along with the parenteral trace-element requirements (7). Most trace-element mixtures do not contain iron, but iron administration is not advisable on a routine basis because of its pro-oxidant actions (8).

II. CREATING A TPN REGIMEN

The following stepwise approach demonstrates how to create a TPN regimen for an individual patient. At each step along the way, a sample TPN regimen will be created for a 70 kg adult patient.

A. Daily Requirements

The first step is to estimate the daily protein and calorie requirements. The simple predictive equations below should suffice in most patients (see Chapter 36).

$$\text{Calories (kcal/day)} = 25 \times \text{wt (kg)} \qquad (38.1)$$

$$\text{Protein (g/day)} = (1.2 - 1.6) \times \text{wt (kg)} \qquad (38.2)$$

The body weight in these equations should be ideal or lean body weight. The range (1.2–1.6) in the protein estimation represents the degree of metabolic stress (1.2 is mild, 1.4 is moderate, and 1.6 is severe stress).

1. *Sample Regimen*

For a 70 kg adult with a moderate degree of metabolic stress:

a. The daily calorie requirement is 25 x 70 = 1750 kcal.

b. The daily protein requirement is 1.4 x 70 = 98 grams.

B. Volume of TPN Mixture

The next step is to determine the volume of TPN mixture (amino acid-dextrose mixture) that will provide the estimated protein requirement. This is a function of the protein concentration in the TPN mixture (g/L):

$$\text{Volume (L/day)} = \frac{\textbf{Protein Required (g/day)}}{\textbf{Protein Content (g/L)}} \quad \text{(38.3)}$$

Because equal volumes of amino acid solution and dextrose solution are mixed together, the final concentration of protein is 50% of the protein concentration in the amino acid solution. For example, a mixture of 10% amino acids (500 mL) and 50% dextrose (500 mL), which is designated as A_{10}-D_{50}, has a protein concentration of 50 grams/liter.

1. *Sample Regimen*

   For our 70 kg adult with a daily protein requirement of 98 grams

   a. An equal mixture of A_{10}-D_{50} will provide the needed protein at a daily volume of: 98/50 = 1.9 liters.

   b. The infusion rate of this mixture should be 1900 mL/24 hours = 81 mL/hour (or 81 microdrops/minute).

C. Carbohydrate Calories

The next step is to determine the calories provided by carbohydrates (CHO). This is equivalent to the product of the daily volume of the TPN mixture (in liters), the dextrose concentration in the amino acid-dextrose mixture (g/L), and the caloric yield from dextrose (3.4 kcal per gram).

$$\textbf{CHO calories} = \textbf{Volume} \times \textbf{[Dextrose]} \times \textbf{3.4} \quad \text{(38.4)}$$
$$\textbf{(kcal/day)} \qquad \textbf{(L)} \qquad \textbf{(g/L)} \quad \textbf{(kcal/g)}$$

The dextrose concentration in the amino acid-dextrose mixtures is 50% of the dextrose concentration in the additive solution; i.e., a TPN mixture of A_{10}-D_{50} has a dextrose concentration of $500/2 = 250$ g/L.

1. *Sample Regimen*

   For the 70 kg adult with a daily protein requirement of 98 grams who receives a TPN mixture of A_{10}-D_{50} at a volume of 1.9 liters daily,

   a. The calories provided by carbohydrates are 1.9 x 25 x 3.4 = 1615 kcal/day

   b. The remaining calorie requirement is 1750−1615 = 135 kcal/day.

D. Lipid Calories

A lipid emulsion is used to provide the remainder of the daily calorie requirement not provided by dextrose.

1. *Sample Regimen*

   For our 70 kg adult who has an estimated daily calorie requirement of 1750 calories and will receive 1615 kcal/day from carbohydrates.

   a. The remaining calorie requirement of 1750−1615 = 135 kcal/day can be provided by a 10% lipid emulsion (1 kcal/mL) at a volume of 135 ml/day. Because the lipid emulsion is available in unit volumes of 50 mL, the volume can be adjusted to 150 mL/day to avoid wastage. The maximum infusion rate is 50 mL/hr.

E. TPN Orders

1. *Sample Regimen*

   The orders for our sample TPN regimen will include the following:

   a. A_{10}–D_{50} to run at 80 mL/hour.

   b. 10% Intralipid: 150 mL daily to infuse over 4–6 hours.

Electrolyte, vitamin, and trace element mixtures are added to the amino acid-dextrose mixture in amounts determined by patient needs.

III. METABOLIC COMPLICATIONS

A. Hyperglycemia

Glucose intolerance is one of the most common (and most troublesome) complications of TPN, and often requires the addition of insulin. It is important to emphasize that *insulin adsorbs to all plastics and glass used in intravenous infusion sets*. The amount lost to adsorption varies with the amount of insulin added, but an average loss of 20 to 30% should be expected (8). The following observations about hyperglycemia are relevant.

1. Hyperglycemia is associated with heightened neurologic deficits after ischemic stroke (9).

2. Strict glycemic control to prevent hyperglycemia is associated with a decreased morbidity and mortality in ICU patients (10,11).

As a result of the latter observation, most ICUs have adopted (or should adopt) protocols for preventing hyperglycemia with aggressive use of insulin. (See Reference 12 for a useful flow sheet designed for strict glycemic control.)

B. Hypophosphatemia

Another common consequence of TPN is a progressive decline in serum phosphorus levels (see Chapter 29, Figure 29.2). This effect is due to enhanced cellular uptake of phosphorus (which is linked to enhanced glucose uptake). The phosphorus is used to form thiamine pyrophosphate, a cofactor in glycolysis.

C. Hypercapnia

Overfeeding (i.e., providing calories in excess of the daily energy expenditure) results in excessive production of CO_2, and this can promote CO_2 retention in patients with respiratory insufficiency. Although originally attributed to excess carbohydrate calories, this effect seems to be a reflection of overfeeding in general and not specific overfeeding with carbohydrates (13).

REFERENCES

1. Andris DA, Krzywda EA. Nutrition support in specific diseases: back to basics. Nutr Clin Pract 1994; 9:28–32.

2. Dechelotte P, Hasselmann M, Cynober L, et al. L-alanyl-L-glutamine dipeptide-supplemented total parenteral nutrition reduces infectious complications and glucose intolerance in critically ill patients: the French controlled, randomized, double-blind, multicenter study. Crit Care Med 2006; 34:598–604.

3. Heyland DK, Dhaliwal R, Drover JW, et al. Canadian clinical practice guidelines for nutrition support in mechanically ventilated, critically ill adult patients. J Parenter Enteral Nutr 2003; 27:355–373.

4. Barr LH, Dunn GD, Brennan MF. Essential fatty acid deficiency during total parenteral nutrition. Ann Surg 1981;193:304–311.

5. Borgsdorf LR, Cada DJ, Cirigliano M, et al. Drug facts and comparisons. 60th ed. St. Louis, MO: Wolters Kluwer, 2006.

6. Scheiner JM, Araujo MM, DeRitter E. Thiamine destruction by sodium bisulfite in infusion solutions. Am J Hosp Pharm 1981; 38:1911–1916.

7. Teasley-Strausburg KM, Cerra FB, Lehmann SL, Shronts EP, eds. Nutrition support handbook. Cincinnati: Harvey Whitney Books, 1992:120.

8. Trissel LA. Handbook on injectable drugs. 13th ed. Bethesda, MD: Amer Soc Health System Pharmacists, 2005.

9. Alvarez-Sabin J, Molina CA, Montaner J, et al. Effects of admission hyperglycemia on stroke outcome in reperfused tissue plasminogen activator-treated patients. Stroke 2003; 34:1235–1241.

10. van der Berghe G, Woutens P, Weekers F, et al. Intensive insulin therapy in critically ill patients. N Engl J Med 2001; 345:1359–1367.

11. Finey SJ, Zekveld C, Elia A, Evans TW. Glucose control and mortality in critically ill patients. JAMA 2003; 290:2041–2047.

12. Krinsley JS. Effect of an intensive glucose management protocol on the mortality of critically ill adult patients. Mayo Clin Proc 2004; 79:992–1000.

13. Talpers SS, Romberger DJ, Bunce SB, et al. Nutritionally associated increased carbon dioxide production: Excess total calories vs. high proportion of carbohydrate calories. Chest 1992; 102:551–555.

Chapter 39

ADRENAL AND THYROID DYSFUNCTION

Adrenal and thyroid disorders often act as catalysts for serious, life-threatening conditions while escaping notice themselves. This chapter explains how to unmask an underlying or occult disorder of adrenal or thyroid function and how to treat each disorder appropriately.

I. ADRENAL INSUFFICIENCY

Adrenal insufficiency can be a primary disorder (caused by adrenal dysfunction) or a secondary disorder (caused by hypothalamic-pituitary dysfunction). The description that follows pertains to primary AI, and how it behaves in the critically ill patient (1–4).

A. Prevalence

1. The incidence of AI is about 30% in randomly selected ICU patients (1), and up to 60% in patients with septic shock (1,2). Most of these cases are asymptomatic, and the diagnosis is based on biochemical evidence of impaired adrenal responsiveness.

2. Several conditions that are common in ICU patients can predispose to primary AI. These include major surgery, circulatory failure, septic shock, severe coagulopathy, and human immunodeficiency virus (HIV) infection (1,3).

B. Clinical Manifestations

1. A common manifestation of AI in critically ill patients is *hypotension that is refractory to vasopressors* (1,3). Other features of AI (e.g., electrolyte abnormalities) are either uncommon or nonspecific.

2. The hemodynamic profile in acute AI is similar to septic shock; i.e., low cardiac filling pressures, high cardiac output, and low systemic vascular resistance (3,4).

C. Rapid ACTH Stimulation Test

1. The diagnostic test of choice for primary AI is the rapid adrenocorticotropic hormone (ACTH) stimulation test (2). This test measures the adrenal release of cortisol in response to a bolus injection of synthetic ACTH, and it can be performed at any time of day or night.

2. To perform the test, an initial blood sample is obtained for a plasma cortisol level. Synthetic ACTH (250 μg) is then injected intravenously, and a repeat serum cortisol level is measured 30 and 60 minutes later.

3. The interpretation of the ACTH stimulation test is outlined in Table 39.1.

    a. The diagnosis of AI is supported by a baseline cortisol below 15 μg/dL (415 nmol/L), or an increment in cortisol that is less than 9 μg/dL (250 nmol/L).

4. CAVEAT. Most (90%) of the cortisol in plasma is bound to corticosteroid-binding proteins, while only 10% is in the free or biologically active form (3,5). The cortisol assay used in most clinical laboratories measures total cortisol levels in plasma. Since cortisol transport proteins are often decreased in critically ill patients (5), abnormally low plasma cortisol levels (using standard assays) may not represent AI in critically ill patients.

TABLE 39.1 Interpreting the ACTH Stimulation Test

Plasma Cortisol in µg/dL[†]		Probability of Adrenal Insufficiency
Baseline	Increment	
<15	⟶	Very High
15–34	<9	High
15–34	>9	Low
>34	⟶	Very Low

†To convert µg/dL to nmol/L, multiply by 27.6.
From Reference 3.

D. Steroid Therapy

For patients with suspected AI and severe or refractory hypotension, *steroids can be started before the ACTH stimulation test is performed*. Steroid administration can proceed as follows:

1. **Dexamethasone** (Decadron) will not interfere with plasma cortisol assay and can be given before or during the ACTH stimulation test. The initial dose is 2 mg (as an IV bolus), which is equivalent to 54 mg of hydrocortisone (see Table 39.2) (6).

2. After the ACTH stimulation test is completed, empiric therapy can begin with **hydrocortisone** (Solu-Cortef). The dose is 50 mg IV every 6 hours until the test results are available.

3. If the ACTH stimulation reveals primary AI, hydrocortisone should be continued at 50 mg IV every 6 hours until the patient is no longer in a stressed condition (3). At this point, the daily dose of hydrocortisone should be reduced to 20 mg (equivalent to the amount of cortisol secreted daily by the adrenal glands).

TABLE 39.2 Corticosteroid Comparison Chart

Corticosteroid	Equivalent Doses	AIA Rank[†]	MCA Rank[‡]
Hydrocortisone	20 mg	4	1
Prednisone	5 mg	3	2
Methylprednisolone	4 mg	2	3
Dexamethasone	0.75 mg	1	4

[†]Antiinflammatory activity (1 = best, 4 = worst).
[‡]Mineralocorticoid activity (1 = best, 4 = worst).
From Reference 5.

II. HYPOTHYROIDISM

Laboratory tests of thyroid function can be abnormal in 70% of hospitalized patients and up to 90% of critically ill patients (7). In most cases, this represents an adaptive response to systemic illness and is not a sign of thyroid dysfunction (7,8). True hypothyroidism is uncommon in hospitalized patients

A. Euthyroid Sick

1. Plasma levels of thyroxine (T_4) and its biologically active form, triiodothyronine (T_3), can be abnormally low in systemic conditions such as sepsis and multisystem trauma. The initial abnormality is a decrease in free T_3 levels, and this is followed by a decrease in free T_4 levels as the illness severity increases. These abnormalities are not associated with abnormal function of the thyroid gland or clinical hypothyroidism, and they disappear when the systemic illness subsides (7,8).

   a. When plasma levels of thyroid hormones are decreased

as a result of nonthyroidal illness, the condition is known as *euthyroid sick* (7).

b. Inflammatory mediators may be responsible for this condition by suppressing the conversion of T_4 to T_3 and enhancing degradation of T_4.

3. Plasma levels of thyroid-stimulating hormone (TSH) are normal or slightly reduced in most patients with nonthyroidal illness (7,9), and this distinguishes the euthyroid sick condition from primary hypothyroidism, where plasma TSH levels are increased (see later).

TABLE 39.3 Manifestations of Thyroid Dysfunction

Hyperthyroidism	Hypothyroidism
Cardiovascular	**Effusions**
Sinus tachycardia	Pericardial effusion
Atrial fibrillation	Pleural effusion
Neurologic	**Miscellaneous**
Agitation	Hyponatremia
Lethargy	Skeletal muscle myopathy
Fine tremors (elderly)	Elevated creatinine
Thyroid Storm	**Myxedema Coma**
Fever	Hypothermia
Hyperdynamic shock	Dermal infiltration
Depressed consciousness	Depressed consciousness

B. Clinical Manifestations

The clinical manifestations of hypothyroidism are nonspecific (see Table 39.3).

1. The most common cardiovascular manifestation is pericardial effusion (24), which develops in about 30% of cases (10). These effusions are exudates caused by increased cap-

illary permeability. They usually accumulate slowly and do not cause tamponade.

2. Other manifestations include hyponatremia and a skeletal muscle myopathy.

3. Advanced cases of hypothyroidism are accompanied by hypothermia and depressed consciousness. This condition is called *myxedema coma*, even though frank coma is uncommon (11).

   a. The edematous appearance in myxedema is due to intradermal accumulation of proteins and does not represent edema fluid (11).

C. Diagnosis

Hypothyroidism can be the result of thyroid dysfunction (primary hypothyroidism) or hypothalamic-pituitary dysfunction (secondary hypothyroidism).

1. Most cases represent primary hypothyroidism (10) and are characterized by a decrease in plasma free T_4 and an increase in plasma TSH levels. The latter abnormality is due to enhanced hypothalamic release of thyrotropin-releasing hormone (TRH) in response to the decreased thyroid hormone levels in plasma.

2. Secondary hypothyroidism is characterized by a decrease in both free T_4 and TSH levels in plasma. These cases can be difficult to distinguish from the 30% of euthyroid sick patients who have a decrease in plasma TSH (7).

D. Management

Thyroid replacement therapy is achieved with **levothyroxine**, which can be given orally or intravenously.

1. *Oral Therapy*

   Mild to moderate hypothyroidism is treated with oral levothyroxine in a single daily dose of 50 to 200 µg (12). The initial dose is usually 50 µg/day, which is increased in 50 µg/day increments every 3 to 4 weeks until the TSH level returns to normal (0.5 to 3.5 mU/L). In 90% of cases, this occurs with a levothyroxine dose of 100 to 200 µg/day (12).

2. *Intravenous Therapy*

Intravenous levothyroxine is often used (at least initially) for severe cases of hypothyroidism because reduced gastrointestinal motility can impair drug absorption. The intravenous regimen can proceed as follows: 250 µg on the first day, 100 µg on the second day, and 50 µg daily thereafter until oral therapy is possible (12).

III. HYPERTHYROIDISM

Most cases of hyperthyroidism are due to primary thyroid disorders (e.g., Graves' disease, autoimmune thyroiditis).

A. Clinical Manifestations

Some of the notable manifestations of hyperthyroidism are listed in Table 39.3. The following conditions deserve special mention.

1. *Apathetic Thyrotoxicosis*

Elderly patients with hyperthyroidism may be lethargic rather than agitated (*apathetic thyrotoxicosis*), and this is a source of missed diagnoses. The combination of lethargy and unexplained atrial fibrillation is characteristic of apathetic thyrotoxicosis in the elderly (13).

2. *Thyroid Storm*

An uncommon but severe form of hyperthyroidism known as *thyroid storm* can be precipitated by acute illness or major surgery. This condition, which is characterized by fever, severe agitation, and high-output heart failure, can progress to hypotension and coma, and is uniformly fatal if overlooked and left untreated.

B. Diagnosis

Hyperthyroidism is diagnosed by an elevated free T_4 and free T_3 level in plasma. Because hyperthyroidism is almost always caused by primary thyroid disease, the plasma TSH level is not necessary for the diagnosis.

C. Management

1. *β-Receptor Antagonists*

Intravenous **propranolol** (1 mg every 5 minutes until desired effect is achieved) can be used for troublesome tachyarrhythmias. Oral maintenance therapy (20 to 120 mg every 6 hours) can be used until antithyroid drug therapy is effective.

2. *Antithyroid Drugs*

Two drugs are available for suppressing thyroxine production: methimazole and propylthiouracil (14,15). Both are given orally.

a. **Methimazole** is usually preferred because it causes a more rapid decline in serum thyroxine levels and has fewer troublesome side effects. The starting dose is 10 to 30 mg once daily.

b. **Propylthiouracil** is given at a starting dose of 75 to 100 mg every 8 hours. Reports of drug-induced agranulocytosis have limited the popularity of this drug.

c. The dose of both drugs is reduced by 50% after 4 to 6 weeks of therapy.

3. *Iodide*

In severe cases of hyperthyroidism, iodide (which blocks thyroxine release from the thyroid gland) can be added to antithyroid drug therapy. Iodide can be given orally as

Lugol's solution (4 drops every 12 hours) or intravenously as **sodium iodide** (500 to 1000 mg every 12 hours). If the patient has an iodide allergy, lithium (300 mg orally every 8 hours) can be used as a substitute (16).

4. *Thyroid Storm*

   a. In addition to the above measures, the treatment of thyroid storm often requires aggressive volume infusion (to replace fluid losses from vomiting, diarrhea, and heightened insensible fluid loss).

   b. Thyroid storm can accelerate glucocorticoid metabolism and create a relative adrenal insufficiency. In cases of thyroid storm associated with severe or refractory hypotension, **hydrocortisone** (300 mg IV as a loading dose, followed by 100 mg IV every 8 hours) is advised (16).

REFERENCES

1. Marik PE, Zaloga GP. Adrenal insufficiency in the critically ill: a new look at an old problem. Chest 2002; 122:1784–1796.
2. Annane D, Sebille V, Troche G, et al. A 3-level prognostic classification in septic shock based on cortisol levels and cortisol response to corticotropin. JAMA 2000; 283:1038–1045.
3. Cooper MS, Stewart PM. Corticosteroid insufficiency in acutely ill patients. N Engl J Med 2003; 348:727–734.
4. Dorin RI, Kearns PJ. High output circulatory failure in acute adrenal insufficiency. Crit Care Med 1988; 16:296–297.
5. Hamrahian AH, Oseni TS, Arafah BM. Measurements of serum free cortisol in critically ill patients. N Engl J Med 2004; 350:1629–1638.
6. Zeiss CR. Intense pharmacotherapy. Chest 1992; 101(Suppl):407S–412S.
7. Umpierrez GE. Euthyroid sick syndrome. South Med J 2002; 95:506–513.
8. Peeters RP, Debaveye Y, Fliers E, et al. Changes within the thyroid axis during critical illness. Crit Care Clin 2006; 22:41–55.
9. Burman AD, Wartofsky L. Thyroid function in the intensive care unit setting. Crit Care Clin 2001; 17:43–74.
10. Roberts CG, Ladenson PW. Hypothyroidism. Lancet 2004; 363:793–803.
11. Myers L, Hays J. Myxedema coma. Crit Care Clin 1991; 7:43–56.

12. Toft AD. Thyroxine therapy. N Engl J Med 1994; 331:174–180.
13. Klein I. Thyroid hormone and the cardiovascular system. Am J Med 1990; 88:631–637.
14. Franklyn JA. The management of hyperthyroidism. N Engl J Med 1994; 330:1731–1738.
15. Cooper DS. Hyperthyroidism. Lancet 2003; 362:459–468.
16. Migneco A, Ojetti V, Testa A, et al. Management of thyrotoxic crisis. Eur Rev Med Pharmacol Sci 2005; 9:69–74.

Chapter 40

DISORDERS OF MENTATION

Abnormal mental function is one of the most recognizable signs of serious illness. This chapter focuses on the following disorders of mental function: altered consciousness, delirium, coma, and brain death.

I. STATES OF CONSCIOUSNESS

A. States of Consciousness

1. Consciousness has two components: *arousal* and *awareness*. Arousal is the ability to recognize your surroundings (i.e., wakefulness), and awareness is the ability to understand your relationship to the surroundings (i.e., responsiveness).

2. Arousal and awareness can be used to define the different states of consciousness, as shown in Table 40.1

B. Altered Consciousness

Altered consciousness is an abnormality in arousal and/or awareness. There are a multitude of conditions that can cause altered consciousness, and these can be organized as follows:

1. Conditions that cause direct brain injury, which can be ischemic, traumatic, or infectious in origin.

2. Conditions that cause a global brain disorder (i.e., encephalopathy) and are extrinsic to the brain. These conditions

can be infectious (e.g., septic encephalopathy), metabolic (e.g., uremia), or drug-related in origin.

3. One survey of medical ICU patients revealed that ischemic brain injury was the most common cause of altered consciousness on admission to the ICU, and septic encephalopathy was the most common cause after admission to the ICU (1).

TABLE 40.1 States of Consciousness

Aroused & Aware	Aroused & Unaware	Unaroused & Unaware
Anxiety	Delirium	Sleep
Lethargy	Dementia	Coma
	Psychosis	Brain Death
	Vegetative State	

II. DELIRIUM

Delirium is the most common manifestation of altered consciousness in ICU patients (2,3), and as many as two-thirds of these cases go unnoticed (4).

A. Clinical Features

The clinical features of delirium are summarized in Figure 40.1 (2).

1. *Characteristics*

Delirium is a cognitive disorder characterized by attention deficits and either disordered thinking or an altered level of consciousness. The most characteristic features of delirium are its acute onset and fluctuating clinical course.

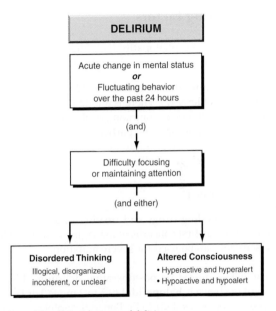

FIGURE 40.1 The clinical features of delirium.

2. *Hypoactive Delirium*

   There is a tendency to consider delirium as a state of agitation (as in delirium tremens), but there is a *hypoactive form of delirium that is characterized by lethargy* (see Figure 40.1). In fact, hypoactive delirium is the most common form of delirium in the elderly (5).

3. *Delirium vs. Dementia*

   Delirium and dementia are distinct disorders that are easily confused because of overlapping clinical features (e.g., attention deficits and abnormal thinking). Furthermore, the two conditions can co-exist (6), which adds to the confusion. The features of delirium that distinguish it from dementia are the abrupt onset and the fluctuating clinical course.

B. Predisposing Factors

1. Any type of encephalopathy (i.e., infectious, metabolic, or drug-related) can produce a state of delirium.

2. Drugs are implicated in as many as 40% of cases of delirium in the elderly (7). There is a long list of potential offenders, but the most common are alcohol (withdrawal), benzodiazepines, opioids (particularly meperidine), digitalis, corticosteroids (high dose), and histamine H_2-receptor antagonists (3,7).

C. Management

Removing offending drugs and treating underlying conditions are obvious first concerns in managing delirium. Short-term sedation can be used for severe agitation.

1. For ICU-acquired or postoperative delirium, the treatment of choice is **haloperidol** (0.5 to 2 mg PO or IV every 4–6 hours as needed) (3,7). Benzodiazepines should be avoided because they can aggravate the delirium (3).

2. For the delirium of alcohol withdrawal, **benzodiazepines** are preferred. (See Table 43.2 for information about benzodiazepine dosing). Haloperidol should be avoided because it can aggravate the delirium and does not prevent the seizures associated with alcohol withdrawal (8).

III. COMA

Because of the vast reserves of the brain, extensive brain injury is required to produce coma , and less than 10% of patients survive coma without significant disability (9). Persistent coma (lasting longer than 6 hours) is most often the result of cardiac arrest or conditions that raise intracranial pressure (e.g., intracerebral hemorrhage).

A. Bedside Evaluation

The bedside evaluation of coma can help to identify the underlying cause, locate the area of brain injury, and determine the likelihood of a satisfactory recovery.

TABLE 40.2 Conditions That Affect the Pupils

Size	Reactive	Nonreactive	
Dilated	Amphetamines Atropine (low) Dopamine	Uncial herniation (unilateral) Post-CPR Brainstem injury Ocular trauma Hypothermia (<28°C)	*High-Dose Drugs:* Amphetamines Atropine Dopamine Phenylephrine Tricyclic antidepressants
Mid-position	Toxic/metabolic encephalopathy Sedative overdose	Brain death Midbrain lesions Barbiturates (high dose)	
Constricted	Toxic/metabolic encephalopathy Pontine injury Opioids	Opioids (high dose) Pilocarpine eyedrops	

1. *Pupils*

   The conditions that affect pupil size and light reactivity are shown in Table 40.2 (10). The following observations deserve mention.

   a. Neuromuscular blocking drugs do not affect pupil size or reactivity (11).

   b. Systemic atropine administration during CPR will dilate the pupils, but they usually remain reactive (12).

   c. High-dose dopamine can cause fixed, dilated pupils (13).

   d. If the pupils remain nonreactive for longer than 6–8 hours after resuscitation from cardiac arrest, the chances of a satisfactory neurologic recovery are poor (14,15).

2. *Ocular Reflexes*

The ocular reflexes are used to evaluate the functional integrity of the brainstem (see Figure 40.2) (16).

a. The *oculocephalic reflex* is evaluated by rotating the head from side-to-side. When the lower brainstem is intact, the eyes will deviate away from the direction of rotation. When lower brainstem function is impaired, the eyes will follow the direction of head rotation.

b. The *oculovestibular reflex* is performed by injecting 50 ml of cold saline into the external auditory canal. When brainstem function is intact, both eyes will deviate slowly toward the irrigated ear. This conjugate eye movement is lost when brainstem function is impaired.

3. *Sensorimotor Exam*

The following findings can have diagnostic or prognostic significance in the presence of coma.

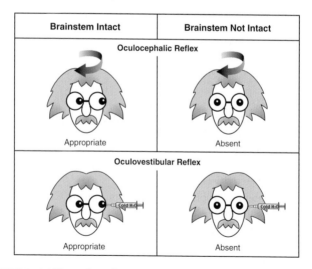

FIGURE 40.2 The ocular reflexes.

a. Clonic movements elicited by flexion of the hands or feet (asterixis) is a sign of metabolic encephalopathy (17), but is not specific for any type of metabolic encephalopathy.

b. A focal motor or sensory defect in the extremities suggests (but does not prove) the presence of a structural lesion.

c. With injury to the thalamus, painful stimuli provoke flexion of the upper extremity. This response is called *decorticate posturing*, and it carries a poor prognosis.

d. With injury to the midbrain and upper pons, the arms and legs extend and pronate in response to pain. This is called *decerebrate posturing*, and it carries a *very* poor prognosis.

B. The Glasgow Coma Score

1. *Description*

The Glasgow coma scale, shown in Table 40.3, is a tool for evaluating the severity of impaired consciousness (18).

a. Points are awarded for performance in three areas: eye opening, verbal communication, and response to verbal and noxious stimuli (18).

b. Points awarded in each area are summed to derive the *Glasgow coma score*. The lowest score is 3 points, and the highest score is 15 points. For intubated patients, who cannot be evaluated for verbal communication, the highest score is 11 points.

2. *Clinical Applications*

The Glasgow coma score (GCS) can be used as follows (14,18,19):

a. To define coma (GCS ≤8).

b. To stratify the severity of head injury; i.e., mild=13–15, moderate=9–12, severe ≤8.

c. To identify candidates for intubation (GCS ≤8).

d. To predict the likelihood of recovery from coma; e.g., in comatose survivors of cardiac arrest, there is virtually no chance of a satisfactory neurologic recovery if the GCS is less than 6 at 72 hours post-arrest (14).

TABLE 40.3 The Glasgow Coma Scale and Score

Eye Opening	Points
Spontaneous	4
To speech	3
To pain	2
None	1 ☐ Points
Verbal Communication	
Oriented	5
Confused conversation	4
Inappropriate but recognized words	3
Incomprehensible sounds	2
None	1 ☐ Points
Motor response	
Obey commands	6
Localizes to pain	5
Withdraws to pain	4
Abnormal flexion (decorticate response)	3
Abnormal extension (decerebrate response)	2
No movement	1 ☐ Points
Glasgow Coma Score (Total points)*	☐ Points

*Lowest score is 3 points, highest score is 15 points (or 11 points with endotracheal intubation).

IV. BRAIN DEATH

Brain death is a condition of irreversible cessation of function in all areas of the brain, with permanent loss of automatic breathing. This condition is most often the result of traumatic head injury, intracerebral hemorrhage, and cardiac arrest.

A. Diagnosis

1. *Overview*

A checklist for the determination of brain death is shown in Table 40.4 (20,21). The clinical diagnosis of brain death requires: 1) irreversible coma, 2) absence of brainstem reflexes, and 3) absence of spontaneous breathing efforts. Two confirmatory evaluations (6 to 8 hours apart) are usually required and additional testing may be necessary in certain situations (see later).

2. *The Apnea Test*

The basis for the apnea test is to observe the patient for spontaneous breathing efforts in the presence of hypercapnia (a powerful respiratory stimulant). The test is performed as follows:

a. After a period of breathing 100% O_2, the patient is separated from the ventilator, and O_2 is insufflated into the endotracheal tube (to prevent hypoxemia during the apnea period).

b. The patient is observed for spontaneous breathing efforts while off the ventilator. If none is evident after 8 to 10 minutes, an arterial blood gas sample is obtained and ventilatory support is resumed. (The arterial PCO_2 will rise an average of 2–3 mm Hg for each minute of apnea.)

c. If the arterial PCO_2 increases by at least 20 mm Hg without breathing efforts, the test confirms the diagnosis of brain death.

d. The period of apnea is not without risk. Hypotension is reported in 25% of apnea tests (22), and life-threatening cardiac arrhythmias can also appear. The apnea test should be aborted if any of these complications develops.

e. Because of the risks involved, the apnea test is usually not repeated if it confirms the diagnosis of brain death.

TABLE 40.4 Checklist for the Diagnosis of Brain Death

When Steps 1, 2, and 3 are confirmed, the patient is declared brain dead.

	Check (✓) Item if Confirmed
Step 1: Prerequisite to Exam	
Establish that the following conditions are not present, and are not contributing to the loss of consciousness.	❏

  1. Hypotension (mean arterial pressure <60 mm Hg)
  2. Hypothermia (core temperature <32°C or <90°F)
  3. Metabolic disturbances (e.g., hypoglycemia)
  4. Contributory drugs or medications
  5. Confounding conditions (e.g., hypothyroidism)

Establish that the cause of coma (known or suspected) is sufficient to account for brain death, or that neuroimaging tests are consistent with brain death.   ❏

Step 2: Absence of Brain and Brainstem Function

Involves 2 exams, usually performed 6 hours apart	1st Exam	2nd Exam
Coma: No cerebral motor response in all extremities *and* face to noxious stimuli[†]	❏	❏
Absent Brainstem Reflexes:		
Pupils: • Size: midposition to dilated (4–9 mm)	❏	❏
• No response to bright light	❏	❏
No corneal reflex (touch edge of cornea)	❏	❏
No gag reflex (stimulate pharynx)	❏	❏
No cough response to tracheal suction	❏	❏
Ocular Reflexes: • Absent oculocephalic reflex[*]	❏	❏
• Absent oculovestibular reflex	❏	❏

Step 2a: Consider Confirmatory Test
if Steps 1 or 2 cannot be completed or adequately interpreted.

Step 3: Absence of Respiratory Effort

Positive Apnea Test: No breathing efforts when arterial PCO_2 >20 mm Hg above baseline   ❏

Step 3a: Consider Confirmatory Test
if Step 3 cannot be completed or adequately interpreted.

Adapted from References 20 & 21. [*]Perform only if cervical spine is stable.
[†]Nail-bed and supraorbital ridge pressure.

3. *Spontaneous Movements*

One source of confusion during the brain death evaluation is the appearance of brief, spontaneous movements of the head, torso, or upper extremities, particularly during the apnea test. These movements (called *Lazarus' sign*) are the result of neuronal bursts from the cervical spine (23) and are not manifestations of functional brain activity.

4. *Confirmatory Tests*

A clinical diagnosis of brain death may not be possible in patients with the following conditions:

a. Severe facial trauma or cervical spinal cord injury.

b. Pre-existing pupillary abnormalities.

c. End-stage pulmonary disease with severe hypercapnia.

d. Significant levels of drugs that can interfere with the clinical evaluation (e.g., neuromuscular blockers).

The diagnosis of brain death in these conditions may require confirmatory tests such as electroencephalography, brain scan with technetium-99m, transcranial doppler, or somatosensory evoked potentials (20,21).

B. The Potential Organ Donor

The following measures can enhance organ viability in the potential organ donor (24,25).

1. *Hemodynamics*

a. Hypotension or reduced urinary output (<1 mL/kg per hour) should prompt volume resuscitation to a CVP of 10–15 mm Hg.

b. Persistent hypotension can be managed with dopamine, preferably in the range of 5–15 μg/kg/min to avoid α-adrenergic vasoconstriction (which can further compromise perfusion of the vital organs).

c. Hemodynamic instability should prompt an evaluation for pituitary failure, as described next.

2. *Pituitary Failure*

More than 50% of patients with brain death will develop pituitary failure with *diabetes insipidus* and secondary *adrenal insufficiency* (25). Both conditions can lead to hemodynamic instability and compromised organ perfusion.

a. The diagnosis and management of diabetes insipidus can proceed as described in Chapter 26, Section IV.

b. The diagnosis of secondary adrenal insufficiency can be difficult because the ACTH stimulation test (for primary adrenal insufficiency) is not useful in this condition. If adrenal insufficiency is suspected because of persistent hypotension, intravenous **hydrocortisone**, 50 mg every 6 hours, is warranted.

REFERENCES

1. Bleck TP, Smith MC, Pierre-Louis SJ, et al. Neurologic complications of critical medical illnesses. Crit Care Med 1993; 21:98–103.
2. Ely EW, Margolin R, Francis J, et al. Evaluation of delirium in critically ill patients: validation of the Confusion Assessment Method for the Intensive Care Unit (CAM-ICU). Crit Care Med 2001; 29:1370–1379.
3. Inouye SK. Delirium in older persons. N Engl J Med 2006; 354:1157–1165.
4. Inouye SK. The dilemma of delirium: clinical and research controversies regarding diagnosis and evaluation of delirium in hospitalized elderly medical patients. Am J Med 1994; 97:278–288.
5. Ely EW, Shintani A, Truman B, et al. Delirium as a predictor of mortality in mechanically ventilated patients in the intensive care unit. JAMA 2004; 291:1753–1762.
6. Fick DM, Agostini JV, Inouye SK. Delirium superimposed on dementia: a systematic review. J Am Geriatr Soc 2002; 50:1723–1732.
7. Brown TM, Boyle MF. Delirium. BMJ 2002; 325:644–647.
8. Kosten TR, O'Connor PG. Management of drug and alcohol withdrawal. N Engl J Med 2003; 348:1786–1795.

9. Hamel MB, Goldman L, Teno J, et al. Identification of comatose patients at high risk for death or severe disability. JAMA 1995; 273:1842–1848.

10. Stevens RD, Bhardwaj A. Approach to the comatose patient. Crit Care Med 2006; 34:31–41.

11. Gray AT, Krejci ST, Larson MD. Neuromuscular blocking drugs do not alter the pupillary light reflex of anesthetized humans. Arch Neurol 1997; 54:579–584.

12. Goetting MG, Contreras E. Systemic atropine administration during cardiac arrest does not cause fixed and dilated pupils. Ann Emerg Med 1991; 20:55–57.

13. Ong GL, Bruning HA. Dilated fixed pupils due to administration of high doses of dopamine hydrochloride. Crit Care Med 1981; 9:658–659.

14. Edgren E, Hedstrand U, Kelsey S, et al. Assessment of neurological prognosis in comatose survivors of cardiac arrest. BRCT I Study Group. Lancet 1994; 343:1055–1059.

15. Zandbergen EG, de Haan RJ, Koelman JH, et al. Prediction of poor outcome in anoxic-ischemic coma. J Clin Neurophysiol 2000; 17:498–501.

16. Bateman DE. Neurological assessment of coma. J Neurol Neurosurg Psychiatry 2001; 71:i13–17.

17. Kunze K. Metabolic encephalopathies. J Neurol 2002; 249:1150–1159.

18. Teasdale G, Jennett B. Assessment of coma and impaired consciousness: A practical scale. Lancet 1974; 2:81–84.

19. Sternbach GL. The Glasgow coma scale. J Emerg Med 2000; 19:67–71.

20. Practice parameters for determining brain death in adults (summary statement): The Quality Standards Subcommittee of the American Academy of Neurology. Neurology 1995; 45:1012–1014.

21. Wijdicks EF. The diagnosis of brain death. N Engl J Med 2001; 344:1215–1221.

22. Goudreau JL, Wijdicks EF, Emery SF. Complications during apnea testing in the determination of brain death: predisposing factors. Neurology 2000; 55:1045–1048.

23. Ropper AH. Unusual spontaneous movements in brain-dead patients. Neurology 1984; 34:1089–1092.

24. Wood KE, Becker BN, McCartney JG, et al. Care of the potential organ donor. N Engl J Med 2004; 351:2730–2739.

25. Detterbeck FC, Mill MR. Organ donation and the management of the multiple organ donor. Contemp Surg 1993; 42:281–285.

Chapter 41

DISORDERS OF MOVEMENT

There are three movement disorders that you may encounter in the ICU: (1) involuntary movements (seizures), (2) weak or ineffective movements (neuromuscular weakness), and (3) no movements (drug-induced paralysis). Each of these conditions is described briefly in this chapter.

I. SEIZURES

Seizures are second only to metabolic encephalopathy as the most common neurologic complication that follows admission to the ICU (1). The incidence of new-onset seizures in ICU patients is 0.8 to 3.5% (1, 2).

A. Types of Seizures

Seizures are classified by the extent of brain involvement (generalized vs. partial seizures), the presence or absence of abnormal movements (convulsive vs. nonconvulsive seizures), and the type of movement abnormality (tonic, clonic, or myoclonic movements).

1. *Abnormal Movements*

The movements associated with seizures can be *tonic* (caused by sustained muscle contraction), *clonic* (rhythmic movements with a regular amplitude and frequency) or *myoclonic* (irregular movements that vary in amplitude and frequency) (3). Some movements are familiar (e.g., chewing) but repetitive; these are called *automatisms*.

2. *Generalized Seizures*

Generalized seizures arise from synchronous electrical discharges that involve the entire cerebral cortex, and they are always associated with loss of consciousness (3). The following statements pertain to generalized seizures in the ICU patient population.

a. Most generalized seizures produce abnormal movements (convulsive seizures), and include both tonic and clonic movements (4).

b. Generalized seizures associated with myoclonic movements have been reported in comatose survivors of cardiac arrest (5), and these seizures carry a poor prognosis for recovery if they persist for longer than 24 hours post-resuscitation (6).

b. As many as 25% of generalized seizures are nonconvulsive; i.e., are not accompanied by abnormal movements (4). According to one clinical study, *nonconvulsive seizures are responsible for 10% of cases of unexplained coma* (7). An EEG is required to uncover nonconvulsive seizures.

3. *Partial (Focal) Seizures*

Partial seizures arise from localized areas of electrical discharge, and they produce abnormal motor activity in areas served by the involved region of the brain. These seizures may or may not result in impaired consciousness, and the abnormal movements can be tonic-clonic, myoclonic, or automatisms. The following partial seizures deserve mention:

a. *Temporal lobe seizures* often produce a motionless stare, accompanied by repetitive chewing or lip smacking (automatisms).

b. *Epilepsia partialis continua* is characterized by persistent tonic-clonic movements of the facial and limb muscles on one side of the body.

4. *Status Epilepticus*

Status epilepticus is defined as more than 30 minutes of continuous seizure activity or recurrent seizure activity without an intervening period of consciousness (4). Any variety of seizure can be involved, and 10% of the convulsive seizures can be refractory to conventional therapy (8).

B. Predisposing Conditions

A variety of conditions can produce seizures in critically ill patients (see Table 41.1). In one survey of seizures in the ICU setting, the most common predisposing conditions were drug intoxication, drug withdrawal, and metabolic abnormalities (e.g., hypoglycemia) (2).

TABLE 41.1 Possible Causes of Seizures in the ICU

Ischemic	**Traumatic**
Acute stroke	Contusion
Cardiac arrest	Intracerebral hemorrhage
Circulatory shock	Intracranial hypertension
	Subdural hematoma
Infectious	
Abscess	**Drug Toxicity**
Meningoencephalitis	Amphetamines
Septic emboli	Cocaine
Toxoplasmosis	Imipenem
	Isoniazid
Metabolic	Meperidine
Hypoglycemia	Theophylline
Hyponatremia	Tricyclics
Hypoxia	
Uremia	**Drug Withdrawal**
Liver failure	Barbiturates
	Benzodiazepines
Hematologic	Ethanol
DIC	Opiates
TTP	

DIC = disseminated intravascular coagulopathy.
TTP = thrombotic thrombocytopenia purpura.

C. Acute Management

Treating and removing the cause of seizures is the obvious treatment of choice. The acute management of convulsive seizures can proceed as summarized in Figure 41.1 (9-13).

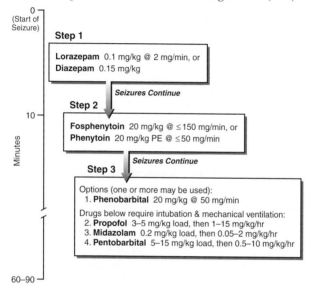

FIGURE 41.1 A stepwise approach to the acute management of convulsive seizures. *PE* = phenytoin equivalents.

1. *Benzodiazepines*

   Intravenous benzodiazepines will terminate 65–80% of convulsive seizures within 2 to 3 minutes (10,11).

   a. **Lorazepam** (Ativan) is currently the agent of choice. A single intravenous dose of 0.1 mg/kg IV is effective for 12 to 24 hours (9,11).

   b. **Diazepam** (Valium) in an intravenous dose of 0.15 mg/kg is as effective as lorazepam for aborting convulsive seizures, but the effects last only 15 to 30 minutes (9,11), so there is a risk of recurrence. Diazepam should be followed immediately by phenytoin to prevent seizure recurrence.

2. *Phenytoin*

Phenytoin is used for seizures that are refractory to benzodiazepines or likely to recur.

   a. The standard intravenous dose is 20 mg/kg in adults; a smaller dose of 15 mg/kg is recommended in the elderly (12). If the initial dose of phenytoin is unsuccessful, additional doses can be given to a total cumulative dose of 30 mg/kg (11).

   b. A maximum infusion rate of 50 mg/min is advised to reduce the risk of cardiovascular depression (caused by the drug and the *propylene glycol* used as a solubilizer) (11).

3. *Fosphenytoin*

Fosphenytoin (Cerebyx) is a water-soluble phenytoin surrogate that produces less cardiovascular depression than phenytoin because it does not contain propylene glycol. As a result, fosphenytoin can be infused three times faster than phenytoin (150 mg/min vs. 50 mg/min) (14). Fosphenytoin is a prodrug (must be converted to phenytoin), and is given in the same doses as phenytoin.

4. *Refractory Status Epilepticus*

Ten percent of patients with convulsive status epilepticus are refractory to first- and second-line anticonvulsants (8). The options for these patients are shown in Figure 41.1.

   a. **Pentobarbital** is the most effective agent for this condition (15). Hypotension is common but often responds to volume resuscitation.

   b. At this stage, consulting a neurologist is probably the best option.

TABLE 41.2 Comparative Features of Myasthenia Gravis and Guillain-Barré Syndrome

Features	Myasthenia Gravis	Guillain-Barré Syndrome
Ocular weakness	Yes	No
Fluctuating weakness	Yes	No
Bulbar weakness	Yes	Yes
Deep tendon reflexes	Intact	Depressed
Autonomic instability	No	Yes
Nerve conduction	Normal	Slowed

II. NEUROMUSCULAR WEAKNESS

The following is a description of clinical disorders that can produce life-threatening muscle weakness.

A. Myasthenia Gravis

Myasthenia gravis (MG) is an autoimmune disease produced by antibody-mediated destruction of acetylcholine receptors on the postsynaptic side of neuromuscular junctions (16).

1. *Predisposing Conditions*
   a. MG can be triggered by major surgery or a concurrent illness. Thymic tumors are responsible for up to 20% of cases, and hyperthyroidism is the culprit in 5% of cases.
   b. Several drugs can precipitate or aggravate MG (17). The principal offenders are antibiotics (e.g., aminoglycosides, ciprofloxacin) and cardiac drugs (e.g., beta-adrenergic blockers, lidocaine, procainamide, quinidine).

2. *Clinical Features*

   The weakness in MG typically worsens with activity and improves with rest.

a. Weakness is first apparent in the eyelids and extraocular muscles, and limb weakness follows in 85% of cases (18).

b. Progressive weakness often involves the chest wall and diaphragm, and rapid progression to respiratory failure, called *myasthenic crisis*, occurs in 15–20% of patients (18).

c. The deficit in myasthenia is purely motor, and deep tendon reflexes are preserved (see Table 41.2).

3. *Diagnosis*

The diagnosis of MG is based on the following findings:

a. The characteristic pattern of muscle weakness; i.e., eyelid or extraocular muscle weakness made worse by repeated use.

b. Increased muscle strength after the administration of **edrophonium** (Tensilon), an acetylcholinesterase inhibitor.

c. The presence of acetylcholine receptor antibodies in the blood. These antibodies are found in 85% of cases of MG (16), and their presence secures the diagnosis.

4. *Treatment*

a. The first line of therapy is an acetylcholinesterase inhibitor like **pyridostigmine** (Mestinon), which is started at an oral dose of 60 mg every 6 hours and can be increased to 120 mg every 6 hours if necessary. Pyridostigmine can be given intravenously to treat myasthenic crisis: the IV dose is 1/30th of the oral dose (19,20).

b. Immunotherapy is added if needed using either **prednisone** (1-1.5 mg/kg/day), **azathioprine** (1 to 3 mg/kg/day), or **cyclosporine** (2.5 mg/kg twice per day) (20).

c. Surgical thymectomy is often advised in patients under 60 years of age to reduce the need for long-term immunosuppressive therapy (20).

5. *Advanced Cases*

In advanced cases requiring mechanical ventilation, clearing pathologic antibodies from the bloodstream by **plasmapheresis** or neutralizing the antibodies with **immunoglobulin G** (0.4 or 2 g/kg/day IV for 2 to 5 days) are equally effective therapies (18,20). However, plasmapheresis produces a more rapid response (20).

B. Guillain-Barré Syndrome

The Guillain-Barré syndrome is an *acute inflammatory demyelinating polyneuropathy* that often follows an acute infectious illness (by 1 to 3 weeks) (21,22). An immune etiology is suspected.

1. *Clinical Features*
   a. The presenting features include paresthesias and symmetric limb weakness that evolves over a period of a few days to a few weeks.
   b. Progression to respiratory failure occurs in 25% of cases (21), and autonomic instability can be a feature in advanced cases (23).
   c. The condition resolves spontaneously in about 80% of cases, but residual neurologic deficits are common (21).

2. *Diagnosis*

   Some distinguishing features of Guillain-Barré syndrome are shown in Table 41.2. The diagnosis is based on clinical presentation, nerve conduction studies (evidence of neuropathy), and cerebrospinal fluid analysis (elevated protein in 80% of cases) (21).

3. *Treatment*

   Treatment is mostly supportive, but in cases with respiratory failure, **plasmapheresis** and intravenous **immunoglobulin G** (0.4 g/kg/day for 5 days) are equally effective in producing short-term improvement. Immunoglobulin G is often preferred because it is easiest to administer.

C. Critical Illness Polyneuropathy & Myopathy

Critical illness polyneuropathy (CIP) and critical illness myopathy (CIM) are secondary disorders and most often accompany severe sepsis and other conditions that trigger progressive systemic inflammation (see Chapter 33, Table 33.2) (24). Both disorders can occur in the same patient, and they usually become apparent when patients fail to wean from mechanical ventilation.

1. *Critical Illness Polyneuropathy*

   a. CIP is a diffuse sensory and motor axonal neuropathy that is reported in at least 50% of patients with severe sepsis (24,25). The onset is variable, occurring from 2 days to a few weeks after the onset of the inciting illness.

   b. Nerve conduction studies are necessary to establish the diagnosis.

   c. There is no specific treatment. Complete recovery is expected in 50% of cases (26) and can take months.

2. *Critical Illness Myopathy*

   a. CIM is a spectrum of muscle disorders. Predisposing conditions include systemic inflammation and prolonged treatment with steroids and neuromuscular blocking agents (25,27). CIM has also been reported in one-third of patients with status asthmaticus, particularly those receiving high-dose steroids (27).

   b. The diagnosis of CIM is supported by electromyography (shows evidence of myopathy) and muscle biopsy (shows atrophy and loss of myosin filaments) (27).

   c. There is no treatment for CIM. If the precipitating condition has resolved, most patients with CPM recover fully within a few months (27).

III. NEUROMUSCULAR BLOCKERS

A. General Features

Drug-induced paralysis is occasionally needed to manage ventilator-dependent patients who are agitated and difficult to ventilate (28,29). However, this practice is frowned upon for reasons stated later.

1. *Mechanisms*

Neuromuscular blocking agents act by binding to acetylcholine receptors on the postsynaptic side of the neuromuscular junction. Once bound, there are two different modes of action.

a. The *depolarizing agents* act like acetylcholine and produce a sustained depolarization of the postsynaptic membrane.

b. The *nondepolarizing agents* act by inhibiting depolarization of the postsynaptic membrane.

B. Drugs

A comparison of neuromuscular blocking drugs is shown in Table 41.3. All three agents in this table are nondepolarizing blockers.

1. **Pancuronium** (Pavulon) has over 35 years of clinical use, but its popularity has dwindled because of its relatively long duration of action (1 to 2 hours) and its tendency to produce tachycardia. Although it can be given by continuous infusion, pancuronium is usually given as intermittent bolus doses (0.1 mg/kg every 1–2 hrs) to decrease the risk of drug accumulation. Dose adjustments are necessary in renal failure.

2. **Rocuronium** (Zemuron) is shorter acting than pancuronium and does not produce tachycardia in usual doses.

Dose reductions are necessary in liver failure.

3. **Cisatracurium** (Nimbex) is also short acting and devoid of cardiovascular side effects. It is considered an improved version of its parent drug **atracurium** because it generates less laudanosine, a metabolite that can cause neuroexcitation (30). Dose adjustments are not necessary in renal and hepatic failure.

TABLE 41.3 Comparison of Neuromuscular Blocking Agents

	Pancuronium	Rocuronium	Cisatracurium
Initial dose (mg/kg)	0.1	0.6–1.0	0.1–2.0
Duration of effect (min)	60–100	30–40	35–50
Infusion (µg/kg/min)	1–2	10–12	2.5–3
Risk of tachycardia	Yes	Minimal	No
Dose adjustment in renal failure	Yes	No	No
Dose adjustment in hepatic failure	No	Yes	No

4. **Succinylcholine** (Anectine) is an ultra-short acting depolarizing agent, and is used only to facilitate endotracheal intubation. An intravenous dose of 1–2 mg/kg produces paralysis within 60 seconds, and the effect lasts for about 5 minutes.

   a. The depolarization of muscle cells leads to potassium efflux, and this can raise the serum K^+ by about 0.5 mEq/L (31).

   b. Life-threatening hyperkalemia can occur when succinylcholine is given in the presence of denervation injury (e.g., head or spinal cord injury), rhabdomyolysis, hemorrhagic shock, thermal injury, and chronic immobility.

C. Monitoring

The standard method of monitoring drug-induced paralysis is to apply a series of four low-frequency (2 Hz) electrical pulses to the ulnar nerve at the forearm and observe for adduction of the thumb. Total absence of thumb adduction is evidence of excessive block. The desired goal is 1 or 2 perceptible twitches, and the drug infusion is adjusted to achieve that endpoint (28).

D. Disadvantages

1. Paralysis is an extremely frightening and even painful experience, and it is imperative to keep patients heavily sedated during the entire period of paralysis. However, it is not possible to evaluate the adequacy of sedation while a patient is paralyzed. Patients often awaken while paralyzed (32), and this alone is reason enough to avoid paralysis whenever possible.

2. Prolonged periods of paralysis can be associated with the following complications:

    a. Critical illness myopathy (described earlier).

    b. Pneumonia (due to pooling of respiratory secretions in dependent lung regions).

    c. Venous thromboembolism (due to prolonged immobilization).

    d. Pressure ulcers on the skin (also due to prolonged immobilization).

REFERENCES

1. Bleck TP, Smith MC, Pierre-Louis SJ, et al. Neurologic complications of critical medical illnesses. Crit Care Med 1993; 21:98–103.

2. Wijdicks EF, Sharbrough FW. New-onset seizures in critically ill patients. Neurology 1993; 43:1042–1044.

3. Chabolla DR. Characteristics of the epilepsies. Mayo Clin Proc 2002; 77:981–990.

4. Marik PE, Varon J. The management of status epilepticus. Chest 2004; 126:582–591.

5. Wijdicks EF, Parisi JE, Sharbrough FW. Prognostic value of myoclonus status in comatose survivors of cardiac arrest. Ann Neurol 1994; 35:239–243.

6. Morris HR, Howard RS, Brown P. Early myoclonic status and outcome after cardiorespiratory arrest. J Neurol Neurosurg Psychiatry 1998; 64:267–268.

7. Towne AR, Waterhouse EJ, Boggs JG, et al. Prevalence of nonconvulsive status epilepticus in comatose patients. Neurology 2000; 54:340–345.

8. Mayer SA, Claassen J, Lokin J, et al. Refractory status epilepticus: frequency, risk factors, and impact on outcome. Arch Neurol 2002; 59:205–210.

9. Manno EM. New management strategies in the treatment of status epilepticus. Mayo Clin Proc 2003; 78:508–518.

10. Treiman DM, Meyers PD, Walton NY, et al. A comparison of four treatments for generalized convulsive status epilepticus. N Engl J Med 1998; 339:792–798.

11. Lowenstein DH, Alldredge BK. Status epilepticus. N Engl J Med 1998; 338:970–976.

12. Epilepsy Foundation of America's Working Group on Status Epilepticus. Treatment of convulsive status epilepticus. Recommendations of the Epilepsy Foundation of America's Working Group on Status Epilepticus. JAMA 1993; 270:854–859.

13. Bassin S, Smith TL, Bleck TP. Clinical review: status epilepticus. Crit Care 2002; 6:137–142.

14. Fischer JH, Patel TV, Fischer PA. Fosphenytoin: clinical pharmacokinetics and comparative advantages in the acute treatment of seizures. Clin Pharmacokinet 2003; 42:33–58.

15. Claassen J, Hirsch LJ, Emerson RG, et al. Treatment of refractory status epilepticus with pentobarbital, propofol, or midazolam: a systematic review. Epilepsia 2002; 43:146–153.

16. Vincent A, Palace J, Hilton-Jones D. Myasthenia gravis. Lancet 2001; 357:2122–2128.

17. Wittbrodt ET. Drugs and myasthenia gravis. An update. Arch Intern Med 1997; 157:399–408.

18. Drachman DB. Myasthenia gravis. N Engl J Med 1994; 330: 1797–1810.

19. Berrouschot J, Baumann I, Kalischewski P, et al. Therapy of myasthenic crisis. Crit Care Med 1997; 25:1228–1235.

20. Saperstein DS, Barohn RJ. Management of myasthenia gravis. Semin Neurol 2004; 24:41–48.

21. Hughes RA, Cornblath DR. Guillain-Barre syndrome. Lancet 2005; 366:1653–1666.

22. Hund EF, Borel CO, Cornblath DR, et al. Intensive management and treatment of severe Guillain-Barre syndrome. Crit Care Med 1993; 21:433–446.

23. Pfeiffer G, Schiller B, Kruse J, et al. Indicators of dysautonomia in severe Guillain-Barre syndrome. J Neurol 1999; 246:1015–1022.

24. Hund E. Neurological complications of sepsis: critical illness polyneuropathy and myopathy. J Neurol 2001; 248:929–934.

25. Bolton CF. Neuromuscular manifestations of critical illness. Muscle & Nerve 2005; 32:140–163.

26. van Mook WN, Hulsewe-Evers RP. Critical illness polyneuropathy. Curr Opin Crit Care 2002; 8:302–310.

27. Lacomis D. Critical illness myopathy. Curr Rheumatol Rep 2002; 4:403–408.

28. Murray MJ, Cowen J, DeBlock H, et al. Clinical practice guidelines for sustained neuromuscular blockade in the adult critically ill patient. Crit Care Med 2002; 30:142–156.

29. Coursin DB, Prielipp RC. Use of neuromuscular blocking drugs in the critically ill patient. Crit Care Clin 1995; 11:957–981.

30. Fodale V, Santamaria LB. Laudanosine, an atracurium and cis-atracurium metabolite. Eur J Anaesthesiol 2002; 19:466–473.

31. Koide M, Waud BE. Serum potassium concentrations after succinylcholine in patients with renal failure. Anesthesiology 1972; 36:142–145.

32. Parker MM, Schubert W, Shelhamer JH, et al. Perceptions of a critically ill patient experiencing therapeutic paralysis in an ICU. Crit Care Med 1984; 12:69–71.

Chapter 42

ACUTE STROKE

The focus of this chapter is a cerebrovascular disorder that has suffered through a variety of poorly descriptive names like apoplexy, cerebrovascular accident (what accident?), stroke, and brain attack. Considering that this disorder is the third leading cause of death in the United States, and the leading cause of long-term disability (1, 2), it deserves a better name.

I. DEFINITIONS

According to the National Institute of Neurological Disorders and Stroke, stroke is "an acute brain disorder of vascular origin accompanied by neurological dysfunction that persists for longer than 24 hours" (3).

A. Types of Stroke

Stroke is classified according to the immediate cause of brain injury; i.e., ischemia or hemorrhage (1,3).

1. *Ischemic stroke* accounts for 80 to 88% of all strokes.

   a. *Thrombotic stroke* accounts for 80% of ischemic strokes and is caused by atherosclerotic disease.

   b. *Embolic stroke* accounts for 20% of ischemic strokes. Most emboli originate from thrombi in the left atrium (from atrial fibrillation) or left ventricle (from acute MI), but some originate from venous thrombi in the legs that reach the brain through a patent foramen ovale (4).

2. *Hemorrhagic stroke* accounts for 12–20% of all strokes.

   a. Intracerebral hemorrhage accounts for 75% of hemorrhagic strokes, and subarachnoid hemorrhage accounts for the remaining 25%.

b. Epidural and subdural hematomas are not classified as strokes (3).

B. Transient Ischemic Attack

1. A transient ischemic attack (TIA) is an acute episode of focal loss of brain function that is caused by ischemia and lasts less than 24 hours (3).

2. The one feature that distinguishes TIA from stroke is the *reversibility of clinical symptoms*. Reversibility of cerebral injury is not a distinguishing feature because one-third of TIAs are associated with cerebral infarction (5,6).

II. THE EVALUATION

A. Avoiding Delays

Prompt recognition of acute stroke is mandatory for the following reasons:

1. Each minute of ongoing infarction causes the destruction of 1.9 million neurons and *7.5 miles of myelinated nerves* (7).

2. The benefit of thrombolytic therapy in ischemic stroke is confined to the first 3 hours after symptom onset (8a,8b).

B. Bedside Evaluation

Stroke is primarily a clinical diagnosis (9). The presentation is characterized by one or more focal neurologic deficits corresponding to the region of brain injury. The clinical findings and corresponding regions of ischemic brain injury are shown in Figure 42.1.

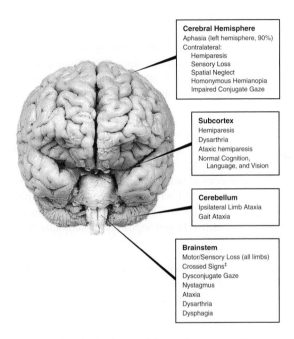

Cerebral Hemisphere
Aphasia (left hemisphere, 90%)
Contralateral:
  Hemiparesis
  Sensory Loss
  Spatial Neglect
  Homonymous Hemianopia
  Impaired Conjugate Gaze

Subcortex
Hemiparesis
Dysarthria
Ataxic hemiparesis
Normal Cognition,
  Language, and Vision

Cerebellum
Ipsilateral Limb Ataxia
Gait Ataxia

Brainstem
Motor/Sensory Loss (all limbs)
Crossed Signs[‡]
Dysconjugate Gaze
Nystagmus
Ataxia
Dysarthria
Dysphagia

FIGURE 42.1 Neurologic abnormalities and corresponding areas of ischemic brain injury. ‡Signs on same side of face and other side of body.

1. *Consciousness*

   Most cerebral infarctions are unilateral, and thus loss of consciousness is not a common finding (10). When focal neurologic deficits are accompanied by coma, the most likely diagnoses are intracerebral hemorrhage, massive cerebral infarction with cerebral edema, brainstem infarction, or nonconvulsive seizures.

2. *Aphasia*

The left cerebral hemisphere is the dominant hemisphere for speech in 90% of subjects.

a. Injury in the left cerebral hemisphere produces a condition known as aphasia, which is defined as a disturbance in the comprehension and/or formulation of language.

b. Patients with aphasia can have difficulty in verbal comprehension (*receptive aphasia*), difficulty in verbal expression (*expressive aphasia*), or both (*global aphasia*).

3. *Sensorimotor Function*

The hallmark of injury involving one cerebral hemisphere is weakness and sensory loss on the contralateral side of the face and body.

a. The presence of hemiparesis supports the diagnosis of TIA or stroke, but is not specific for these conditions.

b. Hemiparesis has also been described in metabolic encephalopathy (11) and septic encephalopathy (12).

4. *Other Findings*

a. As many as 50% of patients admitted for stroke will have swallowing dysfunction (13).

b. Fever (>37.5°C) develops in 40% cases of acute stroke and usually appears in the first 24 hours after symptom onset (14,15).

c. Seizures are uncommon (5%) in the first 2 weeks after ischemic stroke (16).

B. Diagnostic Evaluation

1. *Candidates for Thrombolytic Therapy*

If a stroke is suspected based on the bedside evaluation, further diagnostic evaluation is influenced by whether the patient is a candidate for thrombolytic therapy. Table 42.1 shows a checklist that can be used to determine if thrombolytic therapy is appropriate for an individual patient.

TABLE 42.1 Checklist for Thrombolytic Therapy

1. *Check the **indications** below that apply:*
   - ❏ Patient is 18 years of age or older
   - ❏ Time of symptom onset can be identified accurately
   - ❏ Thrombolytic therapy can be started within 3 hrs of symptom onset

2. *If all the boxes in Step 1 are checked, then review the **absolute contraindications** below and check the ones that apply:*
   - ❏ Head CT scan today shows intracranial bleeding
   - ❏ Head CT scan today shows no intracranial bleeding, but the clinical presentation is suspicious for subarachnoid hemorrhage
   - ❏ Head CT scan today shows multilobar infarction (hypodense area >1/3 the area of the cerebral hemisphere)
   - ❏ Any of the following within the past 3 months: intracranial or intraspinal surgery, serious head trauma, or a witnessed seizure
   - ❏ Witnessed seizure since the onset of symptoms
   - ❏ Blood pressure >186 mm Hg (systolic or >110 mm Hg (diastolic)
   - ❏ Arterial puncture at noncompressible site within past 7 days

   Risk of Hemorrhage
   - ❏ Evidence of active internal bleeding
   - ❏ Patient has arteriovenous malformation, aneurysm, or neoplasm
   - ❏ Prior history of intracranial bleeding
   - ❏ Laboratory evidence of a coagulopathy (e.g., platelet count <100,000/µL)
   - ❏ Patient on coumadin and INR ≥1.7, or patient received heparin in past 48 hr and aPTT above normal range

3. *If none of the boxes in Step 2 is checked, review the **relative contraindications** below and check any that represent an unacceptable risk:*
   - ❏ Major surgery or serious trauma in past 14 days
   - ❏ Gastrointestinal or urinary tract bleeding within past 21 days
   - ❏ Acute MI in past 3 months or post-MI pericarditis
   - ❏ Blood glucose <50 mg/dL or >400 mg/dL

If all boxes in Step 1 are checked, and no boxes in Steps 2 and 3 are checked, then give thrombolytic therapy.

From 2005 American Heart Association Guidelines for Cardiopulmonary Resuscitation and Emergency Cardiovascular Care. Part, Adult Stroke. Circulation 2005; 112:IV111-120.

1. *Computed Tomography*

   a. The principal role of CT imaging in suspected stroke is to identify hemorrhage, which is an absolute contraindication to thrombolytic therapy (see Table 42.1). The sensitivity of CT scans for intracerebral hemorrhage is almost 100% (5).

   b. CT imaging should not be used to confirm the diagnosis of ischemic stroke because one-half of cerebral infarcts are not apparent on CT scan (13), and the diagnostic yield is even less in the first 24 hours after symptom onset (5). Figure 42.2 demonstrates the non-value of CT imaging in the early diagnosis of ischemic stroke (17).

2. *Magnetic Resonance Imaging*

   Magnetic resonance imaging (MRI) can detect 90% of is-

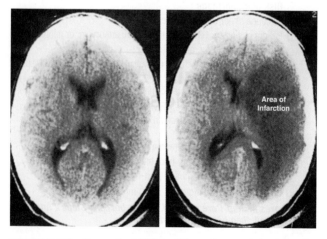

FIGURE 42.2 The diagnostic yield from CT scans in acute ischemic stroke. The CT image on the left was obtained within 24 hours after symptom onset and is unrevealing. The CT image on the right was obtained 3 days later in the same patient, and shows a large hypodense area (infarction) with mass effect in the left cerebral hemisphere. From Reference 17.

chemic strokes in the first 24 hours after symptom onset (5). Because of the superior diagnostic yield, MRI is likely to replace CT imaging for the early evaluation of suspected stroke.

3. *Echocardiography*

   Echocardiography is useful in the following situations:

   a. When stroke is associated with atrial fibrillation, acute MI, or left-sided endocarditis (to identify a source of cerebral embolism).

   b. When stroke occurs in patients with no risk factors, or in patients with venous thromboembolism (to identify a patent foramen ovale).

III. ANTITHROMBOTIC THERAPY

A. Thrombolytic Therapy

1. Thrombolytic therapy is indicated if it can be started within 3 hours of symptom onset and there are no contraindications (8a,8b). The absolute and relative contraindications for thrombolytic therapy are included in the checklist in Table 42.1

2. **Tissue plasminogen activator** (tPA) is the only thrombolytic agent approved for use in acute stroke. The dose is 0.9 mg/kg infused over 1 hr, with a maximum dose of 90 mg (18).

B. Aspirin

Aspirin is recommended for all cases of acute ischemic stroke (unless there are contraindications) (8a, 8b, 13).

   a. When thrombolytic therapy is given, aspirin should be started on the following day. Otherwise, the first dose of aspirin should be given after intracranial hemorrhage is ruled out by neuroimaging.

b. The recommended dose of aspirin is 160–300 mg initially (orally or per rectum), followed by 75–150 mg daily.

C. Heparin

1. Anticoagulation with heparin has been a traditional practice for patients with acute ischemic stroke who show progression of symptoms. However, the results of clinical trials do not support this practice (19).

2. The only role for heparin in acute ischemic stroke is for prophylaxis of venous thromboembolism (see Chapter 3).

IV. MEDICAL MANAGEMENT

The importance of medical management in acute ischemic stroke is demonstrated by reports showing that medical complications are responsible for close to 50% of deaths following acute stroke (2). The following is a brief description of the most troublesome medical problems in stroke victims.

A. Hypertension

1. An increase in blood pressure is common in acute stroke, but the pressure usually returns to baseline within a few days (20).

2. Despite the transient nature of the rise in blood pressure, the American Stroke Association recommends antihypertensive treatment in acute stroke if the systolic pressure is above 220 mm Hg or the diastolic blood pressure is above 140 mm Hg (8a, 8b).

3. The acute decrease in blood pressure should not exceed 10–15% to avoid troublesome decreases in cerebral blood flow (cerebral autoregulation is impaired in acute stroke, so cerebral blood flow will vary directly with changes in cerebral perfusion pressure).

4. For acute control, intravenous **labetalol** (10–20 mg) or **nicardipine** (5 mg/hr) is preferred because these agents tend to preserve cerebral blood flow (8a, 8b). Sublingual nifedipine can produce a rapid fall in blood pressure, and should be avoided.

B. Hyperglycemia

1. Hyperglycemia is common in severe stroke and is associated with a poor neurologic outcome (21,22).

2. Current guidelines recommend that blood glucose be kept below 300 mg/dL (8a, 8b). Tighter glycemic control has been advocated (22), but care must be taken to avoid hypoglycemia, which can also worsen the neurologic outcome (8a).

C. Fever

1. Patients who develop a fever in association with acute stroke have greater neurologic deficits and a higher mortality (23,24).

2. Current guidelines recommend antipyretic therapy for all patients with fever in the early period following acute stroke (8a, 8b).

3. **Acetaminophen** is favored for antipyretic therapy (8a, 8b, 25), but it can only be given orally or by rectal suppository. The antipyretic dose is 325 to 650 mg every 4 to 6 hours.

4. Intravenous antipyretic therapy is possible with **ibuprofen** (a nonsteroidal antiinflammatory agent). An intravenous dose of 10 mg/kg (up to 800 mg) every 6 hours has been used in ICU patients with sepsis (26).

5. Fever in the early period after ischemic stroke can be infectious in origin (27), so the concern about fever should not end with antipyretic therapy.

REFERENCES

1. Thom T, Haase N, Rosamond W, et al. Heart disease and stroke statistics—2006 update: A report from the American Heart Association Statistics Committee and Stroke Statistics Subcommittee. Circulation 2006; 113:e85–151.
2. Brott T, Bogousslavsky J. Treatment of acute ischemic stroke. N Engl J Med 2000; 343:710–722.
3. Special report from the National Institute of Neurological Disorders and Stroke. Classification of cerebrovascular diseases III. Stroke 1990; 21:637–676.
4. Kizer JR, Devereux RB. Clinical practice: Patent foramen ovale in young adults with unexplained stroke. N Engl J Med 2005; 353: 2361–2372.
5. Culebras A, Kase CS, Masdeu JC, et al. Practice guidelines for the use of imaging in transient ischemic attacks and acute stroke. A report of the Stroke Council, American Heart Association. Stroke 1997; 28:1480–1497.
6. Ovbiagele B, Kidwell CS, Saver JL. Epidemiological impact in the United States of a tissue-based definition of transient ischemic attack. Stroke 2003; 34:919–924.
7. Saver JL. Time is brain—quantified. Stroke 2006; 37:263–266.
8a. Adams HP, Jr., Adams RJ, Brott T, et al. Guidelines for the early management of patients with ischemic stroke: A scientific statement from the Stroke Council of the American Stroke Association. Stroke 2003; 34:1056–1083.
8b. Adams H, Adams R, Del Zoppo G, et al. Guidelines for the early management of patients with ischemic stroke: 2005 guidelines update a scientific statement from the Stroke Council of the

American Heart Association/American Stroke Association. Stroke 2005; 36:916–923.

9. Hand PJ, Kwan J, Lindley RI, et al. Distinguishing between stroke and mimic at the bedside: The brain attack study. Stroke 2006; 37:769–775.

10. Bamford J. Clinical examination in diagnosis and subclassification of stroke. Lancet 1992; 339:400–402.

11. Atchison JW, Pellegrino M, Herbers P, et al. Hepatic encephalopathy mimicking stroke: A case report. Am J Phys Med Rehabil 1992; 71:114–118.

12. Maher J, Young GB. Septic encephalopathy. Intensive Care Med 1993; 8:177–187.

13. Warlow C, Sudlow C, Dennis M, et al. Stroke. Lancet 2003; 362:1211–1224.

14. Georgilis K, Plomaritoglou A, Dafni U, et al. Aetiology of fever in patients with acute stroke. J Intern Med 1999; 246:203–209.

15. Boysen G, Christensen H. Stroke severity determines body temperature in acute stroke. Stroke 2001; 32:413–417.

16. Bladin CF, Alexandrov AV, Bellavance A, et al. Seizures after stroke: a prospective multicenter study. Arch Neurol 2000; 57:1617–1622.

17. Graves VB, Partington VB. Imaging evaluation of acute neurologic disease. In: Goodman LR Putman CE, eds. Critical care imaging. 3rd ed. Philadelphia: WB Saunders, 1993: 391–409.

18. The National Institute of Neurological Disorders and Stroke rt-PA Stroke Study Group. Tissue plasminogen activator for acute ischemic stroke. T N Engl J Med 1995; 333:1581–1587.

19. Rothrock JF, Hart RG. Antithrombotic therapy in cerebrovascular disease. Ann Intern Med 1991; 115:885–895.

20. Semplicini A, Maresca A, Boscolo G, et al. Hypertension in acute ischemic stroke: A compensatory mechanism or an additional damaging factor? Arch Intern Med 2003; 163:211–216.

21. Bruno A, Levine SR, Frankel MR, et al. Admission glucose level and clinical outcomes in the NINDS rt-PA Stroke Trial. Neurology 2002; 59:669–674.

22. Bruno A, Williams LS, Kent TA. How important is hyperglycemia during acute brain infarction? Neurologist 2004; 10:195–200.

23. Reith J, Jorgensen HS, Pedersen PM, et al. Body temperature in acute stroke: relation to stcroke severity, infarct size, mortality,

and outcome. Lancet 1996; 347:422–425.

24. Hajat C, Hajat S, Sharma P. Effects of poststroke pyrexia on stroke outcome: a meta-analysis of studies in patients. Stroke 2000; 31:410–414.

25. Dippel DW, van Breda EJ, van Gemert HM, et al. Effect of paracetamol (acetaminophen) on body temperature in acute ischemic stroke: a double-blind, randomized phase II clinical trial. Stroke 2001; 32:1607–1612.

26. Bernard GR, Wheeler AP, Russell JA, et al. The effects of ibuprofen on the physiology and survival of patients with sepsis. N Engl J Med 1997; 336:912–918.

27. Grau AJ, Buggle F, Schnitzler P, et al. Fever and infection early after ischemic stroke. J Neurol Sci 1999; 171:115–120.

Chapter 43

ANALGESIA AND SEDATION

Our principal role in caring for the sick is not to save lives (since this is impossible on a consistent basis) but to relieve pain and suffering. The analgesic and sedative drug regimens described in this chapter will allow you to serve in this role.

I. OPIOIDS

A. Overview

Pain relief in ICU patients is achieved almost exclusively with *opioids*, which are natural derivatives of opium that produce their effects by stimulating discrete opioid receptors in the central nervous system (1,2)

1. Stimulation of opioid receptors can produce a variety of beneficial and adverse effects (3).
   a. The beneficial effects include analgesia, sedation, and euphoria.
   b. The adverse effects include respiratory depression, bradycardia, hypotension, and reduced bowel motility.
2. The analgesic effects of opioids are accompanied by mild sedation but no amnesia (4).

B. Intravenous Opioids

The most frequently used intravenous opioids are **morphine**, **fentanyl**, and **hydromorphone**. A comparison of these agents is shown in Table 43.1 (1,2,5).

TABLE 43.1 Comparative Features of Intravenous Opioids

	Morphine	Hydromorphone	Fentanyl
Loading dose	5–10 mg	1–1.5 mg	50–100 µg
Onset of action	10–20 min	5–15 min	1–2 min
Duration (after bolus)	2–3.5 hrs	2–3 hrs	30–60 min
Infusion rate†	1–5 mg/hr	0.2–0.5 mg/hr	50–350 µg/hr
PCA			
Demand (bolus)	0.5–3 mg	0.1–0.5 mg	15–75 µg
Lockout interval	10–20 min	5–15 min	3–10 min
Lipid solubility	x	0.2x	600x
Active metabolites	Yes	Yes	No
Histamine release	Yes	No	No
Dose adjustment in renal failure*	Decrease 50%	None	Decrease 50%

†Initial infusion rate. May need further adjustment.

*From Aronoff GR, Bennet WM, Berns JS, et al., eds. Drug prescribing in renal failure. 5th ed. Philadelphia: American College of Physicians, 2007:18-19.

1. *Morphine vs. Fentanyl*

   Morphine is the most frequently used opioid in ICUs (6), but fentanyl may be preferred for the following reasons:

   a. Fentanyl is faster acting than morphine (because it is much more lipid soluble), which allows more rapid dose titration.

   b. Morphine promotes the release of histamine, which can cause vasodilation and hypotension, but fentanyl is devoid of this effect (7). This makes fentanyl the better choice for patients with hemodynamic compromise.

   c. Opioids are metabolized in the liver, and their metabolites are excreted in the urine. Morphine has active metabolites that can accumulate in patients with renal dysfunction (8), while fentanyl has no active metabolites.

2. *Fentanyl Accumulation*

The only caveat for fentanyl is the tendency for the drug to accumulate in the brain (because of its high lipid solubility), which can result in prolonged drug effects after just 4 hours of continuous infusion. For this reason, fentanyl infusions may be less appealing for long-term pain control. Fentanyl dosing in renal failure may need adjustment because of increased sensitivity to opioids.

B. Meperidine

1. Meperidine (Demerol, Pethidine) is an opioid analgesic with a significant risk of toxicity. One of the products of meperidine metabolism (normeperidine) is slowly excreted by the kidneys, and accumulation of this metabolite produces neuroexcitation with agitation, delirium, and seizures (9).

2. Accumulation of the toxic metabolite occurs with repeated dosing and is more likely to occur in ICU patients who often have renal dysfunction. As a result, the routine use of meperidine is not advised in ICU patients.

3. Although meperidine has been favored over other opioids for pain relief in cholecystitis and pancreatitis, experimental studies show that meperidine and morphine are equivalent in their ability to promote spasm of the sphincter of Oddi and increased intrabiliary pressure (10).

4. Meperidine is still preferred for control of shivering. In the rewarming period following cardiac surgery, low doses of meperidine (25 mg IV) can stop shivering within minutes.

C. Patient-Controlled Analgesia

For patients who are awake and aware of their surroundings, *patient-controlled analgesia* (PCA) can achieve more effective pain control and greater patient satisfaction than traditional methods of opioid administration (11).

1. *Method*

   The PCA method uses an electronic infusion pump that can be activated by the patient. At the first sense of discomfort, the patient presses a button connected to the pump and receives a bolus dose of the opioid. After each bolus, the pump is disabled for a mandatory time period called the *lockout interval*, to prevent overdosing. This interval is a function of the time to achieve peak drug effect (11).

2. *PCA Regimens*

   Table 43.1 includes recommendations for PCA dosing, including the bolus drug doses and lockout intervals for each opioid. A loading dose may be needed at the start of PCA if the patient has not been receiving opioids.

C. Adverse Effects

There are a variety of adverse effects attributed to opioids, The following are the ones of most concern in the ICU.

1. *Respiratory Depression*

   Opioids produce a centrally-mediated, dose-dependent decrease in both respiratory rate and tidal volume (12,13), but clinically significant respiratory depression and hypoxemia are surprisingly uncommon (14). Troublesome respiratory depression is more likely in patients with sleep apnea syndrome or chronic hypercapnia (13).

2. *Cardiovascular Effects*

   a. Opioids can cause a mild decrease in blood pressure and heart rate from reduced sympathetic activity (sedative effect) and increased parasympathetic activity, but these effects are usually mild and well tolerated, at least in the supine position (13). Some opioids (e.g., morphine) release histamine, and this can add to the hypotensive effect.

b. Decreases in blood pressure can be pronounced in conditions like hypovolemia or heart failure, where increased sympathetic activity plays an important role in blood pressure support.

c. Opioid-induced hypotension usually responds to volume infusion and placing the patient in a supine position.

3. *Bowel Motility*

a. Reduced peristalsis from stimulation of opioid receptors in the bowel can lead to problems such as impaired tolerance to enteral feedings and postoperative ileus (15).

b. Opioid-induced bowel dysfunction might benefit from drugs that block opioid receptors in the bowel. One such drug is **alvimopan**, which has been shown to reduce the incidence of postoperative ileus when given orally in a dose of 6 to 12 mg twice daily (beginning 2 hours before surgery) (16).

II. NON-OPIOID ANALGESIA

The only non-opioid analgesic approved for parenteral use in the United States is ketorolac.

A. Ketorolac

Ketorolac is a nonsteroidal antiinflammatory drug (NSAID) that is 350 times more potent than aspirin as an analgesic (17). It does not cause respiratory depression, but other toxic effects limit its use (see later). It is usually given as an adjunct to opioids for postoperative analgesia and has an *opioid-sparing effect*.

1. *Dose Regimens*

   Ketorolac can be given intravenously or by IM injection.

   a. For patients under 65 years of age, the initial dose is 30 mg IV or 60 mg IM, followed by 30 mg (IM or IV) every 6 hours (maximum of 120 mg/day) for up to 5 days.

   b. For patients ≥65 years of age, under 50 kg, or with renal dysfunction, the initial dose is 15 mg IV or 30 mg IM, followed by 15 mg (IM or IV) every 6 hours (maximum of 60 mg/day) for up to 5 days.

   c. Intramuscular injection of ketorolac can cause hematoma formation, and the IV route is preferred (18). Continuous IV infusion (5 mg/hr) produces the best results (18).

   d. Drug use should be limited to 5 days (see below).

2. *Adverse Effects*

   Ketorolac inhibits platelet aggregation and should not be used in patients with a high risk of bleeding (18).

   a. When ketorolac is given for more than 5 days, there is an increased risk of bleeding (GI and operative site) (19).

   b. Ketorolac inhibits renal prostaglandin synthesis and can impair renal function, but the risk of renal toxicity is minimal if drug therapy does not exceed 5 days.

III. SEDATION WITH BENZODIAZEPINES

Benzodiazepines are popular sedatives in the ICU because they are generally safe to use, and the sedation is accompanied by amnesia (20).

A. General Features

The following characteristics of benzodiazepines deserve mention.

1. All benzodiazepines are lipid soluble and will accumulate

in the brain with continued use. This produces prolonged (and unwanted) sedation after the drug is discontinued.

2. The effective dose of benzodiazepines is lower in elderly patients and in patients with heart failure and hepatic insufficiency.

TABLE 43.2 Comparative Features of Intravenous Benzodiazepines

	Midazolam	Lorazepam[1]	Diazepam[2]
Loading dose (IV) (mg/kg)	0.02–0.1	0.02–0.06	0.05–0.2
Onset of action	1–5 min	5–20 min	2–5 min
Duration (after bolus)	1–2 hrs	2–6 hrs	2–4 hrs
Maintenance[†] infusion (mg/kg/hr)	0.04–0.2	0.01–0.1	Rarely used
Dose adjustment in renal failure*	Decrease 50%	None	None

Use ideal body weight for dose calculations.
[1]Lorazepam (Abbott Labs) contains propylene glycol (830 mg/mL)
[2]Diazepam (Abbott Labs) contains propylene glycol (400 mg/mL)
Adapted from References 1,20–23.

B. Drug Comparisons

Three (of 13) benzodiazepines can be given intravenously: midazolam, lorazepam, and diazepam. The comparative properties of these agents are shown in Table 43.2. Because of the tendency to accumulate in fatty tissues, benzodiazepine dosing should be based on *ideal body weight* (21).

1. **Midazolam** (Versed) is the benzodiazepine of choice for

short-term sedation because it has the fastest onset and shortest duration of action (21–23). Because of its short duration of action, midazolam is usually given by continuous infusion. However, infusions of midazolam lasting longer than a few hours *can produce prolonged sedation* (because of rapid accumulation in the brain) (21).

2. **Lorazepam** (Ativan) has the slowest onset of action of the IV benzodiazepines. Because of its long duration of action, lorazepam is used for prolonged sedation (e.g., ventilator-dependent patients) (1). However, prolonged use of lorazepam carries a risk of propylene glycol toxicity (see next section).

3. **Diazepam** (Valium) is the least favored of the IV benzodiazepines because of the risk for oversedation and propylene glycol toxicity (see next section).

C. Adverse Effects

Excessive dosing and accumulation of benzodiazepines can lead to hypotension, respiratory depression and excessive sedation (24). (See Chapter 46, Section II for more on benzodiazepine toxicity). The following are some additional concerns.

1. *Propylene Glycol Toxicity*

   Intravenous preparations of lorazepam and diazepam contain the solvent propylene glycol to enhance drug solubility. Prolonged administration of propylene glycol can produce a toxidrome characterized by agitation, metabolic acidosis, hypotension, and seizures.

   a. Propylene glycol toxicity has been reported in 19% to 66% of ICU patients receiving high-dose lorazepam or diazepam for more than 2 days (25,26).

   b. Switching to midazolam will eliminate the risk of propylene glycol toxicity.

2. *Withdrawal Syndrome*

Abrupt termination following prolonged benzodiazepine administration can produce a withdrawal syndrome consisting of agitation, disorientation, hallucinations, and seizures (27). The risk of withdrawal is difficult to predict.

3. *Drug Interactions*

a. Several drugs can inhibit the metabolism of diazepam and midazolam, including erythromycin, fluconazole, diltiazem, verapamil, and omeprazole (28). However, the only significant interaction may be the one between erythromycin and midazolam: these two drugs should not be used in combination. The metabolism of lorazepam is unaffected by other drugs (28).

b. Theophylline antagonizes the sedative effect of benzodiazepines (possibly by blocking adenosine receptors), and IV aminophylline (110 mg over 5 min) has been used to promote awakening from benzodiazepine sedation (29).

IV. OTHER SEDATIVES

A. Propofol

Propofol (Deprivan) is a rapidly–acting sedative that is used for induction and maintenance of general anesthesia. In the ICU, it can be used for short-term sedation (i.e., for procedures), but more widespread use is not advised because of adverse effects.

1. *Preparation and Dosage*

a. Propofol is suspended in a 10% lipid emulsion that is almost identical to 10% Intralipid used in parenteral nutrition formulas (and has the same energy yield of 1.1 kcal/mL).

b. The bolus and infusion doses of propofol are shown in Table 43.3 (30,31). Propofol should be dosed according to *ideal body weight*, and no dose adjustment is needed for renal failure or hepatic insufficiency (31).

2. *Adverse Effects*

a. Propofol is well known for producing respiratory depression, and the drug should be used only during controlled ventilation.

b. Decreased blood pressure is frequently observed following a bolus dose of propofol, and hypotension is most likely to occur in patients who are elderly, have heart failure, or are hypovolemic (31).

c. Anaphylactoid reactions to propofol are uncommon but can be severe (31).

d. The lipid emulsion can cause hypertriglyceridemia after prolonged use (>72 hrs).

3. *Propofol Infusion Syndrome*

Propofol can cause a rare but often lethal idiosyncratic reaction characterized by the abrupt onset of bradycardia, heart failure lactic acidosis, hyperlipidemia, and rhabdomyolysis (32). This is called the *propofol infusion syndrome,* and it is usually associated with prolonged, high-dose propofol infusions (>4–6 mg/kg/hr for longer than 24 to 48 hrs). The mortality is high (>80%), even when the drug is discontinued.

B. Dexmedetomidine

Dexmedetomidine is a highly-selective α_2-adrenergic agonist that produces sedation without respiratory depression (33). The properties of this drug are shown in Table 43.3. Because of the short duration of action, dexmedetomidine is usually given by continuous infusion.

1. *Clinical Uses*

Due to the lack of respiratory depression, dexmetomidine

has been recommended for sedation during weaning from mechanical ventilation (34). However, the 24-hour limit on drug use (see next section) limits the utility of this drug.

2. *Adverse Effects*

Dexmedetomidine infusions can produce hypotension (30%), and bradycardia (8%) (33). There is also a risk for agitation and "sympathetic rebound" following drug withdrawal. To minimize this risk, infusions should not be continued for longer than 24 hours.

TABLE 43.3 Intravenous Nonbenzodiazepine Sedatives

	Propofol[1]	Dexmedetomidine
Loading dose	0.25–1 mg/kg	1 µg/kg over 10 min
Onset of action	<1 min	1–3 min
Time to arousal	10–15 min	6–10 min
Maintenance infusion (µg/kg/min)	25–75	0.2–0.7
Respiratory depression	Yes	No
Adverse effects	Hypotension Hyperlipidemia Contamination/ Sepsis Propofol Infusion syndrome	Hypotension Bradycardia Sympathetic rebound

[1]Propofol dosage should be based on ideal body weight.

Adapted from References 1,30–33.

C. Haloperidol

The advantage of haloperidol (Haldol) as a sedative is lack of cardiorespiratory depression. Intravenous delivery is not approved by the FDA, but IV haloperidol is safe and effective (35) and is recommended in the practice guidelines of the Society of Critical Care Medicine (1).

TABLE 43.4 Intravenous Haloperidol for Sedation

Severity of Anxiety	Dose
Mild	0.5–2 mg
Moderate	5–10 mg
Severe	10–20 mg

1. Administer dose by IV push.
2. Allow 10–20 minutes for response:
   a. If no response, double the drug dose, *or*
   b. Add lorazepam (1 mg)
3. If still no response, switch to another sedative.
4. Give 25% of the initial dose every 6 hours to maintain sedation.

Adapted from References 1,35.

Table 43.4 contains recommendations on the IV administration of haloperidol.

1. *Clinical Uses*

   a. Because of the delayed onset of action (10 to 20 min), haloperidol is not suitable for immediate control of anxiety.

   b. Haloperidol is preferred for sedation of the patient with delirium.

   c. The lack of respiratory depression makes haloperidol well suited for sedation during weaning from mechanical ventilation (35).

2. *Adverse Effects*

   a. Extrapyramidal reactions are a well-known side effect of haloperidol, but these reactions are uncommon when the drug is given intravenously (36). Haloperidol should not be used in patients with Parkinson's disease.

   b. Haloperidol prolongs the QT interval and can precipitate a polymorphic ventricular tachycardia known as *torsades de pointes* (see Chapter 15, Section VI). This arrhythmia has been reported in 3–4% of patients receiving intravenous haloperidol (37). As a result, haloperidol should never be used in patients with a prolonged QT interval.

c. Another adverse effect of haloperidol is the *neuroleptic malignant syndrome* (38), an idiosyncratic reaction that is described in Chapter 32, Section II-E. Unexplained fever in a patient receiving haloperidol should always raise suspicion for this disorder.

V. INTERRUPTING SEDATIVE INFUSIONS

Prolonged infusions of sedatives (and opioids) results in progressive drug accumulation and persistent sedation after the drug infusion is discontinued. This can delay weaning from mechanical ventilation and prolong the ICU stay. When patients have been maintained on sedative drug infusions for longer than 24 hours and are beginning to recover, daily interruptions of drug infusions until the patient begins to awaken are advised (39).

TABLE 43.5 Modified Ramsay Scale for Scoring Sedation

Score	Description
1	Anxious and agitated, or restless, or both
2	Cooperative, orientated and tranquil
3	Drowsy, but responds to commands
4	Asleep, brisk response to light glabellar tap or loud auditory stimulus
5	Asleep, sluggish response to light glabellar tap or loud auditory stimulus
6	Asleep and unarousable

Adapted from Reference 40.

A. Monitoring Sedation

1. Current guidelines recommend routine monitoring of sedation (1), which reduces the risk of oversedation.

2. The original scoring system for sedation, the *Ramsay scale*, is shown in Table 43.5 (40). This scale is well suited for evaluating oversedation because it has four levels of sedation (score 3 to 6) but only one level of agitation (score = 1).

3. There are other more elaborate scoring systems for sedation (41), but there is no evidence that they perform any better that the simple scoring system in Table 43.5.

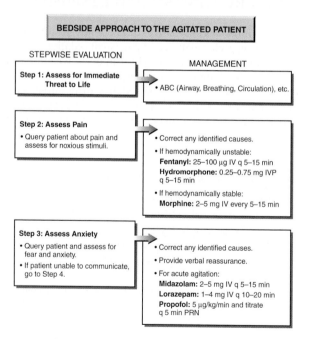

FIGURE 43.1 An organized approach to the patient with acute agitation. Adapted from Reference 1.

VI. THE AGITATED PATIENT

A common scenario in the ICU is a nurse informing you that your patient has suddenly become agitated. The stepwise approach in Figure 43.1 might prove useful in this situation.

REFERENCES

1. Jacobi J, Fraser GL, Coursin DB, et al. Clinical practice guidelines for the sustained use of sedatives and analgesics in the critically ill adult. Crit Care Med 2002; 30:119–141.

2. Murray MJ, Plevak DJ. Analgesia in the critically ill patient. New Horizons 1994; 2:56–63.

3. Pasternak GW. Pharmacological mechanisms of opioid analgesics. Clin Neuropharmacol 1993; 16:1–18.

4. Veselis RA, Reinsel RA, Feshchenko VA, et al. The comparative amnestic effects of midazolam, propofol, thiopental, and fentanyl at equisedative concentrations. Anesthesiology 1997; 87:749–764.

5. Quigley C. A systematic reviw of hydromorphone in acute and chronic pain. J Pain Symptom Manag 2003; 25:169–178.

6. Soliman HM, Melot C, Vincent JL. Sedative and analgesic practice in the intensive care unit: The results of a European survey Br J Anaesth 2001; 87:186–192.

7. Rosow CE, Moss J, Philbin DM, et al. Histamine release during morphine and fentanyl anesthesia. Anesthesiology 1982; 56:93–96.

8. Smith MT. Neuroexcitatory effects of morphine and hydromorphone: Evidence implicating the 3-glucuronide metabolites. Clin Exp Pharmacol Physiol 2000; 27:524–528.

9. Latta KS, Ginsberg B, Barkin RL. Meperidine: A critical review. Am J Ther 2002; 9:53–68.

10. Lee F, Cundiff D. Meperidine vs morphine in pancreatitis and cholecystitis. Arch Intern Med 1998; 158:2399.

11. White PF. Use of patient-controlled analgesia for management of acute pain. JAMA 1988; 259:243–247.

12. Bowdle TA. Adverse effects of opioid agonists and agonist-antagonists in anaesthesia. Drug Safety 1998; 19:173–189.

13. Schug SA, Zech D, Grond S. Adverse effects of systemic opioid analgesics. Drug Safety 1992; 7:200–213.

14. Bailey PL. The use of opioids in anesthesia is not especially associated with nor predictive of postoperative hypoxemia. Anesthesiology 1992; 77:1235.

15. Kurz A, Sessler DI. Opioid-induced bowel dysfunction: pathophysiology and potential new therapies. Drugs 2003; 63:649–671.

16. Delaney CP, Wolff BG, Viscusi ER, et al. Alvimopan for postoperative ileus following bowel resection. Ann Surg 2007; 245:355–363.

17. Buckley MM, Brogden RN. Ketorolac: A review of its pharmacodynamic and pharmacokinetic properties, and therapeutic potential. Drugs 1990; 39:86–109.

18. Ready LB, Brown CR, Stahlgren LH, et al. Evaluation of intravenous ketorolac administered by bolus or infusion for treatment of postoperative pain: A double-blind, placebo-controlled, multicenter study. Anesthesiology 1994; 80:1277–1286.

19. Strom BL, Berlin JA, Kinman JL, et al. Parenteral ketorolac and risk of gastrointestinal and operative site bleeding: A postmarketing surveillance study. JAMA 1996; 275:376–382.

20. Young CC, Prielipp RC. Benzodiazepines in the intensive care unit. Crit Care Clin 2001; 17:843–862.

21. Fragen RJ. Pharmacokinetics and pharmacodynamics of midazolam given via continuous intravenous infusion in intensive care units. Clin Ther 1997; 19:405–419.

22. Reves JG, Fragen RJ, Vinik HR, et al. Midazolam: pharmacology and uses. Anesthesiology 1985; 62:310–324.

23. Barr J, Zomorodi K, Bertaccini EJ, et al. A double-blind, randomized comparison of i.v. lorazepam versus midazolam for sedation of ICU patients via a pharmacologic model. Anesthesiology 2001; 95:286–298.

24. Gaudreault P, Guay J, Thivierge RL, et al. Benzodiazepine poisoning: Clinical and pharmacological considerations and treatment. Drug Safety 1991; 6:247–265.

25. Wilson KC, Reardon C, Theodore AC, Farber HW. Propylene glycol toxicity: A severe iatrogenic illness in ICU patients receiving IV benzodiazepines. Chest 2005; 128:1674–1681.

26. Arroglia A, Shehab N, McCarthy K, Gonzales JP. Relationship of continuous infusion lorazepam to serum propylene glycol concentration in critically ill adults. Crit Care Med 2004; 32:1709–1714.

27. Moss JH. Sedative and hypnotic withdrawal states in hospitalised patients. Lancet 1991; 338:575.

28. Dresser GK, Spence JD, Bailey DG. Pharmacokinetic-pharmaco-dynamic consequences and clinical relevance of cytochrome P450 3A4 inhibition. Clin Pharmacokinet 2000; 38:41–57.

29. Hoegholm A, Steptoe P, Fogh B, et al. Benzodiazepine antagonism by aminophylline. Acta Anaesthesiol Scand 1989; 33:164–166.

30. Angelini G, Ketzler JT, Coursin DB. Use of propofol and other nonbenzodiazepine sedatives in the intensive care unit. Crit Care Clin 2001; 17:863–880.

30. McKeage K, Perry CM. Propofol: a review of its use in intensive care sedation of adults. CNS Drugs 2003; 17:235–272.

32. Kang TM. Propofol infusion syndrome in critically ill patients. Ann Pharmacother 2002; 36:1453–1456.

33. Bhana N, Goa KL, McClellan KJ. Dexmedetomidine. Drugs 2000; 59:263–268.

34. Venn RM, Hell J, Grounds RM. Respiratory effects of dexmedeto-midine in the surgical patient requiring intensive care. Crit Care 2000; 4:302–308.

35. Riker RR, Fraser GL, Cox PM. Continuous infusion of haloperi-dol controls agitation in critically ill patients. Crit Care Med 1994; 22:433–440.

36. Sanders KM, Minnema AM, Murray GB. Low incidence of ex-trapyramidal symptoms in the treatment of delirium with intra-venous haloperidol and lorazepam in the intensive care unit. J Intensive Care Med 1989; 4:201–204.

37. Sharma ND, Rosman HS, Padhi ID, et al. Torsades de pointes associated with intravenous haloperidol in critically ill patients. Am J Cardiol 1998; 81:238–240.

38. Sing RF, Branas CC, Marino PL. Neuroleptic malignant syndrome in the intensive care unit. J Am Osteopath Assoc 1993; 93:615–618.

39. Kress JP, Pohlman AS, O'Connor MF, et al. Daily interruption of sedative infusions in critically ill patients undergoing mechani-cal ventilation. N Engl J Med 2000; 342:1471–1477.

40. Ramsay MA, Savege TM, Simpson BR, et al. Controlled sedation with alphaxalone-alphadolone. Br Med J 1974; 2:656–659.

41. Ely EW, Truman B, Shintani A, et al. Monitoring sedation status over time in ICU patients: reliability and validity of the Richmond Agitation-Sedation Scale (RASS). JAMA 2003; 289:2983–2991.

Chapter 44

ANTIMICROBIAL THERAPY

This chapter presents the intravenous antibiotics you are most likely to use in the ICU. Each is presented in the order shown below.

1. Aminoglycosides (gentamicin, tobramycin, amikacin)

2. Antifungal agents (amphotericin B, fluconazole, capsofungin)

3. Carbapenems (imipenem, meropenem)

4. Cephalosporins (ceftriaxone, ceftazidime, cefepime)

5. Fluoroquinolones (ciprofloxacin, levofloxacin, gatifloxacin, moxifloxacin)

6. Penicillins (pipericillin-tazobactam)

7. Vancomycin and its replacements (linezolid, daptomycin)

I. AMINOGLYCOSIDES

The aminoglycosides include **gentamicin** (introduced in 1966), **tobramycin** (introduced in 1975), and **amikacin** (introduced in 1981). These drugs were once the antibiotics of choice for serious gram-negative infections, but their popularity has waned because of renal toxicity (1).

A. Activity & Clinical Uses

1. The aminoglycosides are active against aerobic gram-neg-

ative bacilli, and amikacin has the greatest activity (see Figure 44.1) (2).

2. Aminoglycosides can be used to treat any serious infection caused by gram-negative bacilli, but their use is generally reserved for infections caused by *Pseudomonas* species.

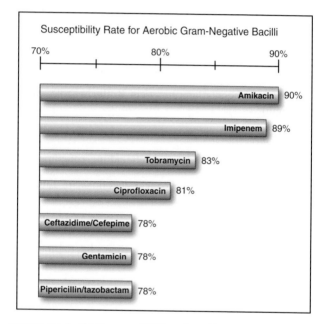

FIGURE 44.1 Antibiotic susceptibilities of aerobic gram-negative bacilli isolated from 35,790 culture specimens obtained from ICU patients. Adapted from Reference 2.

B. Dosing

1. Aminoglycoside dosing is based on body weight and renal function (see Table 44.1) (1,3). These drugs are poorly distributed in adipose tissue, so ideal body weight should be

used for normal or overweight patients, while actual body weight is more appropriate for underweight patients (1).

2. Once-daily dosing is preferred for aminoglycosides because these antibiotics have a concentration-dependent bactericidal effect (1), so one large daily dose will produce more effective tissue concentrations than multiple smaller doses.

3. The dose adjustment in renal failure is achieved by increasing the dosing interval (see Table 44.1), which preserves the concentration-dependent bactericidal effects of these antibiotics.

TABLE 44.1 Aminoglycoside Dose Recommendations

Drug	Usual Dose	Renal Failure[†]	HD[†]
Amikacin	15 mg/kg q24 h		1/2 the normal dose after each dialysis
Gentamicin	5 mg/kg q24 h	q48–72 h	
Tobramycin	5 mg/kg q 24 h		

HD = hemodialysis.   [†]From Reference 3.

C. Adverse Effects

1. Aminoglycosides are referred to as *obligate nephrotoxins* because renal impairment will eventually develop in all patients (1). The serum creatinine usually begins to rise after one week of drug therapy.

   a. Nephrotoxic effects are enhanced by hypovolemia, advanced age, renal impairment, hypokalemia, and concurrent therapy with loop diuretics and vancomycin (1,4).

2. Aminoglycoside-induced ototoxicity can produce irreversible hearing loss and vestibular damage, but these effects are almost never apparent clinically (1).

3. Aminoglycosides can block acetylcholine release from presynaptic nerve terminals. This effect almost never produces muscle weakness *de novo* (5), but it can aggravate the muscle weakness in myasthenia gravis (6).

D. Comment

Because of the substantial risk of renal damage, it's always wise to *avoid using aminoglycosides* whenever possible. Other less toxic antibiotics are available for effective gram-negative coverage (e.g., the carbapenems).

II. ANTIFUNGAL AGENTS

A. Amphotericin B

Amphotericin B (AmB) is the most effective antifungal agent in clinical use, but is also the most toxic antifungal agent as well.

1. *Clinical Uses*

   AmB is the drug of choice for all life-threatening fungal infections and for empiric antimicrobial therapy in neutropenic patients with persistent fever.

2. *Dosage and Administration*

   AmB is given once daily in an intravenous dose of 0.5 to 1 mg/kg. The dose is initially delivered over a 4-hour time period, but this can be reduced to a one-hour infusion if tolerated. The total AmB dose is 0.5 to 4 grams and is determined by the type and severity of the fungal infection.

   a. Central venous cannulation is preferred for AmB infusions to reduce the risk of infusion-related phlebitis (7).

3. *Infusion-Related Inflammatory Response*

   Infusions of AmB are accompanied by fever, chills, nausea, vomiting, and rigors in about 70% of instances (8).

This reaction is most pronounced with the initial infusion, and often diminishes in intensity with repeated infusions. The following measures can reduce the intensity of this reaction (8):

a. Thirty minutes before the infusion, give acetaminophen (10 to 15 mg/kg orally) and diphenhydramine (25 mg orally or IV). If rigors are a problem, premedicate with meperidine (25 mg IV).

b. If the above regimen does not give full relief, add hydrocortisone to the AmB infusate (0.1 mg/mL).

4. *Nephrotoxicity*

a. AmB produces an injury in the renal tubules that clinically resembles a renal tubular acidosis (distal type), with increased urinary excretion of potassium and magnesium (9). Hypokalemia and hypomagnesemia are common consequences.

b. Azotemia is reported in 30 to 40% of patients during daily infusions of AmB (9). An increase in serum creatinine above 3.0 mg/dL should prompt cessation of AmB infusions for a few days or a switch to the liposomal AmB preparation, described next (8).

5. *Liposomal Amphotericin B*

Specialized lipid preparations of AmB have been developed to reduce binding to mammalian cells (thereby reducing the risk of renal injury).

a. Clinical trials have shown that *liposomal AmB* (AmBisome) is as effective as standard AmB but causes fewer cases of renal dysfunction (7,10).

b. The daily dose of liposomal AmB is 5 mg/kg, which is 5 times higher than the dose of standard AmB (7).

B. Fluconazole

Fluconazole is a less toxic alternative to AmB for *Candida* infections.

1. *Activity & Clinical Uses*

   a. Fluconazole is used to treat invasive candidiasis. (11). It does not adequately cover *Candida krusei*, but this organism is involved in only 5 to 10% of cases of invasive candidiasis (12).

   b. Fluconazole can be used alone in immunocompetent patients (10), and it can be used after an initial course of AmB in immunocompromised patients (12).

2. *Dosing*

   Fluconazole can be given orally or IV in a single daily dose of 400 to 800 mg (the same dose is used for oral and IV delivery). If the creatinine clearance is less than 50 mL/min, the dose should be reduced by 50% (7).

3. *Adverse Effects*

   a. Fluconazole can impair the hepatic metabolism of phenytoin, cisapride (Propulsid), and the statins (lovastatin, atorvastatin) (7). It should not be used with cisapride and the statins, and phenytoin doses should be adjusted according to serum phenytoin levels (7).

   b. Fluconazole is safe to use in most patients, but it has been implicated in cases of severe and even fatal hepatic injury in HIV patients (13).

C. Capsofungin

1. Capsofungin may be superior to fluconazole for treating invasive candidiasis because it is active against all *Candida* species, has fewer drug interactions, and does not require dose modification in renal failure (12). It has proven comparable to AmB for treating invasive candidiasis (14) and for empiric therapy of neutropenic patients with fever (12).

2. For invasive candidiasis, the IV dose of capsofungin is 70 mg initially, then 50 mg daily thereafter.

III. CARBAPENEMS

The carbapenems (imipenem and meropenem) have *the broadest spectrum of activity of any antibiotics currently available* (16).

A. Imipenem

Imipenem is the original carbapenem (introduced in 1985) and the one that has been studied the most.

1. *Activity & Clinical Uses*
    a. Imipenem is active against all common bacterial pathogens except methicillin-resistant *Staph. aureus* (MRSA).
    b. As demonstrated in Figure 44.1, imipenem is one of the most active agents for aerobic gram-negative bacilli. It also provides good coverage for gram-positive cocci (including pneumococci, methicillin-sensitive *Staph. aureus*, and *Staph. epidermidis*), and anaerobes (including *Bacteroides fragilis* and *Enterococcus faecalis*).
    c. Imipenem can be used for virtually any infection that does not involve MRSA. It can also be used as a single agent for empiric antibiotic coverage in neutropenic patients with fever (16).

2. *Preparation & Dosing*
    a. Imipenem is inactivated by enzymes on proximal renal tubules, so it is not possible to achieve high drug levels in urine. To overcome this problem, the commercial preparation of imipenem (Primaxin) contains an enzyme inhibitor, cilastatin.
    b. The recommended dose of imipenem is 500 mg every 6 hours (15). The daily dose should be reduced 50% in renal insufficiency and 75% in renal failure (3).

3. *Adverse Effects*
    The major adverse effect is *generalized seizures*, which occur in 1.5% of patients (15). Contributing factors in-

clude a history of seizure disorder, an intracranial mass, or renal failure. With appropriate dose adjustments in renal insufficiency, the incidence of imipenem-induced seizures is *less than 1%* (15).

B. Meropenem

1. Meropenem (introduced in 1996) is similar to imipenem in spectrum of antibacterial activity, but it *does not produce seizures* (15).

2. The usual intravenous dose is 500 mg to 1 gram every 8 hours, and a 50% daily dose reduction is required in renal failure (3).

C. Comment

The carbapenems are ideal antibiotics because they are relatively safe to use and they cover most ICU-associated pathogens except MRSA. Meropenem is favored by many because of the reduced seizure risk, but there is little risk of seizures with imipenem if the dose is adjusted for renal dysfunction.

IV. CEPHALOSPORINS

There are more than 25 cephalosporins available for clinical use (17), but only a few are useful for treating serious infections in ICU patients.

A. Useful Cephalosporins

The cephalosporins that are used most often in the ICU are listed in Table 44.2, along with dosing recommendations for each drug.

1. **Cefazolin** (Ancef) can be used to treat infections caused by susceptible strains of staphylococci. However, this

agent is not active against MRSA or *Staph. epidermidis,* and this limits its use in the ICU.

2. **Ceftriaxone** (Rocephin) is used to treat serious community-acquired pneumonias because it is active against penicillin-resistant pneumococci and *Hemophilus influenza.*

3. **Ceftazidime** (Fortaz) and **cefepime** (Maxipime) are used to treat infections caused by aerobic gram-negative bacilli, including *Pseudomonas aeruginosa.* Both of these agents have been recommended for empiric antibiotic coverage in neutropenic patients with fever (18). However, these agents are not the most active against common gram-negative isolates (see Figure 44.1).

TABLE 44.2 Cephalosporin Dose Recommendations

Drug	Serious Infections	Renal Failure*
Cefazolin	1 g every 6 h	1 g every 24 h
Ceftriaxone	2 g every 12 h	2 g every 12 h
Ceftazidime	2 g every 8 h	2 g every 48 h
Cefepime	2 g every 8 h	2 g every 24 h

*From Reference 3.

B. Toxicity

Cephalosporins are relatively free of serious adverse effects. There is a 5 to 15% incidence of cross antigenicity with penicillin, so these agents should not be used in patients with a history of anaphylactic reactions to penicillin.

V. FLUOROQUINOLONES

The fluoroquinolones can be separated into early generations (e.g., **ciprofloxacin**) and later generations (e.g., **levofloxacin**, **gatifloxacin**, and **moxifloxacin**) (19).

A. Activity & Clinical Uses

1. Ciprofloxacin was extremely popular when first introduced (in 1987) because of its activity against aerobic gram-negative bacilli, including *Pseudomonas aeruginosa*. However, this activity has diminished over the years (see Figure 44.1), and ciprofloxacin is no longer considered a first-line agent for serious gram-negative infections.

2. The newer fluoroquinolones (e.g., levofloxacin, gatifloxacin, moxifloxacin) retain the gram-negative coverage of ciprofloxacin (except less activity against *P. aeruginosa*), but provide added coverage for streptococci, pneumococci (including penicillin-resistant strains) and "atypical" organisms like *Mycoplasma pneumoniae* and *Hemophilus influenza*.

   a. These agents are used primarily for community-acquired pneumonias and uncomplicated urinary tract infections.

   b. They can also be used for early-onset (within 5 days of admission) ventilator-associated pneumonias in selected patients (see Chapter 34, Section III-A, and Table 34.3).

   c. More widespread use of these antibiotics in the ICU is limited by the lack of activity against MRSA and the limited activity against *P. aeruginosa*.

B. Dosing

1. Table 44.3 shows the recommended intravenous doses for four fluoroquinolones. The newer agents have longer half-lives than ciprofloxacin and require only once-daily dosing.

2. Dose adjustments are required in renal failure for all the agents except moxifloxacin, which is metabolized in the liver.

TABLE 44.3 Fluoroquinolone Dose Recommendations

Drug	Serious Infections	Renal Failure*
Ciprofloxacin	400 mg every 8 h	400 mg every 18 h
Levofloxacin	500 mg every 24 h	250 mg every 48 h
Gatifloxacin	400 mg every 24 h	200 mg every 24 h
Moxifloxacin	400 mg every 24 h	400 mg every 24 h

*From Reference 3.

C. Adverse Effects

1. Ciprofloxacin interferes with the hepatic metabolism of theophylline and warfarin and can potentiate the actions of both drugs. The newer fluoroquinolones do not share these drug interactions (20).

2. Neurotoxic reactions (confusion, hallucinations, seizures) have been reported in 1 to 2% of patients receiving quinolones (21).

3. Prolongation of the QT interval and polymorphic ventricular tachycardia (*torsades de pointes*) have been reported in association with all quinolones except moxifloxacin (22).

VI. THE PENICILLINS

Penicillin use in the ICU is restricted mostly to the extended-spectrum penicillins.

A. Extended-Spectrum Penicillins

The penicillin analogues that are active against aerobic gram-negative bacilli include the aminopenicillins (ampicillin and amoxicillin), the carboxypenicillins (carbenicillin and ticarcillin), and the ureidopenicillins (azlocillin, mezlocillin, and pipericillin). The latter two groups are active against *P. aeruginosa* (23) and are called *antipseudomonal penicillins*. The most widely used antipseudomonal penicillin is **pipericillin**, which is available in a combination product (see next).

1. *Pipericillin-Tazobactam*

Pipericillin is usually given in combination with tazobactam, a β-lactamase inhibitor that is synergistic with pipericillin. The pipericillin-tazobactam preparation (Zosyn) contains pipericillin in an 8:1 ratio with tazobactam.

a. The recommended dose of pipericillin-tazobactam is 3.375 grams (3 grams pipericillin and 375 mg tazobactam) IV every 4 to 6 hours. In patients with renal impairment, the dose should be reduced to 2.25 grams every 8 hours (24).

c. Pipericillin-tazobactam is used mostly for urinary tract infections and intraabdominal sepsis. It has also been recommended for empiric therapy of febrile neutropenia (18).

VII. VANCOMYCIN

Vancomycin is the most frequently used antibiotic in the ICU, but concerns about emerging resistance have prompted a general mandate to curtail its use.

A. Activity & Clinical Uses

1. Vancomycin is active against all gram-positive cocci, including all strains of *Staphylococcus aureus* (coagulase-positive, coagulase-negative, methicillin-sensitive, meth-

icillin-resistant) as well as aerobic and anaerobic strepto-cocci (including pneumococcus and enterococcus) (25).

2. Vancomycin is the drug of choice for infections caused by methicillin-resistant *Staphylococcus aureus* (MRSA), *Staphylococcus epidermidis, Enterococcus faecalis,* and penicillin-resistant pneumococci.

3. As much as 2/3 of the vancomycin use in ICUs is not directed at a specific pathogen, but is used for empiric antibiotic coverage of gram-positive pathogens (26).

B. Dosing

1. The usual intravenous dose of vancomycin is 1 gram every 12 hours (29). Each dose must be infused slowly (no faster than 10 mg/min) to prevent infusion reactions (see below).

2. Dose reduction is necessary with impaired renal function and is accomplished by increasing the dosing interval. In renal insufficiency (creatinine clearance = 10 to 50 mL/min), the dosing interval is 1 to 3 days, and in renal failure (creatinine clearance <10 mL/min), the dosing interval is 4 to 7 days (3). A supplemental dose after hemodialysis is not necessary (3).

3. Serum drug levels can be monitored to limit toxicity and maintain efficacy. Peak levels should be below 40 mg/L to reduce the risk of ototoxicity, and trough levels should be above 5 mg/L to maintain antibacterial activity (27).

C. Adverse Effects

1. *Red Man Syndrome*

Rapid infusions of vancomycin can be accompanied by vasodilation, flushing, and hypotension (*red man sydrome*) as a result of histamine release from mast cells (25). Slowing the infusion rate to less than 10 mg/min usually corrects the problem.

2. *Ototoxicity*

Vancomycin can cause reversible hearing loss for high-frequency sounds when serum drug levels exceed 40 mg/L (27). Permanent deafness has been reported when serum levels exceed 80 mg/L (26).

3. *Nephrotoxicity*

Renal insufficiency is reported in 5% of patients receiving vancomycin (27). There is no apparent relationship to the dose of vancomycin, but the incidence is higher when aminoglycosides are given concurrently. Renal function usually returns to normal after stopping the drug.

D. Vancomycin Replacements

Over the last decade, there has been a steady rise in the prevalence of vancomycin-resistant stains of enterococci and staphylococci (particularly MRSA) (28). This has led to a search for antibiotics to replace vancomycin, particularly for the treatment of multidrug-resistant gram-positive organisms. Two possible replacements are described next.

1. *Linezolid*

Linezolid (Zyvox) was introduced in 2000 to treat infections caused by multidrug-resistant gram-positive organisms (29). It is intended for cases where vancomycin is ineffective or not tolerated but may become a replacement for vancomycin. One study comparing vancomycin and linezolid for the treatment of MRSA pneumonia showed better results with linezolid (30), probably because linezolid penetrates into respiratory secretions, while vancomycin does not.

   a. The intravenous dose is 600 mg every 12 hours, and no dose adjustment is needed in renal failure.

b. Linezolid can cause a pancytopenia if given for more than 2 weeks (29), and an optic neuropathy can appear (rarely) after one month of drug therapy (31).

2. *Daptomycin*

Daptomycin (Cubicin) has proven successful in treating bacteremias caused by MRSA and coagulase-negative staphylococci (32).

a. The intravenous dose is 4 to 6 mg/kg once daily (the higher dose is for bacteremias). The dosing interval should be increased to 48 hours in patients with impaired renal function (3).

b. No serious side effects have been reported, but drug use has been limited.

REFERENCES

1. Turnidge J. Pharmacodynamics and dosing of aminoglycosides. Infect Dis Clin N Am 2003; 17:503–528.

2. Neuhauser MM, Weinstein RA, Rydman R, et al. Antibiotic resistance among gram-negative bacilli in U.S. intensive care units. JAMA 2003; 289:885–888.

3. Aronoff GR, Bennett WM, Berns JS, et al. Drug prescribing in renal failure. 5th ed. Philadelphia: American College of Physicians, 2007:49–70.

4. Wilson SE. Aminoglycosides: assessing the potential for nephrotoxicity. Surg Gynecol Obstet 1986; 171(Suppl):24–30.

5. Lippmann M, Yang E, Au E, Lee C. Neuromuscular blocking effects of tobramycin, gentamicin, and cefazolin. Anesth Analg 1982; 61:767–770.

6. Drachman DB. Myasthenia gravis. N Engl J Med 1994; 330:179–1810.

7. Groll AH, Gea-Banacloche JC, Glasmacher A, et al. Clinical pharmacology of antifungal compounds. Infect Dis Clin N Am 2003; 17:159–191.

8. Bult J, Franklin CM. Using amphotericin B in the critically ill: a new look at an old drug. J Crit Illness 1996; 11:577–585.

9. Carlson MA, Condon RE. Nephrotoxicity of amphotericin B. J Am Coll Surg 1994; 179:361–381.

10. Walsh TJ, Finberg RW, Arndt C, et al. Liposomal amphotericin B for empirical therapy in patients with persistent fever and neutropenia. N Engl J Med 1999; 340:764–771.

11. Pappas PG, Rex JH, Sobel JD, et al. Guidelines for treatment of candidiasis. Clin Infect Dis 2004; 38:161–189.

12. Perfect JR. Management of invasive mycoses in hematology patients: current approaches. J Crit Illness 2004; 19:3–12.

13. Gearhart MO. Worsening of liver function with fluconazole and a review of azole antifungal hepatotoxicity. Ann Pharmacother 1994; 28:1177–1181.

14. Mora-Duarte J, Betts R, Rotstein C, et al. Comparison of capsofungin and amphotericin B for invasive candidiasis. N Engl J Med 2002; 347:2020–2029.

15. Hellinger WC, Brewer NS. Carbapenems and monobactams: imipenem, meropenem, and aztreonam. Mayo Clin Proc 1999; 74:430–434.

16. Freifield A, Walsh T, Marshall D, et al. Monotherapy for fever and neutropenia in cancer patients: a randomized comparison of ceftazidime versus imipenem. J Clin Oncol 1995; 13:165–176.

17. Marshall WF, Blair JE. The cephalosporins. Mayo Clin Proc 1999; 74:187–195.

18. Hughes WT, Armstrong D, Bodey GP, et al. 2002 Guidelines for the use of antimicrobial agents in neutropenic patients with fever. Clin Infect Dis 2002; 34:730–751.

19. O'Donnell JA, Gelone SP. Fluoroquinolones. Infect Dis Clin N Am 2000; 14:489–513.

20. Walker RC. The fluoroquinolones. Mayo Clin Proc 1999; 74:1020–1037.

21. Finch C, Self T. Quinolones: recognizing the potential for neurotoxicity. J Crit Illness 2000; 15:656–657.

22. Frothingham R. Rates of torsades de pointes associated with ciprofloxacin, oflaoxacin, levofloxacin, gatifloxacin, and moxifloxacin. Pharmacotherapy 2001; 21:1468–1472.

23. Wright AJ. The penicillins. Mayo Clin Proc 1999; 74:290–307.

24. McEvoy GK, ed. AHFS drug information, 2001. Bethesda, MD: American Society of Hospital Pharmacists, 2001:419–422.

25. Lundstrom TS, Sobel. Antibiotics for gram-positive bacterial infections: vancomycin, quinapristin-dalfopristin, linezolid, and daptomycin. Infect Dis Clin N Am 2004; 18:651–668.

26. Ena J, Dick RW, Jones RN. The epidemiology of intravenous vancomycin usage in a university hospital. JAMA 1993; 269:598–605.

27. Saunders NJ. Why monitor peak vancomycin concentrations? Lancet 1994; 344:1748–1750.

28. Courvalin P. Vancomycin resistance in gram-positive cocci. Clin Infect Dis 2006; 42(Suppl):S25–S34.

29. Birmingham MC, RaynerCR, Meagher AK, et al. Linezolid for the treatment of multidrug-resistant gram-positive infections: Experience from a compassionate use program. Clin Infect Dis 2003; 36:159–164.

30. Wunderink RG, Rello J, Norden C, et al. Linezolid vs. vancomycin: Analysis of two double-blind studies of patients with methicillin-resistant *Staphylococcus aureus* pneumonia. Chest 2003; 124:1789–1795,

31. Rucker JC, Hamilton SR, Bardenstein D, et al. Linezolid-associated toxic optic neuropathy. Neurology 2006; 66:595–598.

32. Sakoulas G, Golan Y, Lamp KC, et al. Daptomycin in the treatment of bacteremia. Am J Med 2007; 120:S21–S27.

Chapter 45

HEMODYNAMIC DRUGS

This chapter describes five drugs that are used for circulatory support: dobutamine, dopamine, nitroglycerin, nitroprusside, and norepinephrine. Each is presented in alphabetical order.

I. DOBUTAMINE

Dobutamine is a synthetic catecholamine that is used to augment cardiac output.

A. Actions

1. Dobutamine is a potent β_1-receptor agonist and a weak β_2-receptor agonist: the β_1 stimulation produces positive inotropic and chronotropic effects, and the β_2 stimulation produces peripheral vasodilation (1–3).

2. As demonstrated in Figure 45.1, dobutamine causes a dose-dependent increase in stroke volume (upper graph) accompanied by a decrease in cardiac filling pressure (lower graph) (4). Heart rate may be increased, decreased, or unchanged.

3. Dobutamine-induced increases in stroke output are accompanied by proportional decreases in systemic vascular resistance; as a result, the arterial blood pressure usually remains unchanged (1,3).

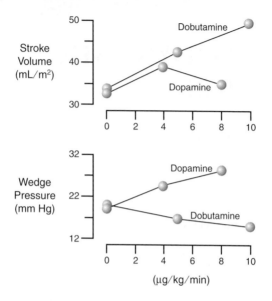

FIGURE 45.1 Effects of dobutamine and dopamine on stroke volume (upper graph) and left ventricular filling pressure (lower graph) in patients with severe heart failure. Adapted from Reference 4.

B. Clinical Uses

1. Dobutamine is used primarily for cases of decompensated systolic heart failure associated with a normal blood pressure. The drug is effective in both right-sided and left-sided systolic failure.

2. Because dobutamine does not raise the blood pressure, it is not recommended (at least as monotherapy) in cardiogenic shock.

3. Like all positive inotropic agents, dobutamine is *contraindicated* in patients with hypertrophic cardiomyopathy (1).

C. Administration

1. Dobutamine dosing is weight-based (there is no clear preference for ideal or actual body weight). The initial dose rate is 3 to 5 µg/kg/min, which is then titrated to achieve the desired cardiac output or stroke volume. (Dobutamine infusions require a pulmonary artery catheter to monitor the desired endpoints).

2. The usual dose range is 5 to 15 µg/kg/min (1), but higher dose rates may be needed, particularly in elderly patients (5). Dose rates as high as 200 µg/kg/min have been used safely (6).

D. Adverse Effects

The principal side effects of dobutamine are tachycardia and ventricular ectopic beats (1).

1. The tachycardia is usually mild.

2. Malignant tachyarrhythmias are rare.

II. DOPAMINE

Dopamine is an endogenous catecholamine that serves as a neurotransmitter and a precursor for norepinephrine synthesis. When given as an exogenous agent, dopamine activates a variety of receptors in a dose-dependent manner (see next) (7).

A. Actions

1. *Low Dose Rates*

   At low dose rates (≤3 µg/kg/min), dopamine selectively activates dopamine-specific receptors in the renal and splanchnic circulations, resulting in increased blood flow in these regions (2).

2. *Intermediate Dose Rates*

At intermediate dose rates (3 to 10 μg/kg/min), dopamine stimulates β-receptors in the heart and peripheral circulation, producing an increase in myocardial contractility, an increase in heart rate, and peripheral vasodilation. The overall result is an increase in cardiac stroke output, which is demonstrated in Figure 45.1 (upper graph).

3. *High Dose Rates*

At high dose rates (>10 μg/kg/min), dopamine produces a progressive activation of α-receptors in the systemic and pulmonary circulations, resulting in progressive pulmonary and systemic vasoconstriction. This vasopressor effect counteracts the cardiac stimulation produced by intermediate-dose dopamine. This is demonstrated in Figure 45.1 (upper graph), which shows the loss in augmentation of stroke volume as the dose rate of dopamine is progressively increased.

4. *Wedge Pressure*

Dopamine causes a dose-dependent increase in the pulmonary capillary wedge pressure, as shown in Figure 45.1 (lower graph). This effect is believed to result from dopamine-induced vasoconstriction in pulmonary veins. This ability to constrict pulmonary veins makes the pulmonary capillary wedge pressure an unreliable measure of left-ventricular filling pressure during dopamine infusions. (See Chapter 8 for a description of the wedge pressure.)

B. Clinical Uses

1. Low-dose dopamine is often used in an attempt to increase the glomerular filtration rate in acute renal failure, but this is inappropriate (see Chapter 25, Section II-B).

2. Intermediate-to-high dose dopamine is used in situations where both cardiac stimulation and peripheral vasoconstriction are desired. The classic example of this is *cardiogenic shock*.

3. Dopamine is also used to correct the hypotension in septic shock, but norepinephrine may be the preferred vasopressor in this condition (see later).

C. Dose Administration

1. Because of its vasoconstrictor actions, dopamine should always be infused through large, central veins.

2. Dopamine dosing is weight-based, and *ideal body weight* is preferred to actual body weight (2,7). The initial dose rate is usually 3 to 5 µg/kg/min, and dose rates are subsequently increased to achieve the desired effect.

   a. Dose rates of 3 to 10 µg/kg/min are optimal for augmenting cardiac output.

   b. Dose rates above 10 µg/kg/min are usually needed to raise the blood pressure.

D. Adverse Effects

1. *Tachyarrhythmias* are the most common adverse effect of dopamine infusions. Sinus tachycardia is common (7), but rarely is severe enough to prompt a change in drug or dose rate. Malignant tachyarrhythmias (e.g., multifocal ventricular ectopics, ventricular tachycardia) can also occur but are uncommon.

2. Other adverse effects of dopamine include:

   a. Gangrene of the digits (7).

   b. Increased intraocular pressure (8).

   c. Delayed gastric emptying (9).

III. NITROGLYCERIN

Nitroglycerin (NTG) is an organic nitrate (glyceryl trinitrate) that relaxes vascular smooth muscle and produces a generalized vasodilation.

A. Actions

1. *Vasodilator Effects*

   The conversion of NTG to nitric oxide is responsible for the relaxation of vascular smooth muscle (10). The vasodilator effects are dose-dependent and involve both arteries and veins (11,12).

   a. Venous vasodilator effects are prominent at low dose rates (<40 µg/min), and arterial vasodilator effects predominate at high dose rates (>200 µg/min).

   b. At low dose rates, NTG produces a decrease in cardiac filling pressures with little or no change in cardiac output. As the dose rate is increased through the intermediate dose range, the cardiac output begins to rise as a result of progressive arterial vasodilation. Further increases in the dose rate will eventually produce a drop in blood pressure.

2. *Antiplatelet Effects*

   Nitrates inhibit platelet aggregation, and nitric oxide is believed to mediate this effect as well (13). The antiplatelet actions of NTG have been proposed as the mechanism for the antianginal effects of the drug (13).

B. Clinical Uses

1. Intravenous NTG has two principal uses:

   a. Augmenting cardiac output and reducing edema formation in patients with acute, decompensated heart failure.

   b. Relieving chest pain in patients with unstable angina.

    c. Treating hypertensive emergencies (see Table 45.1)

2. NTG should *not* be used in patients who have taken a phosphodiesterase inhibitor for erectile dysfunction within the past 24 hours (because of the risk of hypotension).

TABLE 45.1 Vasodilator Therapy of Hypertensive Emergencies	
Drug	**Dose Regimen**
Esmolol	500 µg/kg loading dose over 1 min, then infuse at 25–50 µg/kg/min and increase by 25 µg/kg/min every 10–20 min to a maximum of 300 µg/kg/min
Labetalol	20 mg initial bolus, then infuse at 2 mg/min to maximum dose of 300 mg in 24 hrs
Nitroglycerin	Start at 5 µg/min and increase 5 µg/min every 5–10 min as needed
Nitroprusside	Start at 0.52 µg/kg/min and increase if needed to maximum rate of 2 µg/kg/min

From Marik PE, Varon J. Hypertensive crises. Chest 2007; 131:1949–1962.

C. Administration

1. *Adsorption to Plastic*

    a. As much as 80% of the NTG in infusates can be lost by adsorption to polyvinylchloride (PVC) in standard intravenous infusion systems (12).

    b. NTG does not bind to glass or hard plastics like polyethylene (PET), so drug loss via adsorption can be eliminated by using glass bottles and PET tubing.

2. *Dosing*

NTG should be started at a dose rate of 5 to 10 µg/min. The rate is then increased in 5 µg/min increments every 5 minutes until the desired effect is achieved. The dose requirement should not exceed 100 µg/min in most patients. High dose requirements (>350 µg/min) are often the result of drug loss via adsorption or nitrate tolerance (see later).

D. Adverse Effects

1. *Hemodynamics*
    a. NTG-induced increases in cerebral blood flow can lead to increased intracranial pressure (14).
    b. In patients with ARDS, the vasodilation from NTG can increase intrapulmonary shunt and aggravate hypoxemia (15).
    c. NTG-induced venodilation can promote hypotension in patients with hypovolemia or right heart failure.

2. *Methemoglobinemia*

    The metabolism of NTG produces inorganic nitrites, and accumulation of nitrites can lead to methemoglobin formation (by oxidizing the heme-bound iron moieties in hemoglobin). However, an increase in methemoglobin levels to clinically significant levels is an infrequent consequence of NTG infusions, and requires excessive dose rates for prolonged periods of time (14).

3. *Solvent Toxicity*

    NTG does not readily dissolve in aqueous solutions, and nonpolar solvents such as ethanol and propylene glycol are required to keep the drug in solution. These solvents can accumulate during prolonged infusions.
    a. Both ethanol intoxication (16) and propylene glycol toxicity (17) have been reported as a result of NTG infusions.
    b. Propylene glycol toxicity may be more common than suspected because this solvent makes up 30 to 50% of some NTG preparations (14). Signs of toxicity include agitation, coma, seizures, lactic acidosis, and hypotension.

E. Nitrate Tolerance

1. Tolerance to the vasodilator and antiplatelet actions of NTG can appear after only 24 hours of continuous drug administration (14). The underlying mechanism is unclear.

2. The most effective measure for preventing or reversing nitrate tolerance is a daily drug-free interval of at least 6 hours (14).

IV. NITROPRUSSIDE

Nitroprusside is a rapidly acting vasodilator that is favored for the treatment of severe hypertension. The use of this drug should be restricted because of the risk of cyanide intoxication (see later).

A. Actions

1. The vasodilator actions of nitroprusside, like those of nitroglycerin, are mediated by nitric oxide (10). Nitroprusside dilates both arteries and veins, but it is less potent than nitroglycerin as a venodilator and more potent as an arterial vasodilator.

2. Nitroprusside has variable effects on cardiac output when cardiac function is normal (18), but it augments cardiac output in decompensated heart failure (19).

B. Clinical Uses

1. The major use of nitroprusside is for hypertensive emergencies (see Table 45.1).

2. Nitroprusside can also be used to treat decompensated heart failure (19) and is effective in treating heart failure due to aortic stenosis (20), a condition where vasodilatory therapy is usually discouraged.

C. Dose Administration

1. Thiosulfate must be added to the nitroprusside infusate to limit cyanide accumulation (see later). About 500 mg of thiosulfate should be added for every 50 mg of nitroprusside (21).

2. Nitroprusside should be started at a low dose rate (0.2 μg/kg/min) and then titrated upward every 5 minutes to the desired result.

3. Satisfactory control of hypertension usually requires dose rates of 2 to 5 μg/kg/min, but the dose rate should be kept below 3 μg/kg/min, if possible, to limit cyanide accumulation (21). In renal failure, the dose rate should be kept below 1 μg/kg/min to limit thiocyanate accumulation (21).

4. The maximum allowable dose rate is 10 μg/kg/min for 10 minutes.

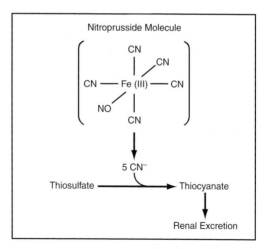

FIGURE 45.2 Mechanism for clearing the cyanide ions (CN^-) released by nitroprusside.

D. Cyanide Accumulation

Cyanide accumulation is common during therapeutic infusions of nitroprusside (14,21,22). The origin of the cyanide is the nitroprusside molecule, which is a ferricyanide complex that contains 5 cyanide atoms bound to an oxidized iron core (see Figure 45.2).

1. *Cyanide Clearance*

   When nitroprusside disrupts to release nitric oxide and exert its actions, the cyanide is released into the bloodstream. The cyanide is normally cleared by the transfer of sulfur from a donor molecule (thiosulfate) to cyanide to form a thiocyanate compound, which is then cleared by the kidneys (see Figure 45.2).

   a. Normally there is enough thiosulfate to detoxify 68 mg of nitroprusside (14). At a nitroprusside infusion of 2 μg/kg/minute (therapeutic range) in an 80 kg adult, the 68 mg capacity is reached in 500 minutes (8.3 hrs).

   b. Once the capacity for cyanide removal is exceeded, the free cyanide will combine with the oxidized iron in cytochrome oxidase (which blocks the utilization of O_2 in mitochondria).

2. *Cyanide Intoxication*

   The signs of cyanide intoxication are shown in Table 45.2. One of the early signs is nitroprusside tachyphylaxis (14). Signs of impaired oxygen utilization (e.g., lactic acidosis) do not appear until the late stages of cyanide intoxication (23).

   a. Whole-blood cyanide levels can be used to document cyanide intoxication (see Table 45.2), but the results are not available for 3 to 4 hours. Therefore, immediate decisions about cyanide intoxication are often based on clinical signs. *A gradual increase in the effective nitroprusside dose rate (tachyphylaxis) is an important early marker of cyanide accumulation.*

3. *Treatment*

Treatment of cyanide intoxication should begin with the inhalation of 100% oxygen. The Cyanide Antidote Kit (Eli Lilly & Co.) can be used as described in Table 45.2 (24). This kit uses: 1) nitrates and nitrites (which promote methemoglobin formation) to facilitate cyanide binding to methemoglobin, and 2) thiosulfate to clear cyanide from the bloodstream.

TABLE 45.2 Diagnosis and Treatment of Cyanide Intoxication		
Clinical Signs	Early Stages	Behavioral changes
		Impaired O_2 extraction
		Nitroprusside tachyphylaxis
	Late Stages	Coma
		Generalized seizures
		Lactic acidosis
Laboratory Test	**Toxicity**	**Blood Cyanide Level**
	Mild	0.5–2.5 µg/mL
	Severe	>2.5 µg/mL
	Fatal	>3.0 µg/mL
Cyanide Antidote Kit	Amyl nitrate inhaler for one minute, *or*	
	Sodium nitrite: 300 mg IV over 15 min *plus*	
	Sodium thiosulfate: 12.5 g IV over 15 min	

From References 14.,23,24.

E. Thiocyanate Toxicity

1. When renal function is impaired, thiocyanate can accumulate and produce a toxic syndrome that is distinct from cyanide intoxication. The clinical features include anxiety, pupillary constriction, tinnitus, hallucinations, and generalized seizures (14,21).

2. The diagnosis is established by the serum thiocyanate level. Normal levels are below 10 mg/L, and levels above 100 mg/L are associated with clinical toxicity (24).

3. Thiocyanate intoxication can be treated by hemodialysis.

V. NOREPINEPHRINE

Norepinephrine is a vasopressor that promotes vasoconstriction more readily than dopamine.

A. Actions

1. Norepinephrine is a prominent α-receptor agonist and a mild β_1-receptor agonist. The overall effect is widespread systemic vasoconstriction with variable effects on cardiac output (25).

2. The vasoconstrictor response to norepinephrine is usually accompanied by a decrease in organ blood flow, particularly in the kidneys. This is not the case in septic shock, where norepinephrine tends to preserve renal blood flow (17,26).

B. Clinical Uses

1. Norepinephrine is often used as a second-line vasopressor behind dopamine because of the greater tendency to promote vasoconstriction and hypoperfusion of vital organs.

2. Norepinephrine may be the preferred vasopressor in septic shock because of the tendency to preserve renal blood flow.

3. Despite the ability to correct hypotension, norepinephrine (like all vasopressors) does not improve survival in septic shock or any other type of circulatory shock (27).

C. Dose Administration

1. Because of its vasoconstrictor actions, norepinephrine should always be infused through a large, central vein.

2. Norepinephrine infusions are started at a dose rate of 0.2 µg/kg/min (10 to 20 µg/min for a 70 kg patient) and titrated upward to the desired effect.

3. The effective dose range is usually between 0.2 and 1.3 µg/kg/min. In refractory cases of hypotension, dose rates as high as 5 µg/kg/min may be required (27).

D. Adverse Effects

The most undesirable side effect of norepinephrine is vasoconstriction and organ hypoperfusion. However, whenever a vasoconstrictor drug is required to correct hypotension, it is often difficult to distinguish between adverse drug effects and adverse disease effects.

REFERENCES

1. Dobutamine monograph. Mosby's Drug Consult, 2006. Available at www.mdconsult.com. Accessed on 2/3/2006.

2. Bayram M, De Luca L, Massie B, Gheorghiade M. Reassessment of dobutamine, dopamine, and milrinone in the management of acute heart failure syndromes. Am J Cardiol 2005; 96(Suppl): 47G–58G.

3. Romson JL, Leung JM, Bellows WH, et al. Effects of dobutamine on hemodynamics and left ventricular performance after cardiopulmonary bypass in cardiac surgical patients. Anesthesiology 1999; 91:1318-1327.

4. Leier CV, Heban PT, Huss P, et al. Comparative systemic and regional hemodynamic effects of dopamine and dobutamine in patients with cardiomyopathic heart failure. Circulation 1978; 58: 466–475.

5. Rich MW, Imburgia M. Inotropic response to dobutamine in elderly patients with decompensated congestive heart failure. Am J Cardiol 1990; 65:519–521.

6. Hayes MA, Yau EHS, Timmins AC, et al. Response of critically ill patients to treatment aimed at achieving supranormal oxygen delivery and consumption: Relationship to outcome. Chest 1993; 103:886–895.

7. Dopamine monograph. Mosby's Drug Consult, 2006. Available at www.mdconsult.com. Accessed on 2/4/2006.

8. Brath PC, MacGregor DA, Ford JG, Prielipp RC. Dopamine and intraocular pressure in critically ill patients. Anesthesiology 2000; 93:1398–1400.

9. Johnson AG. Source of infection in nosocomial pneumonia. Lancet 1993; 341:1368 (Letter)

10. Anderson TJ, Meredith IT, Ganz P, et al. Nitric oxide and nitrovasodilators: similarities, differences and potential interactions. J Am Coll Cardiol 1994; 24:555–566.

11. Nitroglycerin. In: McEvoy GK, ed. AHFS Drug Information, 2001. Bethesda, MD: American Society of Health System Pharmacists, 2001:1832–1835.

12. Elkayam U. Nitrates in heart failure. Cardiol Clin 1994; 12:73–85.

13. Stamler JS, Loscalzo J. The antiplatelet effects of organic nitrates and related nitroso compounds in vitro and in vivo and their relevance to cardiovascular disorders. J Am Coll Cardiol 1991; 18:1529–1536.

14. Curry SC, Arnold-Cappell P. Nitroprusside, nitroglycerin, and angiotensin-converting enzyme inhibitors. Crit Care Clin 1991; 7:555–582.

15. Radermacher P, Santak B, Becker H, Falke KJ. Prostaglandin F1 and nitroglycerin reduce pulmonary capillary pressure but worsen ventilation–perfusion distribution in patients with adult respiratory distress syndrome. Anesthesiology 1989; 70:601–606.

16. Korn SH, Comer JB. Intravenous nitroglycerin and ethanol intoxication. Ann Intern Med 1985; 102:274.

17. Demey HE, Daelemans RA, Verpooten GA, et al. Propylene glycol-induced side effects during intravenous nitroglycerin therapy. Intensive Care Med 1988; 14:221–226.

18. Nitroprusside. In: McEvoy GK, ed. AHFS Drug Information, 2001. Bethesda, MD: American Society of Health System Pharmacists, 2001:1816-1820.

19. Guiha NH, Cohn JN, Mikulic E, et al. Treatment of refractory heart failure with infusion of nitroprusside. N Engl J Med 1974; 291:587–592.

20. Khot UN, Novaro GM, Popovic ZB, et al. Nitroprusside in critically ill patients with left ventricular dysfunction and aortic stenosis. N Engl J Med 2003; 348:1756–1763.

21. Hall VA, Guest JM. Sodium nitroprusside-induced cyanide intoxication and prevention with sodium thiosulfate prophylaxis. Am J Crit Care 1992; 2:19–27.

22. Robin ED, McCauley R. Nitroprusside-related cyanide poisoning: Time (long past due) for urgent, effective interventions. Chest 1992; 102:1842–1845.

23. Hall AH, Rumack BH. Clinical toxicology of cyanide intoxication. Ann Emerg Med 1986; 15:1067–1072.

24. Kirk MA, Gerace R, Kulig KW. Cyanide and methemoglobin kinetics in smoke inhalation victims treated with the Cyanide Antidote Kit. Ann Emerg Med 1993; 22:1413–1418.

25. Norepinephrine bitartrate. In: McEvoy GK, ed. AHFS Drug Information, 2001. Bethesda, MD: American Society of Health System Pharmacists, 2001:1258–1261.

26. Desairs P, Pinaud M, Bugnon D, Tasseau F. Norepinephrine therapy has no deleterious renal effects in human septic shock. Crit Care Med 1989; 17:426–429.

27. Beale RJ, Hollenberg SM, Vincent J-L, Parrillo JE. Vasopressor and inotropic support in septic shock: An evidence-based review. Crit Care Med 2004; 32(Suppl):S455–S465.

Chapter 46

PHARMACEUTICAL TOXINS & ANTIDOTES

This chapter describes the manifestations and management of overdose with the following pharmaceutical agents: acetaminophen, benzodiazepines, β-blockers, and opioids. Each is presented in alphabetical order.

I. ACETAMINOPHEN

Acetaminophen is a popular analgesic that is included in over 600 commercial drug preparations. It is also a hepatotoxin, and is the *leading cause of acute liver failure in the United States* (1). The general public seems unaware of acetaminophen's toxic potential because almost one third of overdoses are unintentional (2).

A. Toxic Metabolite

The toxicity of acetaminophen is related to its hepatic metabolism.

1. A small fraction (5–15%) of acetaminophen is metabolized to a toxic metabolite that can promote oxidant injury in hepatic parenchymal cells. This metabolite is normally inactivated by conjugation with glutathione, an intracellular antioxidant.

2. The metabolic burden created by acetaminophen overdose can deplete hepatic glutathione reserves. When this occurs, the toxic metabolite accumulates and promotes hepatocellular injury (4).

B. Clinical Presentation

The period following acetaminophen overdose can be divided into 3 stages (3,5,6).

1. In the initial stage (the first 24 hours), symptoms are either absent or nonspecific (e.g., nausea), and there is no laboratory evidence of hepatic injury.

2. In the second stage (24–72 hours after drug ingestion), clinical signs of toxicity continue to be minimal or absent, but laboratory evidence of hepatic injury begins to appear. Elevated aspartate aminotranferase (AST) is the most sensitive marker of acetaminophen toxicity; the rise of AST precedes the hepatic dysfunction, and peak levels are reached at 72–96 hours.

3. In severe cases, a third stage (after 72–96 hours) occurs where there is clinical and laboratory evidence of progressive hepatic injury (e.g., encephalopathy, coagulopathy). Death from hepatic injury usually occurs within 3 to 5 days.

C. Prognostic Markers

Patients often present within 24 hours of the toxic ingestion, when there are no manifestations of hepatic injury. The principal task at this time is to identify patients who are likely to develop life-threatening hepatotoxicity. Two variables have prognostic value.

1. *Ingested Dose*
   a. The hepatotoxic dose of acetaminophen can vary in individuals, but an ingested dose of 8 grams or higher is considered hepatotoxic (3–5).
   b. Chronic ethanol ingestion increases susceptibility to acetaminophen hepatotoxicity (4).

2. *Plasma Drug Levels*

   a. The most reliable predictor of hepatotoxicity is the plasma acetaminophen level.

   b. The standard nomogram in Figure 46.1 predicts the risk of hepatotoxicity based on plasma acetaminophen levels at 4 to 24 hours after drug ingestion (4). A plasma level that falls in the high-risk area (≥60% risk of hepatotoxicity) warrants treatment with *N*-acetylcysteine (see next).

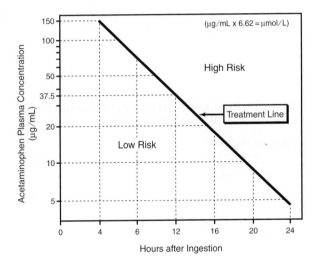

FIGURE 46.1 Nomogram for predicting the risk of of acetaminophen hepatotoxicity. From Reference 4.

D. Activated Charcoal

Acetaminophen is completely absorbed from the gastrointestinal tract in the first few hours after drug ingestion (5), and activated charcoal (1 g/kg body weight) is recommended only in the first 4 hours after toxic ingestion (5,7).

E. Antidote Therapy

The antidote for acetaminophen hepatotoxicity is **N-acetyl-cysteine** (NAC), a glutathione surrogate that inactivates the toxic acetaminophen metabolite.

1. *Timing*

NAC is indicated only when therapy can be started within 24 hours after acetaminophen overdose (4–6,8). It is most effective when started in the first 8 hours after ingestion.

TABLE 46.1 Treatment of Acetaminophen Overdose with N-Acetylcysteine (NAC)

Intravenous Regimen[1]

Use 20% NAC (200 mg/mL) for each of the doses below and infuse in sequence:

1. 150 mg/kg in 200 mL D_5W over 60 min
2. 50 mg/kg in 500 mL D_5W over 4 hrs
3. 100 mg/kg in 1,000 mL D_5W over 16 hrs

Total dose: 300 mg/kg over 21 hrs

Oral Regimen[2]

Use 10% NAC (100 mg/mL) and dilute 2:1 in water or juice to make a 5% solution (50 mg/mL).

Initial dose: 140 mg/kg
Maintenance dosage: 70 mg/kg every 4 hrs for 17 doses

Total dose: 1,330 mg/kg over 72 hrs

---

[1]From Cumberland Pharmaceuticals, Acetadote Package Insert. 2006.

[2]From Reference 8.

2. *Therapeutic Regimens*

NAC can be given intravenously or orally using the dosing regimens shown in Table 46.1. Both regimens are considered equally effective (9), but the IV regimen is preferred because drug delivery is more reliable, and the treatment is more agreeable to patients (see next).

3. *Adverse Effects*

a. Oral NAC has a very disagreeable taste (often described as rotten eggs) due to the sulfur content of NAC. This often incites vomiting, and a nasogastric tube may be required to complete the oral regimen.

b. Oral NAC also produces diarrhea in about 50% of patients, but this resolves with continued therapy in over 90% of patients (8,10).

c. Intravenous NAC can trigger anaphylactic reactions (11). Although rare, fatal reactions have been reported in atopic patients (12)

II. BENZODIAZEPINES

Benzodiazepines are the second most frequently overdosed prescription drugs in the United States and are second only to analgesics as the leading cause of medication-related death (13).

Overdose of benzodiazepines can also occur in the ICU, where prolonged infusions of benzodiazepines can lead to troublesome drug accumulation (see Chapter 43, Section III).

A. Clinical Toxicity

1. Benzodiazepines produce a dose-dependent depression in the level of consciousness.

2. Respiratory depression is uncommon, but has been re-

ported in ICU patients receiving prolonged infusions of benzodiazepines (14,15).

B. Antidote Therapy

The antidote for benzodiazepine overdose is **flumazenil**, a pure antagonist that binds to benzodiazepine receptors in the central nervous system but does not elicit agonist effects (16). Flumazenil is effective in reversing the sedative effects of benzodiazepines, but it does not consistently reverse the respiratory depression (14,15).

1. *Drug Administration*

   a. Flumazenil is given as an intravenous bolus. The initial dose is 0.2 mg, and this can be repeated every few minutes if necessary to a cumulative dose of 1 mg.

   b. The response is rapid, with onset in 1–2 minutes and peak effect at 6–10 minutes. The effect lasts about one hour (16).

   c. Since flumazenil has a shorter duration of action than the benzodiazepines, recurrence of sedation is common. To avoid this risk, the bolus dose(s) of flumazenil can be followed by a continuous infusion at 0.3–0.4 mg/hr (17).

2. *Adverse Reactions*

   Flumazenil has few side effects. It can precipitate a benzodiazepine withdrawal syndrome in chronic users, but this is uncommon (18).

3. *Use in the ICU*

   Flumazenil has been used to reverse oversedation from benzodiazepines in ventilator-dependent patients (17), and this can hasten weaning from mechanical ventilation (19). However, interruption of benzodiazepine infusions to prevent drug accumulation (see Chapter 43, Section V) is a better approach to the problem of oversedation.

III. ß-RECEPTOR ANTAGONISTS

Like benzodiazepines, β-blocker toxicity can originate in the ICU as well as the community because β-blockers are used to manage a number of conditions in ICU patients (e.g., hypertension, tachyarrhythmias, and acute coronary syndromes).

A. Clinical Toxicity

1. *Cardiovascular Toxicity*

   a. The most common manifestations of β-blocker toxicity are bradycardia and hypotension (20,21). The bradycardia is usually sinus in origin and is well tolerated. The hypotension can be due to peripheral vasodilatation (renin blockade), or a decrease in cardiac output ($β_1$-receptor blockade). Sudden or refractory hypotension is an ominous sign (22).

   b. β-blockers can also prolong atrioventricular (AV) conduction via a membrane-stabilizing effect that is independent of β-receptor blockade (23).

2. *Neurotoxicity*

   Most β-blockers are lipid soluble and accumulate in lipid-rich organs like brain. As a result, β-blocker overdoses are often accompanied by neurotoxic effects; i.e., depressed consciousness and generalized seizures. These effects are the result of the membrane-stabilizing actions of β-blockers, and are not caused by β-receptor antagonism.

B. Antidote Therapy

The treatment of choice for reversing the cardiovascular depression from β-blockers is the regulatory hormone **glucagon**.

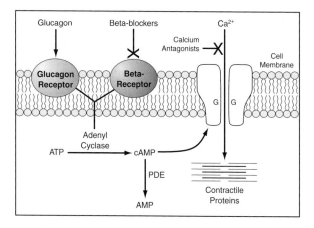

FIGURE 46.2 The mechanism of action of drugs that affect the strength of cardiac contraction. Abbreviations: ATP = adenosine triphosphate, cAMP = cyclic adenosine monophosphate, PDE = phosphodiesterase, AMP = adenosine monophosphate.

1. *Mechanism of Action*

   As shown in the diagram in Figure 46.2, glucagon activates receptors on the surface of the heart that are independent of cardiac β-receptors but share the same mechanism of action. This allows glucagon to produce β-like effects that are independent of β-receptor blockade.

2. *Indications*

   a. Glucagon is indicated for the treatment of hypotension and symptomatic bradycardia associated with toxic exposure to β-blockers.

   b. Glucagon is *not* indicated for reversing the prolonged AV conduction or neurotoxicity in β-blocker overdose because these effects are not mediated by β-receptor blockade.

   c. When used appropriately, glucagon produces a favorable response in 90% of cases (24).

3. *Dosage*

Glucagon is given as an IV bolus: the initial dose is 3 mg (or 0.05 mg/kg), and this can be followed by a second dose of 5 mg (or 0.07 mg/kg) if necessary (21,24,25). The effect can be short-lived (5 minutes), and a favorable response should be followed by a continuous infusion (5 mg/hr).

4. *Adverse Effects*

a. Nausea and vomiting are common at glucagon doses above 5 mg/hr.

b. Mild hyperglycemia is common and is due to glucagon-induced glycogenolysis.

c. Glucagon promotes the adrenal release of catecholamines, and this can raise the blood pressure in hypertensive patients. This response is exaggerated in pheochromocytoma, and glucagon is contraindicated in this condition.

IV. OPIOIDS

The adverse effects of opioid analgesics are described in Chapter 43 (see Section I-E). The material presented here focuses on the treatment of opioid intoxication with **naloxone**.

A. Naloxone

Naloxone is a pure opioid antagonist that binds to endogenous opioid receptors but does not elicit agonist responses. It is most effective in blocking opioid receptors that are responsible for analgesia, sedation, and respiratory depression (26).

1. *Routes of Administration*

Naloxone is usually given as an intravenous bolus injection (onset 2–3 minutes). However, it can also be given by intramuscular injection (onset 15 minutes) (27), by bolus endotracheal injection (28), or by intralingual injection (29).

2. *Dosing Regimens*

Reversal of depressed consciousness usually requires smaller doses of naloxone than reversal of the respiratory depression. The dosing recommendations for naloxone in each of these conditions is shown in Table 46.2.

TABLE 46.2 Naloxone Reversal of Opioid Intoxication

For Depressed Consciousness:
1. Administer 0.4 mg naloxone as an IV bolus.
2. Repeat in 2 min, if necessary.
3. A response should be apparent after the second dose if the depressed consciousness is opioid-related.
4. For patients with known opioid dependency, reduce the bolus dose of naloxone to 0.1 or 0.2 mg.

For Respiratory Depression:
1. Administer 2 mg naloxone as an IV bolus.
2. Repeat every 2 min if necessary to a total dose of 10 mg.

Naloxone Infusion:
If there is a favorable response to naloxone, start a continuous infusion:
1. Infuse naloxone for 6 hrs (in 250 mL isotonic saline) using an hourly dose that is 2/3 the strength of the effective dose.
2. 30 min after the start of the infusion, give a bolus dose of naloxone using half the strength of the effective dose. This reduces the time to reach steady-state drug levels..

From References 18 and 30.

---

3. *Naloxone Infusion*

The effects of naloxone last about 60 to 90 minutes, which is less than the duration of action of most opioids. Therefore, a favorable response to naloxone should be followed by a continuous naloxone infusion. This infusion should adhere to the guidelines in Table 46.2

4. *Adverse Effects*

Naloxone has few side effects. The most common adverse effect is the opioid withdrawal syndrome (anxiety, abdominal cramps, and vomiting). Adverse effects that occur rarely include acute pulmonary edema and generalized seizures (18).

REFERENCES

1. Larson AM, Polson J, Fontana RJ, et al. Acetaminophen-induced acute liver failure: Results of a United States multicenter, prospective study. Hepatology 2005; 42:1364–1372.

2. Schiodt FV, Rochling FA, Casey DL, et al. Acetaminophen toxicity in an urban county hospital. N Engl J Med 1997; 337:1112–1117.

3. Hendrickson RG, Bizovi KE. Acetaminophen. In: Flomenbaum NE, et al., eds. Goldfrank's toxicologic emergencies. 8th ed. New York: McGraw-Hill, 2006: 523–543.

4. Rumack BH. Acetaminophen hepatotoxicity: the first 35 years. J Toxicol Clin Toxicol 2002; 40:3–20.

5. Anker AL, Smilkstein MJ. Acetaminophen: Concepts and controversies. Emerg Med Clin North Am 1994; 12:335–349.

6. Rumack BH, Peterson RC, Koch GG, et al. Acetaminophen overdose. 662 cases with evaluation of oral acetylcysteine treatment. Arch Intern Med 1981; 141:380–385.

7. Spiller HA, Krenzelok EP, Grande GA, et al. A prospective evaluation of the effect of activated charcoal before oral N-acetylcysteine in acetaminophen overdose. Ann Emerg Med 1994; 23:519–523.

8. Smilkstein MJ, Knapp GL, Kulig KW, et al. Efficacy of oral N-acetylcysteine in the treatment of acetaminophen overdose: Analysis of the national multicenter study (1976 to 1985). N Engl J Med 1988; 319:1557–1562.

9. Buckley NA, Whyte IM, O'Connell DL, et al. Oral or intravenous N-acetylcysteine: Which is the treatment of choice for acetaminophen (paracetamol) poisoning? J Toxicol Clin Toxicol 1999; 37:759–767.

10. Howland MA. N-Acetylcysteine. In: Flomenbaum NE, et al., eds. Goldfrank's toxicologic emergencies. 8th ed. New York: McGraw-Hill, 2006: 544–549.

11. Sunman W, Hughes AD, Sever PS. Anaphylactoid response to intravenous acetylcysteine. Lancet 1992; 339:1231–1232.

12. Appelboam AV, Dargan PI, Knighton J. Fatal anaphylactoid reaction to N-acetylcysteine: caution in patients with asthma. Emerg Med J 2002; 19:594–595.

13. Watson WA, Litovitz TL, Rodgers GC, Jr., et al. 2004 Annual report of the American Association of Poison Control Centers Toxic Exposure Surveillance System. Am J Emerg Med 2005; 23:589–666.

14. Shalansky SJ, Naumann TL, Englander FA. Effect of flumazenil on benzodiazepine-induced respiratory depression. Clin Pharm 1993; 12:483–487.

15. Gross JB, Weller RS, Conard P. Flumazenil antagonism of midazolam-induced ventilatory depression. Anesthesiology 1991; 75:179–185.

16. Howland MA. Flumazenil. In: Flomenbaum NE, et al., eds. Goldfrank's toxicologic emergencies. 8th ed. New York: McGraw-Hill, 2006: 1112–1117.

17. Bodenham A, Park GR. Reversal of prolonged sedation using flumazenil in critically ill patients. Anaesthesia 1989; 44:603–605.

18. Doyon S, Roberts JR. Reappraisal of the "coma cocktail": Dextrose, flumazenil, naloxone, and thiamine. Emerg Med Clin North Am 1994; 12:301–316.

19. Pepperman ML. Double-blind study of the reversal of midazolam-induced sedation in the intensive care unit with flumazenil (Ro 15–1788): effect on weaning from ventilation. Anaesth Intensive Care 1990; 18:38–44.

20. Newton CR, Delgado JH, Gomez HF. Calcium and beta receptor antagonist overdose: A review and update of pharmacological principles and management. Semin Respir Crit Care Med 2002; 23:19–25.

21. Weinstein RS. Recognition and management of poisoning with beta-adrenergic blocking agents. Ann Emerg Med 1984; 13:1123–1131.

22. Lane AS, Woodward AC, Goldman MR. Massive propranolol overdose poorly responsive to pharmacologic therapy: use of the intra-aortic balloon pump. Ann Emerg Med 1987; 16:1381–1383.

23. Henry JA, Cassidy SL. Membrane stabilising activity: a major cause of fatal poisoning. Lancet 1986; 1:1414–1417.

24. Kerns W 2nd, Kline J, Ford MD. Beta-blocker and calcium channel blocker toxicity. Emerg Med Clin North Am 1994; 12:365–390.

25. Howland MA. Glucagon. In: Flomenbaum NE, et al., eds. Goldfrank's toxicologic emergencies. 8th ed. New York: McGraw-Hill, 2006: 942–945.

26. Howland MA. Opioid antagonists. In: Flomenbaum NE, et al., eds. Goldfrank's toxicologic emergencies. 8th ed. New York: McGraw-Hill, 2006: 614–619.

27. Naloxone hydrochloride. In: McEvoy GK Litvak K, eds. AHFS Drug Information. Bethesda, MD: American Society of Hospital Systems Pharmacists, 1995; 1418–1420.

28. Tandberg D, Abercrombie D. Treatment of heroin overdose with endotracheal naloxone. Ann Emerg Med 1982; 11:443–445.

29. Maio RF, Gaukel B, Freeman B. Intralingual naloxone injection for narcotic-induced respiratory depression. Ann Emerg Med 1987; 16:572–573.

30. Goldfrank L, Weisman RS, Errick JK, et al. A dosing nomogram for continuous infusion intravenous naloxone. Ann Emerg Med 1986; 15:566–570.

UNITS AND CONVERSIONS

The units of measurements in the medical sciences are taken from the metric system (centimeter, gram, second) and the Anglo-Saxon system (foot, pound, second). The metric units were introduced during the French Revolution and were revised in 1960. The revised units are called Système Internationale (SI) units and are currently the worldwide standard.

Units of Measurement in the Système Internationale (SI)

Parameter	Dimensions	Basic SI Unit (Symbol)	Equivalencies
Length	L	Meter (m)	1 inch $= 2.54$ cm
Area	L^2	Square meter (m^2)	1 square centimeter (cm^2) $= 10^4$ m^2
Volume	L^3	Cubic meter (m^3)	1 liter (L) $= 0.001$ m^3 1 milliliter (mL) $= 1$ cubic centimeter (cm^3)
Mass	M	Kilogram (kg)	1 pound (lb) $= 453.5$ g 1 kg $= 2.2$ lbs
Density	M/L^3	Kilogram per cubic meter (kg/m^3)	1 $kg/m^3 = 0.001$ kg/dm^3 Density of water $=$ 1.0 kg/dm^3 Density of mercury $=$ 13.6 kg/dm^3
Velocity	L/T	Meters per second (m/sec)	1 mile per hour (mph) $= 0.4$ m/sec
Acceleration	L/T^2	Meters per second squared (m/sec^2)	1 $ft/sec^2 = 0.03$ m/sec^2
Force	M x (L/T^2)	Newton (N) $=$ kg x (m/sec^2)	1 dyne $= 10^{-5}$ N

(Continued)

Units of Measurement in the Système Internationale (SI) *(Continued)*

Parameter	Dimensions	Basic SI Unit (Symbol)	Equivalencies
Pressure	$\dfrac{M \times (L/T^2)}{L^2}$	Pascal (Pa)=N/m²	1 kPa=7.5 mm Hg =10.2 cm H₂O 1 mm Hg = 1 x 10⁻⁹ torr (See conversion table for kPa and cm H₂O)
Heat	M x (L/T²) x L	Square meter (m²) (cm²)=10⁴ m²	1 square centimeter
Temperature	None	Kelvin (K)	0°C=−273 K (See conversion table for °C and °F)
Viscosity	M, 1/L, 1/T	Newton x second per square meter (N • sec/m²)	Centipoise (cP)= 10⁻³ N • sec/m²
Amount of a substance	N	Mole (mol)= molecular weight in grams	Equivalent (Eq)=mol x valence

Converting Units of Solute Concentration

1. For ions that exist freely in an aqueous solution, the concentration is expressed as milliequivalents per liter (mEq/L). To convert to millimoles per liter (mmol/L):

$$\frac{mEq/L}{valence} \;=\; mmol/L$$

   a. For a univalent ion like potassium (K⁺), the concentration in mmol/L is the same as the concentration in mEq/L.

   b. For a divalent ion like magnesium (Mg⁺⁺), the concentration in mmol/L is one-half the concentration in mEq/L.

2. For ions that are partially bound or complexed to other molecules (e.g., plasma Ca⁺⁺), the concentration is usually expressed as milligrams per deciliter (mg/dL). To convert to mEq/L:

$$\frac{mg/dL \times 10}{mol\ wt} \;\times\; valence \;=\; mEq/L$$

where mol wt is molecular weight, and the factor 10 is used to convert deciliters (100 mL) to liters.

EXAMPLE: Ca⁺⁺ has a molecular weight of 40 and a valence of 2, so a plasma Ca⁺⁺ concentration of 8 mg/dL is equivalent to: (8 x 10/40) x 2=4 mEq/L.

Converting Units of Solute Concentration *(Continued)*

3. The concentration of uncharged molecules (e.g., glucose) is also expressed as milligrams per deciliter (mg/dL). To convert to (mmol/L):

$$\frac{mg/dL \times 10}{mol\ wt} = mmol/L$$

EXAMPLE: Glucose has a molecular weight of 180, so a plasma glucose concentration of 90 mg/dL is equivalent to: $(90 \times 10/180) = 5$ mmol/L.

4. The concentration of solutes can also be expressed in terms of osmotic pressure, which determines the distribution of water in different fluid compartments. Osmotic activity in aqueous solutions (called osmolality) is expressed as milliosmoles per kg water (mosm/kg H_2O or mosm/kg). The following formulas can be used to express the osmolality of solute concentrations (n is the number of nondissociable particles per molecule).

$$mmol/L \times n = mosm/kg$$

$$\frac{mEq/L}{valence} \times n = mosm/kg$$

$$\frac{mg/dL \times 10}{mol\ wt} \times n = mosm/kg$$

EXAMPLE:

a. A plasma Na^+ concentration of 140 mEq/L has the following osmolality:

$$\frac{140}{1} \times 1 = 140\ mosm/kg$$

b. A plasma glucose concentration of 90 mg/dL has the following osmolality:

$$\frac{90 \times 10}{180} \times 1 = 5\ mosm/kg$$

The sodium in plasma has a much greater osmotic activity than the glucose in plasma because osmotic activity is determined by the number of particles in solution and is independent of the size of the particles (i.e., one sodium ion has the same osmotic activity as one glucose molecule).

Apothecary and Household Conversions

Apothecary	Household
1 grain = 60 mg	1 teaspoonful = 5 mL
1 ounce = 30 mg	1 tablespoonful = 15 mL
1 fluid ounce = 30 mL	1 wineglassful = 60 mL
1 pint = 500 mL	1 teacupful = 120 mL
1 quart = 947 mL	

Temperature Conversions

Corresponding Scales

(°C)	(°F)	Conversions
100	212	Conversions are based on the corresponding
41	105.8	temperatures at the freezing point of water:
40	104	$0°C = 32°F$
39	102.2	and the temperature ranges (from freezing
37	98.6	point to boiling point of water:
36	96.8	$100°C = 180°F$ or $5°C = 9°F$
35	95	The above relationships are then combined
34	93.2	to derive the conversion formulas:
33	91.4	$°F = (9/5°C) + 32$
32	89.6	$°C = 5/9 (°F − 32)$
31	87.8	
30	86	
0	32	

Pressure Conversions

mm Hg	kPa	mm Hg	kPa	mm Hg	kPa
41	5.45	61	8.11	81	10.77
42	5.59	62	8.25	82	10.91
43	5.72	63	8.38	83	11.04
44	5.85	64	8.51	84	11.17
45	5.99	65	8.65	85	11.31
46	6.12	66	8.78	86	11.44
47	6.25	67	8.91	87	11.57
48	6.38	68	9.04	88	11.70
49	6.52	69	9.18	89	11.84
50	6.65	70	9.31	90	11.97
51	6.78	71	9.44	91	12.10
52	6.92	72	9.58	92	12.24
53	7.05	73	9.71	93	12.37
54	7.18	74	9.84	94	12.50
55	7.32	75	9.98	95	12.64
56	7.45	76	10.11	96	12.77
57	7.58	77	10.24	97	12.90
58	7.71	78	10.37	98	13.03
59	7.85	79	10.51	99	13.17
60	7.98	80	10.64	100	13.90

Kilopascal (kPa) = 0.133 x mm Hg   mm Hg = 7.5 x kPa

French Sizes

French Size	Outside Diameter*		Device
	Inches	**mm**	
1	0.01	0.3	Vascular catheters
4	0.05	1.3	
8	0.10	2.6	Small-bore feeding tubes
10	0.13	3.3	
12	0.16	4.0	
14	0.18	4.6	Nasogastric tubes
16	0.21	5.3	
18	0.23	6.0	
20	0.26	6.6	Chest tubes
22	0.28	7.3	
24	0.31	8.0	
26	0.34	8.6	
28	0.36	9.3	
30	0.39	10.0	
32	0.41	10.6	
34	0.44	11.3	
36	0.47	12.0	
38	0.50	12.6	

*Diameters can vary with manufacturers. However, a useful rule of thumb is OD (mm) x 3 = French size.

Gauge Sizes

Gauge Size	Outside Diameter*		Device
	Inches	**mm**	
26	0.018	0.45	Butterfly devices
25	0.020	0.50	
24	0.022	0.56	
23	0.024	0.61	
22	0.028	0.71	Peripheral vascular catheters
21	0.032	0.81	
20	0.036	0.91	
19	0.040	1.02	
18	0.048	1.22	Central venous catheters
16	0.040	1.62	
14	0.080	2.03	Introducer catheters
12	0.104	2.64	
10	0.128	3.25	

*Diameters can vary with manufacturers.

SELECTED REFERENCE RANGES

Reference Ranges for Selected Clinical Laboratory Tests

Substance	Fluid*	Traditional Units	x k =	SI Units
Acetoacetate	P,S	0.3–3.0 mg/dL	97.95	3–30 µmol/L
Alanine amino-transferase (SGPT)	S	0–35 U/L	0.016	0–0.58 µkat/L
Albumin	S	4–6 g/dL	10	40–60 g/L
	CSF	11–48 mg/dL	0.01	0.11–0.48 g/L
Aldolase	S	0–6 U/L	16.6	0–100 nkat/L
Alkaline phosphatase	S	(F) 30–100 U/L	0.016	0.5–1.67 µkat/L
		(M) 45–115 U/L		0.75–1.92 µkat/L
Ammonia	P	10–80 µg/dL	0.587	5–50 µmol/L
Amylase	S	0–130 U/L	0.016	0–2.17 µkat/L
Aspartate amino-transferase (SGOT)	S	0–35 U/L	0.016	0–0.58 µkat/L
β-Hydroxybutyrate	S	<1.0 mg/dL	96.05	<100 µmol/L
Bicarbonate	S	22–26 mEq/L	1	22–26 mmol/L
Bilirubin:Total	S	0.1–1.0 mg/dL	17.1	2–18 µmol/L
Conjugated	S	≤0.2 mg/dL		≤4 µmol/L
Blood urea nitrogen (BUN)	P,S	8–18 mg/dL	0.367	3.0–6.5 mmol/L
Calcium:Total	S	8.5–10.5 mg/dL	0.26	2.2–2.6 mmol/L
Ionized	P	2.2–2.3 mEq/L	0.49	1.1–1.15 mmol/L
Chloride	P,S	95–105 mEq/L	1	95–105 mmol/L
	CSF	120–130 mEq/L		120–130 mmol/L
	U	10–200 mEq/L		10–200 mmol/L
Creatinine	S	0.6–1.5 mg/dL	0.09	0.05–0.13 mmol/L
	U	15–25 mg/kg/24 h	0.009	0.13–0.22 mg/kg/24 h
Cyanide: Nontoxic	WB	<5 µg/dL	3.8	<19 µmol/L
Lethal		>30 µg/dL		>114 µmol/L

(Continued)

Reference Ranges for Selected Clinical Laboratory Tests *(Continued)*

Substance	Fluid*	Traditional Units	x k =	SI Units
Fibrinogen	P	150–350 mg/dL	0.01	1.5–3.5 g/L
Fibrin split products	S	<10 µg/dL	1	<10 mg/L
Glucose (fasting)	P	70–100 mg/dL	0.06	3.9–6.1 mmol/L
	CSF	50–80 mg/dL		2.8–4.4 mmol/L
Lactate: Resting	P	<2 mEq/L	1	<2 mmol/L
Exercise	S	<4 mEq/L		<4 mmol/L
Lactate dehydrogenase (LDH)	S	50–150 U/L	0.017	0.82–2.66 µkat/L
Lipase	S	0–160 U/L	0.017	0–2.66 µkat/L
Magnesium	P	1.8–3.0 mg/dL	0.41	0.8–1.2 mmol/L
		1.5–2.4 mEq/L	0.5	0.8–1.2 mmol/L
Osmolality	S	280–296 mosm/kg	1	280–296 mmol/kg
Phosphate	S	2.5–5.0 mg/dL	0.32	0.8–1.6 mmol/L
Potassium	P,S	3.5–5.0 mEq/L	1	3.5–5.0 mmol/L
Total protein	P,S	6–8 g/dL	10	60–80 g/L
	CSF	<40 mg/dL	0.01	<0.4 mmol/L
	U	<150 mg/24 h	0.01	<1.5 g/24 h
Sodium	P,S	135–147 mEq/L	1	135–147 mmol/L
Thyroxine:Total	S	4–11 µg/dL	12.9	51–142 nmol/L
Free		0.8–2.8 mg/dL	0.49	10–36 pmol/L
Triiodothyronine (T_3)	S	75–220 ng/dL	0.015	12–3.4 nmol/L

*P=Plasma, S=serum, U=urine, WB=whole blood, CSF=cerebrospinal fluid.

Adapted from the New England Journal of Medicine SI Unit Conversion Guide. Waltham, MA; Massachusetts Medical Society, 1992.

Reference Ranges for Vitamins and Trace Elements

Substance	Fluid*	Traditional Units	x k =	SI Units
Chromium	S	0.14–0.15 mg/mL	17.85	2.5–2.7 mmol/L
Copper	S	70–140 µg/dL	0.16	11–22 µmol/L
Folate	RBC	140–960 ng/mL	2.26	317–2169 nmol/L
Iron	S	(M) 80–180 µg/dL (F) 60–160 µg/dL	0.18	(M) 14–32 µmol/L (F) 11–29 µmol/L
Ferritin	P,S	(M) 20–250 ng/mL (F) 10–120 ng/mL	1	(M) 20–250 µg/L (F) 10–120 µg/L
Manganese	WB	0.4–2.0 µg/dL	0.018	0.7–3.6 µmol/L
Pyridoxine	P	20–90 ng/mL	5.98	120–540 nmol/L
Riboflavin	S	2.6–3.7 µg/dL	26.57	70–100 nmol/L
Selenium	WB	58–234 µg/dL	0.012	0.7–2.5 µmol/L
Thiamine (total)	P	3.4–4.8 µg/dL	0.003	98.6–139 µmol/L
Vitamin A	P,S	10–50 µg/dL	0.349	0.35–1.75 µmol/L
Vitamin B$_{12}$	S	200–1,000 pg/mL	0.737	150–750 pmol/L
Vitamin C	S	0.6–2 mg/dL	56.78	30–100 µmol/L
Vitamin D	S	24–40 ng/mL	2.599	60–105 nmol/L
Vitamin E	P,S	0.78–1.25 mg/dL	23.22	18–29 µmol/L
Zinc	S	70–120 µg/dL	0.153	11.5–18.5 µmol/L

*P=Plasma, S=serum, U=urine, WB=whole blood, RBC=red blood cell.

Adapted from the New England Journal of Medicine SI Unit Conversion Guide. Waltham, MA; Massachusetts Medical Society, 1992.

Desirable Weights for Adults*

Height		Males		
Feet	Inches	Small Frame	Medium Frame	Large Frame
5	2	128–134	131–141	138–150
5	3	130–136	133–143	140–153
5	4	132–138	135–145	142–156
5	5	134–140	137–148	144–160
5	6	136–142	139–151	146–164
5	7	138–145	142–154	149–168
5	8	140–148	145–157	152–172
5	9	142–151	148–160	155–176
5	10	144–154	151–163	158–180
5	11	146–157	154–166	161–184
6	0	149–160	157–170	164–188
6	1	152–164	160–174	168–192
6	2	155–168	164–178	172–197
6	3	158–172	167–182	172–202
6	4	162–176	171–187	181–207
		Females		
4	10	102–111	109–121	112–131
4	11	103–113	111–123	120–134
5	0	104–115	113–126	122–137
5	1	106–118	115–129	125–140
5	2	108–121	118–132	128–143
5	3	111–124	121–135	131–147
5	4	114–127	124–138	134–151
5	5	117–130	127–141	137–155
5	6	120–133	130–144	140–159
5	7	123–136	133–147	143–163
5	8	126–139	136–150	146–167
5	9	129–142	139–153	149–170
5	10	132–145	142–156	152–173
5	11	135–148	145–159	155–176
6	1	138–151	148–162	158–179

*Unclothed weights associated with the longest life expectancies. From the statistics bureau of the Metropolitan Life Insurance Company, 1983.

Body Fluid Distribution in Healthy Adults

Parameter	Males	Females
Total body water	600 mL/kg	500 mL/kg
Interstitial fluid	120 mL/kg	100 mL/kg
Blood volume (BV)	70 mL/kg	65 mL/kg
Erythrocyte volume	33 mL/kg	27 mL/kg
Plasma volume	37 mL/kg	38 mL/kg
Hematocrit	40–54%	37–47%

From Documenta Geigy Scientific Tables, 7th ed. Basel, Switzeraland: JR Geigy SA, 1970.

Electrolyte Content of Body Fluids

	mEq/L			
Body Fluid	Na$^+$	K$^+$	HCO$_3^-$	CL$^-$
CSF	140	4	25	130
Saliva	112	20	10–20	30
Sweat	50	10	—	45
Gastric	60	15	0.2	140
Bile	140	6	30–50	90
Pancreatic	130	6	100	60
Small bowel	120	8	20–40	100
Stool	30	60	20–60	40

Peak Expiratory Flow Rates for Healthy Males

	mEq/L			
Age (yr)	Ht: 60"	65"	70"	75"
20	602	649	693	740
25	590	636	679	725
30	577	622	664	710
35	565	609	651	695
40	552	596	636	680
45	540	583	622	665
50	527	569	607	649

(Continued)

Peak Expiratory Flow Rates for Healthy Males *(Continued)*

Age (yr)	Ht:	60"	65"	70"	75"
			mEq/L		
55		515	556	593	634
60		502	542	578	618
65		490	529	564	603
70		477	515	550	587

Peak Flow (L/min) = [3.95 − (0.0151 x Age)] x Ht (cm)

Regression equation from Leiner GC et al. Am Rev Respir Dis 1963; 88:646.

Peak Expiratory Flow Rates for Healthy Females

Age (yr)	Ht:	55"	60"	65"	70"
			mEq/L		
20		309	423	460	496
25		385	418	454	490
30		380	413	448	483
35		375	408	442	476
40		370	402	436	470
45		365	397	430	464
50		360	391	424	457
55		355	386	418	451
60		350	380	412	445
65		345	375	406	439
70		340	369	400	432

Peak Flow (L/min) = [2.93 − (0.0072 x Age)] x Ht (cm)

Regression equation from Leiner GC et al. Am Rev Respir Dis 1963; 88:646.

ADDITIONAL FORMULAS

This section includes formulas that deserve mention but are not included in any of the chapters.

Measures of Body Size

Ideal Body Weight*

Males: IBW (kg) = 50 + 2.3 (Ht in inches − 60)

Females: IBW (kg) = 45.5 + 2.3 (Ht in inches − 60)

Body Mass Index[†]

$$BMI = \frac{Wt \text{ (in lbs)}}{Ht \text{ (in inches)}^2 \times 703}$$

Body Surface Area

Dubois Formula[‡]

BSA (m^2) = Ht (in cm) + Wt (in kg)$^{0.425}$ × 0.007184

Jacobson Formula[§]

$$BSA \text{ (m}^2\text{)} = \frac{Ht \text{ (in cm)} + Wt \text{ (in kg)} - 60}{100}$$

*Devine BJ. Drug Intell Clin Pharm 1974; 8:650.

[†]Matz R. Ann Intern Med 1993; 118:232.

[‡]Dubois EF. Basal metabolism in health and disease. Philadelphia: Lea & Febiger, 1936.

[§]Jacobson B. Medicine and clinical engineering. Englewood Cliffs, NJ: Prentice-Hall, 1977.

Drug Infusion Rates

The following relationship defines the infusion rate of a drug solution that is needed to achieve a desired dose rate:

$$\text{Infusion Rate (mL/min)} = \frac{\text{DR (µg/min)}}{\text{C (µg/mL)}}$$

where:
        DR is the dose rate of the drug
        C is the concentration of the drug in the infusion

Because the volume infused per minute is often small, drug infusions are usually delivered through a microdrip apparatus (60 microdrops = 1 mL). To convert the infusion rate to microdrops per minute:

$$\text{microdrops/min} = \text{mL/min} \times 60$$

Measures of Gas Exchange

A. Alveolar-arterial PO$_2$ Gradient

$$\text{A-a PO}_2 = [\text{FiO}_2 \times (P_B - P_{H_2O}) - (\text{PaCO}_2/\text{RQ})] - \text{PaO}_2$$

where:
    FiO_2 = Fractional concentration of inhaled oxygen (0.2–1)
    P_B = Barometric pressure (760 mm Hg at sea level)
    P_{H_2O} = Partial pressure of water vapor (47 mm Hg at 37°C)
    RQ = Respiratory quotient (usually 0.8)
  PaCO_2 = Arterial PCO$_2$
   PaO_2 = Arterial PO$_2$

B. Dead Space Ventilation

$$V_D/V_T = \frac{\text{PaCO}_2 - \text{P}_E\text{CO}_2}{\text{PaCO}_2}$$

where:
  PaCO_2 = Arterial PCO$_2$
  P_ECO_2 = Mean expired PCO$_2$

Evaluating Diagnostic Tests

The following grid demonstrates the relationships between the results of a diagnostic test and the presence or absence of disease:

	Disease is Present	Disease is Absent
Test is Positive	**a** True Positive	**b** False Positive
Test is Negative	**c** False Negative	**d** True Negative

These relationships are used to derive the following measures of test performance.

Parameter	Derivation	Description
Sensitivity	$\dfrac{a}{a + c}$	Probability that the test is positive when the disease is present
Positive Predictive Value	$\dfrac{a}{a + b}$	Probability that the disease is present when the test is positive
Specificity	$\dfrac{d}{d + b}$	Probability that the test is negative when the disease is absent
Negative Predictive Value	$\dfrac{d}{d + c}$	Probability that the disease is absent when the test is negative

Index

A

Abciximab, as adjunct to reperfusion therapy, 222, 223*t*
Abdomen, sepsis from. *See under* Sepsis
Abdominal abscess, 555
Abscess, abdominal, 555
Acalculous cholecystitis, 554
ACE inhibitors. *See* Angiotensin-converting-enzyme inhibitors
Acetaminophen
  as antipyretic, 202–203, 518, 649
  lactic acidosis and, 365
  toxicity of, 705–709
    activated charcoal, 707–708
    antidote therapy, 708–709, 708*t*
    clinical presentation, 706
    prognostic markers, 706–707, 707*f*
    toxic metabolite, 705
Acetazolamide, for treatment of chloride-resistant alkalosis, 388
Acetoacetate
  alcoholic ketoacidosis and, 372
  diabetic ketoacidosis and, 367*f*, 368
Acetylcholine, 636
N-Acetylcysteine (NAC)
  mucolytic therapy with, 320–321, 320*t*
  for treatment of acetaminophen toxicity, 708–709, 708*t*
  for treatment of contrast-induced renal failure, 399
Acid-base disorders, 350–351, 351*t*
Acid-base interpretations, 349–362, 354–357
anion gap, 357–360, 359*f*
compensatory responses, evaluating, 356–357
gap-gap, 360–361
hydrogen ion concentration, 349–350, 350*t*
metabolic acidosis, evaluating, 357
predictive equations, 351–354, 352*f*
  metabolic acid-base disorders, 352–353
  respiratory acid-base disorders, 353–354
primary acid-base disorder, identifying, 355–356
scheme for, 354–357
types of acid-base disorders, 350–351, 351*t*
Acid-base parameters, 144–145
  arterial base deficit, 144–145
  blood lactate, 145
Acidosis
  as cause of hyperkalemia, 434
  lactic. *See* Lactic acidosis
  metabolic. *See* Metabolic acidosis
  mixed metabolic alkalosis and respiratory, 356
  partially compensated respiratory, 356
  respiratory, 350, 351*t*, 352*f*, 354
Acid-suppressing drugs, bowel sepsis and, 550
ACLS. *See* Advanced life support
Activated charcoal, after toxic ingestion of acetaminophen, 707–708
Acute aortic dissection, 227–229
  chest pain, 227

Acute aortic dissection *(continued)*
  clinical findings, 227–228
  diagnosis, 228
  management, 228–229
  treating hypertension in, 228, 229*t*
Acute coronary syndromes (ACS), 209–232
  acute aortic dissection, 227–229, 229*t*
  definitions, 209
  early complications, 224–227
    arrhythmias, 225
    cardiac pump failure, 226–227, 226*t*
    mechanical, 224–225
  pathogenesis, 209–210
  reperfusion therapy, 214–220
    adjuncts to, 220–224, 221*t*, 223*t*
    coronary angioplasty, 219–220
    thrombolytic therapy, 214–218, 215–216*t*
  routine measures, 210–214, 211*t*
    angiotensin-converting-enzyme inhibition, 211*t*, 213–214
    antiplatelet therapy, 211*t*, 212
    β-receptor blockade, 211*t*, 213
    relieving chest pain, 210–212, 211*t*
Acute heart failure(s), 173–188
  B-type natriuretic peptide, 178–179
  hemodynamic alterations, 173–178
    progressive heart failure, 173–175, 174*f*, 175*t*
    right heart failure, 178
    systolic *vs.* diastolic heart failure, 175–178, 177*t*
  management strategies, 179–186
    left-sided diastolic heart failure, 185–186

  left-sided systolic heart failure, 180–185, 181*f*
  right heart failure, 186
Acute hemolytic reactions, red blood cell transfusions and, 486–487
Acute inflammatory demyelinating polyneuropathy, 634
Acute interstitial nephritis (AIN), 399–400
  drugs that can cause, 400*t*
Acute lung injury, red blood cell transfusions and, 489–490
Acute mitral regurgitation, 225
Acute renal failure. *See* Oliguria and acute renal failure
Acute respiratory alkalosis with secondary metabolic alkalosis, 357
Acute respiratory distress syndrome (ARDS), 255–268, 524, 537
  clinical manifestations, 257, 257*f*
  continuous positive airway pressure for, 312
  diagnosis, 258–260, 258*t*
  hydrostatic pulmonary edema *vs.*, 258–260
  lung recruitment in, 309*f*
  management, 260–267
    blood transfusions, 265
    fluid management, 264–265
    low-volume ventilation, 262–264, 263*t*
    misdirected, 266–267
    pharmacotherapy, 265–266
    ventilator-induced lung injury, 260–261, 261*f*
  mortality rate, 266*f*
  pathogenesis, 255
  PEEP for, 310–311
  predisposing conditions, 255–256, 256*t*
Acute stroke, 641–652
  antithrombotic therapy, 647–648
  embolic, 641

evaluation, 642–647
  avoiding delays, 642
  bedside evaluation, 642–644
  diagnostic evaluation,
    644–647, 646*f*
hemorrhagic, 641–642
ischemic, 641, 643*f*
medical management, 648–650
risk categories for embolic,
    241–242
risk of thromboembolism and,
    33–34
thrombotic, 641
transient ischemic attack, 642
types of stroke, 641–642
Acute tubular necrosis (ATN), 392
Additives, to total parenteral nu-
    trition solutions, 595–596
Adenosine, for treatment of AV
    nodal re-entrant tachycar-
    dia, 245–246, 246*t*
ADH. *See* Antidiuretic hormone
Adhesive dressings, for in-
    dwelling vascular
    catheters, 77
Adjusted-dose warfarin, for
    thromboprophylaxis, 39*t*, 40
Adrenal insufficiency, 603–605,
    606*t*
  clinical manifestations, 604
  pituitary failure and, 624
  prevalence, 603
  rapid ACTH stimulation test,
    604, 605*t*
  steroid therapy, 605, 606*t*
Adults. *See also* Men; Women
  body fluid distribution in, 729
  daily energy requirements in,
    564, 565*t*
  desirable weights for, 728
  endogenous fuel stores in, 567*t*
Advanced life support (advanced
    cardiac life support,
    ACLS), 191–199
  antiarrhythmic agents, 198–199
  defibrillation, 191–195, 192–193*f*
  drug administration routes,
    195–196

vasopressor drugs, 196–198,
    197*t*
AEDs. *See* Automated external
    defibrillators
Aerosol drug therapy for asthma,
    271–273
  intermittent *vs.* continuous,
    273–274, 274*f*
AF. *See* Atrial fibrillation
AG. *See* Anion gap
Age, body temperature and, 505
Agitated patient, bedside ap-
    proach to, 666*f*, 667
AIN. *See* Acute interstitial nephri-
    tis
Airborne illness, protective barri-
    ers and, 8–10, 9*f*
Airway patency, 189
AKA. *See* Alcoholic ketoacidosis
Albumin, anion gap and, 359–360
Albumin solutions, 164–165
Albuterol
  for treatment of anaphylaxis,
    531
  for treatment of asthma, 273,
    275*t*
  for treatment of chronic ob-
    structive pulmonary dis-
    ease, 277
Alcoholic ketoacidosis (AKA),
    367*f*, 371–373
Alcohol-related illness, hypomag-
    nesemia and, 447
Alcohol(s)
  as antiseptic agent, 2, 2*t*
  toxic, 373–376
Alimentary decontamination, 550,
    551*t*
Alkali therapy
  for treatment of diabetic keto-
    acidosis, 371
  for treatment of lactic acidosis,
    366
Alkalosis
  acute respiratory, with second-
    ary metabolic alkalosis, 357
  as cause of ionized hypocal-
    cemia, 459–460

Alkalosis *(continued)*
  metabolic. *See* Metabolic alkalosis
  mixed respiratory acidosis and metabolic, 356
  partially compensated respiratory, 356
  respiratory, 350, 351*t*, 352*f,* 354
Allergic reactions
  to latex, 6–7
  to platelet transfusions, 503
  to red blood cell transfusions, 488–489
Alteplase
  for restoring catheter patency, 81, 81*t*
  for thrombolytic therapy, 49, 216*t*, 217, 218
Altered consciousness, 613–614, 615*f*
Alveolar-arterial PO$_2$ gradient, 732
Alveolar dead space, in venous thromboembolism, 43
Alveolar disruption, 321–325
  clinical manifestations, 321
  pleural drainage system, 323–325, 325*f*
  pneumothorax, 321–323, 323*f*
Alvimopan, to block opioid receptors in bowel, 657
American Stroke Association, 648
Amikacin, 671
  for treatment of pneumonia, 543*t*
Amino acid solutions, 591–593, 592*t*
Aminoglycosides, 671–674
  activity and clinical uses, 671–672, 672*f*
  adverse effects, 673–674
  dosing, 672–673, 673*t*
  for treatment of pneumonia, 543*t*
Amiodarone
  for treatment of atrial fibrillation, 240*t*, 241

for treatment of cardiac arrest, 197*t*, 198
  for treatment of ventricular tachycardia, 250
Amoxicillin-clavulanate, for treatment of chronic obstructive pulmonary disease, 279*t*
Amphetamines, neuroleptic malignant syndrome and, 510*t*
Amphotericin
  drug fever and, 509*t*
  Ringer's solution and, 159
Amphotericin B, 674–675
  for digestive decontamination, 551*t*
  for disseminated candidiasis, 93
  infusion-related inflammatory response, 674–675
  liposomal, 675
  nephrotoxicity of, 675
  for oral decontamination, 545
  for treatment of candiduria, 559
  for treatment of catheter-related septicemia, 91*t*
Ampicillin
  Ringer's solution and, 159
  for treatment of catheter-related septicemia, 91*t*
Ampicillin-sulbactam, for treatment of abdominal abscess, 555
Analgesia, 653–658
  non-opioid, 657–658
  opioids, 653–657
    adverse effects, 656–657
    intravenous, 653–655, 654*t*
    meperidine, 655
    patient-controlled analgesia, 656
Anaphylactic shock, 530, 531–532
Anaphylaxis, 529–532
  anaphylactic shock, 530, 531–532
  clinical presentation, 530
  management, 530–531

response to platelet transfusions, 503
in response to red blood cell transfusion, 489
Anemia, 477–481. *See also* Erythrocyte transfusions
contributing factors, 478–479
correcting, 153
of critical illness, 477
systemic oxygenation and, 479–481, 480*f*
tolerance to, 480–481
Anemia of chronic disease, 477
Angina. *See* Unstable angina
Angiotensin-converting-enzyme (ACE) inhibitors, for treatment of acute cardiac syndromes, 213–214
Anion gap (AG), 357–360
defined, 358
determinants of, 360*t*
influence of albumin on, 359–360
interpreting, 358–359, 359*t*
lactic acidosis and, 363
reference range, 358
reliability, 359
Antiarrhythmic agents, for treatment of cardiac arrest, 197*t*, 198–199
Antibiotic lock therapy, 90–92
Antibiotic therapy
as cause of acute interstitial nephritis, 400*t*
drug fever and, 509
magnesium deficiency and, 446–447
for oral decontamination, 545
for treatment of catheter-related septicemia, 88–90, 89*f*
for treatment of chronic obstructive pulmonary disease, 278–279, 297, 297*t*
for treatment of urinary tract infections, 557–558
Anticholinergic agents, for treatment of asthma, 274–276, 275*t*

Anticoagulation, 47–49, 48*t*
Antidiuretic hormone (ADH)
diabetes insipidus and, 417–418
in hyponatremia, 421
Antidotes
for acetaminophen, 708–709, 708*t*
for benzodiazepines, 710
for β-receptor antagonist toxicity, 711–713
Antiemetic agents, neuroleptic malignant syndrome and, 510*t*
Antifungal agents, 674–676
amphotericin B, 674–675
capsofungin, 676
fluconazole, 675–676
for treatment of candiduria, 559
Antimicrobial-impregnated catheters, 57
Antimicrobial ointment, for indwelling vascular catheters, 78
Antimicrobial therapy, 516, 671–687
aminoglycosides, 671–674, 673*t*
antifungal agents, 671, 674–676
carbapenems, 671, 677–678
cephalosporins, 671, 678–679, 679*t*
fluoroquinolones, 671, 679–681, 681*t*
penicillins, 671, 681–682
for treatment of pneumonia, 541–543, 541–544, 542–543*t*
for treatment of severe sepsis and septic shock, 528
vancomycin, 682–685
vancomycin replacements, 671, 684–685
Antioxidant vitamins, 573
Antiperistaltic agents, *C. difficile* colitis and, 553
Antiplatelet effects, of nitroglycerin, 694
Antiplatelet therapy
for treatment of acute cardiac syndromes, 211*t*, 212

Antiplatelet therapy *(continued)*
for treatment of atrial fibrillation, 242*t*
Antipseudomonal penicillins, 682
Antipsychotic agents, neuroleptic malignant syndrome and, 510*t*
Antipyretic therapy, 516–518
Antiretroviral drugs, indications for following HIV exposure, 12*t*
Antiseptic agents, 1–3, 2*t*
Antiseptics, 1
Antithrombotic therapy, 47–49
anticoagulation, 47–49, 48*t*
thrombolytic therapy, 49
for treatment of atrial fibrillation, 241–242, 242*t*
for treatment of stroke, 647–648
Antithyroid drugs, 610
Apathetic thyrotoxicosis, 609
Aphasia
evaluation of stroke and, 644
expressive, 644
global, 644
receptive, 644
Apnea test, 621
Apothecary and household conversions, 721
ARDS. *See* Acute respiratory distress syndrome
Argatroban, for treatment of heparin-induced thrombocytopenia, 496, 496*t*
Arginine, enteral tube feeding and, 582
Arousal, 613, 614*t*
Arrhythmias, 225
in hypokalemia, 431
magnesium depletion and, 448
Arterial base deficit, 144–145
Arterial PCO_2, in spontaneous breathing trial, 337, 339*f*
Arterial pulse and pressure, monitoring during CPR, 199–201, 200*f*
Arteriovenous hemofiltration, 405

Aspiration, in enteral tube feeding, 588
Aspirin
as adjunct to reperfusion therapy, 222
as antipyretic, 518
for treatment of acute cardiac syndromes, 212
for treatment of stroke, 647–648
Assist-control ventilation, 301–303, 303*f*
Assisted ventilation, 302
Asthma, acute exacerbations of, 269–277
drug therapy for, 271–277, 275*t*
aerosol drug therapy, 271–273, 274*f*
anticholinergic agents, 274–276
beta-receptor agonists, 273–274
corticosteroids, 276–277
management protocol, 272*f*
intrinsic PEEP and, 327
lactic acidosis and acute, 365
peak expiratory flow rate, 269–271, 270*f*
Atelectasis, 537
fever and, 506–507
Atenolol, for treatment of acute cardiac syndromes, 213
ATN. *See* Acute tubular necrosis
Atrial activity, diagnosis of tachycardia and, 235–236, 236*f*
Atrial fibrillation (AF), 233, 237–243
acute rate control, 239–241, 240*t*
adverse consequences, 237–238
antithrombotic therapy, 241–242, 242*t*
DC cardioversion, 238
lone, 237
pharmacologic cardioversion, 238–239
predisposing factors, 237
Wolff-Parkinson-White syndrome, 243

Atrial flutter, 233
Atrial tachycardias, 233
Atrial thrombosis, atrial fibrillation and, 238
Atrium, catheter tip in right, 73–74
Atropine
    for treatment of cardiac arrest, 197*t*, 199
    via endotracheal route, 196
Autoimmune thyroiditis, 609
Automated external defibrillators (AEDs), 195
Automatisms, 627
Autotransfusion maneuver, 150
AV dissociation, 248
AV nodal re-entrant tachycardia (AVNRT), 233, 236*f*, 245–247
    adenosine for, 245–246, 246*t*
AVNRT. *See* AV nodal re-entrant tachycardia
Awareness, 613, 614*t*
Azathioprine, for treatment of myasthenia gravis, 633
Azithromycin, for treatment of chronic obstructive pulmonary disease, 279*t*

B
Bacillus anthracis, skin hygiene and, 3
Bacterial respiratory infections, precautions for, 9*f*
Bacterial transmission, platelet transfusions and, 502
Bacteroides fragilis, imipenem for, 677
BAL. *See* Bronchoalveolar lavage
Balloon, pulmonary artery catheter, 100–101
Balloon flotation method, 97
Barotrauma, 261
Basal energy expenditure (BEE), 564–565

BEE. *See* Basal energy expenditure
Benzodiazepines
    adverse effects, 660–661
    drug comparisons, 659–660, 659*t*
    drug interactions, 661
    sedation with, 658–661, 659*t*
    toxicity of, 709–710
    for treatment of delirium, 616
    for treatment of seizures, 630–631
β-agonist bronchodilators, as cause of hypokalemia, 429
β-hydroxybutyrate
    alcoholic ketoacidosis and, 367*f*, 372
    diabetic ketoacidosis and, 367*f*, 368
β-receptor agonists
    as cause of hypophosphatemia, 468
    for treatment of asthma, 273–274, 275*t*
β-receptor antagonists (β-blockers)
    antidote therapy, 711–713
    as cause of hyperkalemia, 434*t*, 435
    milrinone and, 183
    toxicity of, 711–713
    for treatment of acute aortic dissection, 229, 229*t*
    for treatment of atrial fibrillation, 239–240, 240*t*
    for treatment of hyperthyroidism, 610
β-receptor blockade, 213
Biphosphonates, for treatment of hypercalcemia, 465*t*, 466
Bleeding
    platelet transfusions and, 500
    thrombolytic therapy and, 218
Blood
    calcium and phosphorus in, 458*t*

Blood *(continued)*
  oxygen content of, 125–126, 127*t*
Blood-borne infections, 10–16
  hepatitis B virus, 13–15, 15*t*
  hepatitis C virus, 15–16
  HIV, 11–13, 12*t*
  needlestick injuries, 10
Blood cultures, 515
  in evaluation of pneumonia, 537
  quantitative, 86–87, 86*t*
    choice of methods, 87–88
Blood lactate, 135–136, 145
  severe sepsis and, 135–136
Blood loss, classification of, 140–141
Blood pressure, management of heart failure and, 182–184
Bloodstream infections, pathogens in, 513*t*
Blood transfusions. *See also* Erythrocyte transfusions; Platelet transfusions
  as cause of ionized hypocalcemia, 460
  treatment of acute respiratory distress syndrome and, 265
Blood volume, 139, 140*t*
BNP. *See* B-type natriuretic peptide
Body fluids
  distribution of, 139–140, 140*t*, 729
  electrolyte content of, 729
  sodium concentration in lost, 414*t*
Body mass index, 731
Body size, measures of, 731
Body surface area, 731
Body temperature. *See also* Fever
  normal, 505
Body water, 139, 140*t*
Body weight
  ideal, 659, 662, 693, 731
  predicted, 262, 288–289
Bowel motility, opioids and, 657

Bowel sepsis, 549–551
  gastric colonization, 549
  mucosal disruption, 549–550
  preventive measures, 550, 551*t*
Brain death, 620–624
  diagnosis, 621–623, 622*t*
    apnea test, 621
    confirmatory tests, 623
    spontaneous movements, 623
  potential organ donor, 623–624
Breathing, intrinsic PEEP and increased work of, 328
Bronchoalveolar lavage (BAL), 539–540
  for distinguishing acute respiratory distress syndrome and hydrostatic pulmonary edema, 259–260
  without bronchoscopy, 540
Bronchodilator aerosols, 271–273
Bronchodilator responsiveness, 294
Bronchodilators
  for treatment of anaphylaxis, 531
  for treatment of chronic obstructive pulmonary disease, 277–278
Bronchoscopy
  bronchoalveolar lavage without, 540
  fever and, 508
B-type natriuretic peptide (BNP), 178–179
  diagnostic value, 179
  role in ICU, 179
BUN (blood urea nitrogen)/creatinine ratio, 395–396
Butyrophenones, neuroleptic malignant syndrome and, 510*t*

C
Calcitonin, for treatment of hypercalcemia, 465–466, 465*t*
Calcium, 457–467
  in blood, 458*t*

hypercalcemia, 463–467, 465t
ionized hypocalcemia, 459–463, 461–462t
in plasma, 457–459
total *vs.* ionized, 457–458, 458f, 458t
Calcium-channel blockers
for treatment of AV nodal re-entrant tachycardia, 247
Wolff-Parkinson-White syndrome and, 243
Calcium chloride
for treatment of hyperkalemia, 437–438, 438t
for treatment of ionized hypocalcemia, 462
Calcium gluconate
for treatment of hypermagnesemia, 454
for treatment of ionized hypocalcemia, 462
Calcium oxalate, 373
Calcium replacement therapy, 461–463, 462t
Caloric density, of feeding formulas, 578–579, 579t
Calorie requirements, in enteral tube feeding, 583
Calorimetry, indirect, 565–566
Candida albicans, 513t, 557, 558
Candida infections
capsofungin for, 676
fluconazole for, 675, 676
Candida krusei, 676
Candida spp.
as cause of catheter-related septicemia, 89, 91t, 92
skin hygiene and, 1
Candidiasis, disseminated, 93–94
Candiduria, 558–559
antifungal therapy for, 559
Capillary hydrostatic pressure, wedge pressure *vs.*, 119–120
Capsofungin, 676
for treatment of candiduria, 559
for treatment of catheter-related septicemia, 91t

for treatment of disseminated candidiasis, 93
Carbapenems, 677–678
imipenem, 677–678
meropenem, 678
for treatment of pneumonia, 543t
Carbohydrates, 566
thiamine and metabolism of, 570
in total parenteral nutrition, 597–598
Carbon dioxide retention, chronic, 381
Cardiac arrest, 189–207
induced hypothermia following, 203t
life support
advanced, 191–199
basic, 189–191
monitoring during CPR, 199–202
post-resuscitation concerns, 202–205
Cardiac filling pressures, 113–122, 114t, 143–144
reliability, 120–122
venous pressures in the thorax, 113–115
wedge pressure, 116–120, 116f, 118f
Cardiac index (CI), 105t, 106
Cardiac output
continuous measurements of, 103–104
intrinsic PEEP and reduced, 328
in PEEP, 310, 311f
phosphate depletion and, 469
promoting, 149–152, 151f
weaning from mechanical ventilation and low, 340
Cardiac performance, during positive-pressure ventilation, 285–287, 286f
Cardiac pump failure, 226–227

Cardiogenic pulmonary edema, 258
  continuous positive airway pressure for, 312
Cardiogenic shock, 693
  hemodynamic patterns in, 110*t*
  hemodynamic support for, 226*t*
  treatment of, 183
Cardiopulmonary resuscitation (CPR), 189
  advanced life support, 191–199
  basic life support, 189–191
  monitoring during, 199–202
  post-resuscitation concerns, 202–205
Cardiovascular effects, of opioids, 656–657
Cardiovascular parameters, 104–108, 105*t*
  cardiac index, 105*t*, 106
  central venous pressure, 104, 105*t*
  pulmonary capillary wedge pressure, 105, 105*t*
  pulmonary vascular resistance index, 105*t*, 107–108
  stroke index, 105*t*, 106–107
  systemic vascular resistance index, 105*t*, 107
Cardiovascular toxicity, of beta-blockers, 711
Cardioversion
  direct-current, 238
  pharmacologic, 238–239
  risk of embolism with, 242
Carnitine, enteral tube feeding and, 582
Catheter blood culture, 88*f*
Catheter colonization, 84
Catheter insertion techniques, 62–63, 64*f*
Catheter-over-needle technique, 62, 62*f*
Catheter position, of central venous catheters, 73–74
Catheter-related septicemia, 84, 85
  catheter tip cultures, 85–86, 86*t*

clinical features, 85
  empiric antibiotic coverage for, 88–90, 89*f*
  persistent sepsis, 92–94
  quantitative blood cultures, 86–88, 88*f*
  treatment of, 90–92, 91*t*
Catheters. *See also* Central venous catheters; Pulmonary artery catheters; Vascular catheters; Vascular catheters, indwelling
  flushing, 78
  heparin-bonded, 56–57
  multilumen, 55
  peripherally-inserted central, 61, 63–65
  volume infusion and size of, 146–147, 147*f*
Catheter tip cultures, 85–86, 86*t*
CDC. *See* Centers for Disease Control and Prevention
Cefazolin, 678–679, 679*t*
Cefepime, 679, 679*t*
  for treatment of catheter-related septicemia, 90
  for treatment of pneumonia, 543*t*
Cefotaxime, for digestive decontamination, 551*t*
Ceftazidime, 679, 679*t*
  for treatment of catheter-related septicemia, 90, 91*t*
  for treatment of gram-negative infections, 516
  for treatment of pneumonia, 543*t*
  for treatment of severe sepsis and septic shock, 528
Ceftriaxone, 679, 679*t*
  for treatment of pneumonia, 541, 543*t*
Cefuroxime. for treatment of chronic obstructive pulmonary disease, 279*t*
Centers for Disease Control and Prevention (CDC)

classification of catheter-related infection, 84

handwashing guidelines, 4*t*

Central diabetes insipidus, 418

Central pontine myelinolysis, 424

Central venous catheters (CVCs), 55–57, 56*t*, 58*f*, 61

antimicrobial-impregnated catheters, 57

catheter position, 73–74

heparin-bonded catheters, 56–57

multilumen catheters, 55

occlusion of, 80–83, 81*t*

replacing, 79–80

Central venous oximetry catheters, 526

Central venous oxygen saturation (ScvO$_2$), in severe sepsis and septic shock, 526–527

Central venous pressure (CVP), 104, 105*t*

measuring, 114–115, 115*f*

Cephalosporins, 678–679

dosing, 679*t*

drug fever and, 509*t*

toxicity, 679

for treatment of pneumonia, 543*t*

Cerebral edema, replacing free water and risk of, 417

Chest compressions, 190–191, 200*f*

Chest pain

in acute aortic dissection, 227

relieving, 210–212

Chlamydia pneumoniae, chronic obstructive pulmonary disease and, 278

Chlarithromycin, for treatment of chronic obstructive pulmonary disease, 279*t*

Chlorhexidine

as antiseptic agent, 2*t*, 3

on catheters, 57

insertion site decontamination with, 62

regime, 545

Chloride-resistant alkalosis, 385, 385*t*

management of, 388

Chloride-responsive alkalosis, 385, 385*t*

Chlorpromazine, torsades de pointes and, 252*t*

Chronic disease, anemia of, 477

Chronic obstructive pulmonary disease (COPD)

acute exacerbations of, 277–279

antibiotic therapy for, 278–279, 279*t*

bronchodilator therapy for, 277–278

corticosteroids for, 278

oxygen therapy for, 279

continuous positive airway pressure for, 312

intrinsic PEEP and, 327

Chvostek's sign, 461

CI. *See* Cardiac index

CIM. *See* Critical illness myopathy

CIP. *See* Critical illness polyneuropathy

Ciprofloxacin, 680, 681*t*

drug interactions, 681

for treatment of pneumonia, 543*t*

for treatment of urinary tract infection, 558

Circulatory shock, lactic acidosis and, 363–364, 364*f*

Cisapride, torsades de pointes and, 252*t*

Cisatracurium, 637, 637*t*

Clarithromycin, torsades de pointes and, 252*t*

Clinical laboratory tests, reference ranges, 725–726

Clonic movement, 627

Clopidogrel, for treatment of acute cardiac syndromes, 212

Clostridia, 513

Clostridium difficile, skin hygiene and, 3

Clostridium difficile colitis, 551–553
  clinical presentation, 552
  diagnosis, 552
  pathogenesis, 551–552
  treatment, 553
Clostridium difficile enterocolitis,
    enteral tube feeding and,
    589
CNS drugs, as cause of acute in-
    terstitial nephritis, 400*t*
CNS stimulants, neuroleptic ma-
    lignant syndrome and,
    510*t*
Cocaine, neuroleptic malignant
    syndrome and, 510*t*
Colistin, for oral decontamina-
    tion, 545
Colitis, *Clostridium difficile,*
    551–553
Colloid fluids, 148, 150, 162–167
  albumin solutions, 164–165
  colloid osmotic pressure, 163
  comparative features of, 164*t*
  cons, 168
  crystalloid fluids *vs.,* 151–152,
    164, 167–168
  dextrans, 166–167
  hydroxyethyl starch, 165–166
  pros, 167–168
  volume effects, 163–164
Colloid osmotic pressure, 163
Colloid resuscitation, 157–171
Colonization
  catheter, 84
  gastric, 549
  oropharynx, 542–543, 544
Coma, 616–620
  bedside evaluation, 617–619
  conditions affecting pupils,
    617*t*
  duration following CPR, 205
  Glasgow coma score, 619–620,
    620*t*
  myxedema, 608
Community-acquired pneumo-
    nia, 541
Compensatory responses,
    350–351

  evaluating, 356–357
Compliance, 290
  "static," 295
  thoracic, 295
  transthoracic, 293
Compression stockings, 35
Computed tomography, in evalu-
    ation of stroke, 646, 646*f*
Conditionally essential nutrients,
    581–582
Consciousness
  altered, 613–614, 614*t*
  evaluation of stroke and, 643
  states of, 613–614, 615*f*
Continuous positive airway pres-
    sure (CPAP), 311–312
Contrast-induced renal failure,
    398–399
Controlled ventilation, 302
Conversions. *See* Units and con-
    versions
Cooling blankets, 518
COPD. *See* Chronic obstructive
    pulmonary disease
Coronary angioplasty, 219–220
  lytic therapy *vs.,* 219
Coronary perfusion pressure
    (CPP), 200–201
Coronary steal syndrome, 182
Corticosteroids
  for treatment of asthma, 275*t,*
    276–277
  for treatment of chronic ob-
    structive pulmonary dis-
    ease, 278
  for treatment of severe sepsis
    and septic shock, 528
Cost, of resuscitation fluids, 167*t*
Coumadin
  interaction with sucralfate, 26
  for treatment of heparin-
    induced thrombocytope-
    nia, 496–497
Countercurrent exchange, 402
CPAP. *See* Continuous positive
    airway pressure
CPP. *See* Coronary perfusion pres-
    sure

CPR. *See* Cardiopulmonary resuscitation
Creatinine clearance, in evaluation of renal failure, 395*t*, 396
Cricothyroidotomy, 317–318
Critical closing pressure, 330
Critical illness, anemia of, 477
Critical illness myopathy (CIM), 341, 635
Critical illness polyneuropathy (CIP), 341, 635
Critical oxygen delivery, 132
Crystalloid fluids, 148, 150, 157–161
    colloid fluids *vs.,* 151–152, 164, 167–168
    comparative features of, 160*t*
    cons, 168
    crystalloid distribution, 157–158
    isotonic saline, 158–159
    lactated Ringer's solution, 159–160
    normal pH fluids, 160–161
    for treatment of hypovolemic hypernatremia, 415
Crystalloid resuscitation, 157–171
Cuff-leak test, 343
CVCs. *See* Central venous catheters
CVP. *See* Central venous pressure
Cyanide accumulation, nitroprusside and, 698*f*, 699–700, 700*t*
Cyanide intoxication, 699–700, 700*t*
Cyanide toxicity, nitroprusside and, 181–182
Cyclosporine, for treatment of myasthenia gravis, 633
Cytopathic hypoxia, 364, 529
Cytoprotective agents, 23*t*, 25–26

D

Daily nutrition requirements, in total parenteral nutrition, 596
Dalteparin, 38–39, 39*t*

Dantrolene sodium
    for treatment of malignant hyperthermia, 508
    for treatment of neuroleptic malignant syndrome, 511
Daptomycin, 685
DC cardioversion. *See* Direct-current cardioversion
D-dimers, in venous thromboembolism, 42–43
Dead space ventilation, 732
Death, brain. *See* Brain death
Decerebrate posturing, 619
Decontamination, 1
    alimentary, 550, 551*t*
    gastrointestinal tract, 551*t*
    oral, 544–545
    oral digestive, 551*t*
Decorticate posturing, 619
Defibrillation, 191–195, 192–193*f*
    automated external defibrillators, 195
    technical considerations, 194
    timing, 191–193
Delayed pneumothorax, 73
Delirium, 614–616, 615*f*
    characteristics, 614
    dementia *vs.,* 615
    hypoactive, 615
    management, 616
    predisposing factors, 616
Dementia, delirium *vs.,* 615
Depolarizing agents, 636
Dexamethasone, for treatment of adrenal insufficiency, 605, 606*t*
Dexmedetomidine, 662–663, 663*t*
Dextrans, 166–167
Dextrose solutions, 161–162, 591, 592*t*
    adverse effects, 162
    protein-sparing effect, 161
    volume effects, 161–162
DI. *See* Diabetes insipidus
Diabetes insipidus (DI), 417–418
    pituitary failure and, 624
Diabetes mellitus, magnesium deficiency and, 447

Diabetic ketoacidosis (DKA), 366–371, 420
  as cause of hypophosphatemia, 469
  clinical features, 367–368
  diagnosis, 368
  management, 368–371, 369*t*
  monitoring acid-base status, 371
  pathogenesis, 366–367, 367*f*
Diagnostic tests, evaluating, 733
Dialysis, for treatment of hypercalcemia, 467
Diarrhea
  enteral tube feeding and, 588–589
  secretory, 447
Diastolic heart failure
  left-sided, 185–186
  systolic heart failure *vs.*, 175–178, 177*t*
Diazepam, 659*t*, 660
  for treatment of seizures, 630–631
DIC. *See* Disseminated intravascular coagulation
Diffusion, 402
Digestive decontamination, 551*t*
Digitalis
  as cause of hyperkalemia, 434*t*, 435, 438*t*
  magnesium deficiency and, 447
Digoxin
  interaction with sucralfate, 26
  Wolff-Parkinson-White syndrome and, 243
Diltiazem
  for treatment of atrial fibrillation, 239, 240*t*
  for treatment of AV nodal reentrant tachycardia, 247
Diphenhydramine, for treatment of anaphylaxis, 530
2,3-Diphosphoglycerate, in red blood cells, 483–484, 484*t*
Direct-current cardioversion, 191
Direct-current (DC) cardioversion, 238

Disinfectants, 1
Disseminated candidiasis, 93–94
Disseminated intravascular coagulation (DIC), 497–498, 498*t*
Dissolved oxygen, 126
Diuretic therapy
  acute interstitial nephritis and, 400*t*
  acute respiratory distress syndrome and, 264–265
  hyperkalemia and, 434*t*
  magnesium deficiency and, 446
  metabolic alkalosis and, 380
  for treatment of heart failure, 182, 183, 184
DKA. *See* Diabetic ketoacidosis
DO_2. *See* Oxygen delivery
Dobutamine, 689–691
  actions, 689, 690*f*
  administration, 691
  adverse effects, 691
  clinical uses, 690
  for treatment of acute heart failure, 180*t*, 182–183, 226*t*
  for treatment of severe sepsis and septic shock, 527
Dopamine, 691–693
  adverse effects, 693
  clinical uses, 692–693
  dose administration, 693
  high dose rates, 692
  intermediate dose rates, 692
  low-dose rates, 691–692
  for treatment of acute heart failure, 180*t*
  for treatment of anaphylactic shock, 531–532
  for treatment of cardiogenic shock, 226*t*
  treatment of oliguria and, 397–398
  for treatment of severe sepsis and septic shock, 527
  wedge pressure, 692
Doxycycline, for treatment of chronic obstructive pulmonary disease, 279*t*

Droperidol
neuroleptic malignant syndrome and, 510*t*
torsades de pointes and, 252*t*
Drug administration routes, 195–196
Drug fever, 509, 509*t*
Drug infusion rates, 732
Drugs. *See also individual drug names and categories*
affecting pupils, 617*t*
associated with acute interstitial nephritis, 400*t*
associated with delirium, 616
associated with hyperkalemia, 434*t*, 435
associated with hypocalcemia, 460, 461*t*
associated with myasthenia gravis, 632
associated with nephrogenic diabetes insipidus, 418
associated with neuroleptic malignant syndrome, 510*t*
associated with seizures, 629*t*
associated with torsades de pointes, 251, 252*t*
lactic acidosis and, 365
magnesium deficiency and, 446–447
neuromuscular blocking, 636–638, 637*t*
Dubois formula, for body surface area, 731
Dysoxia, 132

E

Echocardiography abnormalities
hyperkalemia and, 436–437, 436*f*, 438*t*
hypokalemia and, 431
stroke and, 647
ECV. *See* Extracellular volume
Edema
cardiogenic pulmonary, 258, 312
cerebral, 417

hydrostatic pulmonary, 258–260
laryngeal, 342–345, 344*f*
pulmonary, 537
EDP. *See* End-diastolic pressure
Edrophonium, 633
EDV. *See* End-diastolic volume
EF. *See* Ejection fraction
Effective osmotic activity, 411
Ejection fraction (EF), ventricular, 177–178
Electrolytes
content of body fluids, 729
magnesium depletion and, 448
in total parenteral nutrition, 595
Embolic stroke, 641
Embolism, venous air, 71–72
Emphysema
pulmonary interstitial, 321
subcutaneous, 321, 322
Empiric antibiotic therapy
for treatment of catheter-related septicemia, 88–90, 89*f*
for treatment of urinary tract infections, 557–558
Empiric antimicrobial therapy, 516
for treatment of severe sepsis and septic shock, 528
End-diastolic pressure (EDP), 122
heart failure and, 176
End-diastolic volume (EDV), 120–122
heart failure and, 176–177
End-expiratory air flow, in intrinsic PEEP, 329
End-expiratory occlusion, in intrinsic PEEP, 329
End-expiratory pressure, during ventilator breath, 301
Endocarditis, 92–93
nosocomial, 514
Endogenous fuel stores, 567*t*
Endotracheal intubation, switch to tracheostomy, 317
Endotracheal route, 196

Endotracheal tubes, 287, 315–316
  laryngeal damage, 316
  migration of, 315–316
  paranasal sinusitis, 316
End tidal PCO_2, monitoring during CPR, 201–202, 201f
Energy expenditures, daily, 563–566
  basal, 564–565
  healthy adults, 564, 565t
  ICU patients, 564–565, 565t
  indirect calorimetry, 565–566
  oxidation of nutrient fuels, 563–564, 564t
  predictive equations, 564–565, 565t
  resting, 565–566
Enhanced clearance, treatment of hyperkalemia and, 439
Enhanced potassium cellular release, 434–435
Enoxaparin
  as adjunct to reperfusion therapy, 221
  dosage based on renal function, 221t
  for treatment of venous thromboembolism, 38–39, 39t
Enteral tube feeding, 21, 577–590
  complications, 587–589
    aspiration, 588
    diarrhea, 588–589
    tube occlusion, 587–588
  conditionally essential nutrients, 581–582
  feeding formulas, 578–582
    caloric density, 578–579, 579t
    lipid content, 580–581, 581t
    osmolality, 580
    protein content, 580
  feeding regimen, creating, 582–585, 583t
  initiating, 585–587
    feeding tube insertion, 585, 586f
    gastric residuals, 586–587
    starter regimens, 587
  patient selection, 578
  trophic effects, 577–578
Enterobacter, 513t
Enterococci, 513t
  as cause of catheter-related septicemia, 88, 91t
Enterococcus faecalis
  imipenem for, 677
  vancomycin for, 683
Epilepsia partialis continua, 628
Epinephrine
  lactic acidosis and, 365
  for treatment of anaphylactic shock, 531
  for treatment of anaphylaxis, 530
  for treatment of asthma, 274
  for treatment of cardiac arrest, 196–197, 197t
  for treatment of post-extubation stridor, 345–346
  via endotracheal route, 196–197
Eptifibatide, as adjunct to reperfusion therapy, 222, 223t
Erythrocyte products, 482–486
  leukocyte-poor red cells, 483
  packed cells, 482–483
  storage effects, 483–484, 484t
  washed red cells, 483
Erythrocyte transfusions
  erythrocyte products, 482–486, 484t, 485f
  transfusion risks, 486–490, 487t
  transfusion trigger, 481–482
Erythrocyte transketolase assay, 572–573
Erythromycin
  midazolam and, 661
  torsades de pointes and, 252t
Escherichia coli
  as cause of catheter-related septicemia, 88
  as cause of ICU infections, 513t
  gastric acid suppression and, 24, 25f
Esmalol, for treatment of atrial fibrillation, 240, 240t

Esmolol, 695*t*
 in treatment of acute aortic dissection, 229, 229*t*
Essential trace elements
 daily requirements, 573–574,
  573*t*
 selenium, 574
Ethylene glycol intoxication,
  373–375, 375*f*
Euthyroid sick, 606–607
Exhalation, during ventilator
  breath, 301
Exit-site infection, 84
Expressive aphasia, 644
Extended-spectrum penicillins,
  682
Extracellular volume (ECV),
  413–414
 for treatment of hyponatremia,
  424
Extrarenal potassium loss, 430
Extrinsic PEEP, 326
 adding to intrinsic PEEP, 330
 response to, 329

F
Face masks, 8
Failure to wean from mechanical
  ventilation, 339–341
Famotidine (Pepcid), 22, 23*t*
Feeding formulas, 578–582
 caloric density, 578–579, 579*t*
 immune-modulating, 581*t*
 lipid content, 580–581, 581*t*
 osmolality, 580
 protein content, 580
Feeding tube insertion, 585, 586*f*
Feeding tube occlusion,
  587–588
Femoral vein, as venous access
  site, 66*t*, 68–71
 anatomy, 68, 69*f*, 70*f*
 benefits and risks, 70–71
 locating vessel, 68–69
Femoral vein thrombosis, 83
Fenestrated tracheostomy tube,
  344, 344*f*

Fentanyl, 653, 654*t*
 accumulation of, 655
 morphine *vs.*, 654–655
Fever, 505–520
 as defense mechanism,
  516–517, 517*f*
 defined, 506
 iatrogenic, 511
 initial approach, 515–518
  antipyretic therapy, 516–518
  blood cultures, 515
  empiric antimicrobial therapy, 516
 non-hemolytic, 487–488
 noninfectious sources, 506–511,
  507*t*
  drug fever, 509–, 509*t*
  malignant hyperthermia,
   507–508
  neuroleptic malignant syndrome, 510–511, 510*t*
  postoperative fever, 506–507
 normal body temperature, 505
 nosocomial infections, 511–515,
  512*t*
  necrotizing wound, 513–514
  paranasal sinusitis, 514
  prevalence and pathogens,
   511–512, 513*t*
  surgical wound, 512–513
 platelet transfusions and, 503
 stroke and, 649–650
 suppression of, post-CPR,
  202–203
 when fever is harmful, 517–518
Flecainide, torsades de pointes
  and, 252*t*
Flow rate, in vascular catheters,
  54
Fluconazole, 675–676
 for treatment of candiduria,
  559
 for treatment of catheter-
  related septicemia, 91*t*
Fluid management
 for treatment of acute respiratory distress syndrome,
  264–265

Fluid management *(continued)*
   for treatment of diabetic keto-
      acidosis, 369*t*, 370
Flumazenil, for benzodiazepine
      toxicity, 710
Fluoroquinolones, 679–681
   activity and clinical uses, 680
   adverse effects, 681
   dosing, 680–681, 681*t*
   interaction with sucralfate, 26
   for treatment of chronic
      obstructive pulmonary
      disease, 279*t*
Flushing catheters, 78
Focal seizures, 628
Fomepizole, for treatment of eth-
      ylene glycol intoxication,
      374, 375
Fondaparinux
   dosing regimen, 40
   indications, 41
   for thromboprophylaxis, 40–41
Fosphenytoin, for treatment of
      seizures, 631
Fractional excretion of sodium, in
      evaluation of renal failure,
      394
Frank Starling Law of the Heart, 120
Free water deficit
   in hypovolemic hypernatremia,
      415–416
      replacing, 416–417
   in non-ketotic hyperglycemia,
      419–420
French sizes, 53, 54*t*, 56*t*, 723
Fuel stores, 567*t*
Furosemide
   by continuous infusion,
      184–185
   magnesium deficiency and, 446
   thiamine and, 570
   for treatment of heart failure,
      181, 182, 183, 184
   for treatment of hypercalcemia,
      464–465, 465*t*
   treatment of oliguria and,
      397–398
Fusion beats, 248

G
Gap-gap, 360–361
Gaps, 357
   anion, 357–360, 359*t*
   gap-gap, 360–361
Gas exchange, measures of, 732
Gastric acidity, reduced, 22–25,
      23*t*, 24*t*, 25*f*
   gastric cytoprotection *vs.*, 26–28
   hazards of gastric acid suppres-
      sion, 24–25
Gastric colonization, 549
Gastric cytoprotection, 25–26
   reduced gastric activity *vs.*,
      26–28
Gastric residuals, in enteral tube
      feeding, 586–587
Gastric secretion, metabolic alka-
      losis and loss of, 379
Gastrointestinal tract decontami-
      nation, 551*t*
Gatifloxacin, 680, 681*t*
   torsades de pointes and, 252*t*
   for treatment of chronic ob-
      structive pulmonary dis-
      ease, 279*t*
Gauge sizes, 53, 54*t*, 56*t*, 723
Generalized seizures, 628
   imipenem and, 677–678
General surgery
   risk of venous thromboem-
      bolism and, 31–33, 32*t*
   thromboprophylaxis for, 34*t*
Gentamicin, 671
   for treatment of pneumonia, 543*t*
GFR. *See* Glomerular filtration rate
Glasgow coma score, 205,
      619–620, 620*t*
Global aphasia, 644
Glomerular filtration rate (GFR),
      392, 396, 435
Gloves, 5–7
   handwashing and, 6
   indications, 5–6
   latex allergy, 6–7
   recommendations for use in
      ICU, 7*t*
   for vascular cannulation, 61

Glucagon
for treatment of anaphylactic shock, 531
for treatment of beta-blocker toxicity, 711–713, 712f
Glucose loading, as cause of hypophosphatemia, 467
Glutamine
amino acid solutions enriched with, 593
enteral tube feeding and, 582
Glycemic control, post-CPR, 204
Graded compression stockings, 35
Gram-negative aerobic bacilli
as cause of catheter-related septicemia, 88, 91t
skin hygiene and, 1
Grave's disease, 609
Guidewire technique, 63, 64f
Guillain-Barré syndrome, 632t, 634

H
Hagen-Poisseuille equation, 54
catheter size and infusion rate and, 146
Haloperidol, 663–665, 664t
neuroleptic malignant syndrome and, 510, 510t
torsades de pointes, 252t
for treatment of delirium, 616
Handwashing, 3–5, 4t
gloves and, 6
before vascular cannulation, 61
HBV. See Hepatitis B virus
HCV. See Hepatitis C virus
Heart disease, supraventricular vs. ventricular tachycardia and primary, 248–249
Heart failure. See also Acute heart failure(s)
hemodynamic support for, 226t
left-sided diastolic, 185–186
left-sided systolic, 180–185
right, 186

Hematocrit
detecting blood loss and, 142–143
response to red blood cell transfusions, 484–485
Hemodiafiltration, 405
Hemodialysis, 402–404, 403f
advantages and disadvantages, 404
fever and, 508
method, 402
for treatment of ethylene glycol intoxication, 374–375
for treatment of hyperkalemia, 439
for treatment of hypermagnesemia, 454
for treatment of hyperphosphatemia, 473
vascular access, 402–403
Hemodialysis catheters, 58–59, 59f
Hemodynamic drugs, 689–704
dobutamine, 689–691, 690f
dopamine, 691–693
nitroglycerin, 694–697, 695t
nitroprusside, 697–701
norepinephrine, 701–702
Hemodynamic profiles, 109
Hemodynamics
invasive, 143–144
of nitroglycerin, 696
potential organ donor and, 623
of pulmonary artery catheters, 104–109, 105t
cardiovascular, 104–108, 105t
oxygen transport, 105t, 108–109
Hemodynamic support, for cardiac pump failure, 226–227, 226t
Hemofiltration, 403f, 404–405
advantages and disadvantages, 405
arteriovenous, 405
method, 404
vascular access, 404–405
venovenous, 405

Hemoglobin
  detecting blood loss and, 142–143
  phosphate depletion and, 469
  response to red blood cell transfusions, 484–485
  transfusion trigger, 481–482
Hemoglobin-bound oxygen, 125–126
Hemolysis, hypermagnesemia and, 453
Hemophilus influenza
  ceftriaxone for, 679
  chronic obstructive pulmonary disease and, 278
  fluoroquinolones for, 680
  respiratory precautions for, 9*f*
Hemorrhage and hypovolemia, 139–156, 415
  body fluids and blood loss, 139–141
  clinical evaluation, 141–145
    acid-base parameters, 144–145
    hemoglobin and hematocrit, 142–143
    invasive hemodynamics, 143–144
    vital signs, 141–142, 143*t*
  resuscitation strategies, 149–154
    correcting anemia, 153
    end-points of resuscitation, 153–154
    promoting cardiac output, 149–152, 151*f*
    resuscitation volume, 152–153
  volume infusion, 145–148
    catheter size, 146–147, 147*f*
    type of resuscitation fluid, 148, 149*f*
Hemorrhagic stroke, 641–642
Heparin. *See also* Low-dose heparin; Low-molecular-weight heparin
  as adjunct to reperfusion therapy, 220–221, 221*t*
  for treatment of stroke, 648

weight-based dosing regimen, 48*t*
Heparin-bonded catheters, 56–57
Heparin-induced thrombocytopenia (HIT), 494–497
  acute management, 495–496, 496*t*
  clinical features, 494–495
  diagnosis, 495
  long-term management, 496–497
  pathogenesis, 494
  risk factors, 495
Heparinized flushes, 78
Heparin lock, 78
Hepatic failure, amino acid solutions for, 593
Hepatic insufficiency, lactic acidosis and, 365
Hepatitis B vaccine, 13–14
Hepatitis B virus (HBV), 13–15
  management following possible exposure, 14, 15*t*
  risk of transmission, 14
Hepatitis C virus (HCV), 15–16
  postexposure management, 16
  risk of transmission, 16
Hip surgery, thromboprophylaxis for, 39*t*, 41
Histamine blockers, for treatment of anaphylaxis, 530
Histamine type-2 receptor antagonists (H$_2$ blockers), 22, 23*t*
  dosage adjustment in renal insufficiency, 24*t*
HIT. *See* Heparin-induced thrombocytopenia
HIV. *See* Human immunodeficiency virus
Household and apothecary conversions, 721
Human immunodeficiency virus (HIV), 11–13
  mucous membrane exposure, 11
  percutaneous exposure, 11

postexposure management, 11–13, 12*t*

Hydrochloric acid infusion, for treatment of metabolic alkalosis, 387–388

Hydrocortisone
for treatment of adrenal insufficiency, 605, 606*t*, 624
for treatment of hypercalcemia, 465*t*, 466
for treatment of severe sepsis and septic shock, 528
for treatment of thyroid storm, 611

Hydrogen ion concentration, 349–350, 350*t*

Hydromorphone, 653, 654*t*

Hydrostatic pulmonary edema, acute respiratory distress syndrome *vs.*, 258–260

Hydroxyethyl starch (hetastarch), 165–166

Hypercalcemia, 463–467
clinical manifestations, 463–464
etiologies, 463
management, 464–467, 465*t*

Hypercapnia
permissive, 262, 290
total parenteral nutrition and, 600

Hypercatabolism, amino acid solutions for, 592–593

Hyperchloremic metabolic acidosis, 159, 359

Hyperglycemia
dextrose solutions and, 162
non-ketotic, 419–420
stroke and, 649
total parenteral nutrition and, 599

Hyperkalemia, 433–439
acute management, 437–439, 438*t*
drugs that cause, 434*t*
ECG abnormalities and, 436–437, 436*f*
enhanced cellular release, 434–435

impaired renal excretion, 435–436
pseudohyperkalemia, 433–434

Hyperlactatemia, 135–136
stress, 364

Hypermagnesemia, 452–454
clinical manifestations, 453–454
etiologies, 453
management, 454

Hypernatremia, 412–414. *See also* Hypovolemic hypernatremia
causes of, 412–413, 412*t*
extracellular volume, 413–414
management of, 413*f*

Hypernatremic encephalopathy, 415

Hyperphosphatemia, 472–473

Hypertension
stroke and, 648–649
treating, in acute aortic dissection, 228, 229*t*
vasodilator therapy of hypertensive emergencies, 695*t*

Hyperthermia, malignant, 507–508

Hyperthyroidism, 607*t*, 609–611
apathetic thyrotoxicosis, 609
clinical manifestations, 609–610
diagnosis, 610
management, 610–611
thyroid storm, 609–610

Hypertonic, 411

Hypertonic and hypotonic conditions, 409–426
diabetes insipidus, 417–418
hypernatremia, 412–414, 412*t*, 413*f*
hyponatremia, 420–425, 423*f*
hypovolemic hypernatremia, 414–417, 414*t*
non-ketotic hyperglycemia, 419–420
osmotic activity, 409–411

Hypertonicity, 415

Hypertonic resuscitation, 169–170

Hypervolemic hyponatremia, 422

Hypoactive delirium, 615

Hypocalcemia
  ionized, 459–463, 461–462*t*
  magnesium depletion and, 448
Hypokalemia, 428–433
  clinical manifestations, 430–431
  diagnostic approach, 430*f*
  management, 431–433
  metabolic alkalosis and, 381
  potassium depletion, 429–430, 432*t*
  refractory, 433
  transcellular shift, 428–429
Hypomagnesemia. *See also* Magnesium
  replacement protocols for, 451–452
Hyponatremia, 420–425
  changes in total body sodium and water in, 412*t*
  diagnostic approach, 421–422, 423*f*
  hypervolemic, 422
  hypovolemic, 421–422
  isovolemic, 422
  management, 424–425
  pseudohyponatremia, 420–421
  symptoms, 422–423
Hypophosphatemia, 467–472
  clinical manifestations, 469–471, 470*f*
  etiologies, 467–469
  magnesium depletion and, 448
  phosphorus replacement, 471–472, 471*t*
  total parenteral nutrition and, 599
Hypos, 372
Hypotension, blood loss and, 142, 143*t*
Hypothermia, induced, following cardiac arrest, 203*t*
Hypothyroidism, 606–609, 607*t*
  clinical manifestations, 607–608
  diagnosis, 608
  euthyroid sick, 606–607
  management, 608–609
Hypotonic, 411

Hypoventilation, metabolic alkalosis and, 383*f*, 392–383
Hypovolemia. *See* Hemorrhage and hypovolemia
Hypovolemic hypernatremia, 414–417
  consequences of hypotonic fluid loss, 415
  free water replacement, 415–417
  volume replacement, 415
Hypovolemic hyponatremia, 421–422
Hypovolemic shock, 141, 144
  end-points of volume resuscitation, 153–154
  hemodynamic patterns in, 110*t*
  volume infusion and, 145–146
Hypoxia, cytopathic, 364, 529

I
IABP, for treatment of cardiogenic shock, 226*t*
Iatrogenic fever, 511
Ibuprofen, as antipyretic, 518, 649
Ibutilide
  for pharmacologic cardioversion, 239, 240*t*
  torsades de pointes and, 252*t*
ICU patients, daily energy requirements, 564–565, 565*t*
Ideal body weight, 659, 662, 693, 731
Imipenem, 677–678
  for treatment of abdominal abscess, 555
  for treatment of catheter-related septicemia, 90, 91*t*
  for treatment of pneumonia, 543*t*
  for treatment of urinary tract infection, 558
Immune-modulating enteral feeding formulas, 581*t*
Immune suppression, transfusions and, 490

Immunoglobulin G
  for treatment of Guillain-Barré
    syndrome, 634
  for treatment of myasthenia
    gravis, 634
Immunonutrition, 581
IMV. *See* Intermittent mandatory
    ventilation
Indirect calorimetry, 565–566
Indwelling vascular catheter. *See*
    Vascular catheter, in-
    dwelling
Infarction, fever and, 511
Infection control, 1–17
  blood-borne infections, 10–16
  enteral feeding and, 577–578
  protective barriers, 5–10
  skin hygiene, 1–5
Infections. *See also* Infection con-
    trol; Sepsis; Shock
  catheter-related, 83–94
    catheter tip cultures, 85–86,
      86*t*
    clinical features, 85
    empiric antibiotic coverage,
      88–90, 89*f*
    persistent sepsis, 92–94
    quantitative blood cultures,
      86–88, 88*f*
    routes of, 83–84, 84*f*
    treatment of catheter-related
      septicemia, 90–92, 91*t*
    types of, 84
  inflammation and, 523. *See also*
    Inflammatory injury
Infectious Disease Society of
    America, 558
Inferior vena cava filters, to pre-
    vent pulmonary emboliza-
    tion, 50
Inflammation
  anemia of critical illness and,
    478
  antioxidant vitamins and, 573
Inflammatory injury, 521–524
  clinical conditions, 522
  malignant intravascular inflam-
    mation, 522

multiorgan injury, 523–524, 524*t*
renal, 398
systemic inflammatory re-
    sponse syndrome,
    522–523, 523*t*
Inflammatory response, anaphy-
    laxis and, 529
Infusion rate, of enteral tube feed-
    ing, 584
Inodilators, for treatment of heart
    failure, 182
Inspiratory resistance, 295–296
Insulin-dextrose therapy, for hy-
    perkalemia, 439
Insulin therapy
  for treatment of diabetic keto-
    acidosis, 369, 369*t*
  for treatment of non-ketotic hy-
    perglycemia, 420
Intermittent mandatory ventila-
    tion (IMV), 303–304
Intermittent pneumatic compres-
    sion (IPC) devices, 35
Internal jugular vein, as venous
    access site, 66*t*, 67–68
  anatomy, 67
  anterior approach, 67
  benefits and risks, 68
  posterior approach, 67
Intracardiac shunts, pulmonary
    artery catheter and, 103
Intracellular organisms, in bron-
    choalveolar lavage speci-
    mens, 539–540
Intraosseous (IO) route, 196
Intravascular pressure, trans-
    mural pressure vs., 113
Intravenous route, 195–196
Intrinsic positive end-expiratory
    pressure (intrinsic PEEP),
    190, 326–330, 326*f*
  consequences, 328
  management, 329–330
  monitoring, 328–329
  pathogenesis, 326–327, 326*f*
  predisposing factors, 327
Introducer catheters, 57–58, 58*f*,
    147

Intubation
  tracheal, 287–288
  translaryngeal, 342–343
Inverse ratio ventilation (IRV),
    305–306, 306f
Iodide, for treatment of hyperthy-
    roidism, 610–611
Iodophors, as antiseptic agents,
    2–3, 2t
Ionized calcium, 457–458, 458f,
    458t
Ionized hypocalcemia, 459–463,
    461–462t
  calcium replacement therapy,
    461–463, 462t
  clinical manifestations, 461
  etiologies, 459–461, 461t
IO route. See Intraosseous route
Ipatropium bromide
  for treatment of asthma, 275,
    275t
  for treatment of chronic ob-
    structive pulmonary dis-
    ease, 277–278
IPC devices. See Intermittent
    pneumatic compression
    devices
IRV. See Inverse ratio ventilation
Ischemic stroke, 641, 643f
Isosthenuria, 394
Isotonic, 411
Isotonic saline, 158–159
  adverse effects, 159
  composition, 158–159
Isovolemic hyponatremia,
    422

J

Jacobson formula, for body sur-
    face area, 731

K

Ketoacidosis
  alcoholic, 367f, 371–373
  diabetic. See Diabetic ketoaci-
    dosis

Ketorolac, 657–658
Klebsiella pneumoniae, 513t
  as cause of catheter-related sep-
    ticemia, 88
Knee surgery, thromboprophy-
    laxis for, 39t, 41

L

Labetalol
  for acute control of hyperten-
    sion, 649, 695t
  in treatment of acute aortic dis-
    section, 229
Lactated Ringer's solution, 148,
    159–160
  adverse effects, 159–160
  composition, 159
  drug interaction, 159–160
Lactate production, dextrose solu-
    tions and enhanced, 162
Lactic acidosis, 363–366
  alkali therapy, 366
  clinical presentation, 363
  D-lactic acidosis, 365–366
  etiologies, 363–365, 364f
D-Lactic acidosis, 365–366
Laryngeal damage, 316
Laryngeal edema, 342–345, 344f
Latex allergy, 6–7
Lazarus' sign, 623
LDUH. See Low-dose unfraction-
    ated heparin
Left-sided diastolic heart failure,
    185–186
Left-sided systolic heart failure,
    180–185
Lepirudin, for treatment of he-
    parin-induced thrombocy-
    topenia, 495–496, 496t
Leukocyte-poor red cells, 483
Levofloxacin, 680, 681t
  torsades de pointes and, 252t
  for treatment of chronic ob-
    structive pulmonary dis-
    ease, 279t
  for treatment of pneumonia,
    541, 543t

Levothyroxine, for treatment of hypothyroidism, 608–609

Lidocaine
for treatment of cardiac arrest, 197t, 198
for treatment of ventricular tachycardia, 250
via endotracheal route, 196

Life support
advanced, 191–199
basic, 189–191
airway patency, 189
chest compressions, 190–191
ventilation, 189–190

Linezolid, 684–685
lactic acidosis and, 365
for MRSA or vancomycin-resistant strains, 516, 528
for treatment of catheter-related septicemia, 91t
for treatment of pneumonia, 543, 543t
for treatment of severe sepsis and septic shock, 528
for treatment of urinary tract infection, 558

Linoleic acid, 567

Lipid calories, in total parenteral nutrition, 598

Lipid content, of feeding formulas, 580–581, 581t

Lipid emulsions, 593–594, 594t

Lipids, 567

Liposomal amphotericin B, 675

Lithium, neuroleptic malignant syndrome and, 510t

LMWH. *See* Low-molecular-weight heparin

Lone atrial fibrillation, 237

Loop diuretics, magnesium deficiency and, 446

Lorazepam, 659t, 660
for treatment of seizures, 630

Low-dose heparin
complications, 37
dosing regimen, 36
indications, 36
for thromboprophylaxis, 36–37, 37t

Low-dose unfractionated heparin (LDUH), for thromboprophylaxis, 34t

Low-molecular-weight heparin (LMWH)
as adjunct to reperfusion therapy, 220–221
in antithrombotic therapy, 47–48
risk of heparin-induced thrombocytopenia and, 495
for thromboprophylaxis, 34t, 38–40, 39t

Low-volume ventilation, 288–290
for acute respiratory distress syndrome, 262–264, 263t
PEEP during, 311
protocol for initiating, 289t

Lugol's solution, iodide added to, 611

Lung inflation, during ventilator breath, 300

Lung injury, red blood cell transfusions and acute, 489–490

Lung mechanics, 290–296
inspiratory resistance, 295–296
mechanical properties of the lungs, 290
practical applications, 293–294, 294f
proximal airway pressures, 291–293, 291f, 292f
thoracic compliance, 295

Lung recruitment, 309–310, 309f

Lung scan, for evaluation of venous thromboembolism, 45–46

Lusitropic effects, 186

M

Magnesium, 443–456
hypermagnesemia, 452–454
magnesium balance, 443–445, 444t, 445f

Magnesium (*continued*)
    magnesium deficiency. *See*
        Magnesium deficiency
    preparations, 450–451, 451*t*
    reference ranges for, 444*t*
    serum, 443–444
    thiamine and, 571
    for treatment of cardiac arrest,
        197*t*, 198–199
    for treatment of multifocal
        atrial tachycardia, 243–244
    for treatment of torsades de
        pointes, 252
    urinary, 444, 445*f*
Magnesium deficiency, 445–452
    as cause of ionized hypocal-
        cemia, 459
    clinical manifestations, 447–449
    diagnosis, 449–450
    incidence, 445
    magnesium preparations,
        450–451, 451*t*
    magnesium retention test, 449*t*,
        450
    markers of, 446*t*
    predisposing conditions,
        445–447
    refractory hypokalemia and,
        433
    replacement protocols, 451–452
Magnesium preparations,
    450–451, 451*t*
Magnesium retention test, 449*t*,
    450
Magnesium sulfate, 450–451, 451*t*
Magnetic resonance imaging, in
    evaluation of stroke,
    646–647
Malignant hyperthermia (MH),
    507–508
Malignant intravascular inflam-
    mation, 398, 522
Masks, face, 8
    vascular cannulation and, 61
Maximum inspiratory pressure,
    335–336
MDIs. *See* Metered-dose inhalers
Mean arterial pressure, 200

Measurement
    of body size, 731
    of gas exchange, 732
    units of, in Système Interna-
        tionale, 719–720
Mechanical complications, of
    acute cardiac syndromes,
    224–225
Mechanical compression devices,
    for thromboprophylaxis,
    34*t*, 35
    graded compression stockings,
        35
    pneumatic compression de-
        vices, 35
Mechanical ventilation, 283–297.
    See also Positive-pressure
    breathing; Ventilator-
    dependent patient
    discontinuing, 333–347
        failure to wean, 339–341,
            339*f*, 341*f*
        identifying candidates,
            333–336, 334–335*t*, 336*f*
        post-extubation period,
            345–346
        spontaneous breathing trials,
            336–338
        tracheal decannulation,
            342–345, 344*f*
    initiating, 287–290, 289*t*
    monitoring lung mechanics,
        290–296, 291*f*, 292*t*,
        294*f*
    positive-pressure ventilation,
        283–287, 284*f*, 286*f*
Membrane antagonism, hyper-
    kalemia and, 437–438
Men
    body fluid distribution in, 729
    body fluid volumes in, 139,
        140*t*
    creatinine clearance in, 395*t*
    desirable weights in, 728
    normal peak flow rates for, 270,
        270*f*
    normal range of values for red
        cell parameters in, 478*t*

peak expiratory flow rates for, 729–730

Meningitis, nosocomial, 515

Mentation disorders, 613–625
 brain death, 620–624, 622*t*
 coma, 616–620, 617*t*, 618*f*, 620*t*
 delirium, 614–616, 615*f*
 states of consciousness, 613–614, 614*t*

Meperidine, 655

Meropenem, 678
 for treatment of catheter-related septicemia, 90, 91*t*
 for treatment of gram-negative infections, 516
 for treatment of pneumonia, 542, 543*t*
 for treatment of severe sepsis and septic shock, 528
 for treatment of urinary tract infection, 558

Metabolic acid-base disorders, 350, 351*t*, 352–353, 352*f*

Metabolic acidosis, 350, 351*t*, 352*f*, 353
 anion gap of, 358–359
 hyperchloremic, 359
 mixed, 361
 primary, 355

Metabolic alkalosis, 350, 351*t*, 352*f*, 353, 361, 379–389
 chloride-resistant, 385, 385*t*
 chloride-responsive, 385, 385*t*
 classification of, 384–385, 385*t*
 hypoventilation, 382–383, 383*f*
 management of, 386–388
 neurologic manifestations, 382
 origins of, 379–382
 systemic oxygenation, 383–384, 384*f*

Metaclopramide, neuroleptic malignant syndrome and, 510*t*

Metered-dose inhalers (MDIs), 271–273
 nebulizers *vs.*, 273, 274*f*

Metformin, lactic acidosis and, 365

Methadone, torsades de pointes and, 252*t*

Methanol intoxication, 375–376, 375*f*

Methemoglobinemia, of nitroglycerin, 696

Methicillin-resistant *Staphylococcus aureus* (MRSA)
 antibiotics for, 516, 528, 542, 683
 vancomycin for, 683

Methimazole, for treatment of hyperthyroidism, 610

Methylprednisolone
 for treatment of acute respiratory distress syndrome, 265
 for treatment of adrenal insufficiency, 606*t*
 for treatment of anaphylaxis, 531
 for treatment of asthma, 275*t*, 276
 for treatment of chronic obstructive pulmonary disease, 278

Metoclopramide, for treatment of gastric residuals, 586–587

Metoprolol
 for treatment of acute cardiac syndromes, 213
 for treatment of atrial fibrillation, 240, 240*t*
 for treatment of multifocal atrial tachycardia, 244

Metronidazole, for treatment of C. *difficile* colitis, 553

MG. *See* Myasthenia gravis

MH. *See* Malignant hyperthermia

Midazolam, 659–660, 659*t*
 erythromycin and, 661

Migration, of indwelling endotracheal tubes, 315–316

Mill wheel murmur, 72

Metered-dose inhalers (MDIs), 271–273

Milrinone, for treatment of acute heart failure, 180*t*, 182–183, 186

Minocycline, on catheters, 57
Mitral regurgitation, acute, 225
Mixed metabolic and respiratory acid-base disorder, 355
Mixed respiratory acidosis and metabolic alkalosis, 356
Morphine, 653, 654*t*
    fentanyl *vs.*, 654–655
    for relief of chest pain, 210–212
Mortality rate
    acute respiratory distress syndrome, 255
    multiorgan injury, 524
    severe sepsis and septic shock, 525, 525*f*
    tracheostomy, 318
    ventilator-assisted pneumonia, 536
Movement disorders, 627–640
    neuromuscular blockers, 636–638, 637*f*
    neuromuscular weakness, 632–635
        critical illness polyneuropathy and myopathy, 635
        Guillain-Barré syndrome, 632*t*, 634
        myasthenia gravis, 632–634, 632*t*
    seizures, 627–632
        acute management, 630–631, 630*f*
        predisposing conditions, 629, 629*t*
        types of, 627–629
Movements
    associated with seizures, 627
    spontaneous, brain death and, 623
Moxifloxacin, 680, 681*t*
    for treatment of chronic obstructive pulmonary disease, 279*t*
    for treatment of pneumonia, 541
MRSA. *See* Methicillin-resistant *Staphylococcus aureus*

Mucociliary clearance, 319
Mucolytic agent, 320
Mucolytic therapy, 320–321
    with N-acetylcysteine, 320*t*
Mucosal disruption, 549–550
Multifocal atrial tachycardia, 243–244
Multilobar pneumonia, 258
Multilumen catheters, 55
Multiorgan injury, 523–524
    mortality rate, 524
Muscle weakness, hypophosphatemia and, 469–470
Myasthenia gravis (MG), 632–634, 632*t*
    advanced cases, 633–634
    clinical features, 632–633, 632*t*
    diagnosis, 633
    predisposing conditions, 632
    treatment, 633
Myasthenic crisis, 633
Mycobacterium tuberculosis, respiratory precautions for, 9*f*
Mycoplasma pneumoniae, fluoroquinolones for, 680
Myocardial infarction. *See also* Non-ST-segment elevation myocardial infarction
    risk of thromboembolism and, 33
Myoclonic movement, 627
Myoglobinuric renal failure, 400–401
Myopathy
    critical illness, 341
    steroids and, 276
Myxedema coma, 608

N

NAC. *See* N-Acetylcysteine
Nafcillin, for treatment of catheter-related septicemia, 91*t*
Naloxone, for opioid toxicity, 713–715, 714*t*
Narrow QRS complex tachycardias, 233, 235, 236*f*

National Institute of Neurological Disorders and Stroke, 641

Nebulizers, 271
  metered-dose inhalers *vs.*, 273, 274*f*

Necrotizing wound infections, 513–514

Needles, safety-engineered, 10

Needlestick injuries, 10
  risk of HCV infection from, 16
  risk of HIV infection from, 11

Neisseria meningitidis, respiratory precautions for, 9*f*

Nephrogenic diabetes insipidus, 418

Nephrotoxicity
  amphotericin B and, 675
  vancomycin and, 684

Nesiritide, for treatment of heart failure, 185

Neuroleptic malignant syndrome (NMS), 510–511, 510*t*, 665

Neurologic findings
  in magnesium depletion, 448–449
  in metabolic alkalosis, 382

Neurologic outcome, post-CPR, 204–205

Neuromuscular blockers, 636–638
  disadvantages, 638
  drugs, 636–638, 637*t*
  mechanisms, 636
  monitoring, 638

Neuromuscular excitability, ionized hypocalcemia and, 461

Neuromuscular weakness
  critical illness polyneuropathy and myopathy, 635
  Guillain-Barré syndrome, 632*t*, 634
  myasthenia gravis, 632–634, 632*t*
  weaning from mechanical ventilation and, 341

Neuromuscular weakness syndromes, risk of thromboembolism and, 33–34

Neurotoxicity, of beta-blockers, 711

Nicardipine, for acute control of hypertension, 649

Nitrate tolerance, nitroglycerin and, 697

Nitrogen balance, 568–569
  enteral tube feeding and, 584
  nonprotein calories and, 569, 569*f*

Nitroglycerin (NTG), 694–697, 695*t*
  actions, 694
  administration, 695–696
  adverse effects, 696
  clinical uses, 694–695
  nitrate tolerance, 697
  for relief of chest pain, 210
  for treatment of acute heart failure, 180*t*, 181, 182, 183, 186
  vasodilator therapy of hypertensive emergencies, 695*t*

Nitroprusside, 695*t*, 697–701
  actions, 697
  clinical uses, 697
  cyanide accumulation, 698*f*, 699–700, 700*t*
  dose administration, 698
  lactic acidosis, 365
  thiocyanate toxicity, 700–701
  for treatment of acute aortic dissection, 229*t*
  for treatment of acute heart failure, 180*t*, 181–182

NKH. *See* Non-ketotic hyperglycemia

NMS. *See* Neuroleptic malignant syndrome

Non-depolarizing agents, 636

Non-hemolytic fever, red blood cell transfusions and, 487–488

Non-ketotic hyperglycemia (NKH), 419–420

Non-opioid analgesia, 657–658

Nonprotein calories, 566
  in enteral tube feeding, 583–584

Nonprotein intake, 566–567, 567*t*

Non-recruitable lung, 309
Non-STEMI. *See* Non-ST-segment elevation myocardial infarction
Nonsterile gloves, 5–6
Non-ST-segment elevation myocardial infarction (non-STEMI), 209. *See also* Acute coronary syndromes
  heparin for, 220
  platelet glycoprotein inhibitors for, 223–224
Norepinephrine, 701–702
  for treatment of anaphylactic shock, 532
  for treatment of severe sepsis and septic shock, 527
Normal body temperature, 505
Nosocomial infections, 511–515
  endocarditis, 514
  meningitis, 515
  necrotizing wound, 513–514
  paranasal sinusitis, 514
  prevalence and pathogens, 511–512, 512–513*t*
  spontaneous bacterial peritonitis, 515
  surgical wound, 512–513
NSAIDs
  as antipyretic, 518
  as cause of acute interstitial nephritis, 400*t*
  as cause of hyperkalemia, 434*t*
NTG. *See* Nitroglycerin
Nucleoside reverse transcriptase inhibitors, lactic acidosis and, 365
Nutrient fuels, oxidation of, 563–564, 564*t*
Nutritional requirements, 563–576
  conditionally essential, 581–582
  daily energy expenditure, 563–566, 564–565*t*
  essential trace elements, 573–574
    daily requirements, 573–574, 573*t*
    selenium, 574

  substrate requirements, 566–569
    nonprotein intake, 566–567, 567*t*
    protein intake, 567–569
  vitamin requirements, 570–573
    antioxidant vitamins, 573
    daily, 570, 571*t*
    thiamine deficiency, 570–573, 572*t*

O

Obligate nephrotoxins, 673
Occlusion of catheters, 80–83, 81*t*
  restoring patency, 80–82, 81*t*
  sources of obstruction, 80
Occult PEEP, 327
Ocular reflexes, evaluation of coma and, 618, 618*f*
Oculocephalic reflex, 618, 618*f*
Oculovestibular reflex, 618, 618*f*
O₂ER. *See* Oxygen extraction ratio
Oliguria and acute renal failure, 391–407
  acute interstitial nephritis, 399–400, 400*t*
  categories, 391–393
  causes of, 391–393, 392*t*
  contrast-induced renal failure, 398–399
  definition, 391
  evaluation, 393–397
  immediate concerns, 397–398
  inflammatory renal injury, 398
  myoglobinuric renal failure, 400–401
  prerenal azotemia *vs.*, 393*t*
  renal replacement therapy, 401–405
    hemodialysis, 402–404, 403*f*
    hemofiltration, 403*f*, 404–405
Omega-3 fatty acids, in feeding formulas, 581
Omeprazole (Prilosec), 23, 23*t*
Opioids, 653–657
  adverse effects, 656–657

intravenous, 653–655, 654t
meperidine, 655
patient-controlled analgesia,
656
toxicity of, 713–715, 714t
Opioid-sparing effect, 657
Oral anticoagulation, for treatment of atrial fibrillation,
242t
Oral decontamination, 544–545
colonization of oropharynx, 544
digestive, 551t
regimens, 544–545
Organ donor, potential, 623–624
hemodynamics, 623
pituitary failure, 624
Organic acidoses, 363–378
alcoholic ketoacidosis, 371–373
diabetic ketoacidosis, 366–371,
367f, 369t
lactic acidosis, 363–366, 364f
toxic alcohols, 373–376, 375f
Organic anions, metabolic alkalosis and administration of,
381–382
Organ injury
clinical consequences of inflammatory, 524t
multiorgan, 523–524
Oropharynx, colonization of,
542–543, 544
Orthopedic surgery, risk of venous thromboembolism
and, 33
Osmolality, 410
of feeding formulas, 580
Osmolarity, 410
Osmotic activity, 409–411
definitions, 409–410
effective, 411
of plasma, 410–411
Ototoxicity, vancomycin and, 684
Overfeeding, weaning from mechanical ventilation and,
340–341, 341f
Oxacillin, for treatment of
catheter-related sep-
ticemia, 91t

Oxidation of nutrient fuels,
563–564, 564t
Oxidative energy production, hypophosphatemia and, 469,
470f
Oxygen, in blood, 125–126, 127t
dissolved, 126
hemoglobin-bound, 125–126
total content, 126
Oxygenation. *See* Systemic oxygenation
Oxygen consumption, oxygen uptake and, 128
Oxygen delivery (DO₂), 105t, 108,
127–128, 128t
critical, 132
effect of red blood cell transfusion on, 485, 485f
relation to oxygen uptake,
131–133, 133f
Oxygen extraction
role of, 131
tissue oxygenation and, 134
transfusion trigger and, 482
Oxygen extraction ratio (O₂ER),
105t, 109, 130–131
Oxygen therapy, for chronic
obstructive pulmonary
disease, 279
Oxygen transport
anemia and, 479–480
response to red blood cell
transfusions, 485–486, 485f
severe sepsis and septic shock
and, 528–529, 529f
Oxygen transport parameters,
105t, 108–109
oxygen delivery. *See* Oxygen
delivery
oxygen extraction ratio, 105t,
109
oxygen uptake. *See* Oxygen uptake
Oxygen uptake (VO₂), 105t,
108–109, 108–110,128–131
calculated, 128–129
measured *vs.*, 129–130, 130t
control of, 131–133, 133f

Oxygen uptake *(continued)*
    effect of red blood cell transfusion on, 485–486, 485*f*
    hypovolemia and, 144
    measured, 129
    relation to oxygen delivery, 131–133, 133*f*
    tissue oxygenation and, 134
Oxyhemoglobin dissociation, phosphate depletion and, 469

P
Packed cells, 148, 150, 482–483
Pamidronate, for treatment of hypercalcemia, 465*t*, 466
Pancreatic enzyme, for treatment of feeding tube occlusion, 588
Pancreatitis, as cause of ionized hypocalcemia, 460
Pancuronium, 636, 637*t*
Pantoprazole, 23, 23*t*
Paranasal sinusitis, 316, 514
Parenteral therapy, for asthma, 273–274
Paroxysmal supraventricular tachycardia (PSVT), 244–247
    AV nodal re-entrant tachycardia, 245–247, 246*t*
Partial (focal) seizures, 628
Partially compensated respiratory acidosis, 356
Partially compensated respiratory alkalosis, 356
Pasteurella multocida, influence of temperature on, 517*f*
Pathogens
    in bloodstream infections, 513*t*
    in nosocomial infections, 511, 513*t*
    in ventilator-assisted pneumonia, 535, 536*t*
Patient-controlled analgesia (PCA), 656

Patient selection, for enteral tube feeding, 578
PCA. *See* Patient-controlled analgesia
PCV. *See* Pressure-controlled ventilation
PCWP. *See* Pulmonary capillary wedge pressure
Peak airway pressure, during ventilator breath, 300–301
Peak expiratory flow rate (PEFR), 269–271, 270*f*
    for healthy females, 730
    for healthy males, 729–730
Peak flow meter, 269
Peak pressure, 291, 294*f*
PEEP. *See* Positive end-expiratory pressure;
PEFR. *See* Peak expiratory flow rate
Pelvis, sepsis from. *See under* Sepsis
Penicillins, 681–682
    antipseudomonal, 682
    drug fever and, 509*t*
    extended-spectrum, 682
Pentamidine, torsades de pointes and, 252*t*
Pentobarbital, for treatment of refractory status epilepticus, 631
Peripheral blood culture, 88*f*
Peripherally-inserted central catheters (PICCs), 61, 63–65
Peripheral vein catheters, 55
    replacing, 79
Peripheral veins, for venous access, 63
Permissive hypercapnia, 262, 290
pH, relationship to hydrogen ion concentration in arterial blood, 350, 350*t*
Pharmaceutical toxins and antidotes, 705–717
    acetaminophen, 705–709, 708*t*

benzodiazepines, 709–710
beta-receptor antagonists, 711–713, 712*f*
opioids, 713–715, 714*t*
Pharmacologic cardioversion, 238–241, 240*t*
Phenothiazines, neuroleptic malignant syndrome and, 510*t*
Phenytoin
  drug fever and, 509*t*
  interaction with sucralfate, 26
  for treatment of seizures, 631
pH fluids, normal, 160–161
Phlebotomy, anemia and, 478–479
Phosphate, for treatment of diabetic ketoacidosis, 369*t*, 370–371
Phosphate-binding agents, as cause of hypophosphatemia, 468
Phosphorus, 457, 467–473
  in blood, 458*t*
  hyperphosphatemia, 472–473
  hypophosphatemia, 467–472
Phosphorus replacement, 471–472, 471*t*
PICCs. *See* Peripherally-inserted central catheters
Pipericillin, 682
Pipericillin-tazobactam, 682
  for treatment of gram-negative infections, 516
  for treatment of pneumonia, 543*t*
  for treatment of severe sepsis and septic shock, 528
Pituitary failure, potential organ donor and, 624
Plasma
  calcium in, 457–459, 458*t*
  osmotic activity of, 410–411
Plasma D-dimer levels, in venous thromboembolism, 42–43
Plasma exchange, for treatment of thrombocytic thrombocytopenia purpura, 499

Plasmapheresis
  for treatment of Guillain-Barré syndrome, 634
  for treatment of myasthenia gravis, 634
  for treatment of thrombocytic thrombocytopenia purpura, 499
Plasma retention ratio, 152–153
Plasma volume, 140, 140*t*
Plateau pressure, 291–292, 294*f*
Platelet glycoprotein inhibitors, as adjunct to reperfusion therapy, 222–224, 223*t*
Platelet transfusions, 501–503
  complications, 502–503
  contraindications, 499–500
  random donor platelets, 501
  response to transfused platelets, 501–502
  transfusion trigger, 499–501
Pleural drainage system, 323–325, 325*f*
Pleural evacuation, 322–323
Pleur-Evac Chest Drainage System, 323–325
Plicamycin, for treatment of hypercalcemia, 465*t*, 466–467
Pneumatic compression devices, 35
Pneumocystis jiroveci pneumoniae, 322
Pneumomediastinum, 321
Pneumonia, ICU-acquired, 535–547
  antimicrobial therapy, 541–544, 542*t*
    duration of, 544
    empiric, 541–543, 543*t*
  clinical features, 535–536
  clinical manifestations, 536–537
  community-acquired, 541
  diagnostic evaluation, 537–541
    blood cultures, 537
    bronchoalveolar lavage, 539–540
    choosing culture method, 540–541

Pneumonia, ICU-acquired
    (continued)
    protected specimen brush,
        539
    tracheal aspirates, 537–538,
        538*t*
    oral decontamination, 544–545
    pathogens in, 513*t*, 536*t*
    ventilator-assisted, 535–536,
        536*t*
Pneumoperitoneum, 321
Pneumothorax, 72–73, 321–323,
    323*f*
    delayed, 73
    tension, 322
Polymyxin, for oral decontamina-
    tion, 545
Polymyxin E, for digestive decon-
    tamination, 551*t*
Polyneuropathy, critical illness,
    341
Positive end-expiratory pressure
    (PEEP), 115, 263–264,
        307–311
    cardiac performance, 310, 311*f*
    clinical uses of, 311–311
    extrinsic, 326, 329, 330
    features, 307–308, 308*f*
    intrinsic, 190, 326–330, 326*f*
    during low-volume ventilation,
        290
    lung recruitment, 309–310, 309*f*
    occult, 327
Positive-pressure breathing,
    299–313. *See also* Positive
    end-expiratory pressure
    assist-control ventilation,
        301–303, 303*f*
    assisted ventilation, 302
    continuous positive airway
        pressure, 311–312
    controlled ventilation, 302
    intermittent mandatory ventila-
        tion, 303–304, 303*f*
    inverse ratio ventilation,
        305–306, 306*f*
    pressure-controlled ventilation,
        305, 306*f*
    pressure-modulated ventila-
        tion, 305–307, 306*f*
    pressure-supported ventilation,
        306*f*, 307
    ventilator breath, 299–301, 300*f*
Positive-pressure ventilation,
    283–287
    cardiac performance, 285–287,
        286*f*
    pressure-volume relationships,
        283–284, 284*f*
    pressure *vs.* volume control,
        284–285
Post-extubation stridor, 345–346
Postoperative fever, 506–507
Postrenal obstruction, 392*t*, 393
Potassium, 427–441
    deficits in hypokalemia,
        429–430, 432*t*
    distribution of, 427–428, 428*f*
    hyperkalemia, 433–439, 434*t*,
        436*f*, 438*t*
    hypokalemia, 428–433, 432*t*
    total body *vs.* serum, 427, 428*f*
    for treatment of diabetic ke-
        toacidosis, 369*t*, 370
Potassium chloride, for treatment
    of metabolic alkalosis, 387
Potassium depletion, 429–430
Povidone-iodine, 2
    insertion site decontamination
        with, 62
PPIs. *See* Proton pump inhibitors
Predicted body weight, 262,
    288–289
Prednisone
    for treatment of adrenal insuffi-
        ciency, 606*t*
    for treatment of anaphylaxis,
        531
    for treatment of asthma, 276
    for treatment of chronic ob-
        structive pulmonary dis-
        ease, 278
    for treatment of myasthenia
        gravis, 633
Prerenal azotemia, 396
    acute renal failure *vs.*, 393*t*

Prerenal conditions, 391, 392*t*

Pressure, volume *vs.*, 120–121

Pressure control, volume control *vs.*, 284–285

Pressure-controlled ventilation (PCV), 305, 306*f*

Pressure conversions, 722

Pressure-modulated ventilation, 305–307, 306*f*
  inverse ratio ventilation, 305–306, 306*f*
  pressure-controlled ventilation, 305, 306*f*
  pressure-supported ventilation, 306*f*, 307, 337

Pressure-supported ventilation (PSV), 306*f*, 307, 337

Pressure-volume curves, in systolic and diastolic heart failure, 174*f*, 175–177

Pressure-volume relationships, 283–284, 284*f*

Primary metabolic acidosis, 355

Procainamide
  drug fever and, 509*t*
  torsades de pointes and, 252*t*

Prochlorperazine, neuroleptic malignant syndrome and, 510*t*

Progressive heart failure, 173–175, 174*f*, 175*t*
  cardiac performance in, 175*t*

Propofol, 661–662, 663*t*
  lactic acidosis and, 365

Propofol infusion syndrome, 662

Propranolol, for treatment of hyperthyroidism, 610

Propylene glycol, 631
  lactic acidosis and, 365

Propylene glycol toxicity, 660

Propylthiouracil, for treatment of hyperthyroidism, 610

Protected specimen brush (PSB), 539, 540

Protective barriers, 5–10
  airborne illness, 8–10, 9*f*
  gloves, 5–7, 7*tt*
  masks, 8

Protective dressings, for indwelling vascular catheters, 77

Protein content, of feeding formulas, 580

Protein intake, 567–569
  of enteral tube feeding, 584–585
  estimating daily protein needs, 567–568
  nitrogen balance, 568–569
  nitrogen balance and nonprotein calories, 569, 569*f*

Protein requirements, daily, in enteral tube feeding, 583

Protein-sparing effect, of dextrose solutions, 161

Proton pump inhibitors (PPIs), 22–24, 23*t*

Proximal airway pressures, 291–293, 291*f*, 292*t*

PSB. *See* Protected specimen brush

Pseudohyperkalemia, 433–434

Pseudohyponatremia, 420–421

Pseudomembranous enterocolitis, 551

Pseudomonas, aminoglycosides and, 672

Pseudomonas aeruginosa
  as cause of catheter-related septicemia, 88, 91*t*
  as cause of ICU infections, 513*t*, 514
  as cause of pneumonia, 535, 536*t*, 542, 543
  ceftazidime for, 679
  ciprofloxacin for, 680
  penicillins for, 682

PSV. *See* Pressure-supported ventilation

PSVT. *See* Paroxysmal supraventricular tachycardia

Psychogenic polydipsia, 422, 423*f*

Pulmonary angiography, for evaluation of venous thromboembolism, 47

Pulmonary artery catheters, 59, 97–111

Pulmonary artery catheters
(*continued*)
applications, 109–110
hemodynamic profiles, 109,
110*t*
oxygen uptake, 109–110
design, 97–98, 98*f*
hemodynamic parameters,
104–109, 105*t*
cardiovascular, 104–108, 105*t*
oxygen transport, 105*t*,
108–109
placement, 98–101, 100*f*
principle, 97
thermodilution, 101–104, 102*f*
Pulmonary artery occlusion pressure, 116–120
capillary hydrostatic pressure
vs., 119–120
checking for accuracy, 118–119
principle of, 117–118, 118*f*
wedge pressure tracing,
116–117
Pulmonary capillary wedge pressure (PCWP), 99, 105, 105*t*
for distinguishing acute respiratory distress syndrome
and hydrostatic pul-
monary edema, 258–259
dopamine and, 692
right heart failure and, 186
Pulmonary edema, 537
cardiogenic, 258, 312
hydrostatic, 258–260
Pulmonary embolism
clinical and laboratory findings
in patients with, 42*t*
fever and, 511
Pulmonary interstitial emphysema, 321
Pulmonary vascular resistance
index (PVRI), 105*t*,
107–108
Pupils, evaluation of coma and,
617, 617*t*
Purpura fulminans, 497
PVRI. *See* Pulmonary vascular resistance index

Pyridostigmine, for treatment of
myasthenia gravis, 633
Pyridoxine, for treatment of ethylene glycol intoxication,
375

Q
QRS duration, in diagnosis of
tachycardia, 233
QT interval, torsades de pointes
and, 251
Qualitative cultures of tracheal
aspirates, 537–538
Quantitative cultures
blood, 86–87, 86*t*
choice of methods, 87–88
bronchoalveolar lavage, 539
tracheal aspirate, 538, 538*t*, 540
Quinidine
interaction with sucralfate, 26
torsades de pointes and, 252*t*
Quinolones, for treatment of
pneumonia, 541, 543*t*

R
Radiography
for diagnosis of acute respiratory
distress syndrome, 257*f*
for diagnosis of pneumothorax,
72–73
Radionuclide lung scan, for evaluation of venous throm-
boembolism, 45–46
Ramsay scale for scoring sedation, 665*t*, 666
Random donor platelets, 501
Ranitidine
interaction with sucralfate, 26
reasons to avoid gastric acid
suppression with, 27–28
stress ulcer prophylaxis with,
22, 23*t*, 26–28, 27*f*
Rapid ACTH stimulation test,
604, 605*t*
Rapid-shallow breathing index
(RSBI), 334–335

Reactive central nervous system magnesium deficiency, 449

Readiness criteria, for discontinuing mechanical ventilation, 333, 334*t*

Receptive aphasia, 644

Recruitable lung, 309

Red cell parameters, normal range of values, 478*t*

Red cells, washed, 483

Red man syndrome, 683–684

REE. *See* Resting energy expenditure

Reference ranges, 725–730
  body fluid distribution in healthy adults, 729
  clinical laboratory tests, 725–726
  desirable weights for adults, 728
  electrolyte content of body fluids, 729
  peak expiratory flow rates for healthy females, 730
  peak expiratory flow rates for healthy males, 729–730
  vitamins and trace elements, 727

Refractory hypokalemia, 433

Refractory status epilepticus, 631

Renal disorders, 392, 398–401. *See also* Oliguria and acute renal failure
  acute interstitial nephritis, 399–400, 400*t*
  contrast-induced renal failure, 398–399
  inflammatory renal injury, 398
  myoglobinuric renal failure, 400–401

Renal excretion, impaired, hyperkalemia and, 435–436

Renal failure, 392, 392*t*. *See also* Oliguria and acute renal failure
  amino acid solutions for, 593
  ionized hypocalcemia and, 460

Renal function, quantitative assessment of, 395*t*

Renal insufficiency
  hypermagnesemia and, 453
  magnesium replacement and, 452

Renal potassium loss, 429–430

Renal replacement therapy (RRT), 401–405
  hemodialysis, 402–404, 403*f*
  hemofiltration, 404–405

Renal ultrasound, in evaluation of renal failure, 396–397

Reocclusion, thrombolytic therapy and, 218

Reperfusion therapy, 214–220
  adjuncts to, 220–224
  for cardiac pump failure, 227
  coronary angioplasty, 219–220
  thrombolytic therapy, 214–218, 215–216*t*

Replacement fluids, for hypokalemia, 431–432

Respirators, 8

Respiratory acid-base disorders, 350, 351*t*, 352*f*, 353–354

Respiratory acidosis, 350, 351*t*, 352*f*, 354

Respiratory alkalosis, 350, 351*t*, 352*f*, 354
  as cause of hypophosphatemia, 468

Respiratory depression, opioids and, 656

Respiratory distress, bedside evaluation of, 293

Respiratory precautions, for airborne illness, 9*f*

Respiratory secretions, 318–319
  clearing, 318–321, 320*t*

Resting energy expenditure (REE), 565–566

Resuscitation. *See also* Colloid fluids; Crystalloid fluids
  end-points of, 153–154
  hypertonic, 169–170

Resuscitation fluids
  cost comparison for, 167*t*

Resuscitation fluids (*continued*)
efficacy of, 150–151
flow characteristics, 148, 149*f*
types of, 148
Resuscitation strategies, 149–154
correcting anemia, 153
end-points of resuscitation,
153–154
promoting cardiac output,
149–152, 151*f*
resuscitation volume, 152–153
Resuscitation volume, estimating,
152–153
Reteplase, for thrombolytic therapy, 49, 216*t*, 217, 218
Rhabdomyolysis, as cause of hyperkalemia, 434
Rifampin, on catheters, 57
Right heart failure, 178, 186
Right ventricular end-diastolic
volume (RVEDV), right
heart failure and, 186
Risk categories, for embolic
stroke, 241–242
Rocuronium, 636–637, 637*t*
Roll-plate method, of catheter-tip
cultures, 85–86, 86*t*
R-R intervals, diagnosis of tachycardia and uniformity of,
234–235
RRT. *See* Renal replacement therapy
RSBI. *See* Rapid-shallow breathing index
RVEDV. *See* Right ventricular
end-diastolic volume

S

Safety-engineered needles, 10
Saline, tracheal injections of,
319–320
Saline infusion
for treatment of hypercalcemia,
464
for treatment of metabolic alkalosis, 386
Saline solutions, 148

SBT. *See* Spontaneous breathing
trial
Secretions, clearing
mucolytic therapy, 320–321,
320*t*
respiratory secretions, 318–319
tracheal injections of saline,
319–320
Secretory diarrhea, magnesium
deficiency and, 447
Sedation, 658–669
agitated patient, 666*f*, 667
with benzodiazepines, 658–661,
659*t*
dexmedetomidine, 662–663,
663*t*
haloperidol, 663–665, 664*t*
interrupting sedative infusions,
665–666
monitoring, 665*t*, 666
propofol, 661–662, 663*t*
Seizures, 627–632
acute management, 630–631,
630*f*
generalized, 628
imipenem and generalized,
677–678
lactic acidosis and, 365
partial (focal), 628
predisposing conditions, 629,
629*t*
temporal lobe, 628
types of, 627–629
Seldinger technique, 63, 64*f*
Selenium, 573*t*, 574
Semipermeable dressings, for indwelling vascular
catheters, 77
Sensorimotor function
evaluation of coma and,
618–619
evaluation of stroke and, 644
Sepsis, 522. *See also* Severe sepsis
and septic shock
from abdomen and pelvis,
549–561
abdominal abscess, 555
acalculous cholecystitis, 554

bowel, 549–551
  Clostridium difficile colitis,
    551–553
  urinary tract infections,
    556–559, 557t
  as cause of ionized hypocal-
    cemia, 459
  gastric acid suppression and,
    28
  lactic acidosis and, 364
  persistent, 92–94
Sepsis syndrome, acute respira-
    tory distress syndrome
    and, 256
Septic shock, 28, 522
Serial dilution method, of
    catheter-tip cultures, 86,
    86t
Serum magnesium, 443–444
Serum potassium, 427, 428f
  changes in, 427–428
Severe sepsis and septic shock,
    522, 525–529
  blood lactate and, 135–136
  corticosteroids, 528
  early goal-directed therapy,
    525–527, 526t
  empiric antimicrobial therapy,
    528
  oxygen transport, 528–529, 529f
Shock. *See also* Severe sepsis and
    septic shock
  anaphylactic, 530, 531–532
  cardiogenic, 110t, 183, 226t,
    693
  circulatory, 363–364, 364f
  hemodynamic patterns in, 110t
  hypovolemic, 110t, 141, 144,
    145–146, 153–154
  vasogenic, 110t
SI. *See* Stroke index; Système In-
    ternationale
SIADH. *See* Syndrome of inappro-
    priate ADH
Sinusitis, paranasal, 316, 514
Sinus tachycardia, 233
SIRS. *See* Systemic inflammatory
    response syndrome

Skin hygiene, 1–5
  antiseptic agents, 1–3
  handwashing, 3–5
  soap and water, 1
Sleep apnea, continuous positive
    airway pressure for, 312
Soap and water, skin hygiene
    and, 1
Society of Critical Care Medicine,
    506, 663
Sodium, in lost body fluids, 414t
Sodium deficit, treatment of hy-
    ponatremia and, 425
Sodium iodide, 611
Sodium polystyrene sulfonate, for
    hyperkalemia, 439
Solute concentrations, converting
    units of, 720–721
Solvent drag, 404
Solvent toxicity, nitroglycerin
    and, 696
Sorbitol, diarrhea and, 588–589
Sotalol, torsades de pointes and,
    252t
Spinal cord injuries, risk of
    thromboembolism and, 33
Spiral CT angiography, for evalu-
    ation of venous throm-
    boembolism, 46–47
Spontaneous bacterial peritonitis,
    515
Spontaneous breathing trial
    (SBT), 336–338, 339f
  identifying patients for,
    333–336, 334–335t
Spontaneous movement, brain
    death and, 623
Spore-forming organisms, anti-
    septic agents and, 3
SRMI. *See* Stress-related mucosal
    injury
Standard amino acid solutions, 592
Staphylococcus aureus
  as cause of catheter-related sep-
    ticemia, 89
  as cause of endocarditis, 92
  as cause of ICU infections, 513t,
    514

Staphylococcus aureus (continued)
as cause of pneumonia, 535, 536*t*, 541
imipenem for, 677
skin hygiene and, 1
vancomycin for, 682
Staphylococcus epidermidis, 513*t*
as cause of catheter-related septicemia, 88, 90, 91*t*, 92
imipenem for, 677
skin hygiene and, 1
vancomycin for, 683
"Static" compliance, 295
Status epilepticus, 629
STEMI. *See* ST-segment elevation myocardial infarction
Sterile gloves, 5
for vascular cannulation, 61
Steroid therapy
for treatment of acute respiratory distress syndrome, 265
for treatment of adrenal insufficiency, 605, 606*t*
for treatment of anaphylaxis, 531
for treatment of laryngeal edema, 344–345
Streptococcus pneumoniae, chronic obstructive pulmonary disease and, 278
Streptokinase, 216*t*, 217
Stress hyperlactemia, 364
Stress-related mucosal injury (SRMI), 19–29
clinical manifestations, 20
pathogenesis, 19
predisposing conditions, 20–21
preventive measures, 21–28
enteral tube feedings, 21
gastric cytoprotection, 25–26
gastric cytoprotection *vs.* reduced gastric acidity, 26–28
reduced gastric acidity, 22–25, 23*t*, 24*t*, 25*f*
Stress ulcers, 19. *See also* Stress-related mucosal injury
indications for prophylaxis, 20*t*

Stridor, post-extubation, 345–346
Stroke. *See* Acute stroke
Stroke index (SI), 105*t*, 106–107
ST-segment elevation myocardial infarction (STEMI), 209. *See also* Acute coronary syndromes
heparin for, 220
Subclavian vein, as venous access site, 65–66, 66*t*
Subclavian vein thrombosis, 82–83
Subcutaneous emphysema, 321, 322
Substrate solutions, 591–596
additives, 595–596, 595*t*
amino acid solutions, 591–593, 592*t*
dextrose solutions, 591, 592*t*
lipid emulsions, 593–594, 594*t*
Succinylcholine, 637–638
Sucralfate
as cause of hypophosphatemia, 468
drug interaction, 26
for stress ulcer prophylaxis, 23*t*, 25–27, 27*f*
for treatment of hyperphosphatemia, 472–473
Superior vena cava syndrome, 82
Supply-dependent, 132
Suppurative thrombosis, 92
Supraventricular tachycardia (SVT), 233
ventricular tachycardia *vs.*, 247–249, 248*f*
Surgery, risk of venous thromboembolism and, 31–33, 32*t*
Surgical masks, 8
Surgical wound infections, 512–513, 512*t*
SvO₂. *See* Venous oxygen saturation
SVRI. *See* Systemic vascular resistance index
Syndrome of inappropriate ADH (SIADH), 422, 423*f*
Système Internationale (SI), 719–720

Systemic inflammatory response syndrome (SIRS), 522–523
 diagnostic criteria, 523*t*
 significance, 523
Systemic oxygenation, 125–137
 anemia and, 479–481, 480*f*
 control of oxygen uptake, 131–133
 as end-point of volume resuscitation, 154
 metabolic alkalosis and, 383–384, 384*f*
 systemic oxygen transport, 125–131
  oxygen content of blood, 125–126, 127*t*
  oxygen delivery, 127–128, 128*t*
  oxygen extraction, 130–131
  oxygen uptake, 128–130
 tissue oxygenation, 133–136, 133*t*
  blood lactate, 135–136
  oxygen transport parameters, 134–135
Systemic oxygen transport, 144
Systemic vascular resistance index (SVRI), 105*t*, 107
Systolic heart failure
 diastolic heart failure *vs.*, 175–178, 177*t*
 left-sided, 180–185

T
TA. *See* Tracheal aspirates
Tachyarrhythmias, dopamine infusions and, 693
Tachycardias, 233–254
 atrial fibrillation, 237–243
  acute rate control, 239–241, 240*t*
  adverse consequences, 237–238
  antithrombotic therapy, 241–242, 242*t*

DC cardioversion, 238
 pharmacologic cardioversion, 238–239
 predisposing factors, 237
 Wolff-Parkinson-White syndrome, 243
diagnostic approach, 233–236, 234*f*
 atrial activity, 235–236, 236*f*
 QRS duration, 233, 234*f*
 uniformity of R-R intervals, 234–235
multifocal atrial tachycardia, 243–244
paroxysmal supraventricular tachycardia, 244–247
 AV nodal re-entrant tachycardia, 245–247, 246*t*
 features, 244–245
torsades de pointes, 250–252
 drugs that can trigger, 252*t*
ventricular tachycardia, 247–250
 acute management, 249–250, 249*f*
 supraventricular tachycardia *vs.*, 247–249, 248*f*
Temperature conversions, 722
Temporal lobe seizures, 628
Tenecteplase, 216*t*, 217, 218
Tension pneumothorax, 322
Terbutaline, for treatment of asthma, 274
Tetracycline, interaction with sucralfate, 26
Theophylline
 benzodiazepines and, 661
 ciprofloxacin and, 681
 sucralfate and, 26
Therapeutic hypothermia, 203–204, 203*t*
Thermodilution, 101–104, 102*f*
 confounding conditions, 103
 continuous cardiac output measurements, 103–104
 method, 101
 technical considerations, 102
 variability, 103

Thiamine, for treatment of ethylene glycol intoxication, 375
Thiamine deficiency, 570–573
  carbohydrate metabolism, 570
  clinical manifestations, 571–572
  diagnosis, 572–573
  laboratory evaluation of thiamine status, 572*t*
  lactic acidosis and, 364–365
  predisposing factors, 570–571
Thiazide diuretics, magnesium deficiency and, 446
Thienopyridines, for treatment of acute cardiac syndromes, 212
Thiocyanate toxicity, 700–701
Thiopental, Ringer's solution and, 159
Thioridazine, torsades de pointes and, 252*t*
Thoracic compliance, 295
Thoracic pressure, 113–115
  end of expiration, 114
  positive-end-expiratory pressure, 115
  spontaneous variations, 115
Thorax, venous pressures in, 113–115
Thrombocytic thrombocytopenia purpura (TTP), 498–499
Thrombocytopenia, 493–504
  defined, 493
  etiologies, 493–499, 494*t*
    disseminated intravascular coagulation, 497–498, 498*t*
    heparin-induced thrombocytopenia, 494–497, 496*t*
    thrombotic thrombocytopenia purpura, 498–499
    platelet transfusions, 501–503
    transfusion trigger, 499–501
Thrombolytic agents, 216*t*, 217–218
Thrombolytic therapy, 49, 214–218
  bleeding and, 218
  candidates for, 644, 645*t*
  contraindications to, 215*t*
  coronary angioplasty *vs.*, 219

  fibrinolytic agents, 216*t*, 217–218
  indications, 214–215
  reocclusion and, 218
  timing, 215–216
  for treatment of stroke, 644, 645*t*, 647
Thromboprophylaxis, 35–41, 37*t*
  adjusted-dose warfarin, 39*t*, 40
  after hip and knee surgery, 41
  fondaparinux, 40–41
  for general surgery, 34*t*
  for hip and knee surgery, 39*t*
  low-dose heparin, 36–37, 37*t*
  low-molecular-weight heparin, 34*t*, 37*t*, 38–40, 39*t*
  mechanical compression devices, 34*t*, 35
Thrombosis
  femoral vein, 83
  subclavian vein, 82–83
  suppurative, 92
Thrombotic occlusion, 81–82
Thrombotic stroke, 641
Thyroid dysfunction. *See* Hyperthyroidism; Hypothyroidism
Thyroid storm, 609–610
  treatment of, 611
Thyroxine, interaction with sucralfate, 26
TIA. *See* Transient ischemic attack
Ticlodipine, for treatment of acute cardiac syndromes, 212
Tidal volume, 288
  in spontaneous breathing trial, 338, 339*f*
Tirofiban, as adjunct to reperfusion therapy, 222, 223*t*
Tissue factor, 497
Tissue oxygenation, 133–136
  blood lactate, 135–136
  clinical markers of threatened or impaired, 133*t*
  oxygen transport parameters, 134–135
Tissue plasminogen activator (tPA)

for treatment of acute coronary
    syndromes, 216*t*, 217
for treatment of stroke, 647
Tobramycin, 671
    for digestive decontamination,
        551*t*
    for oral decontamination, 545
    for treatment of pneumonia,
        543*t*
Tonicity, 411
Tonic movement, 627
Torsades de pointes, 250–252
    etiologies, 251
    features, 250–251
    fluoroquinolones and, 681
    haloperidol and, 665
    magnesium depletion and, 448
    management, 198, 251–252,
        252*t*
Total body potassium, 427,
    428*f*
Total inspiratory resistance, 295
Total oxygen content, 126
Total parenteral nutrition (TPN),
    591–601
    creating a regimen, 596–599
        carbohydrate calories,
            597–598
        daily requirements, 596
        lipid calories, 598
        TPN orders, 598–599
        volume of mixture, 597
    hypophosphatemia and, 467,
        468*f*
    metabolic complications,
        599–600
        hypercapnia, 600
        hyperglycemia, 599
        hypophosphatemia, 599
    substrate solutions, 591–596
        additives, 595–596, 595*t*
        amino acid solutions,
            591–593, 592*t*
        dextrose solutions, 591, 592*t*
        lipid emulsions, 593–594,
            594*t*
    thiamine and, 571
    trophic effects, 577

Toxic alcohols, 373–376
    ethylene glycol intoxication,
        373–375, 375*f*
    methanol intoxication, 375–376,
        375*f*
Toxic megacolon, 552
Toxins. *See* Pharmaceutical toxins
    and antidotes; Toxic alco-
    hols
tPA. *See* Tissue plasminogen
    activator
T-piece trials, 337
TPN. *See* Total parenteral nutri-
    tion
Trace elements
    reference ranges, 727
    in total parenteral nutrition,
        595*t*, 596
Tracheal aspirates (TA), 537–538,
    540
    qualitative cultures, 537–538
    quantitative cultures, 538, 538*t*,
        540
Tracheal decannulation, 342–345,
    344*f*
Tracheal injections of saline,
    319–320
Tracheal intubation, 287–288
Tracheostomy, 317–318, 343
TRALI. *See* Transfusion-related
    acute lung injury
Transcellular shift, 428–429
    treatment of hyperkalemia and,
        439
Transfusion-related acute lung in-
    jury (TRALI), 489
Transfusions. *See* Erythrocyte
    transfusions; Platelet
    transfusions
Transfusion trigger
    for erythrocyte transfusion,
        481–482
    for platelet transfusion,
        499–500
Transient ischemic attack (TIA),
    642
Translaryngeal intubation,
    342–343

Translocation, 550
Transmural pressure, 115*f*
    intravascular pressure *vs.*, 113
Transthoracic compliance, 293
Transthoracic pressures, 292
Trauma, risk of venous thrombo-
    embolism and, 33
Trendelenburg position, 150
Tricuspid regurgitation, pul-
    monary artery catheter
    and, 103
Trophic effects, of enteral tube
    feeding, 577–578
Trousseau's sign, 461
TTP. *See* Thrombotic thrombocy-
    topenia purpura
Tubercle bacillus, respirators to
    block transmission of, 8

U

Ulcers, stress, 19. *See also* Stress-
    related mucosal injury
Unfractionated heparin
    as adjunct to reperfusion ther-
        apy, 220–221
    in antithrombotic therapy, 47
    risk of heparin-induced throm-
        bocytopenia and, 495
Units and conversions, 719–723
    apothecary and household con-
        versions, 721
    French sizes, 723
    gauge sizes, 723
    measurement in the SI, 719–720
    pressure, 722
    solute concentration, 720–721
    temperature, 722
Unstable angina (UA), 209. *See
    also* Acute coronary syn-
    dromes
    heparin for, 220
    platelet glycoprotein inhibitors
        for, 223–224
Upper extremity venous access
    sites, 63–65
Urinary magnesium, 444, 445*f*

Urinary tract infection (UTI),
        556–559
    candiduria, 558–559
    diagnostic criteria, 556, 557*t*
    empiric antibiotics, 557–558
    pathogens in, 513*t*
Urine cultures, 556
Urine microscopy
    in evaluation of renal failure,
        395
    in evaluation of urinary tract
        infection, 556
Urine osmolality, in evaluation of
        renal failure, 394–395
Urine sodium, in evaluation of
        renal failure, 393–394
Urticaria, 489, 503
UTI. *See* Urinary tract infection

V

Valsartan, for treatment of acute
        cardiac syndromes, 214
Vancomycin, 682–685
    activity and clinical uses,
        682–683
    adverse effects, 683–684
    dosing, 683
    drug fever and, 509*t*
    for MRSA, 516, 528
    replacements, 684–685
    for treatment of *C. difficile* coli-
        tis, 553
    for treatment of catheter-
        related septicemia, 90, 91*t*
    for treatment of pneumonia,
        542, 543*t*
    for treatment of severe sepsis
        and septic shock, 528
    for treatment of urinary tract
        infection, 558
Vancomycin-resistant strains, an-
    tibiotics for, 516, 528
VAP. *See* Ventilator-assisted pneu-
    monia
Vascular cannulation preparation,
    61–62

Vascular catheters, 53–60
  central venous catheters, 55–57, 56t, 58f
  features, 53–54
  flow rate determinants, 54
  hemodialysis catheters, 58–59, 59f
  introducer catheters, 57–58, 58f
  peripheral vein catheters, 55
  pulmonary artery catheters, 59
  size of, 53, 54t
  types of, 55–59
Vascular catheters, indwelling, 77–96
  catheter-related infections, 83–94
    catheter tip cultures, 85–86, 86t
    clinical features, 85
    empiric antibiotic coverage, 88–90, 89f
    persistent sepsis, 92–94
    quantitative blood cultures, 86–88, 88f
    routes of, 83–84, 84f
    treatment of catheter-related septicemia, 90–92, 91t
    types of, 84
  occluded, 80–83, 81t
  routine care, 77–80
    antimicrobial ointment, 78
    dressings, 77
    flushing catheters, 78
    replacing central venous catheters, 79–80
    replacing peripheral venous catheters, 79
Vasodilator effects, of nitroglycerin, 694
Vasodilators
  for treatment of acute aortic dissection, 229, 229t
  for treatment of heart failure, 226t
Vasogenic shock, hemodynamic patterns in, 110t

Vasopressin
  for treatment of cardiac arrest, 197–198, 197t
  for treatment of diabetes insipidus, 418
  for treatment of severe sepsis and septic shock, 527
  via endotracheal route, 196
Vasopressors
  for treatment of cardiac arrest, 196–198, 197t
  for treatment of severe sepsis and septic shock, 527
Vena cava, catheter tip against wall of, 74
Venipuncture sites, 515
Venous access, establishing, 61–75
  catheter insertion techniques, 62–63, 64f
  catheter position, 73–74
  pneumothorax, 72–73
  preparation for vascular cannulation, 61–62
  venous access sites, 63–71
    femoral vein, 66t, 68–71, 69f, 70f
    internal jugular vein, 66t, 67–68
    subclavian vein, 65–66, 66t
    upper extremity, 63–65
  venous air embolism, 71–72
Venous access sites, 63–71
  femoral vein, 66t, 68–71, 69f, 70f
  internal jugular vein, 66t, 67–68
  subclavian vein, 65–66, 66t
  upper extremity, 63–65
Venous air embolism, 71–72
Venous blood gases, monitoring during CPR, 202
Venous oxygen saturation (SvO_2), 134–135
Venous pressures in the thorax, 113–115, 114t
Venous thromboembolism (VTE), 31–52
  antithrombotic therapy, 47–49, 48t

Venous thromboembolism (VTE)
  (continued)
    diagnostic approach, 41–47,
      42*t*
    clinical evaluation, 42–44, 44*f*
    pulmonary angiography, 47
    radionuclide lung scan,
      45–46
    spiral CT angiography, 46–47
    venous ultrasound, 44–45
  inferior vena cava filters, 50
  patient at risk, 31–34, 32*t*, 34*t*
  thromboprophylaxis, 35–41,
    37*t*, 39*t*
Venous thrombosis, 82–83
  femoral vein thrombosis, 83
  subclavian vein thrombosis,
    82–83
Venous ultrasound, for evaluation
    of venous thromboem-
    bolism, 44–45
Venovenous hemofiltration, 405
Ventilation. *See also* Mechanical
    ventilation; Positive-
    pressure breathing
  cardiopulmonary resuscitation,
    189–190
Ventilator, breathing through,
    336–337
Ventilator-assisted pneumonia
    (VAP), 535–536. *See also*
    Pneumonia
Ventilator breath, 299–301, 300*f*
Ventilator-dependent patient,
    315–331
  alveolar disruption, 321–325,
    323*f*, 325*f*
  clearing secretions, 318–321,
    320*t*
  indwelling endotracheal tubes,
    315–316
  intrinsic PEEP, 326–330, 326*f*
  tracheostomy, 317–318
Ventilator-induced lung injury,
    260–261, 261*f*, 288
Ventricular compliance, 122
Ventricular ejection fraction,
    177–178

Ventricular emptying, during
    positive-pressure ventila-
    tion, 285–286
Ventricular end-diastolic volume,
    measuring, 120–121, 121*f*
Ventricular fibrillation (V-Fib)
  defibrillation for, 191, 192–194*f*
  drugs for treatment of, 198
  therapeutic hypothermia and,
    203
Ventricular filling, during posi-
    tive-pressure ventilation,
    285
Ventricular free wall rupture, 225
Ventricular septal rupture, 225
Ventricular tachycardia (VT,
    V-Tach), 247–250
  acute management, 198,
    249–250, 249*f*
  defibrillation for, 191, 192–193*f*
  supraventricular tachycardia
    vs., 247–249, 248*f*
  therapeutic hypothermia and,
    203
Verapamil, for treatment of multi-
    focal atrial tachycardia,
    244
V-Fib. *See* Ventricular fibrillation
Viruses, respiratory precautions
    for, 9*f*
Vitamins
  C, 573
  E, 573
  reference ranges, 727
  requirements, 570–573
    antioxidant vitamins, 573
    daily requirements, 570, 571*t*
    thiamine deficiency, 570–573,
      572*t*
  in total parenteral nutrition, 595
VO₂. *See* Oxygen uptake
Volume, pressure *vs.*, 120–121
Volume control, pressure control
    vs., 284–285
Volume deficits, correcting in
    oliguria, 397
Volume depletion, metabolic al-
    kalosis and, 380–381

Volume effects
  of albumin solutions,
      164–165
  of colloid fluids, 163–164
  of dextrans, 167
  of dextrose solutions, 161
  of hydroxyethyl starch, 165–166
  of hypertonic resuscitation, 169
Volume infusion, 145–148
  catheter size, 146–147, 147*f*
  for treatment of contrast-
      induced renal failure, 399
  type of resuscitation fluid, 148
Volume replacement, in hypov-
      olemic hypernatremia, 415
Volume resuscitation
  for treatment of anaphylactic
      shock, 531
  for treatment of severe sepsis
      and septic shock, 526–527
Volutrauma, 261
VT. *See* Ventricular tachycardia
V-Tach. *See* Ventricular tachycar-
      dia
VTE. *See* Venous thromboem-
      bolism

W
Warfarin
  in antithrombotic therapy, 49
  ciprofloxacin and, 681
  for thromboprophylaxis, 39*t*, 40
Washed red cells, 483
Water intoxication, 422
Wedged blood PO$_2$, 119
Wedge pressure (pulmonary ar-
      tery occlusion pressure),
      116–120
  capillary hydrostatic pressure
      vs., 119–120
  checking for accuracy, 118–119
  principle of, 117–118, 118*f*
  wedge pressure tracing,
      116–117
Wedge pressure (pulmonary cap-
      illary wedge pressure), 99,
      105, 105*t*
  for distinguishing acute respi-
      ratory distress syndrome
      and hydrostatic pul-
      monary edema, 258–259
  dopamine and, 692
  right heart failure and, 186
Weights, desirable, for adults, 728
Wide QRS complex tachycardia,
      235
Withdrawal syndrome, benzodi-
      azepines and, 661
Wolff-Parkinson-White (WPW)
      syndrome, 243
Women
  body fluid distribution in,
      729
  body fluid volumes in, 139,
      140*t*
  creatinine clearance in, 395*t*
  desirable weights in, 728
  normal peak flow rates for, 270,
      270*f*
  normal range of values for red
      cell parameters in, 478*t*
  peak expiratory flow rates for,
      730
WPW syndrome. *See* Wolff-
      Parkinson-White syn-
      drome

Z
Zoledronate, for treatment of hy-
      percalcemia, 465*t*, 466